Health Visiting

For Elsevier:

Commissioning Editor: Ninette Premdas/Mairi McCubbin
Project Development Manager: Katrina Mather
Project Manager: Emma Riley
Design: George Ajayi

Health Visiting

Specialist Community Public Health Nursing

SECOND EDITION

Edited by

Anne Robotham BA MEd PhD DipN(Lond) CertEd(FE)

Formerly Principal Lecturer in Community Health and
PGD/BSc Community Health (Health Visiting) Course Leader,
University of Wolverhampton, Wolverhampton, UK

Marion Frost BA(Hons) MSc PGCEA DipSoc RGN RHV

Chair of United Kingdom Standing Conference on Health Visitor Education;
Principal Lecturer and Health Visitor Course Director, Faculty of Health and Social Care,
London South Bank University, London, UK

Foreword by

Alison Norman CBE

Director of Nursing and Operations, Christie NHS Trust, Withington, Manchester, UK;
President Community Practitioners and Health Visitors Association

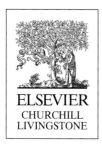

ELSEVIER
CHURCHILL
LIVINGSTONE

EDINBURGH LONDON NEW YORK OXFORD PHILADELPHIA ST LOUIS SYDNEY TORONTO 2005

ELSEVIER
CHURCHILL
LIVINGSTONE

© Harcourt Publishers Limited 2001
© 2005, Elsevier Limited. All rights reserved.

First edition 2000
Second edition 2005

ISBN 0 443 10105 1

British Library Cataloguing in Publication Data
A catalogue record for this book is available from the British Library

Library of Congress Cataloging in Publication Data
A catalog record for this book is available from the Library of Congress

Note
Medical knowledge is constantly changing. Standard safety precautions must be followed, but as new research and clinical experience broaden our knowledge, changes in treatment and drug therapy may become necessary or appropriate. Readers are advised to check the most current product information provided by the manufacturer of each drug to be administered to verify the recommended dose, the method and duration of administration, and contraindications. It is the responsibility of the practitioner, relying on experience and knowledge of the patient, to determine dosages and the best treatment for each individual patient. Neither the Publisher nor the editors or contributors assume any liability for any injury and/or damage to persons or property arising from this publication.

The Publisher

Working together to grow
libraries in developing countries

www.elsevier.com | www.bookaid.org | www.sabre.org

ELSEVIER   BOOK AID International   Sabre Foundation

The
Publisher's
policy is to use
paper manufactured
from sustainable forests

Printed in China

Contents

Contributors

Pat Alexander MSc FPCert Dip Counselling & Interpersonal Skills Dip Aromatherapy Dip Yoga Dip French BSc(Hons) RGN SCM RHV CPT(HV)
Health Visitor/Community Practice Teacher, Nuffield House Clinic, Harlow, UK

Ros Carnwell BA MA PhD RGN RHV CertEd(FE)
Director, Centre for Health and Community Research, North-East Wales Institute, Wrexham, UK

Randa Charles BSc(Hons) RGN RM RHV CPT
Clinical Support Nurse – HV Lead, Newcastle under Lyme PCT, Newcastle under Lyme, UK

Ann Clarridge BSc(Hons) MSc PGCEA DipTh RGN DN PWT
Chair of Association of District Nurse Educators UK
Principal Lecturer, Non-Medical Prescribing Course Director, London South Bank University, London, UK

Joanne Davis MMedSci MA RGN RHV
Health Visitor for Travellers, Balsall Heath Health Centre, Heart of Birmingham Teaching NHS PCT, Birmingham, UK

Marian Evans RGN RM RHV DPSN
Specialist Health Visitor, Heart of Birmingham Teaching NHS PCT, Birmingham, UK

Sarah Forester BSc(Hons) MSc RGN RHV
Co-ordinator Sure Start, London Borough of Wandsworth, Roehampton, London, UK

Janice Frost BSc(Hons) CPT FPCert RGN SCM RHV PGCE Health and Social Care
Health Visitor/Community Practice Teacher North Stoke PCT, Stoke, UK

Marion Frost BA(Hons) MSc PGCEA DipSoc RGN RHV
Chair of United Kingdom Standing Conference on Health Visitor Education, Principal Lecturer and Health Visitor Course Director, London South Bank University, London, UK

Jean Glynn BA MSc SRN RHV CPT FPCert
Clinical Development Manager, North Stoke PCT, Stoke, UK

Anne Higgs BSc(Hons) RGN RHV
Specialist Health Visitor, Heart of Birmingham Teaching NHS PCT, Birmingham, UK

Helen Hoult BSc(Hons) SRN SCM RHV FETC
Health Visitor (formerly for travellers) Wolverhampton PCT, Wolverhampton, UK

Marian Jones BSc(Hons) DPSN RGN DN RHV
Nurse Practitioner for the Homeless, South Birmingham PCT, Birmingham, UK

Joan Leach BSc(Hons) RGN RHV CPT
Health Visitor/Community Practice Teacher/Accident and Emergency Liaison Health Visitor, South Stoke PCT, Stoke, UK

Jane McKears BA MSc RGN RHV CPT
Head of Clinical Governance, Rowley Regis and Tipton PCT, West Midlands, UK

Jane Middleton Dip Management Cert Youth
and Community Work, CQSW
*Sure Start Co-ordinator, Southern Birmingham
Community NHS Trust, Birmingham, UK*

Elizabeth Porter BA MPhil PGCEA RN RM RHV FWT
*Lecturer and Award Leader MSc/BSc (Hons)
Public Health Practice, University of
Southampton, Southampton, UK*

Jane Powell BSc (Econ) MSc PhD
*Programme Leader, MSc Public Health,
University of the West of England, Bristol, UK*

Margaret Reynolds BSc(Hons) RGN RHV CPT
*Designated Nurse Child Protection,
Dudley South NHS PCT, Dudley, UK*

Anne Robotham BA MEd PhD DipN(Lond) CertEd(FE)
*Formerly Principal Lecturer in Community
Health and PGD/BSc Community Health
(Health Visiting) Course Leader, University of
Wolverhampton, Wolverhampton, UK*

Jan Rose MA CertEd(FE)
*Formerly Senior Lecturer, Health Sciences,
University of Wolverhampton,
Wolverhampton, UK*

Doreen Sheldrake BSc
*Formerly Health Visitor/Community Practice
Teacher, Southern Birmingham Community NHS
Trust, Birmingham, UK*

Ruth Wain BA(Hons) MSocSci PhD CertEd Hon.MFPH
*Deputy Director of Public Health, Cotswold and
Vale PCT, Cirencester, UK*

Foreword

I began my journey as a health visitor in 1977.

Since then many things have changed but the essential challenges in health visiting practice remain very familiar.

Society has moved on. Politically there is more hegemony and less of the division that typified the late 70s and 80s. Much of that sharp divide was located in our inner cities and the industrial strife that polarized the nation.

Today, we can take comfort from the fact that there are one million fewer children living in poverty than was the case eight years ago.

Nevertheless large areas of severe post industrial decline mar many towns in the UK. Inner urban and so called 'sink' estates continue to suffer the blight of unemployment, poor housing, crime and substance misuse.

For health visiting, whose origin is deeply embedded in the amelioration of poverty and its gross health effects, this is an enduring continuity with our professional history.

The overt racism and fear of racial violence, which was a real and present shadow over my years of practice in East London, have improved. But, sadly this has now been replaced by a more subtle and focused hatred of discrete groups such as asylum seekers.

At the other end of the social and economic spectrum another set of challenges await. Families struggle to cope with their own and society's high expectations, two jobs, two cars, two kids, cash rich, time poor. For some a merry-go-round to maintain a level of economic viability, for others a desperate search for rest and relaxation.

The cost of this achievement, for many, is measured in social unhappiness, the ever-increasing consumption of anti-depressants and mood enhancers and unprecedented levels of family breakdown.

New national public concerns include fear of terrorism, the adulteration of food and the stalking paedophile. Some of these are legitimate, some less so. Disturbingly, there is an increasing trend to see measures such as immunization, whose purpose is to support the public good, as a conspiracy of the State against individual well being.

Meanwhile we overeat, take too little exercise, continue to smoke and drink more alcohol than ever before.

The purpose of the above is not to render the reader prostrate with anxiety but to make a sharp point about the ongoing and enduring need for a comprehensive and effective health visiting service.

The newly qualified practitioner need not fear limited opportunity for public health work.

Essential to his or her success will be the knowledge and practical advice set out in this important book. The role of the health visitor is to influence personal health and community wellbeing. This text provides an up-to-date guide to the means by which the health visitor can work effectively and efficiently.

The framework of practice through models, use of information and key chapters on discrete issues such as violence and safeguarding children will prove invaluable.

The use of vignettes to illustrate practice brings theory to life in a helpful and clear way. Essentially, this text provides a basis for the practitioner to prioritize and develop a strategic approach to working with individuals and families from a range of different communities and backgrounds.

Health visitors can and do make a difference to the health and wellbeing of their communities. Increasingly this will be through an overt partnership with individuals and groups. The practitioner must also be able to convey health advice and support in a way that appreciates the impact of growing public knowledge (and prejudice) about health matters. Being media 'savvy' is not yet part of the curriculum but perhaps it should be. How else can the health visitor manage discussion about the risks and benefits of MMR, pro's and con's of hormone replacement therapy and the myriad of other health issues covered daily in a newspaper or magazine near you?

Within their introduction the editors of this book do not flinch from drawing attention to concern about the wellbeing and security of the profession.

Notwithstanding the ability of the individual practitioner to work well and effectively, there must be a major onus on employing organizations to lead, develop and deploy the health visiting resource with flair, imagination and clear public health priorities.

The provision of health promotion and prevention services is essential to all communities. Measuring up to this need is our challenge.

My best wishes to all students (and their employers) in succeeding in this vital task.

Manchester, 2005   Alison Norman

Preface to second edition

The second edition of this book has come at the beginning of a period of change for the profession of health visiting, which has not seen its like since health visiting moved from local authority employment to become part of the National Health Service following the National Health Service Reorganization Act in 1973. At that time health visiting felt marginalized and undervalued when the Mayston Committee recommended that health visiting and hospital nursing came under a general division. The health visiting profession fought these proposals vigorously (Robinson 1982), and finally the Nurses, Midwives and Health Visitors Bill was passed in 1979, allowing health visitors to maintain a separate identity within the main body of nursing.

The new Nursing and Midwifery Council of 2002, in determining a new Register (2004), has succeeded in creating the same degree of disappointment and concern within the profession. Health visitors are no longer identified by name and are recognized as being on the third part of the Register, named as Specialist Community Public Health Nurses. It is likely that the greatest battle ahead for health visitors is to be able to persuade their management (who may not be from a nursing background), of the value and breadth of their work abilities.

In many ways this is a greater opportunity for health visitors than in 1979, but it also raises concerns that those areas in which health visiting excels – with families and communities preventing social breakdown, illness and impeded infant development by health education and supportive measures – may be lost under too wide a public health remit.

The editors of this second edition thought long and hard concerning a revised title to this book. We felt that it is extremely important to vigorously encourage the retention of profession of health visiting, and at the same time embrace the opportunity of specialist community public health nursing. Thus this book is for all registrants of the third part of the Register who will be using many of the skills of former health visitors. However, it is also necessary to keep alive on the professional agenda the need to recognize that if the work of health visiting is deleted by an administrative/management stroke of the pen there will be considerable breakdown in child and family health.

We hope that this book will prove of equal value to all practitioners on the third part of the Register, but especially so to health visitors.

London and   Anne Robotham
Wolverhampton, 2005   Marion Frost

Acknowledgements

The Editors wish to acknowledge, with grateful thanks, all the authors and contributors for their time and commitment to this second edition.

Introduction to second edition

Enormous changes have taken place in the 5 years since the publication of the first edition of this textbook. The government is now driving the professions and setting professional agendas, and the rhetoric of ideological change has been a move from a sickness service to a health service. Until 2000 health care tended to be medically driven. With the continual economic problems in the NHS, community and individuals have become the focus for developing health care services. Information is more freely available to enable individuals and communities to make their own choices in health care.

User representatives carry greater responsibility and influence in policy and organizational management discussions, and decision making. Professionals allied to medicine are now increasingly powerful in the health care arena through working in partnership with clients and agencies.

Chapter 1 looks at the specialist community public health nurse, concentrating particularly on health visiting, and also covers professionalism, professional standards and proficiency in practice.

In Chapter 2, Porter focuses on the public health role of health visitors and explores what constitutes this role. Public health has broadened from the medical and epidemiological approach of the 1990s to embrace social, political and environmental issues. Specialist community public health nursing is a small part of a wide agenda embracing many professionals and lay workers in improving the health of populations and reducing inequalities in health.

Chapter 3 is relatively unchanged in this new edition because the models that Carnwell focuses on are so relevant for public health and health promotion in this new health service. The development of models of public health, for example, Beattie's, reflect health visitor education and the requirements for proficiency in specialist community public health practice.

Chapters 4 and 5 seek to explore, analyse and structure the skills that health visitors use in what are essentially two roles: the individual and family, and the wider community and social groups. This reflects the emerging agenda of the Chief Nursing Officer's (2004) report, which recognizes the need for health visitors to work either in the home with children and families, or in the wider community with public health practice.

Within communities and groups there are those members of society who are socially excluded and have difficulty in accessing primary care in the NHS. Chapter 6 discusses the specialist role that health visiting has with travelling families and their health care needs. Marian Jones, Marian Evans and Anne Higgs work principally as first point of contact in enabling access to primary care, and supporting disadvantaged groups who are homeless or seeking asylum.

Leading and managing change is the content of Chapter 7, and this is imperative in creating the dynamism necessary to make effective change in responding to the health needs of clients. This cannot be undertaken without the recognition of a quality framework and clinical governance within the NHS.

The contemporary influences in safeguarding children in Chapters 8 and 9 are explored in relation to the role of government, statutory organizations and appropriately qualified professionals in promoting health and well-being of children and their families. A well-functioning family leads to a vibrant and effectively functioning community. Issues such as developmental screening, child behaviour, accidents and health inequalities are explored as examples of the manner in which health visitors can empower families through support and education.

Chapter 10 focuses on violence, which is increasingly becoming a public health issue in UK society. Violence within homes, schools, the workplace and towards older people has been shown in recent research to be a major factor in health and social breakdown. The chapter explores these issues in raising awareness of the causes of violence and the way in which professional awareness might anticipate and ameliorate the situation.

Chapter 11 acknowledges that reflective practice is now recognized as good professional practice and the use of reflective processes in health care practice enables health visitors to critically examine the content and dynamics of their practice. The skills of negotiating, lobbying and strategy development involved in working with groups and the wider community require health visitors to constantly reflect on the efficacy and effectiveness of their work. Critical thinking, critical analysis, of and in, practice, and critical reflection, have allowed health visitors to articulate practice more clearly and to develop a greater rigour in evidence-based practice.

Reflection on the wider issues of public health soon lead the practitioner to consider ethical issues in health care, and the policies and strategies involved in health care delivery in the UK today can raise ethical dilemmas. Chapter 12 explores these issues in relation to quality and equality health care delivery in

terms of advising, promoting and enabling all citizens to achieve the greatest health and well-being possible. The personal attitudes and values of the professional in conjunction with the political and economic pressures of management require the health visitor of today to be secure in their handling of ethical dilemmas.

The principles of nurse prescribing in practice are now an established part of the specialist community public health nurse role and the qualification of nurse prescribing is a requirement for all health visitors wishing to apply for the third part of the register. Chapter 13 concentrates on the principles of nurse prescribing and the use of the nurses' formulary. Allopathic medicine and complementary therapies have always run alongside each other, but it is becoming a much more acceptable part of normal health care practice.

Although there is limited access to complementary therapy on the NHS, nevertheless Chapter 14 shows the many ways in which health visitors might themselves use, or recommend the use of, other therapies. Alexander currently works as a health visitor using complementary skills in an NHS practice, and her enthusiasm and experience in her work are clearly demonstrated in this chapter.

Health informatics is becoming steadily more important in effective health care systems. Good documentation and recording have always been important but the need to use these within effective clinical governance is now essential. Resource use, risk assessment and seamless communication between acute care and community is dependent on good information and recording systems, and Chapter 15 covers all the issues currently under discussion.

It is likely that all the chapters have discussed or made reference to resource issues, and Chapter 16 on health economics is a very necessary aspect of public health care. Earlier, reference was made to the part that individuals and communities play in the development of effective and collaborative health care. Without an understanding of the principles of health economics, professionals working in the wider arena would find it impossible to work in effective partnership with local policy makers and user groups.

The final chapter of this book explores some of the key debates in government, professional and educational policy that are influencing current and future health visiting practice. Marion Frost suggests that while health visiting has a history of responding and adapting to change, the profession must rise to the current challenges and harness the opportunities available to influence its own future in order to survive. The profession needs to consider its own health as well as the health of its clients.

Chapter 1

The profession of health visiting in the 21st century

Anne Robotham

INTRODUCTION

In the 5 years since this book was first published, a total revision of the Register for Nurses and Midwives has taken place. There have been signs for some time that major change was under way, especially in the light of the continually increasing pressures on all those personnel who make up the National Health Service. The change to the Register is the formation of three separate parts: Nursing, Midwifery and Specialist Community Public Health Nursing. This has meant that there are many former parts to the Register which have now been subsumed under Nursing or Specialist Community Public Health Nursing. This sublimation has meant that nursing personnel who were called, for example, Registered Mental Health Nurses (RMN) are no longer separately identified. In the same way, Health Visitors have become Specialist Community Public Health Nurses – members of a larger part of the Register. As a result many nurses have lost a special name, and thus feel the loss of an identity.

It seems appropriate to explore whether nursing is a profession and how specialist community public health nursing has developed into a specialism that is sufficiently separate from nursing to require a separate entry in the professional register. One of the most important aspects of history is that it enables us to recognize where we are now in our evolutionary process. For that reason no apology is made for starting with the development of medicine as a profession as a precursor to the development of nursing as a profession.

HOW MEDICINE BECAME A PROFESSION

Formed as a result of the 1858 Medical Act, the General Medical Council (GMC) has 104 members elected from the medical profession and the public. The GMC has strong legal powers with which to protect the patient, and it is responsible to the Privy Council for establishing a register of qualified practitioners, defining their qualifications and appointing examiners.

In 1928 Carr-Saunders concluded that medicine and law, as 'established professions', shared two important attributes, namely, that their practice is based on theoretical study of an area of knowledge and that the members feel bound to follow a code of behaviour. There is little evidence to say that Carr-Saunders based his conclusion concerning the 'establishment' of law and medicine as professions other than through the regard by which they were held by the general public, with much of the medical profession's origins being rooted in religion, spiritualism and herbalism. Carr-Saunders and Wilson (1933), however, did stress the virtues of professionalism in medicine as upholding the ideals of service to the client and to the community through the application and advancement of specialized knowledge.

Until the advent of the National Health Service in 1947, the medical profession was a self-employed occupational group considered by their clients to be above reproach. Their practice was unchallenged. When government took a role in the organization and delivery of health care, the British Medical Association was influential in ensuring that doctors were heavily involved in the running of the NHS (Hanlon 2000). For the next two decades or so the medical profession remained relatively undisturbed, though gradually commentators such as Johnson (1972) and Illich (1977) began to challenge professional medical doctors. Johnson particularly identified the medical occupational group as increasing their power by the political strategy of ensuring the autonomy of their professional status, as well as ensuring financial reward, despite their profession of 'service'. Illich in turn saw the use of professionalism (and the medical profession in particular) as a conspiracy to create a dependency in client groups, thereby depriving them of their right and ability to ensure their own welfare and happiness. King (1968) considered that professionalism creates an occupation with a high degree of self-consciousness. Charlatanism and quackery are a creation of professionalism, not the cause of it.

THE DEVELOPMENT OF OTHER PROFESSIONS IN THE WORLD OF HEALTH AND ILLNESS

The natural history of professionalism in the United States has been traced through stages of: emergence of a full-time occupation; establishment of a training school; founding of a professional association; political agitation directed towards the protection of the association by law; and the adoption of a formal code of practice (Wilensky 1964). In the UK, however, as well as including these attributes of a profession, theorists have also tended to focus on the degree of autonomy enjoyed by the occupation; the extent to which practice is based upon theoretical knowledge; and the degree of observation of the ideal of altruistic service (Hickman and Thomas 1969, Johnson 1972).

Related to the notion of a profession is class structure, with the medical profession, on the whole, being drawn consistently from the middle classes, creating a power based on education and patronage. Many of the emerging new professions were developing without the initial power base of medicine. Nursing had its own particular beginnings rooted in the Crimean War with the work of Florence Nightingale. Prior to that time nursing of the sick took place within their families or in hospitals run by religious foundations where, exclusively, nursing was carried out by men. Once women were introduced into nursing it is strongly possible that their gender contributed to their status leaving them subordinate to the male-dominated medical profession. Despite Nightingale's assurances that women entering nursing came from good-class families, the very nature of their work ensured that it was at the direction of the medical profession. In addition, unlike medicine, nursing was seen as a vocation of loving care.

Studying the literature on the rise of professions, it would seem that there were several characteristics which dominated discussions on a profession. First, there was seen to be a distinct domain of knowledge (specialist knowledge or theory of practice). This is associated with the control of admission to the occupational group. Second, there was the establishment of a code of ethics and professional values within the occupational group considered superior to the rules of employment or government. Following on, the occupational group created the power to discipline or debar its members who had transgressed the ethical codes or practice standards. Finally, the development of formal occupational (professional) associations, often with the publication of their own journals, ensured a culture apart from non-professional groups. It is also very obvious from the literature that many of the so-called professions have struggled to develop an identity and continue to do so even until today.

It took almost 60 years from the establishment of the GMC and subsequent registration of medical practitioners, before the statutory requirement for registration of nurses and midwives in the Nursing Registration Act of 1919. The prime movers behind this were, of course, Florence Nightingale and the position of nursing in the First World War. Health visiting was not registered and, until the requirement of a nursing qualification prior to entry to training in 1962, there was no statutory organization for health visitors, who remained under the control of medical officers of health. Health visitors finally formally registered with the advent of the Nursing, Midwifery and Health Visiting Order 1979. Prior to that health visitors were registered with the Council for the Education and Training of Health Visitors (CETHV), established in 1962.

The use of the term 'semi-professions' (Etzioni 1969) in relation to nursing seems to have been based on the fact that their education and training were too short or that there was insufficient obvious autonomy in their work. The term 'professions supplementary to medicine' was a phrase coined in Britain particularly for those occupational groups such as physiotherapists, pharmacists, dieticians and so forth whose work was dependent on the diagnosis of the medical profession. It has only been in the latter half of the 20th century that there has been a noticeable change in the status of the position of the professions supplementary to medicine. Thus recognizing that there is a far greater interdependency between many of the occupational groups and medicine. Today, the new title is 'professions *allied* to medicine', as opposed to *supplementary*. This would appear to be more politically acceptable as well as more accurate. This is particularly apposite for specialist community public health nursing because it is the one main occupation within the broad sense of nursing occupations that practises without any medical diagnosis; indeed there may be little contact with an illness service for the bulk of public health work. The raising of specialist practice qualification to degree status (building on the diploma entry requirements for pre-registration entry) goes some way to mitigating against the term 'semi-profession', although there was some initial disquiet concerning the proposed length of specialist practice courses.

WHAT IS A PROFESSIONAL?

The short answer to the question above is 'anyone who belongs to a profession', but this might categorize the theatre technician and the surgeon as both belonging to the medical profession. They both work in medicine but one may belong to a profession allied to medicine and the other is a professional medical doctor. Johnson (1972) suggests that to become a professional one has to satisfy the criteria for entry to education and training as well as pay a fee to the professional body subsequently in order to practise. To be a professional, therefore, one must adhere to the standards set by the profession. However, there is nothing to say that these standards cannot be sufficiently broad to allow flexibility, and yet concise enough to allow a degree of measurement to ensure quality and rigour, recognizable to outsiders as professional behaviour.

Barber (1963) argues that a professional displays 'professional behaviour', of which he defines four essential attributes:

1. a high degree of general and systematic knowledge

2. primary orientation to the community interest rather than individual self-interest

3. a high degree of self-control of behaviour through codes of ethics internalized in the process of work socialization and through voluntary associations organized and operated by the work specialists themselves

4. a system of awards (monetary and honorary) that is primarily a set of symbols of work achievement and thus ends in themselves, not means to some end of individual self-interest.

Johnson (1972) argues that knowledge provides a powerful tool for use in control over nature and society – hence professional power, which, in relation to specialist community public health nursing, will be discussed in the next section. Parsons (1954) also questions the use of general and systematic knowledge whereby cliques representing specialisms may impose on the profession role, definitions which are geared to maintaining their own dominant position at the expense of the rational application of knowledge. A challenge to the medical profession has been that doctors may only divulge what they consider necessary to divulge about a patient's condition, thus giving inadequate information from which a patient has little opportunity for choice. Again, this argument will be examined in relation to specialist community public health nursing.

Hanlon (2000) considers that, particularly under the 'New Right', professional membership, originally based on a fixed identity and a life-long occupational commitment, is being undermined. There is increasing disagreement between how public sector professionals view their role, how the state views it and how customers/clients view it. In addition there seem to be disagreements between the professionals, with younger professionals seeing greater opportunities created by state interventions than their more conservative older colleagues. This has been very evident in the last 20 years of health visiting when newly qualified students, taking their initiatives from the confidence of their learning from new education courses, have found it difficult to initiate new ways of working alongside older, less well-educated colleagues. Lest this is seen as a pejorative reflection on previous courses, that is not the intention; rather that the organization of health visiting within the field has mitigated against new approaches to practice. This has some relevance to the next paragraph on roles.

The second main area for discussion in relation to *professional* draws from the work of Goffman (1961), in which he discusses professional role definition. Goffman, an American sociologist, illuminates this concept of *professional* through the use of what he called 'role theory'. A 'role' is the activity undertaken by someone 'acting in accord with the normative demands upon someone in his/her position' (Goffman 1961, p. 85). 'Role performance', Goffman suggests, is the actual conduct of the individual while actually carrying out the demands of the position. Further on in his paper, Goffman discusses 'role' in terms of commitment and differentiates between 'role attachment', whereby individuals take on the education and characteristics of the position to which they aspire, and 'role embracement', whereby individuals may take on the demeanour of the role. In exploring the limitations of role theory, Goffman considers that role dysfunction can be too easily explained due to the role expectation (both within and outside the role) that is created by this framework. However, he uses two other descriptors which may have relevance later in this study: namely, 'role distance', supposedly endured by those not willing to embrace the role for diverse reasons, and 'role conflict', relating to the situation professionals may find themselves in when the role conflicts with their personal situation. For the latter Goffman uses the example of a surgeon required to treat a relative impersonally and not as a relation.

The two main approaches discussed above highlight differences and similarities when used for the derivation of the concept of a professional; both are concerned with behaviour, observed and expected. Whereas Barber and Parsons concentrate on epistemological concerns, that is, the knowledge and theory determining the professional, Goffman is more concerned about behaviour which appears to be associated with ontological aspects and is less concerned with epistemology. An ontological approach leads on to the next keyword discussion: professional knowledge.

PROFESSIONAL KNOWLEDGE

Barber (1963) considered a high degree of general and systematic knowledge to be redolent of a professional. 'Trait theory' (the acquisition of a collection of characteristics or traits), discussed by Millerson (1964), included 23 traits, among which are skills based on theoretical knowledge and the provision of education and training. Johnson, in examining Barber's analysis of a professional, argues that the general and systematic knowledge discussed provides a powerful control over society and thus it is important to society that this knowledge is considered to be used in the community interest. Johnson (1972) uses Rueschemeyer to point out that the 'General Practitioner's skills are not even predominantly those of a skilled technician: rather they refer to the ability of the practitioner to relate in a warm and personal way to the patient who is seeking reassurance and a listening ear at least as much as a specific diagnosis and adequate treatment' (Johnson 1972, p. 35). The relevance of this observation appears to be crucial to the debate following the change in the NMC Register.

Eraut (1994) links his characteristics of the professional knowledge-base with the power that these exert mainly through claims to unique forms of expertise not shared by other occupational groups. He particularly focuses on three main ways in which professions present their knowledge-base: carrying the aura of certainty

associated with established scientific disciplines; being sufficiently erudite to justify a long period of training, preferably at degree level or beyond; and different from that of other occupations. Hanlon (1998) is concerned about the weakening of a professional attribute by interference from the state. It remains to be seen whether the notion of a generalist professional education leads to a dilution of ability in many discretely specialist areas, that is, whether specialist community public health nurses who come from health visiting or occupational health will lose their specialist skills if required to show proficiency in public health principles.

The problem about knowledge in practice is that much of it is gained by the means cited – practice, that is, an epistemological process. For instance, when discussing height measurement of a child aged 3 the 'know that' is that children aged 3–4 stand with knees flexed. The 'know how' of measuring is to ask the child to take a deep breath, because in so doing they automatically pull themselves up straight. Yet to ask a child of that age to stand straight may not achieve the desired posture. It is highly unlikely that all aspects of this example will be taught, particularly as part of the course curriculum – they are learnt in practice, often by observation, and it is equally unlikely such aspects will ever be assessed; indeed, they may not be known by some practising health visitors. These are sometimes what are known as the 'wrinkles' of practice. The question then arises: is this knowledge necessary for practice? The answer surely must be no – but may be the difference between specialized knowledge and general knowledge.

THE NEW NURSING AND MIDWIFERY COUNCIL (2001)

The new Nursing and Midwifery Order 2001 passed into statute in December 2001, and in April 2002 the Nursing and Midwifery Council (NMC) replaced the United Kingdom Central Council for Nursing, Midwifery and Health Visiting (UKCC) as the regulatory body. In setting up a new Register the NMC has followed the dominant characteristics of a profession. There is control of admission to the Register through the successful completion of pre-registration courses. A code of ethics has been in place for many years, as has a code of professional conduct, although both will be updated in the light of the new Register. There are standards of proficiency for both pre-registration nursing and midwifery education programmes and these define the overarching principles of practising as a nurse or midwife in the UK, as well as the scope of practice (NMC 2004a). The previous register was cumbersome, having remained extant throughout major educational changes over the years, with new titles merely being added as new parts of the register. The major change mentioned at the beginning of this chapter has been in the naming of a third part of the Register as Registered Specialist Community Public Health Nursing. This is a post-registered part of the Register on to which, at this stage (2004), only health visitors (i.e., those practitioners who have previously been on the register as health visitors), will be eligible for registration. Subsequently, there will be provision for recordable specialist practice qualifications. It is likely that other practitioners who have formerly worked in the community/public health will be admitted to the third part of the register, provided they can show sufficiency of practice in the appropriate standards that are now established. They will, however, be required to show education to at least first degree level.

AN EXPLORATION OF COMMUNITY NURSING ROLES PRIOR TO 2004

Prior to the advent of the new register in 2004, nurses, midwives and health visitors working in the community adhered to the roles that had, by custom and practice, been assigned to the job title. Thus, for example, in the community, district nurses worked in the home and the GP surgery mainly in secondary care and chronic illness, practice nurses worked in the surgery alongside the GP, and health visitors were based in the surgery and worked mainly with under fives and in health promotion in all age groups. In effect there was little cross over of roles and in any one day a family home may have a visit from a district nurse, midwife and health visitor, probably for different family members. The financial and time costs were obviously very high when working this way.

Publication of several key reports (*Primary Care: The Future: Choice and Opportunity* 1996; *Making a Difference* 1999; *The NHS Plan: A Plan for Investment. A Plan for Reform* 2000; *Liberating the Talents* 2002; and others) began a movement whereby major change to the nursing workforce, formerly envisaged, was rapidly developing. A sudden plethora of nursing titles came into being amongst nursing staff who were working in primary care settings. In a study exploring developing roles in primary care in the West Midlands, Carnwell & Daly (2003) examined the roles of Advanced Nurse Practitioners (ANPs) who were working on a practice–strategy continuum. At that time they found that Practice Nurse ANPs' expertise lay in their advanced practical assessment and diagnosis of individual patients, with little opportunity for strategic development. Health Visitor and District Nurse ANPs operated at the strategic end of the practice–strategy continuum, but operated differently at this level. Health Visitors, being community and public health focused, are involved in multi-agency work, practice development and policy formation. District Nurses, on the other hand, work with individual patients/carers and the nursing team; thus their involvement in strategic developments tends to focus predominantly at patient care level, such as protocol and practice developments, although they may work in all three domains. Earlier, Daly & Carnwell (2003) found an abundance of titles, which included:

- Nurse Practitioner
- Clinical Nurse Specialist
- Specialist Practitioner
- Advanced Practitioner
- Nurse Therapist
- Physician's Assistant
- Higher Level Practitioner
- Nurse Consultant.

These titles have developed as the result of reduction in doctors' working hours, staff recruitment and retention problems in some specialities, new personal medical services within Primary Care Teams (PCTs), NHS frameworks and patient demands for greater choice and accessibility. However, there was considerable confusion and ambiguity surrounding these titles and their roles, and the training offered varied from short courses organized locally to postgraduate study. In addition, salary was a contentious issue for many ANPs, with little note taken of the education level of the practitioner. As well as this contention, a further contention arises over the use of clinical skills; some roles created a feeling in the occupant of being deskilled, while others felt they lacked opportunities to develop their broader skills by practising clinically, and felt deskilled if they did not.

THE REASON FOR A NEW REGISTER

The new Register came into being in 2004 and is simplified into three parts – Registered Nurse or Registered Midwife, both by direct entry, and Registered Specialist Community Public Health Nurse – entry being via either of the other parts of the Register.

Mentioned above are some of the reasons for the new Register, but the main and major change has come about, not from nursing and midwifery but from the government's proposals for delivering the *NHS Plan* (DH 2002f). The *NHS Plan* means services should be integrated around the needs of patients and communities. The advent of Primary Care Trusts as the new organizers for delivery of health services in primary care has led to a demand that there should be greater freedom and more flexibility amongst health care workers in primary care. *Liberating the Talents* (DH 2002b) provides primary care organizations with a new framework for planning and delivering nursing services in primary care. The role of nurses and all professionals in primary care is being changed as a result of developments such as PMS pilots, Walk-in-Centres, NHS Direct, GPs with special interests, the 'expert patients programme' and the expansion of support staff and skill mix.

The *NHS Plan* (DH 2001c) requires NHS employers to empower appropriately qualified nurses, midwives and therapists to undertake a wider range of clinical tasks. The Chief Nursing Officer has been instrumental in identifying 10 key roles for nurses in the clinical field (Box 1.1).

Clearly most of these services will be within hospitals or other clinical settings, but they may well lead to the development of an increasing amount of secondary care which, at present, is likely to be in hospital but which will, in the future, be in the community. This secondary care will be mainly the responsibility of nurses. It is very apparent that there will be a need to ensure that any practitioner who undertakes these roles will be competent so to do, and the concerns about maintenance of skills raised by Daly & Carnwell (2003) are extremely important in the light of these changes.

The *NHS Plan* (2002) proposes three core functions to be provided by nurses, midwives and health visitors in primary care (Box 1.2). These appear to be radical changes to the way nurses, midwives and health visitors have been

---

Box 1.1 10 key roles for nurses in the clinical field

- To order diagnostic investigations such as pathology tests and X-rays
- To make and receive referrals direct, e.g. to a therapist or pain consultant
- To admit and discharge patients for specified conditions and within agreed protocols
- To manage patient caseloads, e.g. for diabetes or rheumatology
- To run clinics, e.g. for ophthalmology or dermatology
- To prescribe medicines and treatments
- To carry out a wide range of resuscitation procedures, including defibrillation
- To perform minor surgery and outpatient procedures
- To triage patients using the latest IT to the most appropriate treatment
- To take the lead in the way local health services are organized and run

---

Box 1.2   A new framework for nursing in primary care

Three core functions:

1. first contact/acute assessment, diagnosis, treatment and referral
2. continuing care, rehabilitation, chronic disease management and delivering National Service Frameworks (NSFs)
3. public health/health protection and promotion programmes that improve health and reduce inequalities.

Within this framework there is also the need to:

(a) plan services in a new way through public involvement and choice with services based on needs
(b) develop clinical roles by valuing generalists, developing advanced and specialist skills and aiming for a one-service approach
(c) secure better care by improving the working environment, greater freedom, effective leadership.

NHS Plan (DH 2002f)

---

practising in the community. Yet analyses of the many ways in which some of these professionals have been practising in the last 20 years indicate that this framework is primarily an articulation of what has already been going on. However, because of the formality of this articulation through *Liberating the Talents* (2002) new requirements for pre-registration courses for post-registration specialist practice are required.

REQUIREMENTS FOR ENTRY TO THE THIRD PART OF THE REGISTER – SPECIALIST COMMUNITY PUBLIC HEALTH NURSE

In discussing the meaning of professionalism earlier in the chapter, the point was made concerning the importance of standards of practice and protection of the public. The third part of the Register has been established to ensure that

practitioners are able to work both with individuals and with a population (NMC 2003a). As stated by the NMC:

> *Nurses may make decisions on behalf of a community or population without having direct contact with every individual in that community. Public health nurses need to be able to work along a continuum of practice between clinical work with individuals and interventions at population level. In addition an increasing number of registered practitioners are also required to deliver a public health based nursing service to a range of populations across different health service providers and employers.*
>
> *(NMC 2003a)*

The NMC, in redesigning the Register, recognized that specialist practitioners were likely to come from wide-ranging geographical and organizational backgrounds to specific client groups, as well as according to health needs. The different groups may be families, children, older people, employment groups and those with mental health or learning disabilities, while health needs could include coronary care and long-term illness. A common feature of these practitioners will be that they reflect many, if not all, of the specialist skills outlined in the standards of proficiency for specialist community public health nurses.

The Nursing and Midwifery Order 2001 explicitly requires the NMC to ensure the maintenance of standards. To date (2004) standards have been set for the three parts of the register, namely Pre-registration Nursing, Pre-registration Midwifery and Specialist Community Public Health Nursing. The NMC is in the process of developing consultation documents and meetings for the preparation of standards for the education programmes for pre-registration branches of mental health nursing, learning disabilities nursing, adult nursing and children's nursing. It would seem likely that in due course education guidelines (possibly including competency/proficiency requirements) will be set for health visiting, occupational health nursing and school nursing – specialisms within community public health nursing – although they will be extrapolated from the Standards of Proficiency for Specialist Community Public Health Nurses (NMC 2004a). Nevertheless, any guidelines will probably be loose enough to embrace creativity and flexibility within the curriculum.

STANDARDS OF PROFICIENCY FOR ENTRY TO THE REGISTER FOR SPECIALIST COMMUNITY PUBLIC HEALTH NURSES (2004)

The standards of proficiency (Table 1.1) underpin the 10 key principles of public health practice in the context of specialist community public health

nursing. They are grouped into four domains, which were the original *four principles of health visiting* (Council for the Education and Training of Health Visitors 1977, Twinn & Cowley 1992):

- search for health needs
- stimulation of awareness of health needs
- influence on policies affecting health
- facilitation of health enhancing activities.

These standards have been set for specialist community public health programmes, which at least will ensure that when extant requirements for specialist programmes (e.g., requirements for pre-registration health visitor programmes, 2002) have been modified and approved, practitioners have undertaken a standard

Table 1.1   Standards of proficiency for entry to the Register

Principle	Domain *Search for health needs*
Surveillance and assessment of the population's health and well-being	Collect and structure data and information on health and well-being and related needs of a defined population
	Analyse, interpret and communicate data and information on the health and well-being and related needs of a defined population
	Develop and sustain relationships with groups and individuals with the aim of improving health and social well-being
	Identify individuals, families and groups who are at risk and in need of further support
	Undertake screening of individuals and populations and respond appropriately to findings
Principle	Domain *Stimulation of awareness of health needs*
Collaborative working for health and well-being Working with, and for, communities to improve health and well-being	Raise awareness about health and social well-being and related factors, services and resources
	Develop, sustain and evaluate work
	Communicate with individuals, groups and communities about promoting their health and well-being
	Raise awareness about the actions that groups and individuals can take to improve their health and well-being
	Develop capacity and confidence of individuals and groups, including families and communities, to influence and use available services, information and skills, acting as advocate where appropriate
	Work with others to protect the public's health and well-being from specific risks
Principle	Domain *Influence on policies affecting health*
Developing health programmes and services and reducing inequalities	Work with others to plan, implement and evaluate programmes and projects to improve health and well-being
	Identify and evaluate service provision and support networks for individuals, families and groups

(*Continued*)

Table 1.1 (*Continued*)

Policy and strategy development and implementation to improve health and well-being	Appraise policies and recommend changes to improve health and well-being Interpret and apply health and safety legislation and approved codes of practice with regard for the environment, well-being and protection of those who work within the wider community Contribute to policy development Influence policies affecting health
Research and development to improve health and well-being	Develop, implement, evaluate and improve practice on the basis of research, evidence and evaluation
Principle	**Domain** *Facilitation of health–enhancing activities*
Promoting and protecting the population's health and well-being	Work in partnership with others to prevent occurrence of needs and risks related to health and well-being Work in partnership with others to protect the public's health and well-being from specific risks
Developing quality and risk management within an evaluative culture	Prevent, identify and minimize risk of interpersonal abuse and violence, safeguarding children and other vulnerable people, initiating the management of cases involving actual or potential abuse or violence where needed
Strategic leadership for health and well-being	Apply leadership skills and manage projects to improve health and well-being Plan, deliver and evaluate programmes to improve the health and well-being of individuals and groups.
Ethically managing self, people and resources to improve health and well-being	Manage teams, individuals and resources ethically and effectively

programme for professional practice. This will ensure equality of education to combat the allegations identified by Carnwell & Daly (2003a) earlier in the chapter.

PROFICIENCY AS A UNIT OF MEASUREMENT FOR THE NEW STANDARDS FOR THE THIRD PART OF THE REGISTER

A major change that these standards are setting is that the unit of measurement is set at *proficiency*, unlike previous requirements for education and practice, which used the descriptor *competence*.

To consider the major change that the new standards have set for assessment by using proficiency as a descriptor for the standard, it may be helpful to dwell for a short time on the historical development of nursing theory. From Nightingale until the middle of the 20th century, nursing was described as a vocation built around care of and communication with the patient. Whittington & Boore (1988) describe a

period from the late 1950s until the late 1960s when nursing began to recognize the need to develop a theory of nursing to satisfy a demand for nursing to be seen to truly become a profession. Thus the nursing process commenced which, according to Orlando (1961), consisted of the interactions between patient behaviour, nurse reaction and nurse behaviour on behalf of the patient. These processes became a system and Roy (1970) first described a model. Roy emphasized the existence of biological, psychological and social systems within the person, and suggested that 'feedback loops' exist within each system, the states of which (in the patient and the nurse) the nurse should refer to when planning and implementing care.

These early and rapidly developing moves towards a systems theory of nursing very soon led theorists to recognize that nursing was struggling against other professional groups, for example teaching and social work, in undertaking task analysis studies. Various researchers (Klaus et al 1966, 1968, Urey 1968, Dunn 1970, Schneider 1979, King 1981) worked at task analysis studies to identify a theory of nursing, but it wasn't until Benner (1984) set a taxonomy of descriptors using the Dreyfus & Dreyfus (1980) model of skill acquisition and applied this to nursing that practitioners began to recognize that nursing did not consist of tasks alone. There were differences in the capabilities with which these tasks were carried out. Benner's (1984) stages of ability is now well known:

Novice → Advanced beginner → Competent → Proficient → Expert

Using analyses of nurses in the acute field, Benner suggested that the *competent* nurse has been working in the same job/field for about 3 years and sees the actions of competent nurses in terms of long-range goals or plans of which they are consciously aware. The competent nurse lacks the speed and flexibility of the proficient nurse but does have a feeling of mastery and the ability to cope with and manage the many contingencies of clinical nursing. The conscious deliberate planning that is characteristic of this skill level helps achieve efficiency and organization.

Benner (1984) described the *proficient* nurse as perceiving situations as wholes rather than in terms of aspects, and performance is guided by maxims (principles). The proficient nurse learns from experience what typical events to expect in a given situation and can recognize when the normal picture does not materialise. This improves decision making because the nurse has a perspective on which the many existing attributes and aspects present are the important ones.

NMC (2004a) in the introduction to the standards of proficiency for Specialist Community Public Health Nurses states four key areas of principle. These guiding principles provide the foundation for the standards of proficiency and fitness for practice programmes must show:

● **Preparation**: *fitness for practice* – practice-centred learning, theory and practice integration, evidence-based practice and learning.

● **Service**: *fitness for purpose* – practice orientation, management of community public health practice, professional perspective, service orientation, lifelong learning, quality and excellence.

● **Recognition**: *fitness for award* – level of learning, nature of learning, access and credit, flexibility, integrity and progression, educational quality.

● **Responsibility**: *fitness for professional standing* – adherence to the NMC *code of professional conduct: standards for conduct, performance and ethics*, responsibility and accountability, ethical and legal obligations, respect for individuals and communities.

ASSESSMENT OF STANDARDS

Many commentators (Coit Butler 1978, Dunn et al 1985, Whittington & Boore 1988, Ellis 1988, Runciman 1990, Girot 1993) agree that there is no accepted definition of competence that satisfies all the functional requirements of a profession, and one has to be careful when attempting to define competence to clarify exactly what is meant. Are the competencies of a profession the 'sufficiency of qualification and capacity' as in the dictionary definition, or are they the notion of criterion levels or standards of performance, below which, Ellis (1988) argues, one would be incompetent?

There is little in the literature concerning proficiency except on its premise of competence. In the light of the comments above, and those of other commentators, it is not possible to assess the standards of proficiency as they are articulated in the NMC (2004a) document. As the NMC clearly state, these are standards which reflect a breadth of practice and learning at a level commensurate with the specialist nature of community public health practice. However, NMC have assured the profession (NMC News July 2004) that the various specialist qualifications will not be lost due to the formation of a third branch of the Register. Thus it will be incumbent on the educational development and standards for the professional programmes (Table 1.2).

The NMC have been at pains to point out that the specialist community public health nurse practice has distinct characteristics that require

Table 1.2   Standards of education for specialist community public health programmes

Standard	Guidance
Standard 1	Programmes are required to have an overall length of 52 weeks, of which 45 are programmed weeks
Standard 2	Programmes will comprise practical and theoretical learning transferable to different settings, clients and areas of practice Periods of theory and practice should be distributed throughout the programme
Standard 3	The balance between practice and theory will be 50% practice and 50% theory. A consolidating period of practice equivalent to at least 10 weeks at the end of the programme is required
Standard 4	Where a particular practice route is required students must have completed their consolidated practice experience (minimum 10 weeks) and at least half the remaining practice time (minimum 6.3 weeks) in settings with clients that are central to the responsibilities for that defined area of practice
Standard 5	The minimum academic standard of specialist community public health programmes remains that of a first degree
Standard 6	The contents of the curricula should be that which will enable the achievement of standards of proficiency for safe and effective practice for entry to the third part of the register. Where a student intends to work in a particular area of practice, content must enable sufficient learning to take place within that area to ensure safe and effective practice
Standard 7	Students should be supported in both academic and practice learning environments by appropriately qualified teachers, who hold practice qualifications in the same area of practice as the qualification sought by the students they are supporting
Standard 8	The programme should be arranged so that teaching and learning of both core principles and those specific to particular practice routes are integrated through the whole programme at a level beyond initial registration as a nurse or midwife
Standard 9	In order to provide a knowledge base for practice, contemporary theoretical perspectives and public health standards should be explored
Standard 10	A range of assessment strategies should be used throughout the programme to test knowledge and standards of proficiency in all aspects of the specialist community public health nursing curriculum NMC (2004a)

public protection. These include the responsibility to work with both individuals and a population, which may mean taking decisions on behalf of a community or population without having direct contact with every individual in that community. It is therefore likely that programmes for the individual specialists who will make up the community public health nurse will be based on smaller units of measurement which are more easily measurable as against the holism of proficiency. Currently requirements for the pre-registration health visitor programme (NMC 2002c) will remain extant until 2007. These are stated in terms of domains and competencies using the principles of health visiting (Council for the Education and Training of Health Visitors 1977, Twinn & Cowley 1992) and as such they match very comprehensively the new standards of proficiency.

As there are 148 competencies described in the health visitor pre-registration programme document (NMC 2002c), the single example in Table 1.3 is taken from the domains and competencies and matched against the proficiency standards.

ASSESSMENT OF FIELDWORK PRACTICE

McMullan et al (2003) use Rowntree (1987), Somers-Smith & Race (1997) and Milligan (1998)

Table 1.3 Proficiency standards matched to competence framework for health visiting A1
(NMC 2002c, p. 11)

Principle (proficiency standards)	Domain (search for health needs)
Surveillance and assessment of the population's health and well-being	Develop and sustain relationships with groups and individuals within those groups with the aim of improving health and social well-being
Domain Pre-registration HV programme Develop and sustain relationships with groups and individuals within those groups with the aim of improving health and social well-being	**Competencies** This includes: (a) identifying one's own role and responsibilities and the limits of these (b) communicating in a manner that is appropriate to the needs, context and culture of the group and the individuals within it (c) listening to what people are saying and not saying (d) enabling people to think through their feelings about their health and social well-being (e) actively encouraging people to think about their own health and social well-being and that of others in their group (f) giving people sufficient time and space to think about and say what they want to say (g) enabling every individual within a group to make their own contribution (h) ensuring the confidentiality and security of written, verbal and electronic information that may be used in a professional capacity (i) disclosing information only to those who have a right and a need to know it and only once proof of identity and right of disclosure have been obtained
	Groups and individuals will include: Families – partners, relatives and friends Those brought together by a common interest Those brought together by a common aspect

to make the point that the purpose of assessment is to contribute to the maintenance of professional standards and to facilitate judgements about students' qualities, abilities and knowledge against predetermined criteria. This raises questions about the methods of assessment used, role of the assessor, and validity and reliability of the assessment.

Assessment of fieldwork practice can become an emotionally charged activity where there is resistance and challenge in terms of subjectivity or objectivity. In health visiting, fieldwork assessment relies heavily on the skills of the assessor to tease out and understand the complexities and dynamics of the interpersonal interventions between student and client. Chalmers' (1992) work on the theory of giving and receiving in health visiting practice

highlights this clearly when she discusses the 'pattern of mutual interaction between health visitors and clients in which both parties control the interactions by regulating what they offer and accept from each other'. She goes on to discuss these encounters within three inter-related phases of entry, health promotion and termination. In a similar vein, de la Cuesta (1994) talks of health visitors negotiating and compromising in their dealings with clients, aimed at getting the best solution given the context. The position of the community practice teacher as assessor becomes fraught with difficulties when set within the above contexts. In gaining his or her own experience a community practice teacher will have developed a personal set of skills that will work most effectively in the situations of giving and receiving, negotiating and compromising. Indeed it may take several years to become experienced and effective, and yet the community practice teacher assessor is making a judgement on the abilities of a student to show effectiveness in the early days of practice.

Subjectivity, in the light of the above, would seem to be about the values and beliefs of the assessor and could lead to prejudging of issues within the intervention process between student and client which do not fit the community practice teacher's expectations of how the intervention should be performed. Jarvis & Gibson (1985) make the important observation that the emotion of subjectivity is considerably reduced where it is made very clear that it is the practice that is being commented on, and not the practitioner as an individual. Nevertheless, Jarvis & Gibson also show how using Rowntree's (1987) use of the term 'descriptive assessment', which is objective assessment, namely – the student implemented an interaction with the client in a specific way – must be coupled with a judgement on the effectiveness of the intervention. This intervention may not have been carried out in a way that the community practice teacher might have used, but if the outcome was effective then the subjectivity becomes softened towards objectivity bound up in the outcome observed.

Jarvis (1983, 1987, 1992, 1999) has constantly worried about the philosophical issues underpinning practice education and assessment, and particularly when practice is both taught and assessed in the practicum by the same community practice teacher, unlike longer pre-registration nursing courses where the student will meet a number of assessors during practical/clinical experience. He has considered the philosophical bases for practice education and has shown that through the constant development of processes of peer and self-assessment through reflection, articulated by Schön (1987), reflective thinking is encouraged. However, Jarvis (1999) makes the important point that practice is not only the basis of reflective learning, but it is also the foundation on which theory is constructed.

He goes on to say that once practice is placed at the heart of education then there has to be a recognition of the way in which correct practice is assessed. The nature of assessment needs to be designed in such a way that practical wisdom is examined rather than what the practitioner does – the practitioners' reasoning about their practice, as much as the practice itself. The point is also made that the theory presented in the initial preparation of practitioners is merely information that the practitioners can experiment with in practice.

There are fundamental issues about the conceptual relationship between theory and practice, the links between Argyris and Schön's (1974) suggestions of *espoused theory* and *theory in practice* and Jarvis's suggestions of experimentation of theory during practice. These deserve exploration and it would seem to be important to differentiate between the aspects of practice to which the above can be applied. Where clinical practice demands practical dexterity combined with clinical knowledge there would seem to be a narrow area of focus thus reducing the opportunity for experimentation because of the boundaries of the reductionist (micro) field of expertise. That is, the protocols for practical skills in acute surgery or medicine are laid down by constraints of best practice and quality assurance; thus the student becomes an expert by constant practice along with clearly defined sets of behaviours. Where practice is about teaching, education, advising and supporting – the 'soft skills' – then there would seem to be far greater opportunity for experimentation of theory in practice. Practitioners are unlikely to accept this as experimentation, considering it to be more an application or modification of theory in context. Again, this discussion highlights the difficulties of the assessment of practice, particularly the 'soft skills' of practice.

EVIDENCE FOR COMPETENCE

This is important in the current climate of Clinical Governance (Department of Health 1997a), which has set up a National Institute of Clinical Excellence (NICE) specifically to report on clinically effective treatments; this will inevitably be based on hard science and leave little space for intuition or practical experience

(Robotham 2000). However, Benner & Tanner (1987) argue that a scientist may get agitated at the lack of precision evident in skilled know-how, but the lack of precision is not due to lack of judgement or knowledge. It is due to the inexactitude of the situation and the complex, skilled judgement required to consider the possibilities for each individual patient – in other words, competence in context only.

Intuition plays an important part in health visiting (and nursing), and is identified as part of the process of the use of knowledge from experience. It is also worth considering this statement under the notion of the ideology of a profession. If a profession is challenged for the inexactitude of its science this does not weaken the argument for its professional status. Rather it lends itself to the ideology of the uniqueness of the use of its knowledge and the fact that this knowledge is based on skills which cannot (or choose not to) be analysed from a hard scientific base but from a soft scientific (psychosocial) base. This is dealt with further in the chapter on reflective practice.

Reflective practice is considered at length in Chapter 11 and the skills of specialist community public health nursing–health visiting are considered, again at length, in Chapters 4 and 5. In considering the various discussions so far in this chapter there clearly appear to be two main facets in relation to competence in professional practice: first, the knowledge base on which practice is premised; and second, the skills and techniques whereby practice is carried out in context. In formulating a tool for the assessment of competence and academic grading of fieldwork practice, Robotham (2001) proposed that so-called 'competence' was actually made up of two capabilities: *knowledge capability* and *technical capability*:

- *Knowledge capability* is the professional knowledge in context which underpins and informs practice.
- *Technical capability* is the understanding and appropriate use of the tools of practice, dexterity skills, communication and reflectivity skills and strategy components (Robotham 2001).

There are, fundamentally, three types of tools in use whereby practitioners can consider, in detail, the components of their practice. The first type can be considered to be a reflective journal in which a student can record all their processes of practice experience and education. Within these journals students can be encouraged to reflect on a whole range of issues, including how they might tackle the situation if it occurs again. The value of a reflective practice *journal* over a reflective practice *diary* is that a diary has connotations of privacy and as such this means that a mentor/practice teacher cannot have access to this tool, and thus cannot use discussion and analysis as part of problem-based learning. It could be argued that this is merely semantics and a journal may also be private; however, a working document is also considered to be a journal. It is recommended that a reflective journal remains private to the student and practice teacher/mentor and that course tutors do not see these documents. The following (with the permission of the student and practice teacher) is a comment in the reflective journal of a student in the early days of practice:

Initially I felt apprehensive that I would ever feel confident about visiting clients alone. My knowledge was limited initially and I felt frustrated that I did not know more about health visiting and what it involved. Since Christmas I have felt a big change in myself. My confidence has improved enormously. I do not feel afraid to admit if I am unsure of something and will then set myself a plan to learn about that particular aspect so I will become more knowledgeable and understand more.

It is likely that the writer of this journal comment is not concerned about specific knowledge but more about general knowledge related to the type of clients she is visiting, which she can then modify to suit the situation. In reporting on the abilities of this particular student the practice teacher commented:

B ... is now far more confident than at the end of the first semester. Increased confidence and faith in her own abilities has helped her to become more creative in different aspects of health visiting. If difficulties are encountered B … uses reflective practice to think around the issues, to develop alternative strategies to deal with the situation. An example is, enabling a mother to participate in a sleep programme for her child believing it would work. Previously the mother had been very sceptical.

Further examples and models of reflective practice are to be found in Chapter 11.

The second type of tool to enable the articulation of competence(s) is a portfolio which, in nurse education, is used for both professional and personal development. In the UK portfolios have been part of nursing for many years, particularly as an assessment strategy to integrate theory and practice. Students acquire knowledge and skills, such as problem-solving and critical thinking from academics; however, they acquire and develop equally important practical skills and 'technical capabilities' from clinicians.

The content of a portfolio should be carefully selected examples of the achievements of learning outcomes. The selection depends on the proficiency and creativity level of the student, applicability of past experiences, depth of self-reflection and purpose of the portfolio. Too much information creates an unwieldy collection of documents, too little a sterile exercise. It is important that a portfolio is not just a collection of items in a folder, but that it shows how reflection on these items by the student demonstrates learning (McMullan et al 2003).

The third type of tool to articulate evidence of competence is an assessment document developed by several universities, in which the student provides evidence for the capabilities prescribed. In one such document (Robotham 1994) technical capabilities were assessed by the practice teacher – in effect, a subjective assessment of behavioural practice. In the same document the student was asked to complete the section which articulated a knowledge capability. The student was then asked to provide the evidence to demonstrate acquisition of the capability; the technical capabilities that were used (i.e., the resources and strategies);

the specific knowledge/theories used; and finally, comments on the evidence by the practice teacher. In both sections of the assessment tool the practice teacher and student were asked to negotiate a grade using a grading profile which reflected the grading profile used for academic assignments.

Research (Robotham 2001) using both quantitative and qualitative data and document analysis over four cohorts (about 120 students) showed stability and reliability of the fieldwork tool. Content analysis of the technical grading capability section of the tool showed it to be sufficiently penetrative and comprehensive to summarize the professional and behavioural abilities of the students. Content analysis of the knowledge capabilities section showed that students were able to articulate, through written evidence and reflective processes, what knowledge they used in practice situations.

Both sections of the tool – knowledge capability and technical capability – were graded by student and practice teacher alike, using grading standards commensurate with those for theoretical (academic) work.

SPECIALIST COMMUNITY PUBLIC HEALTH NURSING – HEALTH VISITOR PRACTICE: EXAMINING DOMAINS

Earlier in this chapter (p. 10) Daly & Carnwell (2003) explored a series of role titles found amongst practitioners in the community. In the first edition of this book there was a wide-ranging discussion over the proposed higher-level practitioner. In the event rapid political movements via the *NHS Plan* (2002) intervened in this, but it is clear that the proposals for higher level practice are no longer necessary because the new third part of the Register now allows for a much more flexible approach to practice than former traditional health visiting practice.

The following vignettes from Robotham and Sheldrake (2000) in the first edition have been matched against the domains of the proficiency standards and the health visiting pre-registration programme requirements.

Domain Search for health needs – identify groups and individuals who are at risk or in need of further support

Rita, aged 45 years, has left her husband and is homeless, and has come to lodge with her brother Fred. The council will not rehouse Rita because of a history of unpaid debts and antisocial behaviour. She has a daughter, Dawn, who is 15 years old, and two sons: 4-year-old Dominic and 18-month-old Damien. Dawn has started at the local school but does not like it. She does not attend and instead goes out with her 16-year-old unemployed friend, who gets drunk and takes drugs. Dawn has an 18-year-old boyfriend. She uses no contraception but Rita is sure she is sexually active and wants her to go on the 'pill'. Dawn also told Rita that she has a vaginal discharge and an itch but there is no way she is going to see the doctor. Dominic keeps scratching his head and Rita fears he may have nits, as he has had them in the past. He also has a skin rash, which is itchy. Rita says that she is very depressed because she is unemployed and Fred is hopeless and keeps getting drunk and they are all very overcrowded. She has come to the surgery to see the specialist community health practitioner.

Marie, the specialist community health practitioner with a health visitor qualification, has completed a nurse practitioner course, has been health visiting for 5 years and is also family planning trained. She runs her own clinic in the surgery and patients/clients are given the choice of whether they wish to see Marie or the GP when they make an appointment.

As a specialist practitioner, Marie will use her skills to listen to Rita and hear all her problems. She clearly understands Rita's feelings of hopelessness and spends time initially hearing about her financial problems. It is likely that Rita is getting insufficient income supplement and Marie helps Rita to make an appointment to seek advice from an officer in the social security office. She also telephones the housing office on Rita's behalf to arrange an appointment for Rita to go to see the special needs officer and discuss methods of paying off her unpaid debts. At the time of this visit Marie arranges for a subsequent visit to undertake a health screening for Rita.

Marie encourages Rita to arrange for Dawn to come to the clinic, where Marie will take a vaginal swab and discuss contraception. She gets Rita's permission to discuss Dawn with the GP and explains the need for her clinic discussions with Dawn to remain confidential to herself and Dawn, although she will encourage Dawn to accept the GP's advice once the swab test results are known. Marie asks Rita whether she would be willing for the school nurse to work with Dawn at school. Marie arranges another appointment for the following day, so that Rita can bring Dominic and she can examine him for live head lice and see what treatment she can prescribe for his rash.

After the initial interview Marie sees Rita regularly, either at the surgery or at home. The school nurse has spoken to Dawn and found out that she dislikes school because she is ridiculed for her poor reading skills – the school has arranged supporting sessions to help develop her reading. Dawn has accepted the help of a particular teacher who she thinks is wonderful because she listens to her. Gradually, the family's problems begin to resolve.

The specialist practitioner in this vignette is able to work with this family to help them to resolve their problems and this has been expedited by the following facts:

- Marie's surgery appointments are for half an hour if necessary.

- She is able to take swabs for differential diagnosis and, in the case of Dominic, to prescribe therapeutic cream for his rash and teach Rita how to fine-comb his hair. The GP is happy for Marie to carry out all the consultation and examination for Dawn, and will prescribe oral contraception, with Rita's permission and with Marie keeping a regular check.

- Marie has good links with the housing department and the special needs officer is sympathetic to the situation.

- Marie's knowledge of the benefit system means that, when she advises Rita to go to the benefits office, she knows she is likely to get a positive response.

- Marie's good links with the school nursing service mean that the school nurse is alerted to the situation and can liaise with the school pastoral service to help Dawn. The school nurse also spends some time talking with Dawn about handling her friend's alcohol behaviour and her own attitude towards alcohol.

- When the initial oral contraceptive does not suit Dawn, Marie discusses this with the GP, who changes the prescription, and Dawn is able to change her pills safely.

There are 10 competencies listed under this domain and this vignette would appear to encompass them all. It also calls for a practitioner who has undertaken both former health visiting-type education and training, but also has further developed her clinical skills. It is useful to match the competencies belonging to this domain against the vignette to see all the knowledge, observational, listening, planning, liaising, screening and clinical skills that are part of registration on the third part of the Register.

Domain Facilitation of health-enhancing activities – apply leadership skills and manage projects to improve health and well-being

Jennifer, a health visitor, works closely with her practice nurse colleague, Lynette, in the Sneed & Partners practice. The practice meeting, which all GPs, health visitor, practice nurse and district nurses attend, is looking at the quality of health care interventions. Jennifer and Lynette have been discussing for some time the group of potentially at-risk menopausal women who currently attend the surgery and who are seeking support and information concerning HRT. The practice meeting encourages Jennifer to undertake an audit of all the women receiving HRT. Jennifer designs a questionnaire to circulate to all women registered with the practice who are over the age of 45. The practice team agrees that they should ascertain knowledge of and attitudes towards HRT in this target group and also what the women feel about their HRT treatment. The questionnaire has a high response rate, and indicates that the group contains several important categories of women:

- those who have tried HRT and are not happy with it
- those who have not yet reached the menopause but who wish to know more about HRT
- those who are in the menopause and are undecided about the use of HRT
- a small group of women who have had an artificial menopause treated with HRT.

After consideration with Lynette and the GPs, Jennifer sets up informal discussion groups with the women to respond to their wish for education. Jennifer and Lynette spend time in consultation with the groups and respond to their needs with advice, counselling and health care support. The GPs and Jennifer decide to explore the needs of those women who were unhappy with HRT and establish two or three different therapeutic regimens, which Jennifer carefully monitors with an audit tool. Gradually, the practice establishes an audit cycle – defining best practice, implementing it, measuring and taking action where necessary. Jennifer, Lynette and the GPs are pleased with the results of this initiative and are interested in continuing this, and other practice developments to improve the quality of health in other groups.

The proficient practice demonstrated by the vignette shows the need for clinical leadership towards clinical effectiveness, and in the majority of situations it requires a team approach. This was a clearly defined group in whom the age process may well have adverse health effects to the quality of their life. The health visitor understood the audit process and her knowledge, in conjunction with the practice nurse, of the health needs of a target group within the practice population established a cycle of audit, risk management and clinical effectiveness. Challenging the original therapeutic regimens of the practice in relation to HRT was not without its difficulties, but good methodology in collecting information and establishing the situation soon convinced all the professionals concerned that this was an effective way forward. These are all part of the competencies of this domain and particularly require the skills of planning, liaising, researching, advising, supporting and demonstrating evidence-based practice.

Domain Influence on policies affecting health – work with others to plan, implement and evaluate programmes and projects to improve health and well-being

Sarah, a health visitor, works in a district chosen for a Sure Start trailblazer programme and has been chosen by her Trust to represent it at the local Sure Start planning meeting. The meeting identifies a housing estate that suffers from serious problems with services for children and young families. There is a well-established voluntary organization already running a good project in the area, with some informal drop-in parent groups. Sarah links with the voluntary organization, the local authority, the residents' association and other service providers and together they set up a partnership to widen the scope of activities to include health care, family support and outreach and childminder networks. Sarah liaises and networks to gain information and evidence of interest from many groups, and actively encourages members of the partnership to adopt the same networking framework. They work with the advisers, provided free, to prepare an application and Sarah is identified as the person who will be trained to help as an adviser for another area which wants to put an application in for the next wave. Sarah's group's application is successful and they begin actively developing their plan to transform existing services for the Sure Star programme.

Publicity is given to all parents and parents-to-be in the catchment area and introductory meetings are set up for parents to get access to services. Sarah is part of the organizing group that sets up home visiting sessions for parents who wish to have this facility. She undertakes some visiting herself and draws from a group of nursery nurses, link workers and some parents (who have had induction programmes in supporting) to undertake regular home visiting. Along with other planning group members Sarah sets up parent support groups, crèche facilities, a housing advice centre and a special teenage support group.

The voluntary sector-run family centre offers open-access drop-in services and a play group, as well as a small kitchen and parents' room. With the extra funding received from Sure Start, Sarah is part of the group that plans and develops extra facilities within the extension that has been built, in which there are now meeting rooms, a playgroup and an outdoor play site. Nursery workers for the crèche and day care are employed and further group activities for parents and children are developed.

As time goes on, midwives run regular preconceptual and antenatal clinics in the centre, the health visitors and the GP run regular drop-in health clinics such as well men's and well women's clinics, which are also attended by dietitians and health promotion staff. Cookery classes are set up and social services begin to develop a centre where children who are separated from one or other parent can meet and enjoy a social time together.

(This vignette is based on the examples from Sure Start – A Guide for Trailblazers, Department for Education and Employment 1999b.)

This is a wide-ranging competency under the proficiency principle of 'developing health programmes and services and reducing inequalities'. It involves working collectively with a community and the groups and professionals within it to plan and develop strategies to improve the health and well-being of this deprived population. The competencies involved are eight in number but with further subsets of skills with which to satisfy these competencies.

Domain Influence on policies affecting health – contribute to the development, implementation, evaluation and improvement of practice on the basis of research evidence and evaluation

Jane is part of the nursing forum that has been set up to support the nurse members of the local primary care team (PCT). Jane has an interest in research and is constantly encouraging her colleagues to collect data in relation to the health care needs of their client groups. Jane is particularly interested in hospital discharge care for older people and asks her colleagues to collect evidence of situations that they meet in their regular practice. Collection of this information over 6 months establishes several concerns, particularly about delays in the discharge information reaching appropriate professionals, but also about the number of times elderly clients complain that they have been visited by a series of professionals who do not seem to do anything and about whose function they know nothing. There also seems to be some doubt as to whether the link with the local social services for the elderly adviser is very clearly established. Jane hears of a good system that works in another part of the country and sets out to discover more about it. Her management realizes the value of this work and arranges for her to visit the area concerned. Jane listens closely to all the information she can obtain and makes copious notes to bring back to her colleagues. There is a wide-ranging discussion in the nursing forum and Jane's colleagues are impressed by what they have heard. A small pilot scheme is set up with one of the geriatric rehabilitation units that serves Jane's PCT area and the local

social services adviser is invited to join in the scheme. At the end of 6 months the scheme is evaluated and patients and staff are pleased with the results. The nurse forum, through Jane, asks the nurse representatives on the PCT to discuss the results with the board. This generates interest from the PCT, which establishes a larger pilot scheme to confirm the original results.

Certainly professionals should constantly develop their own practice but it often needs a larger group of the professional team to ultimately enable greater changes to health care practice.

Jane's ability to evaluate and audit practice in relation to both self and others and to take the wider perspective was the trigger factor here. Using the nurse forum as a basis to sound out her ideas and recognizing the need for improvement in this area meant that Jane could network outside her own immediate workgroup with the other organizations involved in elderly discharge planning and implementation. There are a number of competencies within the proficiency principle and they are particularly focused towards the strategic health of specialist community public health nursing.

Domain Influence on policies affecting health – develop, implement, evaluate and improve one's own practice on the basis of research, evidence and evaluation

Jean works as a community staff nurse for the elderly, liaising with other professionals and assistants who care for and support older people in their homes. Jean was originally an enrolled nurse and converted to RGN 5 years ago. She enjoyed the conversion course and learned about reflection, which she uses in her practice. Jean selects a health visitor as her clinical supervisor and the sessions prove very fruitful to both herself and her supervisor. She gains so much from this that she undertakes the clinical supervisor's course run by her trust and then in her turn she acts as a supervisor to two colleagues caring for older people, both of whom are care assistants employed by the trust. Jean feels frustrated because she recognizes that she needs further skills and education to work more effectively with her patients and clients. She applies for sponsorship for health visitor education and, at interview and subsequently, makes it quite clear that she wishes to continue to focus on older clients. Her enthusiasm and determination are recognized and she undertakes and successfully completes the health visitor course, eventually returning to work in her original post. Her confidence is high and she brings to her practice a wider dimension from her recent education. She undertakes some small-scale research with her client group and this is published in a peer-reviewed journal. Jean continues to clinically supervise care assistants and develops within them an enthusiasm for knowledge and self-development. They in turn take up opportunities for short education and development courses. In time, Jean and her colleagues, both in health and social care, set up a large support unit for carers and older people focused on the local community hospital. Jean reflects on her own development and that of her colleagues and recognizes how much they have all progressed through sheer hard work, determination and desire for self-fulfilment.

This may sound almost trite in its positive outcome but it is based on a real situation. The health visitor in the vignette is not a high-flier and her practice is rooted in basic no-nonsense care, support and commitment. What characterizes this scenario is determination. Jean did not have to undertake the health visitor course; indeed she was lucky that she received sponsorship, because she might have been too focused in her approach to health care and illness prevention. The competency aspects of this vignette are that Jean was reflective and self-aware and she was able to develop and use strategies to influence practice. The vignette says nothing about the high regard that patients and their carers have for Jean or how she fits into the wider health visiting team. Nevertheless, there is a great deal of advanced practice in this profile.

Domain Facilitation of health-enhancing activities – lead individual practitioners in improving health and social well-being

Mary works as a health visitor for a community trust that believes in the 'grass roots' approach to introducing new practices. Mary has long wanted to introduce the use of the Edinburgh Postnatal Depression Scale (EPDS) on a regular basis to the health visiting team working in the trust. She discusses this with the development manager, who is very supportive of her ideas and suggests a pilot study. Mary and the two colleagues working in her clinic decide on a strategy:

- All three undertake a literature search about EPDS.

- Discussions are set up with the local midwives to tell them about the intended project and to seek their support and collaboration.

- They write a short paper on how they wish to set up the project and approach the GPs serving the area to seek their support. Two practices are very supportive; one only gives permission to use patients provided it does not interfere with the status quo.

- The manager, who is very supportive, finds some money to fund an evaluation study of the project, to be undertaken by the local university.

- Mary goes to see health visitors in another part of the country who have set up a project similar to the one she and her colleagues are planning.

- Mary and her colleagues contact Professor John Cox (Cox & Holden 1994) to seek any advice that he can give.

- A time-scale is set up, materials are purchased and the project gets under way.

At the end of a year evaluation is undertaken and there are clear advantages to using the scale as a routine health visiting tool with postnatal women. Mary and her colleagues find that their practice with perinatal women has changed and that their clients have benefited greatly from the use of the tool. Mary and her colleagues are encouraged by their manager to disseminate their results to the rest of the health visitors in the trust. (See Ch. 5 for further information about EPDS.)

In wishing to change their practice as the result of research evidence, and in targeting a particular group with health needs, Mary and her colleagues are working towards a domain under the principle of *facilitation of health-enhancing activities, including developing services and programmes, plus working with and for communities.* They have used appropriate strategies to set up a project and have been proactive in managing the change required to alter practice. Not only is strategic planning required and much negotiating and networking, but also there are the 'invisible' changes that have to be planned for. These include aspects such as the changes that will have to be made to their weekly work data input to include a different approach to work, and ensuring that it is correctly coded for the information collection system.

Domain Facilitation of health-enhancing activities – develop partnerships with others to improve the health and social well-being of groups and individuals

John is a health visitor who is also a team leader for the Westerby practice. This practice has reorganized to include a self-managed primary health care team, including district nurses, health visitors, community staff nurses, care assistants and a nursery nurse. The GP practice nurse works closely with John and the team and they consider her to be a member although she is employed by the GPs. John acts as a leader rather than a manager and supports all the team members in their work and self-development. He holds a small budget and ensures that his colleagues can attend conferences or courses, provided they can justify how such attendance will enhance their practice. The budget also allows the employment of bank staff to underpin the study leave. John has worked closely with his colleagues, helping them to develop reflective practice skills, and they have regular sessions to maintain these skills. John is qualified in HIV and AIDS care and has a diploma in asthma care and in diabetic care. John acts as a resource to his colleagues and regularly holds small teaching sessions when they want new information that he can supply. He has actively encouraged his colleagues to produce information material for patients with varying chronic diseases and the team all take part in the approval process. Clinical supervision sessions, originally carried out on a one-to-one basis, have now changed to group sessions and John encourages a rotating clinical supervisor role among the more senior team members. A recent evaluation by the community trust has shown a positive response to this change by all the team members.

This is a clear leadership and development role undertaken by the health visitor. It embraces other disciplines and is facilitative rather than managerial, supportive rather than directive, and encouraging a positive ambience in which his colleagues can develop. Teaching and advice to colleagues in other disciplines and developing a climate conducive to learning and evidence-based practice are clearly working at a higher level, but John also thinks constantly about best practice to meet the needs of patients and clients. A patient/client consultative forum, set up by John, gives this group the opportunity to communicate the needs and aspirations of patients and their carers and the continual two-way communication between clients and professionals covering all manner of information helps to break down barriers and create effective partnerships in the practice.

CONCLUSION

At the beginning of this chapter it was explained how the NMC came into being following the closing down of the UKCC. The NMC (2003a) states that their prime function is to protect the public and in addition to set standards and guidelines for professional behaviour and accountability for all registrants. This chapter has discussed and explored the development and meaning of professionals and professional knowledge. Professionalism and professional knowledge are important in modern nursing and the formation of a third part of the Register has allowed an analysis of the need to be mindful of what it means to be a registered professional. Because specialist community public health nursing has such a wide-ranging brief it is even more important that the professional organization carefully underpins licence to practice. In this chapter some examples have been given of how practitioners may fulfil the domains of practice and these show briefly the level of expertise and knowledge that will be involved in assessing, analysing and providing for health care needs.

The following chapters in this book all contribute towards the goal of proficiency in specialist community public health–health visiting practice. Each chapter will contain many competencies of health visiting which go towards the standards of proficiency for entry to the Register.

Chapter **2**

Public health and health visiting

Elizabeth Porter

INTRODUCTION

This chapter is about public health, and its development with health visiting from the appointment of respectable women by the Ladies Sanitary Reform Association in 1867 to the present day. The public health role of health visiting is not all that simple because it has been influenced by the identification and evolvement of the role and function. These include policy changes in public health and medicine, expectations from others of its place within public health or the National Health Service (NHS) and of professional status and its interface with nursing.

THE 'HEROIC AGE' OF THE LATE 18th CENTURY AND EARLY 19th CENTURY

This was a period of public health concerned with healthy conditions in relation to the basic necessities of life. It was the age of environmental sanitation (1840–1890). The development of the Manchester and Salford Reform Association in 1852 was the origin of health visiting, where the approach adopted was didactic. Sanitary visitors (later to be called health visitors) talked, distributed tracts and gave information to the poor. The age of developments in bacteriology (isolation, disinfection) (1890–1910) saw Florence Nightingale herself as instrumental in setting up the first health visitor training course in Buckinghamshire in the 1890s. Allan & Jolly (1982) state that her vision of health visiting was quite clear: 'it hardly seems necessary to contrast sick nursing with this (health visiting). The needs of home health require different, but not lower, qualifications and are more varied. She (the health visitor) must create a new work and a new profession for women' (p. 92).

PUBLIC HEALTH AND HEALTH VISITING IN THE 19th CENTURY

Public health and health visiting in the 19th century aimed to attack the causes of ill health by controlling elements of the physical environment which were known or thought to be important to health, in particular, improving water, food supplies and housing while developing effective ways of disposal of sewage and controlling working conditions.

This was achieved physically through legislation and supply of administrative resources. It could be argued that the work of public health was dependent on political and administrative change. However, such an approach does not take account of individual behaviours, which are so important in prevention of ill health and management of disease. In order to tackle ignorance and eradicate practices harmful to the health of children in particular, health visiting became established as a state service to educate mothers in matters relating to the care of children and specifically matters of hygiene. The development of health visiting and the role of the state is seen as one of control and influence over the form and content of the health visitors' work, where the context of capitalist and middle-class concerns about the productive labour of the working classes encourages state intervention in the previously private sphere of the working-class home (Dingwall et al 1988).

PUBLIC HEALTH AND HEALTH VISITING IN THE 20th CENTURY

This became the age of education and personal hygiene from 1910 onwards. Health visitors became agents of pastoral power developed as a result of health discourses whose origins were located in the biopolitics, medical and hygiene discourses of 19th-century Britain (Focault 1979). The relationship between power, discourse and

knowledge is expressed in the relationship of the health visitor with the client group. The family is seen as the prime target for intervention and the working-class child as being endangered by disease and corruption and therefore a potential danger to society.

With the high infant mortality rates of 1925 causing concern for the Ministry of Health, the activities of the health visitor were refocused towards reducing infant mortality rates, and all entrants to health visitor training were required to have 6 months training in midwifery. This both limited the numbers of nurses qualified to become health visitors and restricted the profession to women, as only women could practise as midwives at this time. This clearly had an impact on the type of public health activity for health visitors. In the 1930s public health gave way to social medicine and following the Second World War legislation brought many changes to the health and welfare services. The emphasis of the role of health visiting shifted towards the all-purpose family visitor. The work extended to include the School Health Service in 1945, under the School Health Service (Handicapped Pupils) Regulations, and under Section 24 of the National Health Service (NHS) Act 1946 the preventive and social aspects of health visiting were re-established, with more attention paid to the family as a unit.

This role became more focused as a result of the Jameson Report (Ministry of Health 1956). Developed in part to address the high infant mortality rate, Jameson insisted that the course syllabus for trainee health visitors include the development of practical knowledge of home management with much emphasis on family welfare aspects and greater emphasis on social and mental health. The main conclusions and recommendations of the Jameson Report may be summarized as follows:

1. Functions to be primarily health education and social advice.
2. More attention to mental hygiene with some contact with all families where there are children.
3. Play a larger part in health education in schools.

4. Prevention of ill-health among the healthy to extend to include services of health visitors with infectious diseases qualifications.
5. Work with the family doctor where tuberculosis after-care measures are necessary for the recovery of the patient and family.
6. Work with the family doctor offering health education and social advice to whole families, especially mothers and children, old age, handicap, chronic illness.
7. Play an important role in relation to mental health, taking account of psychological factors in helping mothers.
8. Ascertain the social needs of the older person and handicapped person.
9. Supervise children with learning differences.
10. A family visitor, acting as a common point of reference and source of standard information, a common advisor on health teaching, a common factor in family welfare – a general-purpose family visitor.

Studies over the last 30 years have analysed the content of the role of the health visitor and found it to be much the same as in 1956, concentrating on children from birth to 5 years old. It has been suggested that the legacy of this era of health visiting lies 'in the pervasive stereotype of the rigid and authoritarian worker preoccupied with physical health and adhering to dogmatic methods of practice' (Robinson 1982, p. 25).

This view is in sharp contrast to the intention of the 1965 syllabus for education (Council for the Education and Training of Health Visitors (CETHV) 1965) which was to develop the health visitor as a health teacher and counsellor with skills in teaching, counselling, environmental health, knowledge and practice of health visiting, nursing and medicine. Training was based on the view that the work of the health visitor has five main aspects:

1. The prevention of mental, physical and emotional ill health or the alleviation of its consequences.
2. Early detection of ill health and the surveillance of high-risk groups.
3. Recognition and identification of need and mobilization of appropriate resources where necessary.
4. Health teaching.
5. Provision of care; this will include support during periods of stress, and advice and guidance in cases of illness as well as in the care and management of children.

The aim of this focused public health education was to develop skills in establishing interpersonal relationships to provide the basis for constructive work with families and individuals. The health visitor would have enhanced skills of perception of early deviations from the normal course of health and knowledge of the various statutory and voluntary agencies to assist in any particular family situation. Health education and a critical attitude to its use would form the basis for this work.

The skills of perception are seen as essential to identify the root causes of a client's anxiety satisfactorily. The health visitor facilitates clients in taking ownership of their agenda. Contact with clients in the home setting is viewed as enabling the health visitor to gain insight into the clients' perception of their health needs.

The public health activity of health visiting still centres on the family as a unit, concentrating on maternal and child welfare, tuberculosis visiting, control of infectious disease and school health. The term 'family visitor' increasingly becomes a misnomer as visiting is a mixture of control, education, inspection and support focused upon an individual, not a family.

Boundaries for practice are set by the masculine authority of, first, the Medical Officer for Health (1929–1974) and latterly the Community Physician (1974–1988), to whom the female professional was accountable. Men exerted definitional power over the boundaries of the emerging profession of health visiting through their control and management of resources and legitimacy, while the work of the health visitor involved the exercise of limited power over other women within a patriarchal home and family. 'Thus class and gender relations intersected to give health visiting its specific identity within public health' (Symonds 1994), as cited in Health Visitor Association (1994, p. 2).

The success of the health visitors' role, defined as educative and advisory, is in its ability to provide a low-cost method of health surveillance in which health visitors gain status through their association with the Infant Welfare Movement. It is the health visitors' methods of individual health education combined with the search for factors predisposing to disease that appealed to Community Physicians, whose practice was based on epidemiological principle.

The Infant Welfare Movement and the concern of the public about the high infant mortality rate provides health visiting with the legitimacy it needs to intervene in the lives of women and latterly their families. The power of health visitors in defining their own clientele lies within the area of agreement they are able to negotiate with the state. It can be argued that health visiting was created to carry state policies into the previously private sphere of the working-class home. The fact that it was originally intended as a new career for women is important for the limitation of the role in the public sphere and the direction of its work today (Kelly & Symonds 2003).

THE REORGANIZATION OF THE NHS IN 1974 SPLITS THE PUBLIC HEALTH WORKFORCE

This reorganization brought all local authority health services into the NHS, i.e. health visitors, district nurses, community dentistry, podiatry and physiotherapy. This move separates the public health function of health visitors from other public health workers and influences the direction of public health activity from this time. Within the local authority, environmental health officers came into existence in place of public health inspectors. They took over all aspects of food hygiene, pollution, noise radiation, water and sewer inspections, infestation nuisances, and some health and safety work in small and Crown premises.

Medical Officers of Health became District or Area Medical Officers and were sucked into NHS medical administration (many resigned). The new 'community physicians' are supposed to use their knowledge of epidemiology to tackle the epidemic diseases of the late 20th century:

- heart disease
- strokes
- cancers
- smoking-related respiratory and circulatory diseases
- accidents
- chronic disability and handicap.

Infection is thought to be a thing of the past. The Medical Officer of Environmental Health is the Health Authority Community Physician who has the statutory responsibility as 'proper officer' to the local authority for the control of notifiable, infectious diseases and food poisoning.

PUBLIC HEALTH ISSUES OF THE 1980s

The Alma-Ata declaration from the World Health Organization (WHO) in 1978 declared the goal of 'Health for All 2000'. This included designating the 1980s as the decade of safe water, the expanded programme of immunization (against diphtheria, tetanus, polio, whooping cough, tuberculosis and measles) and the Control of Diarrhoeal Disease programme to increase knowledge of the use of oral rehydration programmes in childhood diarrhoeal illness. The increasing momentum and desire for a new public health movement to tackle the health problems of the 21st century found its expression in the WHO 'Global Strategy for Health for All by the Year 2000' (HFA 2000), which was accepted as WHO policy in 1981 (World Health Organization 1981).

'Health for All' was not confined to developing countries, however: in 1985 the European Office of the WHO produced 38 Targets for Health for All in the European Region – from environment (water, housing) through to health care and health research (World Health Organization 1985).

The development of primary health care is seen as being central to the attainment of the goal of Health for All 2000 and it is recognized that the strategy depends on the development of community participation and collaboration between different sectors and agencies. If we remind ourselves of the public health function of the health visitor (list on p. 31) we can see how health visitors, placed within primary care (following the 1974 reorganization of the NHS) are in an ideal position to work towards this goal.

The three main objectives for WHO are:

- prevention of preventable conditions
- promotion of lifestyles conducive to health
- rehabilitation and health services.

In England in 1988, The Acheson Report (Acheson 1988) is the first official inquiry into public health in Britain since the 1871 Report of the Royal Sanitary Commission. In his report, Acheson used the WHO categories to define public health as: 'the science and art of preventing disease, prolonging life and promoting health through organized efforts of society'. This definition, in conjunction with one put forward by Brotherson (1988) – 'the organized application of resources to achieve the greatest health for the greatest number' – gives a fairly comprehensive definition of the philosophical, economic and organizational basis of public health at this time. The Acheson definition of public health has been the most used by health visitors and public health workers during the last 25 years and reflects how public health has been perceived within UK health policy since 1988.

Cowley (2002) suggests that in this definition public health is seen as a social construct based on a population perspective, concerned mainly with ensuring that the health of the public as a whole is sufficiently strong to ensure that society is able to function in a manner that is socially and politically determined as appropriate.

In 1994 the UKCC introduced proposals for the future education of community health care nurses (UKCC 1994a), where the title of health visitor was expanded to 'Public Health Nurse (Health Visitor)' in anticipation that this would encompass a broader function.

The Standing Nursing and Midwifery Advisory Committee report *Making it Happen*

(Department of Health 1995d) goes to some length to show that public health is a worldwide concept and that the Maastricht Treaty (Article 129) provides for European Community action in the field of public health. This action is limited to the principles of taking action if it is more effectively achieved by the Community rather than the member states, or taking action over issues relating to public health but not to delivery of health services. The bovine spongiform encephalopathy (BSE) crisis regulations of the early to mid 1990s, involving mainly the agricultural industry, were nevertheless imposed under principles of public health.

PUBLIC HEALTH IDENTIFIED FOR THE 21st CENTURY

In England the main goals recommended by the WHO are addressed in emerging policy documents. *The New NHS: Modern and Dependable* (Department of Health 1997a) puts public health at the heart of health authorities led by a Director of Public Health, and primary care is enhanced to play a leading role in health improvement and reducing inequalities. Primary Care Groups are introduced; where possible they are coterminous with local authority boundaries and their boards are multi-professional. *Saving Lives: Our Healthier Nation* (Department of Health 1999c) identifies new population health responsibilities to improve the health of all and address health inequality in the local community. Alongside this, the need for new nursing roles in public health is emphasized and the government suggested that in order to take forward its policies health visiting had to modernize its role to encompass working across traditional boundaries with voluntary workers and other professionals. It outlines new ways of public health working for the health visitor and introduces legislation placing a new statutory duty on health authorities to improve the health of their population.

At its heart *The NHS Plan* (Department of Health 2000c) aims to improve health and health care for communities. *Shifting the Balance of Power* installed public health as 'a corporate function' (Department of Health 2001f) and in 'securing good health for the whole population' (Wanless 2004) public health is identified as requiring strong leadership and organization in public health delivery and a national strategy to develop the public health workforce.

These and other major policy documents identify the government's commitment to a strong and effective public health workforce with the emphasis on public health practice (Department of Health 1999a, 1999c, 2000c, 2001e). This poses challenges to current ways of working and, in particular, working across traditional boundaries, networking and developing services in conjunction with service users and other professional and voluntary workers.

All four UK governments have set tough challenges around improving health, reducing social exclusion and joining up public services (Department of Health 1999a, Scottish Executive 1999, National Assembly for Wales 2001, Northern Ireland Office 1999). This acknowledges the need for the public health workforce of the future to be skilled, staffed and resourced to deal with the major task of delivering on health strategy. While health visitors and medically qualified public health staff have played a key part in the development of public health, there is a need to include in the new public health workforce people from a wide range of professional backgrounds. It is anticipated that this will meet the range of public health skills needed to deliver in the future (capability and capacity for public health practice).

The delivery of public health activity in this first decade of the 21st century is more client and team focused. The modernization agenda puts the user of health and social care services at the heart of the reforms (Department of Health 2000c). People who use health and social care services have a contribution to make to service provision, particularly in identifying their needs. This core public health value identified by the World Health Organization (1978) and reinforced in 1995 (World Health Organization 1997) puts community at the centre of the health care system, defining need, setting priorities and planning and evaluating services, embracing notions of health promotion through community empowerment, participation and self-determination.

THE ROLE OF PRIMARY CARE TRUSTS IN PUBLIC HEALTH

Primary Care Trusts (PCTs) were established in the NHS in 1999, with responsibility for providing and commissioning integrated health and social care for a defined local population. By bringing health and social care services together it is envisaged that public health policy within PCTs will develop strategies that address the wider determinants of health and health inequalities which have traditionally been outside the health domain, these to include employment, education, housing, income and the environment, as well as their effect on lifestyle.

Shifting the balance of power (Department of Health 2001f) gave PCTs a key public health role in identifying and responding to health needs and developing plans for health improvement, particularly in partnership with other agencies. The Priorities and Planning Framework (PPF) 2003–2006 confirmed that public health goals are a key part of Local Delivery Plans (LDPs) in improving access to services, breast screening and mental health in prisons, while reducing coronary heart disease death rates, suicides, cancer deaths, deaths from substance misuse, smoking rates and teenage pregnancy.

In responding to the Public Service Agreement and Priorities and Planning Framework, PCTs and Strategic Health Authorities (SHAs) set out priorities and objectives in their LDP. The LDP identifies the time-scale, milestones and delivery mechanism by which the PCT and SHA will achieve the targets in the Priorities and Planning Framework. The SHA develops a comprehensive Local Development Plan for their area, bringing together the NHS Trust Plans and local development plans of each constituent PCT.

The PCT, as the lead NHS organization in assessing need, planning and securing all health services and improving health, is expected to forge new partnerships with local communities and lead the NHS contribution to joint working with local government and other partners.

These local strategic partnerships have the remit to deliver the agenda of improving health and reducing inequalities in health.

In the 2002 Spending Review the Department of Health specified their aim to 'transform the health and social care system so that it produces faster, fairer services that deliver better health and tackle health inequalities' (Wanless 2004, p. 46). Specific objectives and targets are identified within a Public Service Agreement (PSA) as to how to improve service standards, and improve health and social care outcomes for everyone. In summary, the Department of Health delivers its functions through PCTs, SHAs and NHS Hospital Trusts. The PCTs and SHAs set out their priorities and objectives through the Local Delivery Plan.

LOCAL STRATEGIC PARTNERSHIPS

Local Strategic Partnerships (LSPs) were first introduced into neighbourhood renewal areas in 2001, to bring together voluntary, statutory and business sectors with community representatives to provide an action plan to tackle deprivation.

The focus of activity is to deliver services to meet the needs of the local population and the vehicle is partnership working between primary and community care. The aim of the LSP is to prepare and implement a local delivery plan with the aim of promoting or improving economic, social and environmental well-being in consultation with local people, public sector bodies and other organizations whose activities have a local impact.

PCTs have a central role to play in ensuring the decisions relating to both provision and commissioning of the public and key stakeholders. Improving the public's health and reducing inequalities is one of many responsibilities facing PCTs, and a whole systems approach to planning services as part of the LDP involving the community and partner organizations is seen as key to this working.

PCTs coordinate strategic action on inequalities through their LDP, working in partnership with local agencies and communities.

The focus of delivery is through public health teams in the areas covered by local authorities and PCTs. Although no single organization can now claim ownership of public health, the staff making up local public health teams will be from a variety of agencies whose work impacts on the public's health. This to be achieved through:

- multidisciplinary public health
- implementation of strategies to improve health and reduce inequalities
- interdisciplinary working across organizational boundaries.

Over the last decade the public has become more health conscious than ever before and ready to support innovative approaches to health care. PCTs are being challenged to find new ways of providing high-quality, effective, preventive health care for the population as the gap between expectations and reality widens. In setting out the government's strategy in England for closing the gap, the ninth of ten core principles in the *NHS Plan* (Department of Health 2000c) states that 'the NHS will keep people healthy and work to reduce health inequalities' (p. 5). For PCTs this means having good-quality data about the local population for a needs-based approach. Health visitors working alongside PCT public health specialists can play a key role in assessing the needs and profiling the population, while the Public Health Observatories can advise PCTs on accessing lifestyle data. Wanless (2004) advocates that the Commission for Health care Audit and Inspection (CHAI) should develop a robust mechanism for the performance assessment of the public health role of PCTs and SHAs. The test for each PCT is in how they assemble community resources to achieve this goal.

BUILDING CAPACITY AND CAPABILITY

The public health workforce in the PCTs is the key to delivering PCT health improvement targets and delivering on the National Service Frameworks (NSFs). It is felt that capacity and capability can be achieved if the public health workforce in PCTs consists of a mixture of the following:

- Specialists in public health: senior public health professionals (medically qualified and increasingly from backgrounds other than medicine) who work as Directors of Public Health, consultants and other specialists.

- Senior practitioners: public health practitioners who have senior-level expertise in specific areas, e.g. health promotion specialists, health strategy advisors, information specialists.

- Public health practitioners: health professionals working in PCTs who have a public health focus or component to their jobs, e.g. health visitors, school nurses, environmental health officers, community nurses, specialist general practitioners.

- Public health workforce: individuals working in PCTs and agencies who have the potential to make a positive contribution to public health, e.g. voluntary workers, nursery nurses, educationalists, youth and community workers.

This public health workforce can help PCTs maximize effort and resource by:

- 'Using epidemiological and health information analytical skills to provide population based assessment of health needs, and to ensure that resources are targeted to where they will have the most impact.

- Reviewing and providing the evidence to ensure that services are effective, both clinically and economically.

- Minimizing risks to the population through effective health protection measures and screening programmes.

- Providing longer term health improvements and reduced service use through effective health promotion.

- Providing public health leadership by working with other agencies and primary care services to deliver effective public health programmes.

- Good multi-disciplinary working where each occupational group has a sound sense of its own identity, contribution and boundaries, as well as a strong respect for others' (Hampshire and Isle of Wight Public Health Network 2003).

The key threats to future health, identified as smoking, obesity, coronary heart disease and health inequalities, have to be tackled today. Target setting has become the key instrument of public health policy within the PCT and stems from the WHO targets published in Agenda 21 (WHO 1999).

PCTs and local authorities increasingly recognize that health needs assessments are an effective way of gathering data from a community. They also provide opportunities for building partnerships, determining service priorities and identifying staff public health development needs (Public Health Development 2001).

Wanless (2004) makes over 20 recommendations on how to fully engage people in the UK in activities to improve their health, focusing on prevention and the wider determinants of health.

HEALTH IMPROVEMENT AND MODERNIZATION PLAN

This plan provides the main focus for partnership working between the NHS, local agencies and communities and is the local initiative for improving health and health care based on the annual report of the Director of Public Health. PCTs are leading the process, which has a 3-year strategic vision on how the health community, jointly with partners, will address health inequalities, health improvement and NHS modernization. PCTs are the key health organization to represent health within wider partnership working.

Health visitors must ensure they are involved in the planning of these strategies because they require a programme from a health and social focus that will meet the most important health needs of the population. For local planning it is the people working on the ground with the population who should be able to bring forward, or encourage local communities to bring forward, their health concerns.

The actual implementation of the health improvement plan falls into the hands of the management structure of PCTs, but it is the SHA who will monitor the running and effectiveness of the plan. The actual responsibility for commissioning more joint health and social care services to satisfy local health need will belong to PCTs, and these will be built into their service agreements with NHS Trusts. This means that health visitors need to know who their local nurse representatives are on the PCT board and keep in close contact with them to ensure that their voices are heard on behalf of, and with, their clients. It may well be that the nurse members of the local PCT will look to health visitors to provide them with information about the health needs of the local population.

HEALTH NEEDS ASSESSMENT, HEALTH IMPACT ASSESSMENT AND INTEGRATED IMPACT ASSESSMENT

All three approaches to assessment use the same core steps in planning, although they use different language. The main difference is their starting point and the scope of the assessment. The three approaches are used across the NHS, local, regional and national government and voluntary agencies. They offer three decision-making approaches, which are developing rapidly across all the sectors above to help improve health and reduce health inequalities.

HEALTH NEEDS ASSESSMENT

Health needs assessment (HNA) aims to improve the health of a population and reduce health inequalities in order to identify those with most to gain and ensure that the programme targets them. The protection and improvement of the health of populations, communities and individuals (public health) are based on the collection of health and social information in order to draw up accurate profiles on the health needs of the population. Before profiling the health

needs of a community at least three types of information are required:

- Information to describe the basic characteristics of the community (number of individuals, age, sex, etc.)
- Information to describe and monitor the health status of the community
- Information on the determinants of health in the community.

HNA starts with a population, defined by geography, gender, age or ethnicity, service user or issue. It then creates programmes for improving health and reducing health inequalities. It is a systematic and explicit process which identifies the particular health issues affecting a population that can be changed. The result is the identification of clear health priorities for the population from which programmes are planned to tackle them.

Searching for health needs and assisting in meeting them is a legitimate public health activity of health visiting. Responsible for assessment of need and the prescription of a plan of action for clients, health visitors are intimately concerned with the delivery of that plan and the evaluation of the intervention. The Public Health skills audit (Department of Health 2001h) examines health visitor activity and acknowledges the importance of assessing health needs and working in local communities.

Health needs assessment includes three steps:

1. Profiling the community and deciding on a wish list of needs
2. Using identified criteria, systematically deciding on health issues to be tackled by the team
3. Analysing each health problem and deciding on team action (Hooper & Longworth 1998).

This model incorporates aspects of the three main approaches to needs assessment. These include (a) the epidemiological approach, (b) the health economist approach and (c) the rapid appraisal approach.

(a) The epidemiological approach aims to understand causal factors well enough in order to devise interventions to prevent adverse events before they start (prevent initiation of the disease process or prevent injury). It defines needs in terms of morbidity and mortality. It enables health visitors to use both qualitative and quantitative research methods to collect epidemiological data (descriptive epidemiology). Qualitative data can add an important dimension to the understanding of the complex needs of a community. By analysing existing data the health visitor may be able to predict future health trends to inform practice (analytical epidemiology). This can then facilitate the targeting of health needs using appropriate resources (analytical and experimental epidemiology).

(b) The health economist approach defines need in the context of effectiveness and focuses on supply and demand. If areas of need are relative then they can be traded off against each other when there are limited resources. Economic risk is determined by the relationship between financial resources and demand on those resources. The goal of the health economist is to achieve balance, equity and efficiency across the quality, accessibility, continuity and cost of delivering the health service. Each of these is influenced by the demographic, social and political forces. For example:

- demographic forces: an ageing population with increased life expectancy
- social forces: change in leading causes of death like tuberculosis
- political forces: increased regulation and public health policy (see Chapter 16).

(c) The rapid (participatory) appraisal approach involves using the community's own perspective of its needs. It is widely recognized that the main determinants of health encompass a multifaceted nature, with the link between economic and social deprivation and ill health accepted (Leon et al 2001). This approach enables health visitors to try and understand how a community perceives its health needs. A participating community is not only necessary to focus individuals into identifying their health needs but is also a prerequisite for achieving equity and addressing inequalities which are the most important barriers to achieving health

goals (Tones & Tilford 2001). Knowledge acquired from a local community can enable health visitors to provide a vital contribution to the PCT. It can influence decisions which may be made about the development of appropriate health care interventions or services required to meet the needs of the local population. This should be reflected within the PCT Health Improvement Plan, which outlines identified areas of need within the local community. The distribution of resources is then made between areas in proportion to their relative need with different social groups targeted effectively (see Chapter 5).

Basic characteristics of data collection by health visitors

These can include a wide range of data that is all relevant when viewed holistically but whose constituent parts are often overlooked because the relevance is not recognized. Personal data is the most easily accessed by health visitors because of the types of record available in NHS databases: these include age, sex and occupation. However, economic data about the individual that includes employment requires more intensive inquiry to tease out and raise to the surface the hidden problems of industrial disease, deprivation and poverty. It is often difficult to ascertain the numbers of families and individuals who receive family credit and yet this may be fundamental to their health status. Similarly, leisure data and support networks such as religious activities and other community activities, which play an indirect and important part in health status, are less easy to find except on individual inquiry and are often considered difficult to access and therefore unimportant. Data on housing occupancy and condition can be collected fairly easily and the importance is evident, but environmental issues such as noise and pollution can be viewed from different contexts and these are less easy to pursue. For example, noise from traffic or industry is constant, although it may affect sleep and personal thinking space, but noise from neighbour behaviour is variable and possibly more threatening, creating an environment that may ultimately become more prejudicial to health.

The collection of this data is part of public health surveillance which is ongoing and involves the systematic collection, analysis and interpretation of data essential to the planning, implementation, dissemination, application and evaluation of public health practice.

The objectives of public health surveillance can be categorized under the Principles of Health Visiting (CETHV 1977, Twinn & Cowley 1992) as follows:

The search for health needs

- Determine health needs of the local population and identify trends
- Systematically collect, analyse and interpret data in order to create a profile of the local community (e.g. asylum seekers and refugee situation).

The stimulation of an awareness of health needs

- Provide information which enables people to address issues which influence their health (e.g. incidence of tuberculosis or asthma rates in children under 16 years of age)
- Raise awareness of health needs and facilitate a response if required (e.g. tuberculosis screening or providing information on prevention of asthma).

The influence on policies affecting health

- Plan interventions and target resources to meet the health need (e.g. work with PCTs to develop strategies to deal with tuberculosis or contribute to services in a healthy living centre to combat asthma).

The facilitation of health-enhancing activities

- Acting as a health agent, mediating between agencies on behalf of individuals, families or community health status (e.g. working with asylum seekers and refugees and PCTs in developing information for them in a user-friendly format, or mediating with services on behalf of families with children who are asthmatic to improve the air quality in public places), evaluating the effectiveness of the intervention (e.g. demonstrate the effectiveness of all interventions in order to evidence the benefits of public health action).

Certain aspects of health status are easier for health visitors to find out, such as mortality and its causes, and therefore, by implication, morbidity. However, most health workers argue that morbidity cannot ever be completely ascertained and that there are individual personality and coping factors to be considered. Quality of life and well-being assessment is possible both on an individual basis and from a family or community viewpoint, but the tools available vary in reliability and are time consuming to administer. Bowling (1991) argues that recent indices of health status have focused on ill health and were based on negative concepts of health – for example, mortality and morbidity rates, the self-reporting of symptoms, illness and functional ability. Health care professionals and social scientists are now looking more closely at the measurement of health status through the development of tools for positive measures of health. These include concepts of 'social health', 'social well-being' and 'quality of life', which influence the individual as well as the family and community.

Vital statistics are the maps and milestones of public health for health visitors and, in the main, include demographic statistics (population, marriages and births) mortality statistics (numbers and causes of death) and morbidity statistics (illness, injury, incapacity and hospitalization).

The trigger for assessment, action or intervention stems from the analysis of a community population profile and from the needs assessment identified with the client of the health visiting service. The search for health needs is impelled by the principles of non-stigmatizing, expert, purposeful, self-initiated activity (CETHV 1977).

Assessment of health needs is the first step in public health activity. It is fundamental to the planning of health care interventions and sees health visitors able to assess health needs through community profiling and caseload analysis. Health needs assessment has become an integral part of the government's reforms and initiatives, and the importance of accurately assessing identified health needs is well documented.

Epidemiological data in health visiting profiles

Despite the fact that information collection and audit have become increasingly comprehensive, it must be remembered that epidemiological data should always be viewed critically in terms of:

- *Accuracy.* Examples are: (a) hospital records of admissions will log readmission of the same person as a separate admission; (b) death certificates are required by law to state the immediate cause of death followed by the underlying cause of death. In Western countries few deaths are recorded as due to 'mental illness' or 'degenerative joint disease'.

- *Completeness.* Examples are: (a) only those road traffic accidents reported are counted; (b) although doctors are required by law to notify the Public Health Department of infectious diseases and are paid a small fee for doing so, underreporting is common.

- *Timeliness.* How up to date is the information? Collation, analysis and publication can take the National Office of Statistics 2 or 3 years.

- *Validity.* For example, lung cancer morbidity can be based on mortality statistics because most people affected die within a short space of time. For diabetes – a chronic disease – morbidity statistics cannot be based on mortality data.

Concern has been expressed by health visitors working in specialist areas related to public health departments that many of them collect data about the frequency of health problems but this has in the past been glanced at superficially where interventions have not been measured. The new public health audit tools (Department of Health 2001e) offer a more accurate interpretation to enable effective intervention analysis. All health visitors and public health workers need, therefore, to be quite clear about the meanings of epidemiological descriptors and measures.

Measuring the frequency of health problems

Rates

Over the course of 2 years 123 children were seen in a hospital fracture clinic with broken arms following a bicycle accident. Details of the main types of accident were as follows:

- accident with a car – 25 cases
- accident with an immovable obstruction – 23 cases
- accident with a person or animal – 15 cases
- accident on a slippery surface – 10 cases
- accident due to bicycle fault – 20 cases.

Does this mean that children are more likely to be injured while riding on roads alongside motor vehicles?

Answer: It is not possible to make a judgment until further information is available:

- How many bicycle-riding children are there in the area surrounding the particular clinic?
- How many children ride safe or faulty bicycles among cars, people, animals or on slippery surfaces?

To make a valid comparison we need to relate the number of children who ride bicycles, faulty or otherwise, to the number of bicycle-riding children in the area, or to the number of children who ride their bicycles in each set of circumstances. In other words we need to use rates.

A rate is a measure of how frequently an event occurs. All rates are ratios, which means they consist of one number divided by another number:

$$rate = \frac{\textit{number of accidents over a specified time period (numerator)}}{\textit{average population of bicycle-riding children during the time period (denominator)}}$$

The figure is usually multiplied by, for example, 1000 to convert it from a fraction to a whole number.

Incidence and prevalence

A secondary school has 100 children in the third year. On the first day of November, 10 children were away with a cold. Over the month of November, another 18 children developed colds and were away from school.

Assuming that the number of children in the year did not change during November, answer the following questions:

- What proportion of children had a cold on the first day of November? (point prevalence)
- What proportion of children had a cold some time during the month of November? (prevalence)
- What proportion of children who didn't have a cold at the start of November developed a cold during the month of November? (incidence)

Point prevalence refers to the proportion of people in a population with a disease or condition at one point in time: 10% (10/100).

$$prevalence = \frac{\text{total number of cases in a specified time period}}{\text{total population in the time period}}$$
$$= 28\% \, (28/100)$$

$$incidence = \frac{\text{number of new cases in a specified time period}}{\text{population at risk in this time period}}$$
$$= 20\% \, (20/100)$$

Population at risk is important: 90% of the population in this example. It refers to all people who could become new cases as 10 of the 100 children already had a cold on 1 November. Ninety children were at risk. The population at risk can require some careful selection to ascertain true (rather than assumed) numbers.

Example: You are interested in the incidence of testicular cancer in your area. You find out the number of new cases over the past year from the cancer registry. This gives the numerator for calculating the incidence. The denominator is the population 'at risk'. Imagine that you start with the total population of your area for the past year. Make a list of everyone who should be excluded from this to leave you with the true population 'at risk'.

Your list should include women, men who have had testes removed and men who already have diagnosed testicular cancer.

As can be imagined, it is difficult to calculate the size of the population at risk; however, if health visitors aim to work with this population then they must be sure of the validity of their data and the means by which they seek to achieve their ends. The same initial questions are posed for any medical epidemiological problem:

- Consider your 'at risk' population.
- Consider the source of the data and their collection methods.
- Consider the accuracy and validity of the source data.
- Make comparisons with other similar populations.
- Consider relevant social data.

It is reasonable to seek out health problems using medical epidemiology based on available morbidity and mortality statistics and not to consult the community per se. However, most empirical evidence suggests that members of the community are less aware of medical problems and far more concerned about social issues.

Profiling with the community

It is unlikely that a community has only one need that is common to all, and thus various groups will identify different needs depending on factors such as age, socio-economic status, political persuasion and available resources.

Profiling with the community will require constant dialogue with representatives of the many groups and subgroups that contribute to the diversity and richness of community life. Hooper & Longworth (2002) suggest that to profile with the community it is necessary to:

- use clear definitions and unambiguous language
- develop a common understanding of key words from the start

Table 2.1   Three dimensions of a community

Geographic location (includes inner city, rural, suburban)	Social construct (includes subsystem within)	Population (includes all people within the boundaries)
Boundaries	Health of the people	Demography
Access to health services	Family structures	Vital statistics
Geographic features	Economic sustainability	Size of population
Climate	Education provision	Density
Ecology	Religions	Composition
Housing	Local government services	Cultural differences
Local services	Politics	Social class
	Leisure	Occupations
	Communication networks	Mobility

- involve a range of people from differing backgrounds to get as wide a view as possible
- share ideas and discuss them
- engage in debate to share perceptions
- challenge assumptions and generate support for the final outcomes.

Table 2.1 shows three possible dimensions of a community.

HEALTH IMPACT ASSESSMENT AND INTEGRATED IMPACT ASSESSMENT

Health Impact Assessment (HIA) is defined by the Health Development Agency (Quigley et al 2004) as 'an approach that can help identify and consider the health and inequalities impacts of a proposal on a given population' (p. 1) and integrated impact assessment (IIA) as 'an approach that assesses the possible impact of proposals on a range of issues that previously may have been assessed separately' (p. 3); such issues include health, quality of life, economics, and environment and sustainability. Both approaches are seen as key to addressing equality and equity, which are a central dimension for all HIAs and IIAs.

Local strategic partnerships (LSPs), first introduced into neighbourhood renewal areas in 2001, drew together members of statutory, voluntary and business sectors with local community representation in order to provide solutions to the complexities of deprivation. In undertaking an HIA they were able to prepare a proposal (community strategy, for example) to promote or improve the economic, social and environmental well-being of their areas in consultation with local people, public sector bodies and other organizations whose activities have a local impact. The benefit of undertaking an IIA is that it can offer practical ways to enhance the positive aspects of a proposal (community strategy).

These two approaches to assessment are required by current health policy, including National Service Frameworks (NSFs) (Department of Health 2002e), as it is important to review the impact of existing and proposed plans on addressing health and inequalities in health.

The usual starting point for assessments are proposals (policy, programme, strategy, plan, project or other development) that have not yet been implemented. They are then modified so the programme or policies maximize the improvements in health and the reduction of inequalities. This takes account of the important effects of a range of policies across different public and voluntary sectors for a population.

In using the determinants of health as a basis for assessing the proposals, these approaches assess the impact of the determinants on the health of a population and the results provide clear health priorities for a set of activities that affect the health of the target population. Recommendations for changes are then made.

The six steps to HIA are identified by Quigley et al (2004) as:

- screening: is an HIA required
- scoping: if so, how to undertake it
- appraisal: identify and consider the evidence of health impact
- formulate and prioritize recommendations
- ongoing discussion with decision makers
- continuous monitoring and evaluation.

The six steps to IIA are identified by Quigley et al (2004) as:

- objective appraisal: scoping the initiative
- options appraisal: identifying the most sustainable options for delivery
- policy/activity appraisal: draft outline of the detailed activities
- full plan/project appraisal: compatibility of defined activities with policy/activity appraisal
- indicator selection: set indicators for measuring when goals are achieved
- appraisal for feedback/review: monitoring and evaluating how the initiative will be kept on target.

A comparison of these three approaches is offered in Table 2.2.

The concept of risk to poor health refers to the probability within a specified time-frame that a population, community, family or individual may develop an adverse health condition. A high-risk population includes those persons who, because of exposure, lifestyle, family history or other factors, are at greater risk of heart disease, poor mental health or acquiring ill health in their later life than the population at large.

The concept of absolute risk versus relative risk can be helpful in prioritizing scarce resources to identify those at high risk of HIV, for example. As far as we know, all persons are susceptible to HIV infection and subsequent development of AIDS. Therefore, everyone is in the population at risk for HIV/AIDS. Persons who have multiple sexual partners without adequate protection or who use intravenous drugs would be in the high-risk population for HIV infection.

NATIONAL SERVICE FRAMEWORKS

National Service Frameworks (NSFs) have been introduced to target risk in the population and to provide a structural basis on which to tackle inequalities in health and improve health in priority areas. They do so by setting national standards, defining service models and putting in place strategies to support implementation and establishing performance measures against which progress is measured.

Much of the challenge of implementation rests with primary care teams and their local partners. The NSFs to date are:

- Mental Health (Department of Health 1999e)
- Coronary Heart Disease (Department of Health 2000e)
- The Cancer Plan: a plan for investment, a plan for reform (Department of Health 2000f)
- Older People (Department of Health 2001a)
- Diabetes Services (Standards) (Department of Health 2001k)
- The Diabetes Service Delivery Strategy (Department of Health 2002g)
- Acute Children's Framework (Department of Health 2002h)
- Children, young people and maternity service framework (Department of Health 2004d).

The public health involvement in the NSFs sees primary prevention involving interventions aimed at reducing the incidence of disease through promoting health and preventing disease processes from developing. For example, it is well documented that certain high-risk lifestyles have an impact on the development of ill health in the lifespan for some people.

Preventing ill health is seen as a task for everyone, but primary care has a leading role in taking forward preventive action and supporting local initiatives led by non-NHS organizations. Delivering health improvement and achieving the various prevention targets require action by a whole range of local public services, the voluntary and statutory sector and communities themselves.

Table 2.2   Health Needs Assessment, Health Impact Assessment and Integrated Impact Assessment – a comparison

Health Needs Assessment	Health Impact Assessment	Integrated Impact Assessment
Search for health needs: Who is the defined population? Why the assessment? What are the health needs of a given population? How will the HNA happen?	**Screening:** Is an HIA required and what is the possible impact on the health, and in particular, inequalities of health, of the population?	**Objective appraisal:** What is to be achieved and what is the likely impact on economic, social, environmental sustainability, health and well-being and quality of life?
Determine health needs, health assets of the local population and identify trends before proposals are put forward for the development and delivery of improved services/programmes. This is the specific responsibility of the PCT (Department of Health 2001f)	**Scoping:** How to undertake the HIA. For example, using determinants of health (housing, transport, environment, economic activity) as a basis for assessing proposals and how they may impact on the health of a population	**Options appraisal:** Which option is the most sustainable? Assessing sustainability (balanced integration of social, environmental and economic outcomes, or Integration of sector-specific objectives designed to assure joined up planning (Quigley et al 2004)
Systematically collect, analyse and interpret data in order to create a profile of the local community to provide a local picture of inequalities in describing health needs	**Appraisal:** Identify and consider the evidence in detail for health effects. Appraise the impact of those effects, choose priorities and identify affected populations	**Policy/activity appraisal:** Draft the detailed activities of the proposal to ensure quality and coherence of the policy development process
The stimulation of an awareness of health needs: To provide information and implement a programme which enables people to address issues that influence their health. Raise awareness of health needs and facilitate a response if required. Agree who will lead on this	**Formulate/prioritize recommendations:** Agree changes required and choose priorities	**Full plan/project appraisal:** Review the plan to identify whether defined activities are compatible with activity appraisal
Influence on policies affecting health: Findings can be used to inform health equity audits, HIAs and IIAs A multi-agency team to plan action and interventions and target resources to meet the health need	**Ongoing discussion with decision makers:** A wide range of stakeholders may be involved and the HIA is designed to facilitate the inclusion of opinion and views of key players involved in the proposal, as well as evidence from quantitative and qualitative sources	**Indicator selection:** Set indicators for measuring when goals are achieved and ensure that the indicators adequately address inequalities, making best use of evidence available from a range of sources

(Continued)

Table 2.2   (Continued)

Health Needs Assessment	Health Impact Assessment	Integrated Impact Assessment
Facilitation of health enhancing activities: Acting as a health agent, mediating between agencies on behalf of individuals, families or community health status Evaluating the effectiveness of the intervention	**Continuous monitoring/evaluation:** Feedback is especially important when participatory methods have been used. Stakeholders need to understand how their contributions have influenced the recommendations for addressing the identified health inequality Further information is available on Health Development Agency website at http://www.hda.nhs.uk	**Appraisal for feedback and review:** How the initiative will stay on target – monitor and evaluate the best available evidence from a variety of sources

The NSF for children, young people and maternity services is a 10-year programme intended to stimulate long-term and sustained improvement in providing high-quality and integrated health and social care services from pregnancy through to the transition to adulthood. Its aims are to improve services, tackle inequalities and enhance partnerships.

Health visitors and school nurses can target those most at risk and provide services that can help to address these, for example parenting education programmes and general health education programmes for improving diet and physical activity (Liberating the Talents, Department of Health 2002b).

COMMUNITY DEVELOPMENT

A current desire to demonstrate an improvement in health and social care services through the development of collaborative partnerships has led to the growth of public health activity in communities. Community development offers a community focus to address health inequalities. Labonte (1998) describes community development as a process by which the community defines its own health needs and organizes to make known those needs to service providers in order to bring about change.

In developing strategies for public participation, using community development as a key part of a health needs assessment communities can be engaged in solving local health problems in partnership with statutory and voluntary agencies.

Community-based interventions can be less stigmatizing and more effective than individual interventions. Sure Start is the cornerstone of the government's drive to tackle child poverty and social exclusion. Its programmes are multiagency in approach and work in partnership with parents to improve the health and well-being of families and children before and after birth. Sure Start is geographically based and is only accessible to families living within its boundaries. Evidence suggests that home visiting and early intervention with children can reduce child abuse and neglect and improve parenting skills and the quality of mother–child interaction (Olds et al 1998) (see Ch. 8).

HEALTH ACTION ZONES

Health Action Zones (HAZs) introduced to develop local innovative public health strategies to tackle health inequalities, use the language of partnership and empowerment in relation to developing the health of communities and individuals (Powell & Moon 2001). HAZs have been trailblazing new ways of tackling health inequalities and modernizing services in some of the most deprived areas in England. Through partnership working, new ways of integrating health, regeneration, employment, housing, anti-poverty initiatives and education have been set up in areas with some of the worst health records in the country so that poor health is more effectively addressed. This is a response to meeting the needs of the most vulnerable and disadvantaged groups and communities. HAZs have not been set up to create another separate organization dealing with health and care services; they are designed to be a catalyst for encouraging existing organizations to work together, cut across geographical and structural boundaries, tackle health inequalities and deliver measurable improvements in public health and health outcomes. This is achieved with the participation of individuals and communities and results in the modernization of local treatment and care services through consciousness raising and empowerment of the community, with power gravitating to those who solve problems (Freire 1972).

Community participation is seen as a way of expanding accessibility to health services without necessarily increased costs, but outcomes of community development may depend more on whose values count, those of the public or politicians, managers or health visitors and colleagues working in the HAZ. HAZs are expected to act as trailblazers for new ways of working and integrating services between health and local authorities. Good examples can be seen at http://www.haznet.org.uk.

PCTs who sit within a HAZ have taken on the responsibility for funding them. Balancing the prevention and public health agenda against the commissioning of secondary care within the HAZ offers a huge challenge for the prioritizing of services for the PCT. The challenge for the PCT is to ensure funds are available to address inequalities and that this will be seen to be as important as commissioning secondary care. The National Primary Care Trust Development Team has developed an organizational competency framework which includes partnership competency covering areas such as joint working, active partnership with the local authority and joint development. Information is available at http://www.natpact.nhs.uk/home.php.

Within the HAZs are the three main settings identified by government as focal points for health inequalities: healthy schools, healthy workplaces and healthy neighbourhoods.

HEALTHY SCHOOLS

'Healthy schools' is an initiative particularly designed to take the opportunity to encourage healthier lifestyles in children. It is supported by the government's strategy to raise educational achievement and address inequalities. The National Healthy School Standard (Department of Health, Department for Education and Skills 1999) offers a framework for delivering aspects of child-centred public health particularly designed to take the opportunity to encourage healthier lifestyles in children. Health psychology has shown that lifestyle habits taken up during younger and middle childhood will become lifelong habits and thus, if there is a clear focus on health, particularly in relation to healthier eating (National School Fruit Scheme), regular exercise (new opportunity for PE and sport in schools) and a warm and happy environment (specialist support and advice through Sure Start Plus advisors), children will respond positively (Department of Health 2003c). Healthy children have more chance of becoming healthy adults, and much adult disease and many emotional and psychological difficulties may have their roots in childhood. Of particular concern is the effect of inequalities and poverty on the life and health of children and young people. There are a number of initiatives in different schools around the country which have established enterprising approaches to projects such as a breakfast club, healthy tuck shops, homework clubs and latch-key support clubs. All these and other initiatives have been set up as the result of an alliance involving the school, local supermarkets, local business organizations and the children and their parents. School nurses and health visitors have been involved and there are opportunities for them to support the development of further initiatives. Health visitors in particular have knowledge of lonely or isolated people who are free during the day and would be willing to give up some of their time to support these ventures. The upshot of these activities is that, with a continual focus on health, there should be some reversal of the increased development of poorer health behaviours resulting from the modern technological, health-awareness-lacking age. It is important also for health visitors to recognize that inequalities in health will become less obvious among children where healthy eating support ventures ensure that costs are kept to a minimum and that the numbers of children who qualify for free school meals are not reduced by such ventures.

HEALTHY WORKPLACES

Health visitors are in a strong position to raise awareness of the problems of employees who work in smaller organizations and businesses where there is no occupational health department. In particular, women often discuss with health visitors visiting their homes their employment concerns about their partners. These women are concerned about raising awareness of the need to adhere to health and safety regulations, particularly where there are work risk factors that could influence the health of the family. For example, men who work in small units such as car repair garages should be aware of the need to ensure that heavy oils do not seep through their clothing, especially in the groin area, which would put them at risk of testicular cancer. It is useful to work through women to raise awareness of the risk factors that men face, but also for health visitors who are working in the community to make direct approaches to small businesses, offering regular health discussion sessions to minimize risk-taking and build in better health practices. Empirical evidence from health visitors working in areas with small pockets of industrial units has shown that employers welcome help and support through health-teaching programmes and well-person advice sessions. As part of the Bradford Health for Men network, many men who have not been to a GP for several years have benefited from this approach (Arnold 2004).

TRANSPORT INITIATIVES

The government White Paper *A New Deal for Transport: Better for Everyone* (Department of Environment, Transport and the Regions 1998) particularly stresses a new integrated strategy for transport in general, but there are local measures aimed specifically at improving health that health visitors can bring to the attention of the women with whom they are working. It is not suggested that health visitors should take an active role in transport initiatives on a national level, but at a local level they may well be involved in safer routes to school, setting up school crossing patrols or safety initiatives to reduce the incidence of accidents outside the home. Raising awareness in families of ways in which health could be improved might include:

- encouraging more people to walk to work or use cycles
- encouraging safer routes for children to walk or cycle to school
- encouraging mothers to try to keep children in pushchairs away from vehicle exhausts
- encouraging fathers to press employers to introduce green transport plans to help them use alternatives to driving to work alone.

HEALTH INITIATIVES IN BUSINESS

Employers in some areas have allowed small labour forces to have an hour out of the office/shop periodically for discussion of health topics that the employees had themselves requested. Unlike large industrial organizations, in businesses where employees number fewer than 100 there is no requirement for an occupational health service, yet they may face similar health risks, with only health and safety inspections to ensure compliance with regulations and no occupational health promotion or education. Health visitors in some areas of the West Midlands have responded to that need (Department of Health 2002b).

Health visitors also should take up opportunities to link with other offices and businesses who have little or no access to health advice and information. In particular, guidance on handling stress, bullying in the workplace, repetitive strain injury and other problems associated with continued computer use could all be introduced, taught and supported by health visitors. These programmes could be set up as part of the health action zone initiatives and, if necessary, could draw on the lottery funding available.

These healthy workplace initiatives require the skills of professionals such as health visitors who are trained and able to approach a wide network of businesses and organizations, possibly initially through Rotary, Soroptimists, Inner Wheel, the Townswomen's Guild or other business people's organizations. They have access to funds, some charitable, to underpin small health promotion/well-people initiatives but, more importantly, raising awareness of health issues leading to a healthier workforce and workplace would greatly improve the public health.

HEALTHY NEIGHBOURHOODS

A number of initiatives have been developed over the last few years to help to improve environments, particularly in inner city and urban areas. An initiative announced by central government under the Social Exclusion Unit's (1998) report *Bringing Britain Together: A National Strategy for Neighbourhood Renewal* produced a new fund, worth £800 million over 3 years, intended to help the poorest neighbourhoods. These neighbourhoods have severe multiple problems, which usually include:

- poor job prospects
- high levels of crime
- a run-down environment
- no one in charge of managing the neighbourhood and coordinating public services that affect it.

The programme started in 1999 with 17 pilot areas, selected because their problems are particularly severe. Health visitors, with their overview of the neighbourhood area, were able to lobby for changes to be made even if their area was not selected for this developmental money.

Today, monies under the Neighbourhood Renewal fund have meant that many new pockets of housing development and improvement have been set up in run-down and derelict former industrial areas. This type of approach to tackling problems through mainstream services and funding within disadvantaged areas, supported by neighbourhood renewal funds,

could be rolled out to communities beyond these boundaries. Health improvement plans have been identified and money sought from central funding to enable local authorities to tackle regeneration of cities and large towns to bring people and life back into the centre from the suburban fringes where they had moved. Development strategies for cities and large towns now mean that these are safer areas for people to come into, especially at night. Policing and improved lighting, closed-circuit cameras and pedestrian-only zones have meant that personal safety after dark has also been improved. The uptake across the UK has been patchy, with an uneven variety of grassroots work and high-level publicity. Teams of health visitors and community workers throughout the country now have their own budgets to improve health among deprived communities, as part of a £3 million package rolled out by Alan Milburn as Secretary of State for Health in 2001. Matched funding from PCTs and groups give each team a community budget of at least £5000 a year. This funding was first made available alongside the launch of the health visitor and school nurse resource packs, aimed at supporting their widening public health role (http://www.innovate.hda-online.org.uk).

In large, former local authority housing estates and other smaller private estates, local people have come together to introduce Neighbourhood Watch schemes, traffic-calming initiatives and more school crossing patrols to raise levels of safety and reduce fear among residents, especially older people. Surveys among older people have shown that fear of burglary and theft is their greatest anxiety and keeps them trapped in their homes after dark. Health visitors have been instrumental in helping some neighbourhoods to set up such schemes as Neighbourhood Watch, and the networking necessary with local leaders, councillors and organizations does mean that these skills should continue to be taught to and used by health visitors.

HEALTHY LIVING CENTRES

More than 349 healthy living centres have been set up with lottery funds distributed by the

New Opportunities Fund worth £265 million (Cole 2003).

They are a positive endeavour to help people identify and set the agenda for their own health needs. They rank as one of the biggest public health initiatives ever seen in the UK. Most have developed as a mix of capital and revenue schemes that will continue until 2006 and possibly beyond. All projects address the wider determinants of health such as social exclusion and poor access to services, as well as linking into the NHS National Service Framework priorities of reducing heart disease and cancer and improving health in old age. The centres are based in the most deprived parts of a community and have to involve the local community, reflect residents' priorities for action and be accessible to at least 20% of the population. The projects involve the community working with voluntary, public and private sector organizations who design, set up and quality assure the effectiveness of these centres. They offer opportunity for health and fitness facilities for all, as well as meeting rooms for opportunities for raising awareness of good health behaviours. They include initiatives like drop-in centres, development of outreach services and parenting programmes (see Health Development Agency website at www.hda.nhs.uk).

There are opportunities for the health visitor in advising, guiding and delivering the health promotion and education sessions. Working in partnership, they are available to respond to requests from the local community and be actively involved in enabling them to identify their agenda and help them provide a response to it. This could also involve lobbying for funding or provision of statistical evidence in support of the identified need.

The new direction for public health requires new definitions and ways of working. Professional boundaries must change and a refocus in education and service provision to encompass an inter-professional approach to public health is required. The following sections discuss some of the developments emerging from policy, regulation and practice.

REDEFINING PUBLIC HEALTH FOR THE 21st CENTURY

Wanless (2004) proposes a redefined and more appropriate definition for the 21st century where 'the organized efforts of society' are used in the widest sense to include not only government, public and private sector organizations and communities, but also the collective efforts of individuals, their health status and that of their families. He defines public health as:

> The science and art of preventing disease, prolonging life and promoting health through the organized efforts and informed choices of society, organizations, public and private, communities and individuals.
>
> (Wanless 2004, p. 27)

Such a definition enables public health workers to take a 'step change' in public health to deliver the fully engaged scenario envisaged by the 2002 Wanless review.

FAMILY–CENTRED PUBLIC HEALTH ROLE

For years health visitors have recognized that family care is part of community care and that the family is the primary unit of health care. The family in a real sense does not exist today – we have many different forms of family in which relationships are constantly modifying and changing (Allan & Crow 2003).

Health visiting recognizes the dynamic nature and impact of these changes on the public health of individuals within different families. In 1988 Acheson advocated domiciliary health visiting to all families as an essential aspect of public health practice.

The success of this type of public health intervention is demonstrated through the results of 11 randomized control trials which provide scientific results of decreases in postnatal depression, increases in immunization rates and reduction in child abuse (Elkan et al 2000b).

A family-centred public health approach enables health visitors to focus on tackling the causes of ill health, not just responding to the consequences, and to address the wider determinants of health. These include poverty, housing, social exclusion, employment, environmental issues, cultural differences and education. By identifying and modifying risk factors or barriers to healthy living and promoting a healthy lifestyle, a public health approach can optimize health and improve the quality of life. Health visiting shares with social work a concern for social justice, especially in relation to vulnerable and marginalized people, but aims to prevent breakdown and the need for social work intervention.

The current emphasis on partnership working, user involvement and a reduction in inequality has contributed towards the development of health visitors and agencies working together more effectively to pool resources and expertise. Health alliances are developing, for example, agencies such as education, social work and health projects working together. The ability of health visitors to unify and collaborate across the different perspectives suggests that they can be key public health workers in promoting partnerships in the health and social care system (Jinks et al 2003).

The modernization of the role of the health visitor emphasizes the need for health visitors to improve health and tackle health inequality through adopting a family-centred public health role (Department of Health 1999a, 1999b, 2001f). This new role aims to strengthen the community-based, population approach to public health through recognizing the interdependent nature of the different elements of working with individuals, families and communities to promote health. This stance was adopted by the WHO (1999) when they challenged the usefulness of maintaining a division between individually focused practice and public health. They suggested that health care should be seen as a continuous link of activities that all contribute in different ways to enhancing health. The changing political paradigm,

focusing on strengthening communities, makes traditional health visiting activities insufficient for the current agenda.

THE HEALTH VISITOR PRACTICE DEVELOPMENT RESOURCE PACK (DEPARTMENT OF HEALTH 2001e)

This pack demonstrates a continuum for public health practice in health visiting to enable health visitors to see the individual and population elements of their work on a continuous scale rather than at opposing ends of a spectrum of activity.

This resource pack offers a framework for practice and guidance on the public health aspects of the health visitor role and in particular the family-centred public health role. Suggestions for new ways of working are given and projects have been funded by government to provide incentives to refocus practice (see Sure Start Project in Chapter 8).

Health visitors tend to work within two models of health: the medical model and the social model. Working across these two paradigms offers a public health focus that concentrates on prevention which is measured in terms of the absence of disease and the promotion of health, acknowledging the social and economic determinants of health.

There is a shifting ideology of public health in the health service, and its impact on health visiting and nursing will take us through into the next decade of the 21st century.

The development of partnership working by the health service as mainstream activity with local government, and the implementation of Health Improvement Plans and National Service Frameworks (NSFs), have demanded new ways of applying public health knowledge and skills for the health visitor and the nursing profession as a whole.

This is provoking a new form of separation in nursing. Specialists are needed in public health, leadership and management and clinical nursing practice. Power is manifest in the ways in which this specialist knowledge is identified and used by health visitors and nursing.

Historically one of the principal reasons for health visiting and nursing being identified as a semi-profession (Etzioni 1969) has been its inability to develop dominance in discrete areas of knowledge. The streamlining of the professional register for nurses, midwives and health visitors from 15 parts into three distinct categories – nursing, midwifery and specialist community public health nursing (Department of Health 2001j) – could be seen as a way of addressing this. In the 21st century traditional definitions of professionalism appear outdated, failing to reflect the educational, social, political and economic factors influencing the new constructs of professional status evident in the changing division of labour in a post-modern society.

The commitment of the professional ideals of the organization of health visiting, expressed in attitudes and beliefs, have been replaced by a post-modern perspective which requires us to reintroduce knowledge and skills of public health as central to the imposition of power within nursing, health visiting and the NHS. This is reflected in The NHS Plan (Department of Health 2000c), which, as suggested by Donaldson (2001), affirms public health as the mainstream activity for the NHS (Donaldson 2001). It adopts a pragmatic approach covering issues of professional and clinical leadership (modern matron, nurse consultant) and multidisciplinary working (working smarter to make maximum use of the talents of all the NHS workforce) and professional development and quality of care (a statutory duty of quality on all NHS organizations).

The embedding of the 10 occupational standards for public health (Prime R&D Ltd for Skills for Health 2003) with the four principles of health visiting (CETHV 1977, Twinn & Cowley 1992) within the competency framework for the Specialist Community Public Health nurse (SCPHN) register provides nursing with the exclusive rights to perform specialist community public health nursing, to control training for access to this profession and with the right to determine the way the work is performed. The regulated title of health visitor vanishes and the protection of the public is offered through the SCPHN registration (NMC 2004a). Health visiting has never been static as it is influenced by changes and developments in social policy, public health and the overall needs of individuals within society, but its refocus within nursing is not comfortable for its public health role and function.

PUBLIC HEALTH AND THE COMPETENCIES FOR A NEW ROLE FOR SPECIALIST COMMUNITY PUBLIC HEALTH NURSES AND EXISTING REGISTERED HEALTH VISITORS

The established four principles of health visiting (CETHV 1977, Twinn & Cowley 1992) and the 11 Principles of Good Practice developed by Prime R&D Ltd for Skills for Health (2003) form the basis for the development of public health activity across the specialist community public health nursing workforce.

The health visiting principles developed in 1977 by the CETHV underpin the professional practice of health visiting and provide a sound basis for the public health activity of the new SCPHN and existing registered health visitors (*Principles of Health Visiting*, CETHV 1977, Twinn & Cowley 1992):

- the search for health needs
- the stimulation of an awareness of health needs
- the influence on policies affecting health
- the facilitation of health-enhancing activities.

The 11 Principles of Good Practice developed for all public health workers (Prime R&D Ltd for Skills for Health 2003) are embryonic in comparison and have emerged from the work of the Tripartite Steering Group (which comprised the Faculty of Public Health Medicine, the Multidisciplinary Public Health Forum and the Royal Institute of Public Health, plus the health departments of the four UK countries).

These principles are set to underpin the work of all public health practitioners including SCPHNs and existing registered health visitors, and are as follows (Prime R&D Ltd for Skills for Health 2003):

1. Balance people's rights with their responsibilities to others and to wider society, challenging those who affect the rights of others.
2. Promote the values of equality and diversity, acknowledging the personal beliefs and preferences of others and promoting anti-discriminatory practice.
3. Promote and welcome community and individual diversity by working with agencies to reduce social exclusion.
4. Balance the need to share information between agencies to improve health and well-being with the need to maintain confidentiality and manage risk.
5. Recognize the effect of the wider social, political and economic context on health and well-being and on people's development.
6. Enable people to develop to their full potential, to be as autonomous and self-managing as possible and to have a voice and be heard.
7. Recognize and promote health and well-being as a positive concept.
8. Develop and maintain effective relationships with people and maintain the integrity of these relationships.
9. Work in ways that are sustainable and based on evidence of effectiveness.
10. Develop oneself and one's own practice to improve the quality of services offered.
11. Work within statutory and agency frameworks.

The purpose of public health is given under four bullet points in the functional map for the practice of public health (Prime R&D Ltd for Skills for Health 2003, p. 1). These are to:

- improve the health and well-being of the population
- prevent disease and minimize its consequences

- prolong valued life
- reduce inequalities in health.

From the purpose of public health work 10 areas are identified as those aspects which need to be undertaken in order to achieve the purpose of public health. These national occupational standards for public health practice are (Skills for Health, http://www.skillsforhealth.org.uk):

1. Surveillance and assessment of the population's health and well-being
2. Promoting and protecting the population's health and well-being
3. Developing quality and risk within an evaluative culture
4. Collaborative working for health and well-being
5. Developing health programmes and services and reducing health inequalities
6. Policy and strategy development and implementation to improve health and well-being
7. Working with and for communities to improve health
8. Strategic leadership for health and well-being
9. Research and development to improve health and well-being
10. Ethically managing self, people and resources to improve health and well-being.

These form the 10 National Occupational Standards for all public health workers and are developed from the 10 National Occupational Standards for Specialist Practice in Public Health (Specialist Practice in Public Health describes the work of individuals at a level currently comparable to consultants in public health medicine and dental public health).

These occupational standards are mapped to the four principles of health visiting and the domains underlying the competency framework for registration as an SPCPN (NMC 2004a), which enables the SCPHN to demonstrate competence in public health activity and to meet the national occupational standards for public health practice.

SPECIALIST COMMUNITY PUBLIC HEALTH NURSING, 2004 ONWARDS

The functions identified from this for SPCHNs and the existing registered health visitors form the foundation of the public health activity. The specific contribution to the improvement of public health is based on the public health knowledge and skills developed over the last two centuries by health visitors. The new roles place the SCPHN and existing registered health visitors in an ideal position to take a population–individual approach to the improvement of public health and to work with the Wanless (2004) definition of public health. They can empower people to take responsibility for their own health needs and through this activity enable them to prevent and minimize the effects of disease, dysfunction and disability. The role is seen as providing a public health service in an era of increasing specialization in the health care available to individuals, families and communities. In monitoring the health needs and demands of clients they are seen to be contributing to the fulfilment of these needs and facilitating appropriate public health activity and service by working in partnership with the wider public health workforce.

The knowledge that underpins practice is based on the reflective and anti-discriminatory principles, and the origins of good practice are research based. SCPHNs work in a variety of settings and increasingly their role rests in their ability to demonstrate a 'family-centred public health approach'. This involves unsupervised, independent practice with the use of high levels of decision making and complex practice skills involved in motivating individuals, families and communities to seek and maintain a high level of wellness for themselves and others. In preventing disease, promoting health and protecting the client, they act as facilitators, innovators and change agents in the fostering of decision making for achieving optimum well-being. This activity places them in a pivotal public health role.

CONCLUSION

It will be up to future generations of specialist community public health nurses to decide whether their public health activity requires a systematic body of knowledge that is different from nursing, designed to develop a quality of perception, sensitivity to need and a capacity for the organization of public health activity (CETHV 1973).

Health visiting was never nursing care but public health activity, which involves focused interventions designed to promote health and prevent ill health in the well population.

Since the introduction of the Public Health Nurse (Health Visitor) (UKCC 1994a) the role has taken on a more medically focused approach to tackling public health issues. Changing structures of professional practice and the need for health visitors to recognize the scope of practice and the implications for practice are implicit within the requirements for the pre-registration health visitor programme set out by the NMC in 2002. From 2004 (NMC 2004a) this public health activity is owned by nursing. A family-centred public health role is a model of practice developed to enhance the health of families and communities. It is in working with family groups and groups within communities that health visitors have been most effective so far, and continued work with mothers and young families through Sure Start and Health Action Zones is essential. The opportunity to respond to local need through the emergence of flexible initiatives for people in similar circumstances can offer cost-effective and cost–benefit approaches responding to fluctuating circumstantial changes to help and support all young families in an equitable and participatory way.

Chapter **3**

Models for health visiting in specialist community public health nursing

Ros Carnwell

INTRODUCTION

The use of models has followed a different course in health visiting from in nursing. Nursing theorists provided the impetus for nursing to define itself more clearly in conceptual and academic terms. Despite difficulties in the application of models to nursing practice (Kenny 1993), the use of models has provided the nursing profession with a wealth of opportunity to debate its professional development. Most nursing models do not 'fit' health visiting practice, because of such fundamental concepts as self-care deficit (Orem 1985) or disequilibrium (Roy & Andrews 1991). Such concepts arguably imply a state of ill health rather than health, which is irreconcilable with the health emphasis of health visiting. One of the few nursing models that fits well with health visiting (Peplau 1952) provides an ideal framework for understanding the transition of the health visitor–client relationship, but is limited to individual work with families, rather than communities.

The search for suitable models for both nursing and health visiting has not been helped by ambiguity in language. Robinson (1992), for example, argues vehemently that nursing uses such terms as 'model' and 'paradigm' inappropriately. McFarlane (1986), too, comments on the inconsistent terminology and convoluted language used in discussions of nursing models.

Health visiting, then, has probably been wise to reject the drive to use nursing models, most of which would require to be adapted for health visiting. The use of a single model might also reduce complex human characteristics and situations into something that can be conceived within the components of a model. Health visiting does, however, need to consider ways of demonstrating and evaluating its activities. The models discussed in this chapter focus on two important components of health visiting: health promotion and public health. Community work, rather than work with individuals, is therefore the predominant focus of this chapter. Prior to discussing health promotion and public health models in relation to health visiting, it is necessary first to distinguish between concepts, theories and models.

CONCEPTS, THEORIES AND MODELS – DEFINITIONS AND DEVELOPMENT

Concepts can be simply described as labels ascribed to images and objects. Britt (1997) likens concepts to blocks in a Lego set but argues that, unlike the tangible building blocks, concepts are elusive, changeable and tentative. Labelling such elusive concepts fulfils the purpose of categorizing them in order to make sense of experience (Carnwell 1998). Concepts are categorized by grouping things together that have properties in common and separating things that have different properties in common (Britt 1997). The concept of culture, for example, can be derived by grouping together such properties as beliefs, attitudes, norms, religious practices and mores. Properties such as skin colour, stature and other biological characteristics would be separated out, as these are properties associated with race rather than culture. Properties associated with culture and properties associated with race could then be linked to each other to allow deeper understanding of complex issues. This linking together of concepts is fundamental to the development of models.

Models can be defined as: 'organizing devices for a continuing, explicit dialogue between multiple sources of data and assumptions … models summarize what we have learned about the dynamics of phenomena in patterns woven from different contexts, in different historical periods and with different individuals and social groups' (Britt 1997, p. 2).

Britt (1997) also distinguishes between four different types of model: descriptive, interpretative, explanatory and predictive. These categories are cognisant with Akinsanya et al's (1994) view that models describe, explain and predict practice. The capacity of models to fulfil these functions is derived from their development. Most models emerge either from empirical research findings or from the literature. The different types of model could emerge from either qualitative or quantitative findings, or indeed a combination of the two (Britt 1997). A rich description of a culture could, for example, form the basis of a descriptive model. An interpretative model might attempt to make sense of some of the relationships between concepts in more detail. An explanatory model would look for causes of phenomena, such as why certain concepts, rather than others, emerged as important and whether there were causal links between concepts. A predictive model would attempt to anticipate whether the same phenomena would emerge in the same way in the future or in different circumstances.

Although models tend to be theoretical and research based, they do have utility value in that they help practitioners to organize their thoughts and justify how and what they do (McClymont et al 1991). Moreover, according to Fawcett (1992), there is a reciprocal relationship between conceptual models and practice. Models guide practice, for example, while practice provides evidence for the credibility of the model.

Models also guide the development of theory on which practice is based. At a more pragmatic level, health visitors' understanding of a range of models of society enables them to draw on models as appropriate in order to provide effective interventions (Elkan et al 2000a). Britt (1997) views models as more explicit than theories, however, as they help us to understand what aspects of our environment we consider to be important and how these aspects relate to other variables within the environment. Our assumptions about such relationships can then be tested, which is the beginning of theory development. A model, for example, might make propositional statements about relationships between perceptions of health, subsequent health behaviour and health status. An example is models concerning risk perception and optimistic bias (Rutter & Quine 2002). Rutter & Quine (2002) refer to Weinstein's (1980) view that people tend to think they are invulnerable. Thus, he argues, that the more people perceive they can control a negative event, the less likely they perceive they are to be affected by it. This might explain why some people continue smoking despite all the evidence of its deleterious effects. These relationships between variables of individual perception and behaviour could be tested empirically in order to develop a theory around health behaviour and outcomes. The emerging theory might then be used to guide future practice, such as how to deliver health education messages or how to promote health at an organizational level.

It cannot be assumed, however, that because a model has been derived from theory or empirical evidence it has sufficient credibility to benefit practice. For this reason, authors such as Fawcett (1985) and Britt (1997) have developed criteria for the evaluation of models.

EVALUATING MODELS

On the basis of the work of Fawcett (1985) and Britt (1997), 10 criteria for evaluation are proposed (Box 3.1). The criteria are divided into three categories of questions for evaluation: questions concerning the clarity of concepts within the model; questions concerning the accuracy of concepts within the model; and questions concerning application of the model to practice. Unlike Fawcett's criteria, which are nursing-oriented, these criteria are appropriate to models in a wider sphere of professional practice. The criteria will be used, as appropriate, to evaluate the models in this chapter.

Box 3.1   Questions for evaluation

Conceptual clarity

1. Do the concepts within the model appear factually accurate within their context?
2. Do the concepts within the model hang together in a logically congruent way?
3. Are the definition and description of concepts sufficiently detailed to give confidence in the ability of the model to reflect reality?

Conceptual accuracy

4. Do the concepts within the model reflect the reality of the situation and people to whom they apply?
5. Does the model include all expected concepts and are irrelevant concepts avoided?
6. Are the concepts within the model grounded in theory and empirical evidence?

Application to practice

7. Do predicted relationships between concepts accurately depict real life events both in the future and in different contexts?
8. Is there potential contradiction between theories emerging from the model and the reality of practice?
9. Can theories emerging from the model be tested in practice?
10. Does the model have practical significance and offer guidance for future practice?

HEALTH PROMOTION MODELS APPLIED TO HEALTH VISITING

Several concepts characterize models designed to promote health. These include concepts relating to changing behaviour, maintaining behavioural change, understanding individual perceptions and cognitions concerning health, and explaining health behaviour in terms of sociostructural variables. The simplest of these approaches, such as Procaska & DiClemente's (1984) model of change, focuses exclusively on changing and maintaining changes in behaviour. Slightly more complex models (e.g. those of Becker et al 1974, and Pender 1987) locate behavioural change within a societal context. More complex still is an attempt to consider the nature and impact of structural variables on different phases of diagnosis, such as that used in the model of Green et al (1980). Each of these models will be discussed and evaluated in relation to health visiting and public health.

THE TRANSTHEORETICAL MODEL OF CHANGE

Procaska & DiClemente (1984) developed a transtheoretical model based around the process of change. They developed their model specifically for the treatment of addictive behaviours. Their intention was to develop a comprehensive model of change that was applicable to the broad range of ways in which people change a wide array of different behaviours; the various types of treatment available (e.g. therapy programmes, self-help); and the course that people follow when bringing about change. Procaska & DiClemente's model uses the revolving door model of change (Fig. 3.1) developed by McConnaughy et al (1983).

According to Procaska & DiClemente's (1984) model, people at different stages of the change process exhibit different psychosocial characteristics. Thus, as individuals progress around the cycle their own psychosocial characteristics will change. People at the precontemplation stage, for example, are likely to see few benefits and many problems related to changing their

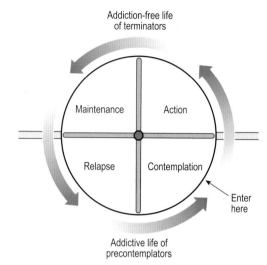

Figure 3.1 The revolving door model of the states of change (redrawn with kind permission from Procaska & DiClemente 1988)

behaviour and are therefore low in self-efficacy in comparison to people who have progressed through to the maintenance stage.

The precontemplation stage is quite crucial, as the efforts of either themselves or other people to persuade them to change their behaviour often fail. This might explain the failure of many attempts made by health visitors to persuade people to change their health behaviour. Traditionally, health visitors would have offered advice to people without necessarily taking into account their personal circumstances or motivation, as will be seen below in the discussion of Beattie's health accounts. Once in the cycle, however, people become motivated by the potential benefits and a successful outcome becomes possible. People may then reach the active or maintenance stage, often regressing to the stage before rather than giving up completely. Thus, once in the cycle of change, such people are receptive to health visiting advice so that health visiting intervention can be construed as successful. It is arguable, however, that such people might have changed their own behaviour without health visiting intervention provided they had access to the appropriate information.

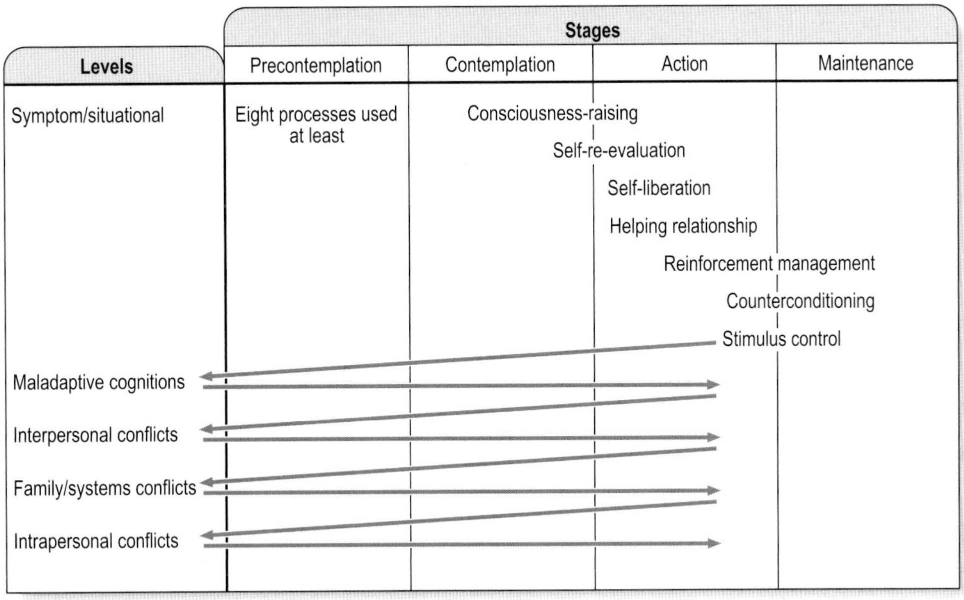

Levels	Stages			
	Precontemplation	Contemplation	Action	Maintenance
Symptom/situational	Eight processes used at least	Consciousness-raising Self-re-evaluation Self-liberation Helping relationship Reinforcement management Counterconditioning Stimulus control		
Maladaptive cognitions				
Interpersonal conflicts				
Family/systems conflicts				
Intrapersonal conflicts				

Figure 3.2   Levels, stages and processes of change (redrawn with kind permission from Procaska & DiClemente 1988)

In addition to the revolving door model of change, Procaska & DiClemente (1988) identify 10 change processes of the transtheoretical approach. Furthermore, they argue that seven of these processes could be exploited during the four different stages of the change cycle (Fig. 3.2).

Consciousness raising, for example, tends to occur when people are contemplating change. During this time they become open to interventions likely to confront the target behaviours. A well-timed visit from the health visitor could enable people to re-evaluate their health behaviour and assess which values they want to work towards (Procaska & DiClemente 1988). During the action phase, a process of self-liberation occurs. This process enables people to relinquish dependence on the therapist and become self-efficacious in bringing about change. The helping relationship is crucial during the action stage in providing the support needed to overcome negative feelings associated with change. During this stage, for example, the health visitor might discuss with the client the negative feelings associated with the change, what situations trigger such feelings and how they could possibly be resolved. As individuals move towards

maintaining change, their management of the changes in their behaviour will need to be reinforced by the health visitor so that they do not relapse to the contemplation stage. Maintaining changes in behaviour also requires counter-conditioning and stimulus control. This would involve the health visitor in discussing the client's circumstances so that the client gains a thorough understanding of the conditions under which they are likely to relapse and the ways of controlling such conditions.

The left-hand side of Figure 3.2 presents five different levels of psychological problem requiring intervention. Procaska & DiClemente (1988) argue that the symptom/situational level represents the primary reason for people entering therapy. They further argue that the lower down the hierarchy, the less aware the person is likely to be of the determinants of the problem and therefore the more resistant to change. Intrapersonal conflicts, for example, could represent unresolved childhood conflicts of which the person may not be fully aware. Such conflicts could include patterns of health behaviour rooted in childhood, which could be resolved through health visiting guidance. Some conflicts, however, might require sensitive counselling and may be beyond the scope of the health visitor. The health visitor in this situation would probably recommend professional counselling prior to working with the client towards changing health behaviours.

Procaska & DiClemente's model is relatively simple. It is designed to respond to complex personal problems requiring therapy. Fundamental to this model is the belief that therapists should be as complex as their clients. This should enable the health visitor to shift the nature of their intervention, focusing on different change processes and levels of intervention during different stages of the change cycle. Although this model does cater for the complex nature of human behaviour, it does so at an individual behavioural level. It does not therefore fully acknowledge societal influences on health behaviour. A model that moves some way to achieving this is the health belief model.

THE HEALTH BELIEF MODEL

A slightly more complex explanation for health behaviour than that offered by Procaska & DiClemente is the health belief model (Becker et al 1974). It is a development of social psychological theories postulated by Lewin (1935). Following Lewin (1935), Rosenstock (1974) developed a theory in which people make decisions about health on the basis of two factors: how severe they perceive an illness to be and what they consider to be the benefits of preventive action. The theory holds that cues to action might bring about changes in these perceptions (Fig. 3.3).

Becker et al (1974) criticized the original model for its emphasis on negative aspects of health such as the threat of disease. They argued instead that positive health motivations exist and account for some portion of health-related behaviour. They also proposed that there is an 'incentive' value of compliance in which the threat of a present illness provides an incentive to reduce the threat. In relating this to the readiness of mothers to take recommended action

when their child is ill, Becker et al suggested that mothers make an estimate of the likelihood of the physician's instructions reducing the threat. In making this estimate mothers take into account their perception of the accuracy of the diagnosis, the usefulness of medication prescribed in the past and the usefulness of modern medical practices.

Becker et al's (1974) health belief model has been used in various health education contexts, such as family-based health visiting (Diment 1991) and school health teaching in primary schools (While 1991). For the purpose of this chapter, the model will be considered in relation to the community context of public health. The value of this model to public health lies in an analysis of modifying factors, which are evident in the central column of the model. The model has been criticized 'for not explaining the nature of the influence of modifying variables upon the individual's perceptions and beliefs and how these are expressed in resultant behaviour' (While 1991, p. 102). This criticism implies that the impact of sociostructural considerations of society on individual perceptions of health and disease is unclear and therefore contentious. Crossing the boundaries between individual perceptions and sociostructural variables is a particular expertise developed in health visiting.

Knowledge of demographic, sociopsychological and structural variables relies on a public health focus. Health visitors using this model use data from community profiling to identify risk variables in a particular community. A high proportion of ethnic minority groups combined with lower social classes in a given population might be indicative of certain conditions such as poor nutrition or substandard housing. These factors, together with poor education, might suggest that a given population would have a lack of perception of susceptibility to, or the severity of, a particular disease. It is at the public health level, therefore, that health visitors would attempt to modify these factors by mass media campaigns.

While (1991) also argues that the model assumes that the individual person is the ultimate unit of analysis. The importance of modifying factors to the model, however, does

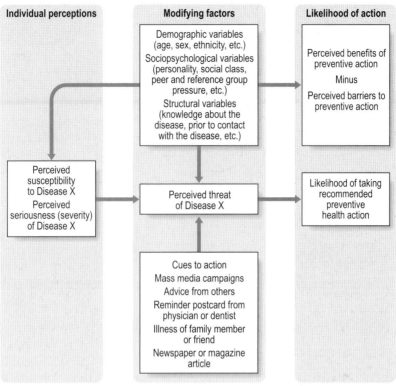

Figure 3.3 The health belief model as a predictor of preventive health behaviour (redrawn with kind permission from Becker et al 1974 A new approach to explaining sick role behaviour in low income populations. Am J Pub Health 64: 205–216, copyright ©1974 American Public Health Association)

counteract this argument. Modifying factors exist outside the individual and impact upon and interact with the individual. Thus the ultimate unit of analysis is arguably the individual within a social context. Individual perceptions, together with the likelihood of action, might also suggest a predominantly individual focus. The model could, however, be applied at a community level. A reminder postcard sent to prompt parents about their children's immunization, for example, has the advantage of increasing the herd immunity of a whole population as well as protecting the individual child. Equally, a 'traffic-calming' campaign in a particular neighbourhood might alert both the public and politicians to the susceptibility of the local population to traffic accidents. It is possible, therefore, for susceptibility to be perceived and acted upon

at a wider level than the individual. Nevertheless, whether susceptibility is an individual or collective perception, the ensuing action will ultimately become collective, if only due to the accumulative action of individual changes in behaviour. It is this collective action that is fundamental to public health initiatives and hence the success of Becker et al's health belief model.

THE HEALTH PROMOTION MODEL

A model that has some similarities with Becker et al's health belief model is the health promotion model (HPM, Pender 1987; Fig. 3.4). The HPM uses social learning theory as its basis, which, like Becker et al's model, is drawn from social psychology.

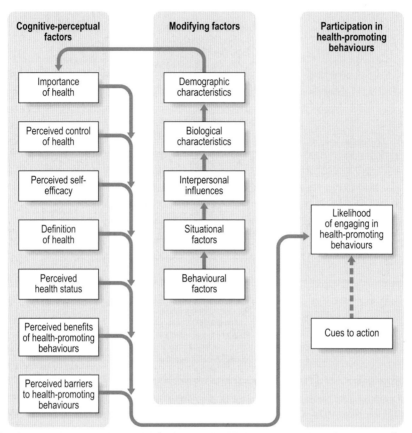

Figure 3.4 Pender's health promotion model (redrawn with kind permission from Pender 1996)

Pender's modifying factors resemble those proposed by Becker et al, while both models focus on cues to action and the likelihood of changing behaviour. Pender (1996), however, argues that, unlike the health belief model, the HPM does not include 'fear' or 'threat' as motivating forces for health behaviour. Pender further argues that avoidance-oriented models are of limited use in motivating healthy lifestyles in some groups.

Two versions of the HPM will be explored in this chapter. The first version (Pender 1987) was developed following the initial formulation in 1982. The second version discussed here (Pender 1996) is the latest version, which was developed on the basis of considerable research and testing of the earlier version.

Pender's 1987 version has its theoretical foundations in expectancy-value theory (Feather 1982) and social cognitive theory (Bandura 1986). Expectancy-value theory holds that individuals are rational and will persist with a given behaviour as long as it produces positive personal value and is likely to produce the desired outcome. Social cognitive theory relies on interaction between the environment, the person and the behaviour, each being capable of modifying the others. Fundamental to the HPM is the belief that individuals play an active role in shaping and maintaining health behaviours and in modifying the environmental context for health behaviour.

The revised HPM (Pender 1996) includes three new variables: activity-related effect; commitment to a plan of action; and immediate competing demands and preferences. The headings at the top of the model (Fig. 3.5) also differ from the original version. Pender

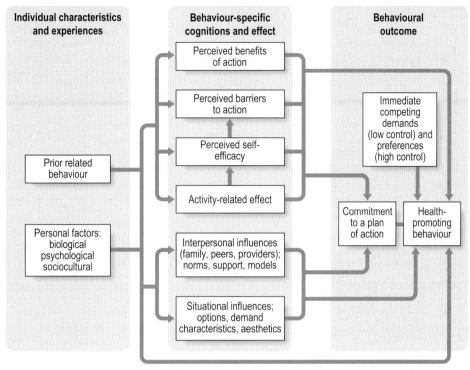

Figure 3.5   Revised health promotion model (redrawn with kind permission from Pender 1996)

divides the model into three discrete sections: individual characteristics and experiences; behaviour-specific cognitions and effect; and behavioural outcome.

Individual characteristics and experiences include prior-related behaviour and personal factors. Drawing on empirical studies, Pender concludes that the best predictor of behaviour is the frequency of the same or similar behaviour in the past. In other words, people who have a habit of engaging in unhealthy behaviours are likely to continue to do so. For Pender, existing bad habits also influence personal perceptions of self-efficacy, as well as perceptions of the benefits of healthy behaviour and barriers to achieving it. Barriers to healthy behaviour experienced in the past are therefore seen as hurdles to overcome. Personal factors include: biological (e.g. age, sex), psychological (e.g. self-esteem, definition of health) and sociocultural (e.g. race, education, socioeconomic status) characteristics. According to Pender (1996), these directly

influence both behaviour-specific cognitions as well as health-promoting behaviour.

Behaviour-specific cognitions and effect are important to Pender's model as they can be modified by health care intervention. These cognitions include certain perceptions that people hold. The benefits of engaging in healthy behaviour, for example, might be sufficient to motivate some people towards healthy behaviour. However, barriers to action, such as unavailability and expense, might decrease the likelihood of engaging in healthy behaviour. Pender concludes that when readiness to act is low and barriers are high, action is unlikely to occur. Thus, health visitors attempting to change behaviour through advice-giving are often unsuccessful because there are too many barriers to action, such as the high cost of nutritious food. Such barriers might maintain a state of low readiness. When readiness to act is high and barriers are low, however, the probability of action is much greater. A person's perception of their own self-efficacy (Bandura 1986) is also important in influencing behaviour. Not only is a feeling of being efficacious likely to encourage future engagement in the target behaviour, but it also lowers the perception of barriers to the target behaviour so that it seems more achievable. Thus, health visitors would be wise to function at a public health level by reducing barriers to action through public health campaigns and collaborative action. This, in turn, would enable people to feel more efficacious in overcoming barriers to healthy behaviour.

Self-efficacy is also influenced by the activity-related affect. This means that the emotion resulting from the health activity, whether it be positive or negative, will influence whether the activity is repeated in future. This, in turn, will influence the person's perception of self-efficacy. A person who experiences pleasure from a health activity, for example, is likely to feel efficacious in relation to that activity and is therefore likely to repeat it. The different individual perceptions discussed above, together with the activity-related effect, will impact on people's decisions to commit themselves to a plan of action.

Other factors likely to influence commitment to a plan of action are interpersonal and situational influences. According to Pender (1996) 'individuals are more likely to undertake behaviours for which they will be admired and socially reinforced' (p. 71). People vary, however, in the extent to which they are susceptible to the influence of others. Situational influences on health behaviour include perceptions of the aesthetic features of the environment in which the health behaviour will take place (Pender 1996). Pender views situational factors as having both direct and indirect influences on health behaviour. A feeling of reassurance and compatibility with an environment, for example, will indirectly influence health behaviour. More direct influences will occur in situations where health behaviours are enforced by rules such as no smoking.

The final component of Pender's (1996) model, behavioural outcome, is predicated upon the commitment to a plan, unless a competing demand or preference intervenes to prevent implementation of the plan. Commitment to a plan needs to be reinforced by a strategy in order for it to reach fruition. Moreover, even well-thought-out strategies for health improvement can be influenced negatively by unexpected demands over which the individual has little control; or by competing preferences over which the individual has more control but that are difficult to resist.

Like the two models previously discussed, Pender's health promotion model focuses on individual behaviour. It does, however, give fuller consideration to the social context in which health behaviour occurs. The three models presented thus far are illustrated in the following vignette.

The health visitor in Deep Hayes village has been working with the practice nurse to encourage breast awareness. In particular, attendance for routine mammography screening in the over–50 age group has been poor and they are concerned to improve the uptake. They begin by interviewing women opportunistically to ascertain their stage in Procaska & DiClemente's transtheoretical model. They discover that some women are at the precontemplation stage, do not see breast screening as a priority and do not believe that it has any benefits. Other women have moved to the contemplation stage, but have been deterred from taking action because, having weighed up the pros and cons of mammography and talked to women who have attended for the procedure, they have decided that the procedure is likely to be too uncomfortable and to have limited benefits. A few women have progressed as far as attending for mammography, but have only attended for one screening. These women are in their mid–fifties and have not been screened for 4 years. They have therefore failed to maintain the screening programme and have relapsed to their preprogramme behaviour. The health visitor and practice nurse want to achieve two outcomes: to increase the attendance for all women and to increase the annual attendance of the same women in order to increase the detection rate of early breast changes.

Procaska & DiClemente's transtheoretical model is useful in enabling them to assess the women's stage in the change cycle, but has limited use in promoting attendance. Indeed, the therapeutic nature of the model makes it more valuable in changing addictive behaviours than in promoting healthy activities. It is unlikely, therefore, that the health visitor and practice nurse would move to a deeper level of therapeutic intervention than focusing on the situational context. Furthermore, the change processes might well be limited to consciousness raising, thus moving the women from precontemplation to contemplation, but no further. The health belief model, however, proves useful in promoting screening.

The health belief model (Becker et al 1974) enables the health visitor and practice nurse to identify perceived susceptibility and the seriousness of the condition. As a cue to action, they target all women over 50 with a breast awareness campaign. They invite the women to group sessions where they discuss the predisposing factors to breast cancer, so that all women can diagnose their own susceptibility. They then invite the women to share with the group their own personal experiences of breast cancer. A former patient also willingly attends to discuss her personal experience of being cured of breast cancer as a result of the breast screening programme. Sharing this knowledge also acts as a modifying factor by increasing women's knowledge of the condition. It is anticipated that, following the campaign, the women will weigh up the benefits of attending for screening, together with the barriers to attendance, and that this will increase the likelihood of attendance.

The campaign proves largely successful in enabling the women to progress through the cycle of change, although there are a number of women who remain resistant to change. Not wishing to give up on these women, the health visitor uses Pender's health promotion model as an aid to analyse the behaviour-specific cognitions and effects that might account for this resistance to change. The health visitor and practice nurse discover a variety of perceptions that explain their behaviour.

For several women, the complex nature of their lives makes breast awareness a low priority. Although they can see the benefits of screening, these are outweighed by the barriers, such as time to attend and lack of transport. A minority of women do not have financial problems but have such a low perception of their own self-efficacy and so little control over their lives that the future and their health status do not matter to them. Two women have other health problems: one suffers from multiple sclerosis and one has a severe heart condition. What all of these women share in common is a sense of health as 'destiny' that is beyond their control. External attempts to control health on their behalf are not considered significant. Furthermore, previous attendance for screening programmes, such as cervical screening, have not been a pleasurable experience either in terms of the effort required to attend or the procedure itself. This activity-related effect, therefore, only served to reinforce their perceived self-efficacy. Interpersonal and situational influences served to reinforce this further. Experiences of screening programmes shared with family and friends concurred with this view of a negative experience, often requiring long waits in crowded, impersonal waiting rooms.

Pender's (1996) HPM revealed some critical factors in explaining health behaviour. The health visitor had a difficult decision to make. She had to balance attempting to raise the self-esteem of some women against interfering with their right to make their own decisions. Moreover, some of their decisions seemed quite reasonable, given the circumstances.

Although both Becker et al's and Pender's model do take into account structural variables, structural factors are not considered from the point of view of their specific impact on health behaviour. This factor could be crucial in developing public health initiatives and is fundamental to Green et al's PRECEDE model, which will be discussed next.

THE PRECEDE MODEL

The PRECEDE model (Green et al 1980) centres on the need to initiate change in behaviour by analysing its preceding causes. Seven phases represent the process through which behavioural change takes place. In phases 1 and 2, to the right of Figure 3.6, an epidemiological and social diagnosis is made. In particular, phase 1 focuses on quality of life indicators such as the individual's or community's own subjective definition of their quality of life. Of particular interest to the health visitor at this stage would be population factors such as age distribution, the percentage of different ethnic minority groups,

the unemployment rate and housing facilities, as well as numerous other social factors. Edet (1991), for example, used phase 1 of Green's model to identify risks associated with adolescent pregnancy. Quality of life is preceded, and therefore predicated upon, by non health-related factors and health problems (phase 2). Health visitors would therefore be particularly aware of the different dimensions (incidence, prevalence, etc.) of different diseases and conditions, and how they impact on and interact with subjectively defined quality of life perceptions as well as objective quality of life indicators. During phase 2 the health visitor would isolate the specific indicators and dimensions that were thought to impact on the subjectively defined quality of life. In an area with an ageing population, for example, the effects of disabling conditions on the quality of life might be identified as important. In Edet's study of adolescent pregnancy phase 2 involved using available data to

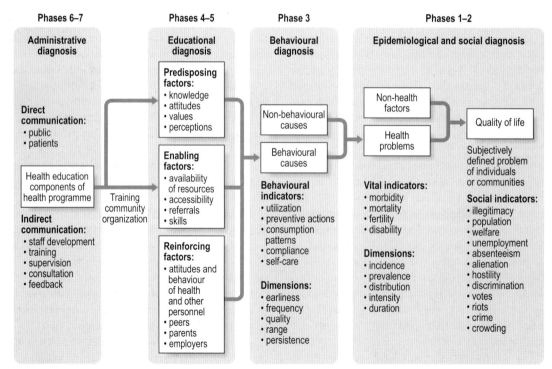

Figure 3.6   Green's PRECEDE model (redrawn from Health Promotion Planning: An Educational and Environmental Approach, Third Edition by Lawrence W Green and Marshall W Kreuter. Copyright ©1999 by Mayfield Publishing Company. Reprinted by permission of the publisher)

identify specific health problems that contribute to adolescent pregnancy, such as high infant and maternal mortality rates associated with adolescent pregnancy.

Phase 3 refers to the behavioural diagnosis needed to identify different causes, both behavioural and non-behavioural, that impact on health problems. Early, frequent and persistent consumption of cigarettes, for example, would represent a behavioural cause of health problems. Non-behavioural causes of health problems could relate to the local environment. Traffic congestion, for example, might increase the incidence of road traffic accidents, or industrial pollution might be responsible for chest diseases. The health visiting response to these two categories of cause would differ considerably. The non-behavioural causes would be addressed through community action and participation, the health visitor engaging in political action by association with relevant local groups. By contrast, Green et al's model would adopt a health education response to the behavioural causes. Phase 3 of Edet's study involved the identification of both behavioural causes such as early exposure to sex, greater sexual freedom and early menarche, and non-behavioural causes such as unemployment and low socioeconomic status.

According to the model (Fig. 3.6), phase 3 is preceded by, and therefore affected by, predisposing, enabling and reinforcing factors represented in phases 4 and 5. Returning to the example of early, frequent and persistent smoking, the educational diagnosis used at phase 4 would identify existing knowledge, attitudes, values and perceptions relating to smoking. Enabling factors, such as support systems to discourage the habit, would also be assessed. Finally, factors that reinforce the habit, such as attitudes of peers and employers, would also be considered. Phase 5 would then involve deciding which of the three classes of factor – predisposing, enabling or reinforcing – should be the focus of attention. The health visitor could, for example, focus on enabling factors by using available support systems to attempt to counteract the effects of predisposing and reinforcing factors.

The final two phases of the model, phases 6 and 7, involve the factors that precede the educational diagnosis. Edet's use of the sixth and seventh phases, for example, involved the implementation and evaluation of the health education programme of sex education. At this stage, then, it is assumed that for an educational diagnosis to take place an administrative diagnosis must first occur and an evaluation strategy be negotiated. This includes communication with the public, training of both the community and the organization staff, staff development, consultation and feedback. Health visitors are particularly effective at this stage, as they work at the interface between health care organizations and the public. Their role therefore includes both direct and indirect communication, as well consultation and feedback.

> A health visitor in Old Town has recently moved to a newly formed post, where she is responsible for developing an outreach service to travelling families on a newly established caravan site.
>
> On examining quality of life non-health factors she discovers that the travelling families are alienated from the local community, which is hostile towards them. The children are regularly absent from school because they are ostracized by their peers. The caravans and the site are overcrowded. Vital indicators of potential health problems include the fact that most families have more than four children and prefer not to use contraception because of their religious convictions. Behavioural causes of this overcrowding, therefore, relate to non-use of birth control. The health visitor appreciates that the predisposing factors leading to this include religious values and beliefs and respects this. The desire for large families could, however, be reinforced by familial norms passed down generations. It is probably at the enabling level that the health visitor has the greatest impact. Using skills of communication she works with the site as a 'community' to discuss the value and norms associated with having children. Through discussion she encourages the families to see the benefits

of limiting family size. She also discusses natural family planning methods and the benefits of this.

In evaluating her performance, the health visitor communicates with both the families themselves and her employer. Clinical supervision is needed to enable her to make good judgements. She could be in danger, for example, of working so closely with the site occupants that she ignores wider health issues such as the alienation and discrimination occurring from the local communities.

The four health promotion models discussed thus far have been successfully applied to health visiting practice in the public health domain. The four models will be evaluated next, before discussing public health models.

EVALUATION OF HEALTH PROMOTION MODELS IN RELATION TO HEALTH VISITING

Using the evaluation criteria listed in Box 3.1, it is evident that all four models discussed thus far have considerable credibility. The three main elements of evaluation – conceptual clarity, conceptual accuracy and application to practice – will be considered separately.

CONCEPTUAL CLARITY

All four models appear to be logical in that clear lines of association exist between concepts. The concepts embraced within Procaska & DiClemente's model and Green's PRECEDE model, however, seem to be less clearly explicated than other models. The transtheoretical model (Procaska & DiClemente 1988) focuses more on processes and theories than on description of concepts. Likewise, Green's PRECEDE model describes different stages without explaining concepts underpinning the derivation of the model. Descriptions of concepts are evident from the original development of the health belief model (Becker et al 1974), the detailed components of which were reviewed by Rosenstock (1966), thus demonstrating the

grounding of the concepts in theory. Supporting empirical evidence for the health belief model can be found in Mitchell's (1969) review of research into Rosenstock's original variables. This revealed that the health belief model provided a satisfactory explanation for most research findings relating to preventive health behaviour. Pender's health promotion model also demonstrates conceptual clarity through the explication of each of the concepts within the revised model.

CONCEPTUAL ACCURACY

The accuracy of the models is depicted in the vignettes, which illustrate the relevance of the models to the people to whom they apply. Pender's and Green et al's models do, however, appear to more accurately reflect complex health behaviours, while Procaska & DiClemente's model of change, and to a lesser extent the health belief model, are limited in this respect. These latter two models, therefore, could arguably be lacking in expected concepts related to causal influences of health behaviour. Green et al's (1980) main value seems to be in its recognition of the impact of causes and factors on health problems and how these can ultimately affect quality of life. The nature of factors preceding other factors is unique to this model and demonstrates the need to always consider what lies behind the evidence presented. The limitation of the model lies in its tendency to focus exclusively on a defined problem to the detriment of other possible problems and solutions. The health visitor in the vignette, for example, chose to focus on family planning rather than alienation or absenteeism. This potentially reductionist approach could result in a narrow focus on identifying problems and the necessary changes in behaviour required to resolve them. The model could therefore be in danger of subordinating autonomy and self-empowerment to its main aim of initiating behaviour change (Naidoo & Wills 1994). Empowering both the local community and the travelling families to meet and discuss their similarities and differences in culture and lifestyle might have relieved alienation and absenteeism at the same time.

Following this, a change in behaviour relating to family planning might be easier to achieve.

Theoretical or empirical grounding of concepts is clearly evident in the health belief model, the health promotion model and the transtheoretical model. The health belief model is grounded in theory of individual perceptions as well as research into how changes in perception can be brought about (Rosenstock 1974). The health promotion model is grounded in theory (social learning theory) as well as in research and testing of the original model. Most of these studies attempted to predict health behaviour from the variables within Pender's original model, such as value of benefits, perceived self-efficacy, perceived barriers and demographic characteristics (Frank-Stromborg et al 1990, Pender et al 1990, Lusk et al 1994, Garcia et al 1995). Pender (1996) concludes from an analysis of these studies that the variables that were most successful in predicting health behaviour were perceived self-efficacy, benefits and barriers. These findings then formed the basis of the revised model. Procaska & DiClemente's model is based on change theory (McConnaughy et al 1983) and, like the other models discussed, is also based in self-efficacy theory (Bandura 1977a).

APPLICATION TO PRACTICE

The predictive ability of the models is dependent on the intended purpose of the model. Green's model is interpretative, rather than predictive, while Procaska & DiClemente's is explanatory. It is therefore not possible to evaluate the predictive ability of these models in relation to time and place. Some support for the predictive value of the health belief model, however, has been found in relation to breast self-examination (Fung 1998) and alcohol consumption (Minugh et al 1998). Certain variables within Pender's health promotion model, too, have proved useful in predicting health behaviour, as indicated above.

The only potential contradiction between theories emerging from the models and the reality of practice occur with Procaska & DiClemente's change cycle and the health belief model, for they arguably provide a limited theory of health behaviour in so far as they omit the entire life context. Nevertheless, the transtheoretical model has proved successful in integrating theory and practice relating to motivating behaviour (Shinitzky & Kub 2001), examining the processes of change in a behaviourally oriented weight loss programme (Suris et al 1998), smoking cessation in pregnancy (Stotts et al 1996) and specific opiate-dependent patients (Tejero et al 1997). The value of this model seems to be, therefore, in planning interventions that target specific stage-dependent causal mechanisms (Pollak et al 1998). An important finding in relation to any model focusing on perceived health status is the capacity for perceived health status to moderate the relations between critical thinking and participation in various types of health behaviours (Settersten & Lauver 2004).

In all cases the models can be tested in practice, as is demonstrated through the two vignettes, as well as the extensive research evidence discussed above. The practical significance of these models can be translated into guidance for health visiting practice. What seems to be evident, however, is that health promotion models are insufficiently complex to take into account the sociocultural constraints that influence people's lives. Recent emphasis on the importance of the role of the health visitor in public health (Hawksley et al 2003, Carr et al 2003, Smith 2004) also indicates the need to consider how this role can be underpinned by public health models. The use of public health and health visiting models might, therefore, prove more worthwhile in guiding health visiting activities.

HEALTH VISITING AND PUBLIC HEALTH FRAMEWORKS AND THEIR APPLICATION TO HEALTH VISITING

The dynamic and unique nature of health visiting, combined with uncertainty about defining and measuring its outcomes, have led to attempts to conceptualize and hence describe and explain health visiting at different stages of its development. Health visitors need to rely on a variety of concepts and models if they are to explain the complexity of their professional activities. The remainder of this chapter will consider a variety of frameworks for health visiting and public health. Beattie's health accounts will provide the predominant framework for this discussion. Other models discussed are Chalmers & Kristajanson's (1989) models of community nursing and Neuman's (1989) systems model. In addition, certain theories and paradigms will be considered, namely Twinn's (1991) paradigms of health visiting and Chalmers' (1992) theory of giving and receiving in health visiting.

Beattie (1993) makes an important contribution to debates about the future of health visiting. He argues that health researchers have made a paradigm shift towards focusing on explanations of health emanating from negotiated meanings through conversational exchanges. This, he argues, is only one way of explaining health and fails to explain what influences people to select particular accounts. This resonates with While's (1991) criticism of the health belief model. Both criticisms seek further explanations than simple structural explanations appear to offer. It was suggested above (see discussion of the health belief model) that applying individual explanations at the community level can integrate individual perceptions with sociocultural considerations of society. Beattie's health accounts develop this argument further by identifying links between what people believe and the social worlds they inhabit.

According to Beattie (1996), what people believe can be defined in terms of two dimensions: modes of thought and focus of attention (Fig. 3.7). Each dimension can be viewed as bipolar. The modes of thought dimension comprise hard (mechanistic) and soft (humanistic) poles. This reflects the seriousness that the professions and society ascribe to different approaches to analysis. Hard approaches, according to Beattie, dominate, as they are in keeping with the natural science tradition. Soft approaches, by contrast, are equated with lay as opposed to expert views and are therefore seen as 'trivial'.

The focus-of-attention dimension comprises the polar opposites of individuals or collectivities. Work in the individual pole focuses on individualist philosophies of health behaviour. Solutions to problems arising from the health behaviour of individuals, therefore, lie either in understanding individual personal biographies in order to explain behaviour or in attempting to correct behaviour. By contrast, work in the collective pole looks for collective causes and solutions relating to health behaviour.

The two dimensions of hard versus soft approaches, and of individual versus collective approaches, reflect the dilemmas of health visiting. Health visitors ascribe to both the soft (humanistic) approach to health care and the hard (mechanistic) approach, depending on the changing and dynamic demands of their work, and their particular orientation. Recent debates concerning the health visitor's public health function represent a return to the hard mechanistic approach to public health and hence a return to the roots of health visiting. However, when this hard mechanistic view is combined with current trends in health visiting towards work with collectivities rather than individuals, then health visiting is firmly located within the reformist rather than the conservative tradition. The soft approach to health visiting remains an important facet of practice, both at the individual and the collective level. At the individual level, health visitors provide counselling within the libertarian tradition. The use of the soft approach within the collective level perhaps marks the most radical shift for health visitors, in which community participation and action occur within the pluralist tradition.

Beattie also identifies four ways of accounting for health: the biopathological model, the ecological model, the biographical model and the communitarian model (Fig. 3.7). The biopathological model, in the top left quadrant, uses a mechanistic mode of thought, focusing on the individual as an organism. At a public health level, the model is exemplified in Chalmers & Kristajanson's (1989) public health model.

According to Chalmers & Kristajanson the public health model identifies at-risk groups in the community, using epidemiological methods. It was developed in the 19th century to respond to threats to health care such as communicable diseases and malnutrition. The goal of public

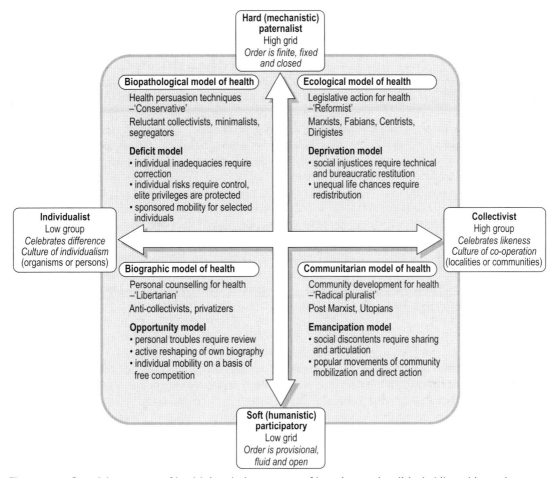

Figure 3.7 Beattie's accounts of health in relation to ways of knowing, sociopolitical philosophies and cultural bias (adapted with kind permission from Beattie 1996)

health at that time was to improve the health of the population by decreasing the spread of disease. According to Chalmers & Kristajanson (1989) the public health model assumes that disease is determined by exposure of a susceptible host (the individual) to the agent (the disease). This interaction between the individual and the environment is known as the host–agent environment interaction. The public health nurse intervenes in this relationship using primary prevention, such as promotion of good nutrition, and secondary prevention, such as screening the population for disease and case finding. In this way the health of the entire population is protected by reducing the spread of disease. During this early stage the emphasis

of health visiting was on defining health problems and providing therapeutic interventions rather than addressing the underlying causes of disease. The agenda, therefore, would have been determined by the 'expert' (Beattie 1979). The focus would also have been on using persuasion techniques, thereby correcting and repairing the 'defective' individual (Beattie 1984). The deficit model would have been prevalent, requiring expert-directed intervention in which the social distance was high (Beattie 1984).

The individualist, paternalistic and conservative characteristics of the top left quadrant can be seen in Twinn's (1991) adaptation of Beattie's model (Fig. 3.8) and in Chalmers' (1992)

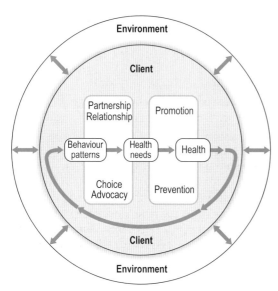

Figure 3.8 Twinn's conceptual framework for health visiting (redrawn with kind permission from Twinn 1991)

theory of health visiting. Twinn used Beattie's four quadrants and some of his dimensions (directive versus non-directive, and collective versus individual) as well as the general principles of the model as the basis for a conceptual framework. For Twinn, intuition and professional artistry, together with professional reflection, are central concepts. Twinn's framework is based on a belief in the client as the central focus in the health visiting strategy. Although this might be seen as endorsing the traditional individualized practice of health visiting, Twinn argues that the client is seen in the context of the community and that 'this does not restrict the framework to an individual or collective paradigm, but is central to the formation of strategies in either setting' (Twinn 1991, p. 971). She further argues that a relationship of partnership must exist between health visitor and client in order to determine strategies that are appropriate to the client's perception of their own health needs. Furthermore, she identifies choice and advocacy as fundamental to both facilitating partnership and responding to the political dimension involved in promoting health and preventing ill health.

Twinn describes health visiting activity in Beattie's top left quadrant as the 'individual

advice giving' paradigm. She argues that individual advice giving is the traditional approach to health visiting practice, involving the provision of advice and health teaching to mothers about the care of infants and young children. This individualist, paternalistic approach to health visiting is also reflected in Chalmers' (1992) theory of giving and receiving in health visiting. Chalmers identified three phases of the health visitor/client relationship:

- the entry phase
- the health promotion phase
- the termination phase.

During the entry phase the health visitor gains access to the client within either an 'open context' (in response to an identified problem or need) or a 'closed context' ('routine' initiation by health visitor). Depending on the context, the health visitor will either make a routine offer of information or will focus on needs identified by the client. In either case the client's perception of the value of the offer will determine whether it is received positively enough to progress to the health promotion phase. Advice and help is offered during this phase to promote health, its success again being determined by its value to the client. Help viewed positively will enable the client to share a range of health issues, which can be addressed throughout the relationship. Alternatively, the client may 'block' any offers not perceived as of value. The interaction between the health visitor and client is therefore regulated by the type of offer made by the health visitor and the perception of its value by the client. The termination phase is characterized by either negotiated or non-negotiated termination. Negotiated termination is characterized by preparation of the client for the termination of visiting. In contrast, visits are terminated without any input from the client in non-negotiated termination.

The top right quadrant of Beattie's model (1993) can also be seen in Twinn's (1991) analysis. Twinn (1991) argues that this public health focus represents the 'environmental control' paradigm of health visiting which she equates with Beattie's ecological model of health. This model represents the hard, mechanistic side of health visiting, concerned with communities rather than individuals. The epidemiological expertise of health visitors is used to analyse the interaction between individuals and the environment so that risks to health can be identified. Twinn (1991) argues, further, that this reflects one of the principles of health visiting: 'the search for health needs' (CETHV 1977). For Twinn, the public health (ecological) model involves health visitors in establishing the health needs of a particular population from a health profile of the community. The findings from the profile would then be used to target priorities and practice. The 'professional' use of health persuasion techniques, evident in early public health initiatives (top left quadrant), gives way to a managerial philosophy that relies on legislative action for health. The agenda, therefore, is determined by bureaucratic rules rather than by the expert (Beattie 1979).

The ecological approach is also similar to Chalmers & Kristajanson's (1989) community participation model. This model differs from the public health model in that it involves the community in the planning and delivery of health services. This radical shift in emphasis changes the power-base from health professionals to the community. In assisting the community to identify its own solutions prior to seeking outside assistance, health visitors encourage communities to identify the causes of health problems as well as solutions. According to Beattie (1984), health professionals working in this quadrant direct their expert power towards custodianship of health, guarding and protecting communities against environmental risks. The community participation model reflects much of health visiting practice, as well as that of other health professionals, during the 1980s and 1990s.

The community participation model is also at the heart of public health initiatives that rely on models of prevention (Caplan 1966). Neuman's (1989) model is particularly suited to the public health role of health visiting as it relies not only on theories of prevention but also on systems theory. The value of systems theory to health visiting and public health lies in its assumption

that a system can only be understood in relation to its totality (Haggart 1993). Health visitors attempt to understand individual clients in relation to their wider environment but also attempt to understand the community within its wider social and political context.

Central to Neuman's theory is a belief that individuals have a defence system, represented as a series of circles referred to as lines of resistance with a normal line of defence and an outer flexible line of defence. According to Neuman (1989), stressors break through this normal line of defence when the outer flexible line of defence fails to protect the individual from stressors. When this occurs the internal lines of resistance attempt to restabilize the individual. The concept of lines of resistance can also be applied at the community level. Communities could be viewed as having an outer flexible line of a defence, which gives the community its geographical or social structure. Stresses can come from both within the community and outside it to threaten the lines of resistance. The community exists within and interacts with the wider system. Neuman identifies intrapersonal, interpersonal and extrapersonal stressors to explicate this interrelationship. From the community perspective, intracommunity stressors would be those stressors arising from within the community, such as crimes against property committed by local youth. Indeed, Haggart (1993) raises the point that some communities 'have lines of resistance and normal lines of defence which may include behaviours or strategies considered by the nurse to be damaging to health' (p. 1919).

Intercommunity stressors arise from interactions between communities. This might occur if a major link road was planned to benefit one community and in doing so disadvantaged another. Extracommunity stressors would occur when stress stems from right outside the community. The development of a new factory would be an example of this.

Neuman's model is also based on assumptions concerning primary, secondary and tertiary prevention (Caplan 1966) and their capacity to prevent stress. This, of course, makes the model particularly pertinent to public health and health visiting. Interventions by the health visitor would therefore take place at three different levels of prevention: primary, secondary and tertiary. At the primary prevention level the health visitor works in partnership with community groups. Through participation with voluntary and statutory organizations the facilities within the community can be continually enhanced in response to the expressed needs of the local population. At the secondary prevention level health visitors work with communities to identify potential problems before they arise. Knowledge of epidemiology enables them to recognize morbidity and mortality trends within the population and to work with communities to identify potential local causes and solutions. The tertiary level of prevention involves working with populations to contain situations to ensure that they do not become worse than they already are, to provide support and monitor the situation. An example of this could be traffic calming measures, which, although they would not reduce the problems caused by traffic, would provide supportive and controlling measures to prevent the worst elements of traffic congestion. Application of Neuman's model to health visiting is illustrated in the following vignette.

High Town is a small community on the outskirts of a large urban city. The town is characterized by a north/south divide. The south side of the town consists predominantly of socio-economic groups I and II. The north side houses mainly people in socio-economic groups IV and V and unemployment is very high. The town is approximately 1 mile from the main city centre. A large ring road has recently been completed, which creates a geographical divide between the north and south sides of the town. This also makes access to the main city more difficult for people on the north side.

One of the health visitors has been working in High Town for some 5 years. He has noticed increasing discontentment and isolation of the population on the north side. In collaboration with a community group he decides to use Neuman's model to assess the stresses within the community, the consequences of these stresses and the preventive action that can be taken to alleviate the problems. Table 3.1 outlines the types of stressor identified within the categories intracommunity, intercommunity and extracommunity.

Table 3.1 Examples of types of stressor and their consequences

Type of stressor	Example	Possible consequences
Intracommunity stressors	High rate of unemployment Local authority housing in poor state of repair Lower than average car ownership Lack of state nursery provision No local facilities for youth	Reduced standards of living Deprivation and poor health Poor access to facilities in city Isolation of women Increased vandalism and crimes by local youth
Intercommunity stressors	Division of single community into two separate communities by ring road Alienation of population on north side from rest of population and from main city	Crime against south side by youth from north side Increased fear of crime
Extracommunity stressors	Shortage of local authority housing Major developments to main city increase traffic flow on ring road and local residential network The Accident and Emergency Department and many wards at local city hospital are to be closed	High incidence of homelessness Increased accident rate Poor access to health care

Having identified the stressors and possible consequences it was possible to consider how the consequences could be limited within the different levels of prevention. Examples of preventive measures are listed in Table 3.2.

The use of Neuman's model in public health provides a useful framework within the bottom right-hand quadrant of Beattie's health accounts. However, health visitors might also adopt both the biographical and communitarian models at different times. Both these models, being at the bottom of Figure 3.7, use soft humanistic approaches, but the biographical model (in the left-hand quadrant) focuses on personal and private troubles, using counselling to facilitate coping. Beattie (1984) describes work within this quadrant as being client centred with low social distance, involving counselling and empowering individuals. Twinn (1991) refers to this as the 'psychological development' paradigm in which health visitors provide personal support. She distinguishes this from the more directive 'advice giving' paradigm by focusing on partnership in which clients participate in decision making. This partnership approach reflects Beattie's (1979) 'consumerist' approach, in which the agenda is determined by the customer. This individualist approach is also evidenced in Chalmers' (1992) theory of giving and receiving. Moreover, it is probable that Chalmers' theory illustrates how health visitors oscillate between Beattie's two left-hand quadrants on the paternalistic (hard) and participatory (soft) approaches to their individual work with clients.

The focus of the communitarian model is on groups and how individuals interact within groups. Health visitors would act as advocates in this context, working with other community workers and campaigns to improve health. Beattie (1979) describes this as a syndicalist approach in which the agenda is determined by collective negotiation between allies. Moreover, as Twinn (1991) points out: 'where health visitors have been successful, they have shared their knowledge and expertise openly, and worked in partnership with community members, making decisions jointly' (p. 968).

This communitarian approach also bears some similarity to Chalmers & Kristajanson's (1989, p. 572) community change model. This model is characterized by an examination of underlying social, political and economic factors affecting health as well as making

Table 3.2   The use of different levels of prevention to alleviate stressors

Level of prevention	Action
Primary prevention	Liaise with local councils to establish job opportunities arising from local city developments Work with local organizations (e.g. schools and voluntary groups) to provide sports facilities and clubs for youth Liaise with local communities to develop Neighbourhood Watch schemes Lobby local council to improve street lighting to reduce fear of crime Lobby local government to improve public transport to main city Lobby local government to improve walking access between the two sides of the ring road and walking access to main city Employ a multi-agency approach to health needs, health education and health promotion
Secondary prevention	Lobby local authority to repair local authority houses and to provide additional housing stock Liaise with local schools to improve nursery school provision Liaise with local authority to increase traffic calming measures in residential areas
Tertiary prevention	Work with local organizations to develop skills training for unemployed and youth Liaise with local groups to monitor provision of services

systemic efforts to alter destructive structures. Thus, all sectors of the community are involved in creating systems that work towards improving health. The emphasis here is not only on community participation, but also on collaboration of different professional and voluntary groups towards a common goal: health improvement. This communitarian model is given legitimacy by the present Labour Government in its White Paper *The New NHS – Modern, Dependable* (Department of Health 1997a). The emphasis on primary care groups within the White Paper, together with health action zones and health improvement programmes, encourages collaboration between professionals and lay people towards health improvement. Such an approach fosters community change through community participation and action.

Central to this belief in community change is the change from health education, which would have involved advice-giving in the early public health model, to health promotion. Health promotion is a much wider concept than health education, involving health visitors in advocacy, mediation and community empowerment. Health promotion thus involves health visitors in political activities in challenging the distribution of power and resource allocation and therefore influencing policies affecting health (CETHV 1977).

Sociopolitical philosophies are also of concern to Beattie (1993) and these too reflect the tensions in health visiting. The dimension of paternalist and participatory (Fig. 3.7) is indicative of the top-down and bottom-up approaches to policy making in health care. One of the principles of health visiting is 'the influence of policies affecting health' (CETHV 1977). This involves health visitors in participatory action. Using the communitarian model enables them to mobilize communities to direct action and is therefore typical of Beattie's radical pluralist philosophy, in which individual problems gain recognition in the public domain.

The final component of Beattie's (1993) analysis to be discussed here is four types of cultural bias (Fig. 3.7). 'Grid' refers to rules and constraints that a culture imposes on its people (Beattie 1996). 'High grid', which is associated with paternalism, refers to a precise definition of roles and statuses and separation of roles. This typifies the public health model described by Chalmers & Kristajanson (1989), in which the power base lies firmly with health professionals. 'Low grid', associated with participation, is characterized by negotiation within a society in which nothing is fixed. The responsiveness of health visitors to the needs and preferences of the client and the client's capacity to choose whether to accept or reject offers of help (Chalmers 1992) are typical of a low-grid culture.

'Group' refers to the boundedness of a group. 'High group' is characterized by a strong sense of belonging to a well-defined social group, to the extent that the interests of the group are more important than individual interests. This, combined with the 'low grid', would characterize the communitarian view of health visiting. In contrast, working with 'low group' characteristics is less typical of contemporary health visiting, although some work with individuals' interests is still carried out.

In tracing the changing nature of health visiting, it is possible to locate the profession within different quadrants of Beattie's accounts at different points in time. The early public health model adopted by health visitors (Chalmers & Kristajanson 1989) seemed to adopt a biopathological model of health, in that advice was given to individuals to enable them to improve their own health and consequently the health of the whole community. This top-down, biopathological approach can also be seen in contemporary health education campaigns aimed at persuading individuals to change their behaviour. Indeed the health belief model (Becker et al 1974), and the transtheoretical model of change (Procaska & DiClemente 1984), are based on this belief. It seems, therefore, that a paternalistic approach has dominated health visiting to some extent throughout its history.

More recently, health visiting has moved towards the collectivist (high group) rather than individualist (low group) pole of Beattie's accounts. The profession continues to struggle with the dilemmas created by working in both ecological and communitarian models. The ecological model is paternalistic and involves health visitors in striving for more formal recognition of their public health role in legislation. This represents a shift from the communitarian model with which they have had some involvement for the past two decades. Beattie's accounts are illustrated in the following vignette.

> The health visitor in Low Town has become aware of the high incidence of smoking during pregnancy. She wants to work with the midwife to set up a Quit Smoking group to help pregnant women to stop. The biopathological model of health can be applied here, in which health behaviour is seen as a deficit in the individual. The conservative philosophy holds that individuals are responsible for their own health and, therefore, that they should be responsible for changing their own behaviour. Using this model it is assumed that, once given the correct information, the women will change their behaviour. This proves difficult, however, as the context of women's lives in Low Town is such that the deprivation and lack of facilities they experience cause undue pressure. The way in which they alleviate their sense of hopelessness is by smoking.

In working with these women the health visitor has to take account of the ecological model of health, which embraces a social reformist rather than a conservative philosophy. This approach therefore assumes that social reform is needed to alleviate deprivation by redistributing life chances and addressing social injustice. It is at this level that health visitors draw on one of the principles of health visiting: 'the influence of policies affecting health' (CETHV 1977). Although they can do this at both macro (societal) and micro (individual/family) level, the collectivist, 'high group' approach within this quadrant would imply that the health visitor would adopt a political stance, working with local communities to improve their facilities.

Working with local communities and instigating political action to shape change also requires the health visitor to adopt the radical pluralist philosophy of the communitarian model. Working closely with the local community enables the health visitor to emancipate the women so that they can help to change the negative forces affecting their own lives. It is only when this process is complete that the health visitor can move to the individualist approach, perhaps addressing personal biographies and how they shape smoking behaviour.

The above vignette has illustrated how health behaviour, and health visiting responses to it, do not happen in a vacuum. Indeed, Beattie's four accounts could be seen as a dynamic cycle, in which health visitors move around and between the four quadrants according to the needs of the individuals and groups with whom they work. It is this dynamic nature of contemporary health visiting that separates it from the different disciplines within nursing and also from specialist branches of medicine and public health.

A review of public health and health visiting models reveals the extent to which health models support and to some extent are built upon Beattie's health accounts. The models discussed above will now be evaluated.

EVALUATION OF HEALTH VISITING AND PUBLIC HEALTH MODELS

The evaluation of health visiting and public health models is complex as most are defined differently from the health promotion models discussed above. With the exception of Neuman's systems model, none of the 'models' discussed above is defined as such by the authors. Chalmers' theory of giving and receiving, for example, is defined as a theory rather than a model. Twinn (1991) describes her analysis of Beattie's work as four conflicting 'paradigms'. Beattie (1993) describes his work as four health accounts. The following evaluation will therefore take into account these differences in definition. The evaluation, as before, will address issues of conceptual clarity, conceptual accuracy and application to practice.

Chalmers' (1992) theory of giving and receiving was probably described as a theory as it emerged from empirical research using a grounded theory methodology. Hence, the theory is high on conceptual clarity since it emerged from empirical interview data from 45 experienced health visitors from 13 different health authorities. Grounding of the theory within the data would ensure that concepts were factually accurate within their context. Chalmers argues that health visitor interactions with clients are influenced by the meaning that events have for them within the context of past experience. This view seems logically congruent both with the theory of giving and receiving and with the reality of health visiting practice. The central concepts within the theory, giving and receiving, reflect the pattern of interaction between health visitors and their clients, and how each controls this interaction. The explanatory nature of the concepts adds conceptual clarity to the theory as the concepts appear factually faithful to the reality of health visiting at the individual level. The concepts are also linked to phases of health visiting and the type of work carried out at each phase. This adds to the congruence and descriptive detail of the theory. It may be concluded, then, that Chalmers' theory of giving and receiving is high on conceptual clarity.

Conceptual accuracy is reflected in the use of grounded theory in Chalmers' research. Use of grounded theory makes it likely that the concepts within the theory reflect the reality of the health visitors studied. Besides being empirically based, the model also has a firm theoretical foundation in concepts from symbolic interactionism (Mead 1934, Blumer 1969). Exchange theory (Homans 1961, Blau 1964) is also used by Chalmers, who suggests that health visitor–client interactions that are not providing any benefits or are creating feelings of lack of self-worth, rejection or powerlessness will be avoided. The use of grounded theory would ensure saturation of the data to the extent that all expected concepts were reflected in the theory. Nevertheless, there can be no guarantee that all possible concepts in client–health visitor interactions were represented within the interviews, or throughout the interpretation of transcripts. Health visiting exchanges within this

theory, for example, are located in only two of Beattie's health accounts. The theory, therefore, is deficient as it does not include all necessary concepts reflecting the public health collective dimension.

Chalmers' theory seems successful in its demonstration of application to practice. A potential contradiction might emerge if health visiting developed its focus on public health to the exclusion of individual work with families. This contradiction also reflects the theory–practice gap, in that some of the work identified by Chalmers is routine and child focused, which is more in keeping with traditional health visiting practice. Chalmers' research was, however, published in 1992, the data possibly being collected in the late 1980s. The theory can be tested in practice and the phases of the health visitor–client relationship are, to some extent, supported by the phases evident in Peplau's (1952) model, which focused on the development of the relationship between mental health nurses and their clients. As a theory grounded in empirical practice, Chalmers' theory provides a good explanatory framework for the reality of practice and thus might offer guidance for future direction.

The three models discussed by Chalmers & Kristajanson (1989), by contrast, are less easy to evaluate. Chalmers & Kristjanson appear to use the term 'model' rather loosely in describing the historical and political changes in public health. The absence of clearly specified concepts results in a lack of conceptual clarity and accuracy. Nevertheless, the changes they identify, although perhaps not overtly testable in practice, do reflect the contemporary dilemmas of health visiting. This grounding of the models (though not concepts) in empirical as well as theoretical evidence, therefore, does ensure that the models have practical significance and therefore contribute to current debates about health visiting practice. The three models are based on existing theories. Biological theories of the host–agent environment and susceptibility, for example, underpin the public health model. Moreover, theories about professional power, cooperation and political activity underpin both community participation and community change models. Furthermore, the three models lend theoretical support to Beattie's (1996) four health accounts as well as Twinn's (1991) four conflicting paradigms in health visiting.

Unlike Chalmers & Kristajanson, Beattie (1996) does not proclaim that the four health accounts are a model. It would therefore be unwise to treat them as such. Beattie does, however, draw on four models of health (deficit, deprivation, opportunity and emancipation), which he subsumes within four broader models of health (biopathological, ecological, biographical and communitarian). These models are derived from Beattie (1991). A variety of philosophies are explicated within the four health accounts, while conceptual clarity is produced through the use of bipolar dimensions. The four quadrants derived from these two different dimensions produce logical congruence, and concepts such as 'high group' versus 'low group' and paternalist versus participatory are sufficiently described to reflect reality. The complex nature of the four quadrants could result in some conceptual inaccuracy, although this needs to be balanced by the danger of omitting concepts that are important to a complex social scene. Like Chalmers & Kristajanson's three models, Beattie's health accounts offer thought for the future of health visiting. It is thus in their practical application that Beattie's health accounts have their greatest power. Beattie's health accounts also proved valuable in forming the basis of Twinn's (1991) conflicting paradigms.

Twinn's four conflicting paradigms of health visiting were used as the basis for a conceptual framework for health visiting. Concepts used included partnership, promotion, choice, advocacy, prevention and health. Despite the obvious use of these concepts, the framework lacks conceptual clarity. The flow of influence between the arrows within the model (Britt 1997), for example, would suggest that health influences health behaviour, which in turn influences health needs, and that the influence of health needs completes the cyclical influence of these concepts upon each other. Twinn does not, however, define health in relation to her framework, nor does she clarify the links between health, health promotion and behaviour patterns or how they relate to partnership, advocacy, promotion and prevention. Instead, she links these concepts to professional artistry and reflection. For these reasons also, the concepts lack logical congruence and there is insufficient description of the concepts to provide confidence in their ability to reflect reality.

Because of the logical incongruence of Twinn's (1991) conceptual framework it is difficult to estimate conceptual accuracy. Some concepts, for example, might be irrelevant, although the model does seem to have had some practical application (Ling & Luker 2000). The lack of conceptual clarity and accuracy within the framework also makes it difficult to develop theories from the model that can be subsequently tested. This conceptual framework is an example of the difficulty experienced in applying models to practice when the defining concepts lack clarity and coherence.

The final model, Neuman's systems model, is typical of many models used in health care. It relies on concepts derived from existing theory, i.e. Seyle's concept of stress (Seyle 1956), which it contextualizes within different levels of personal interaction. This gives conceptual clarity to the model. The categorizing of stressors, for example, enables community groups to enumerate stressors from the perspective of the different stakeholders, and therefore to prioritize the different preventive actions.

Logical congruence is enhanced in Neuman's model by the application of Caplan's (1966) model of prevention. This also provides sufficient confidence in the model's ability to reflect reality. The model was grounded in both theory and empirical evidence and has since been tested in a variety of contexts, including public health nursing (Benedict & Behringer Sproles 1982), mental health, and community nursing (Beitler et al 1980). This lends accuracy to the model.

The evaluation of health visiting and public health models, theories and paradigms suggests that most are valuable tools to analyse contemporary health visiting practice. Although theories and paradigms are defined differently from models they make valuable suggestions for the future of health visiting in public health.

SUMMARY

The models, theories and paradigms discussed in this chapter reveal not only the complex nature of health visiting but also the complexity of defining, evaluating and applying models to health visiting practice. Simple health promotion models have proved useful in explaining health behaviour and possibilities for behavioural change. More complex health promotion models were more successful in explaining behaviour within a cultural milieu. Thus, such models have more value for public health initiatives. Public health models, however, seem to offer a more critical framework for considering future directions in health visiting. Such frameworks offer alternative paradigms for health visiting that may coexist.

The different types of model and framework discussed in this chapter present a challenge for evaluation. Nevertheless, the evaluation criteria developed in this chapter were used successfully in evaluating a range of models, theories and paradigms.

Chapter 4

Skills in specialist community public health nursing–health visiting: working with individuals and families

Anne Robotham

INTRODUCTION

This chapter is designed to discuss the fundamental skills of specialist community public health nursing (SCPHN)–health visiting, which are used to interpret and satisfy the principles and domains outlined for the third part of the Register. Practitioners from many different backgrounds will be working using competencies in the domains and, like them, health visitors will be interpreting and practising using skills, but gained from a different body of knowledge. The main thrust of health visiting practice is in a proactive rather than a reactive forum. The chapter will begin by considering the nature and focus of SCPHN–health visiting practice.

THE NATURE AND FOCUS OF THE PRACTICE OF SCPHN–HEALTH VISITING

In the first edition of this textbook there was a modified example of a model of care (Fig. 4.1). This is reproduced in order to compare it with the new model of public health care which may be defined by the third part of the Register (Fig. 4.2). This model illustrates the breadth of practice which will be SCPHN, and depending on the background or extra education of the

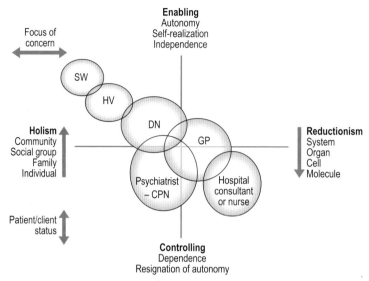

Figure 4.1   Modified example of a model of care (redrawn from Baraclough et al 1983)

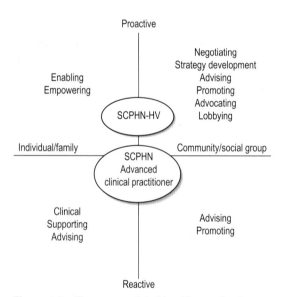

Figure 4.2   The new model of health care for the third part of the Register – Robotham and Frost (based loosely on Twinn's 1991 adaptation of Beattie 1991)

practitioner will determine the main area in which they will focus. Health visiting is in the upper half of the proactive–reactive axis and along the whole of the individual/family–social group/community axis. Health visitors who practise public health care with additional clinical skills acquired through an advanced

specialist clinical course could be working in all four quadrant areas of Model 4.2. Without advanced clinical skills they will be unlikely to be in the practical/clinical quadrant unless in a supporting role towards other members of the family linked to an individual member requiring specialist clinical skills.

THE AMBIENCE OF HEALTH VISITING PRACTICE

Health visiting began with the family unit because it was to work with families in their homes that the forerunners of health visiting came into being. Later when health visitors were required to be nurses, they nevertheless focused their main concern on the family in the home. In the early days of health visiting, work with the family was public health work, communicated through hygiene, family nutrition, health teaching and promotion. Health visitors became accepted as professionals who worked with families, following on from the midwife once delivery and immediate aftercare were completed. Goodwin (1988), discussing the reorganization and refocusing of health visiting, commented that there should be no question of throwing the baby out with the bath water – health visitors are good at working with families and should definitely retain that aspect of their work.

In her seminal work on evaluating health visiting Robinson (1982) collated the research evidence available on the effectiveness of health visiting in relation to the reduction of infant mortality. She cited a study by Ashby (1922), which attempted a controlled trial of health visiting in Birmingham where the Medical Officer of Health found that infant mortality in a selected ward where health visiting was carried out, was below the average for previous years, whereas in the other wards it was above average. This Ashby considered to be a result of health visiting interventions, but other variables at the time – a wet summer, improved sanitation, a mild winter and so forth – must not be ignored.

This expressed caution over the effectiveness of health visiting has been repeated time and again in relation to variables both in the ambience in which the family is living and the type of intervention practised by the health visitors concerned. It is thus important that work that health visitors undertake with families is evaluated for effectiveness before any further examination is made of health visiting and families.

RESEARCH ON HEALTH VISITING IN THE HOME

We are grateful for the work of Robinson (1982) in detailing the activities undertaken by health visitors in four studies: those of the Jameson Committee (Ministry of Health 1956), Jeffreys (1965), Marris (1971) and Clark (1973). The important points from these early studies on health visiting were that although they had a research methodology basis they were concerned about what health visitors did in practice rather than the effectiveness of health visiting. No two of the methodologies for the four studies cited were similar: Jeffreys provided a picture of the work of staff in social welfare services, Clark examined the work of a health visitor in the home, the Jameson Committee focused on the range of health visiting tasks and Marris looked at a 2-week diary of health

visitor activities. Only Clark's (1973) study looked at the characteristics of visits to the home and concluded that the greater number (62%) were initiated by health visitors compared with 12.2% by the client and 5.3% by the general practitioner. All four studies looked at the content of home visits and quantified the time spent on various topic areas. It is interesting to note Robinson's (1982) comment that the shorter visits tended to be those initiated by the health visitor where no particular topic or general advice on practical matters of child rearing were the main concern. Clark particularly commented on the stereotypical health visitor of the day with the didactic authoritarian approach. However, she was able to show that, as there had been a syllabus change during the data collection, there was already a difference in the approach of younger, more recently qualified staff from those of older education status.

Dobby (1986), exploring an assessment of health visiting, used Barker's (1985) comment on the Körner recommendations for data collection to show that process evaluation has little meaning without outcome evaluation. Luker (1978) had also explored this in an earlier discussion and considered that individual interventions with clients when set against their goal attainments could provide a way of looking at outcomes and thus at the effectiveness of health visiting. Again, she urged caution in assuming that health visitor interventions alone were responsible for changes in client behaviour, because of other uncontrollable variables. In a later discussion (1985) Luker revisited this issue of measuring effectiveness of health visiting. She used the principle of the nursing process, with its goal-setting, evaluation and problem-solving approach to care, as appropriate to health visiting. To overcome any criticism that health visitors work with families or individuals who have problems, Luker differentiated between actual problems, which precipitate or arise during a home visit, and potential problems, which are about the preventive aspect of health visiting, such as preparing the family for the mobility of the growing infant in the interests of safety.

In analysing home visiting practice by health visitors, While (1986) demonstrated that during the first year of infant life health visitors made more visits to families from lower social classes, living in local authority accommodation and with social security benefits (family income support). She found a weak link between increased visiting and single parenthood, unplanned pregnancies, paternal unemployment and increasing family size. No other factors appeared to precipitate increased visiting patterns. In the second year of the infant's life, While (1986) found again increased visiting where there was social disadvantage, a single parent, unemployment, lower social class, families on income support and unplanned-pregnancy infants. She found that few families received regular contact during the first 6 months of the infant's life and that during this period any visits undertaken were more likely to be on the basis of a medical model of health, such as an illness problem. In the later months of the infant's first year, While (1986) found that health visitors began to move away from a medical model of health towards a more socially adjusted model of the infant's family life and circumstances. At the end of her study she questioned whether health visiting could be effective. She concluded that such a limited contact by health visitors in the home (once or twice in the second year) would support the belief of the government of the day that child health could be achieved through education of parents.

Moving forward from the valuable work carried out in the late 1970s and early 1980s to more recent evidence of the effectiveness of home health visiting, Robinson (1998) demonstrated the difficulty of using published studies on the effectiveness of home visiting because of the quality of the research evidence. However, Robinson's study group showed home visiting effectiveness results:

- in relation to parents and children
  - improved parenting skills and quality of home environment
  - amelioration of child behaviour problems
  - improved child intellectual and motor development, especially in
    low-birthweight children and failure to thrive
  - increased immunization uptake
  - reduced use of emergency medical services
  - reduced unintentional injury and, to a lesser extent, the prevalence of home hazards
  - improved detection and management of postnatal depression
  - enhanced quality of social support to mothers
  - improved breast-feeding rates
  - initiatives limiting family size
- in relation to special needs, chronic and terminal illness
  - improved psychological functioning of families
  - increased knowledge of asthma and its treatment
- in relation to elderly people and their carers
  - reducing carers' coping stress
  - enhancing carers' quality of life
  - reducing mortality among elderly people
  - reducing hospital admissions.

Robinson (1998) drew on research studies mainly from outside the UK to reach the above conclusions because she was using random controlled trials as the methodology. There is little evidence of this research methodology in relation to either nursing or health visiting studies in the UK literature. What Robinson did find was that the UK literature tended to concentrate on process rather than outcomes. However, as Barker (1985) mentioned, process will lead to outcome. On the basis of the application of this to the UK literature Robinson (1998) suggests that:

- health visitors are remarkably successful in gaining acceptance by a wide range of individuals and their families, who appear to value their interventions highly.

- health visitors are most successful in working in a non-directive, supportive way, encouraging clients to set their individual agendas.

- the health visitor is the only professional who has been trained to integrate successful parenting, bio-psychological and socio-economic factors and the wider environment into the assessment of health need and the planning of appropriate interventions.

- health visitors reach the 'unreachable' – travellers, the homeless, poor, depressed mothers.

- the health visitor is the linchpin in a network of professional and voluntary agencies.

- historically, health visiting has shown effectiveness in the prevention of sudden infant death syndrome and is still modifying advice, on the basis of recent research findings, to further positive effect.

Although Robinson has demonstrated the effectiveness of health visiting in relation to the above topic areas, other aspects of current work appear to be less well demonstrated in the literature. These include:

- the effect of home visiting on the physical development of children
- uptake of other child health services
- incidence of childhood illness
- use of inpatient child health services
- the size of mothers' informal network
- mothers' return to education or the workforce, or use of public assistance
- reducing child abuse and neglect
- inpatient and outpatient service use for asthma
- school absenteeism
- admission of the elderly to long-term institutional care
- elder physical health or functional status
- elder psychological status
- elder well-being or quality of life.

Robinson's (1998) work clearly shows that the effectiveness of health visiting practice is not well evaluated by the scientific approach to research. The basis of medical, and some health and nursing research is on random controlled trials and the difficulty for health visiting research is that the random controlled trial is inappropriate for analysis of any large-scale interventions. This is because of the very nature of trying to combine a bio-psychological and socio-economic approach to health need

and intervention cannot be managed on a large scale and lends itself to small, focused research studies. The other important factor is the ethical dimension in attempting to evaluate effectiveness while manipulating any variable such as intervention processes.

To complete this section it is worth noting that Wright (1998) showed that to develop health visiting practice the use of action research in a small-scale study led the researchers to certain conclusions. While it was appropriate for influencing the development of health visiting practice, the problems were nevertheless very great in relation to the outcome analysis if a researcher (health visitor) moved on and the study was unable to demonstrate whether the desire for practice change remained. Action research, while recognized for its influence during practice and thus on practice, nevertheless would not be recognized for the science of its methodology or control of variables.

Home health visiting intervention was traditionally professionally led. Clients had little say in when and why the health visitor came to see them. Many health visitors in the 1960s–1980s argued cogently for opportunistic visiting, because it allowed them to see families at their potential 'worst'. It was argued that if women had time to clean up the house then the health visitor possibly could not see the circumstances in which children were being reared. There is little wonder that the term 'policing' was used and many health visitors felt uncomfortable with the situation in which they found themselves. Coupled with this was the way in which professionals took their own agenda to the client, with objectives already predetermined, often on a superficial analysis of how the family lived. It is hardly surprising that there was confusion among both health visitors and their clients over their apparent role. Clients saw health visitors in the traditional role of maternal and child health, working with clients in an authoritarian and directive manner, promoting health and preventing ill health by advising and informing in a manner that precluded client participation.

It was during the 1980s that health visiting hit a crisis of confidence over the way forward.

Health visiting practice was challenged by the Early Childhood Development Unit (Barker 1984), Goodwin (1988) and Mayall & Foster (1989) to consider what they were doing in relation to changes in society and the family unit. It was also clear that moves towards a revision of education for general nurses (Project 2000), the raising of academic standards for health visitor education to diploma and ultimately degree level and a number of government reports (Department of Health 1987, 1989c, 1989d) all combined to show health visitors that a fundamental change in the delivery of their work, particularly in homes, was necessary.

Of the changes cited above, the Child Development Programme (Barker 1984) was probably the most influential in changing the way health visitors practised in the home. The aim underpinning the programme was to offer support to families, particularly new-parent families. Although they were often in disadvantaged circumstances the programme was offered to all new parents – arguably a non-stigmatizing intervention. It focused on preparing a parenting programme relevant to the needs of child and parents, using concepts and strategies that were simple and realistic, delivered via a cartoon approach that all parents could relate to, whether highly educated or illiterate. The programme still relied on home visiting as the most effective ambience for health visitors and their clients to work together on an equal basis. It concentrated on changing the immediate caring environment of the child by working with carers to seek their own solutions to problems of child rearing, using health visitors as resources rather than instigators.

The programme was well evaluated and showed considerable improvements in child health through a reduction of the numbers of child protection issues and increased immunization uptake, to name but two measures. It was, however, expensive, relying on materials and organization of health visitors that were seen to be untenable in a cash-strapped, human-resource-limited NHS. In addition, the universality of the programme meant that it was felt by some health visitors to be unnecessary to some populations, demanding as it did the need for extended regular visiting, which some clients did not require.

The White Papers *Working for Patients* (Department of Health 1989d) and *The Patient's Charter* (Department of Health 1991) influenced some Community Trusts to advise health visitors on visiting patterns. Trusts in parts of the West Midlands required that health visitors should visit families with new births for up to a minimum of 6 weeks in the first instance. Other Trusts encouraged midwives to extend their visiting patterns to the length of their traditional remit of 28 days. The fundamental premise behind these directives was that home visiting was more effective than other ways of delivering support to mothers and new babies. It also took into account ethnic groups in the area, especially Asian mothers who are unable to leave the house for 6 weeks after delivery.

UNIVERSAL VERSUS TARGETED HOME VISITING

To promote health visiting as a public health service it must be available to the public in general. Traditionally, health visiting was available universally but to one sector of the population only, namely mothers and babies, although the argument was that by visiting mothers and babies in the home, health visitors gained access to all other family members. That this left a considerable part of the population outside the reach of health visitors was recognized but not responded to except in small pockets, where health visitors began to work with older age groups.

The debate over a universal or a targeted health visiting service continues to rage from the standpoint of cost–benefit analysis and human resource management. In Chapter 16, Powell shows how economic evaluations support home visiting. Robinson (1998), evaluating the effectiveness of domiciliary visiting, particularly focuses on the need to understand the debate and consider how, within public health, the service can seek to reduce health inequalities and improve health status.

Goodwin (1988) proposed a targeted service following a universal initial contact whereby the client is contacted in person or by telephone and the benefits of the service are outlined. Goodwin particularly proposed this in relation to new-birth visits and suggested that clients who wished to take up the service would become the home caseload of health visitors; others would meet the health visitor through the child health clinic. Many health visitors have difficulty in accepting this programme, arguing that vulnerable clients will be missed: circumstances change and if health visiting is not solidly in the background these clients will forget where to turn to for support. This argument seems to contain similar sentiments to those put forward by health visitors wishing to retain their social policing role, albeit disguised by the notion of advice and support.

Targeted health visiting was also behind the use of the dependency rating scales used during the late 1980s and early 1990s and it must also be recognized that health needs profiling is also, in effect, a targeted service. Dependency rating scales for children and their immediate families were based on an 'objective' scoring system against certain criteria. One such scoring system is given in Box 4.1.

This type of system 'scored' the child at the new-birth visit or the next visit and the 'score' changed as situations improved or deteriorated. There was no intention for this to replace normal health visiting practice: it was used as a scoring of extra dependency. Health visiting management thus had an extra tool to use when arguing for resources. This type of dependency rating mirrored the medical/public health approach to population need, which used the Jarman Index (Jarman 1983) or the Scott-Samuel score (Scott-Samuel 1984) and was in many ways an important means of obtaining resources. It was also a way for health visitors to score their caseload in terms of intervention strategies, which could be evaluated depending on score improvements.

At one stage this type of tool was used to measure the effectiveness of targeted visiting. However, it soon became clear that it was simply another subjective means of profiling using criteria whose validity in relation to parenting and child-rearing practices could be challenged. Many of the factors identified were present in

---

Box 4.1   Child dependency rating (the points scored for a positive answer are given in parentheses)

- Abnormal delivery (1)
- Preterm/low birthweight (1)
- Multiple birth (1)
- Low Apgar score – below 3 at 1 minute (1)
- Minor abnormality (1)
- Major abnormality/chronic illness (5)
- Developmental delay (5)

Family factors (minimum 0, maximum 11)

- Parental mental/physical ill health (1)
- Mother under 18 years or over 35 with first child in the household (1)
- Three or more children under 5 in the household (1)
- Chronically sick or handicapped sibling in the household (1)
- History of stillbirth, sudden infant death or other significant bereavement (1)
- Lack of basic amenities (1)
- Unsatisfactory hygiene (1)
- Social isolation (1)
- Unemployment (1)
- Other agencies involved with family (1)
- Inadequate understanding of the English language by mother (1)

Other factors (minimum 0, maximum 10)

- Known family violence (1)
- History of child neglect or abuse of siblings (1)
- This child – known or suspected neglect or abuse (5)
- Registered – yes (3)

---

families about which there was no concern, and indeed it would not be possible to use this tool without the 'universal' approach, reaching every family.

Universal visiting is still not practised by health visitors. It is practised with targeted groups, i.e. antenatal women, the under-fives (and their families) and, in some areas, older people. It is therefore incorrect for health visitors to say that they are a universal service, or indeed that they reach clients that other professionals do not. For home health visiting to be effective, it should remain a universal service to at-risk groups.

To reach other groups in the population health visitors practise in a different way, using health promotion group methods to work with the chronically sick, e.g. asthmatics, to minimize deterioration and maximize potential health gains. Other ways of working include targeting communities through users' groups, liaising with acute units and working in child protection.

INTERVENTION STRATEGIES WITH SPECIFIC CLIENT GROUPS IN THE HOME

How we communicate is of paramount importance to health visiting, and discussions later in the chapter will show how misinterpretation of the health visitor's intentions lead to criticism and rejection of professional intervention. Health visitors are not counsellors but need the counselling skills of listening, attending and reflecting to communicate effectively. Many health visitors use counselling models that they have learned from further development courses and have adapted for use in health visiting, but health visiting is not counselling or casework in the same way as social work or mental health nursing.

In Chapter 3 Carnwell shows how health visitors can use adapted models of nursing care pathways and how Twinn used an adapted health promotion model to provide a structure for health visiting processes. The author of this chapter feels strongly that health visiting should take up a communication approach that covers all aspects of their work along the bio-psycho-socio-economic continuum that does not leave gaps when health visitors are transferring from one counselling model to another.

Despite the research date, the ageless model by Heron (1986), using a philosophical humanist approach, has identified a six-category intervention analysis, which, he argues, transcends any particular theoretical stance adopted by other counselling models. Heron recognizes two basic approaches to intervening and describes these in familiar terms to health visitors as 'authoritative' and 'facilitative'. These two categories are further subdivided into three aspects to each subdivision (Fig. 4.3).

Heron suggested that the two types of intervention – authoritative and facilitative – could be used in a wide range of counselling interventions and he could almost have been thinking of the range of approaches that a health visitor may have to take on in one single client interaction.

It is quite easy to recognize scenarios in which each intervention can be used in health visiting:

- *Prescriptive interventions*. A health visitor gives weaning advice, which is culturally sensitive, to a mother (despite what is otherwise suggested, this is a counselling type of intervention. It is not just telling – mothers have a choice whether to take up the advice or not, so the health visitor takes a directive role and gives advice that is culturally sensitive and based on research evidence).

- *Informative interventions*. A health visitor shares information on the advantages and disadvantages of HRT with a perimenopausal woman (the position of the health visitor here is not a guided/directive role but one of sharing knowledge to increase the choices open to women).

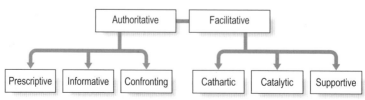

Figure 4.3   Heron's six-category intervention analysis (redrawn with kind permission from Heron 1986)

- *Confronting interventions.* A health visitor says to a mother that she finds it difficult to believe the mother's explanation of her child's bruised face (this is both a challenge and a confrontation – it is stated quietly but with conviction and indicates that the challenge will be repeated if necessary). Heron differentiates between pussyfooting, where the health visitor is vague and unclear and skirts around the point; sledgehammering, where the health visitor becomes aggressive and the intervention becomes an attack on the mother; and confronting, where the health visitor stays calm and keeps to the point.

- *Cathartic interventions.* A woman begins to cry while talking, and the health visitor communicates her empathy (other forms of pent-up emotion such as anger, fear, grief and embarrassment may be dealt with in this way).

- *Catalytic interventions.* A health visitor, approached by 45-year-old Margaret, concerned about her teenage son and daughter's behaviour towards her 70-year-old mother, who lives with them, allows the woman to talk at length about the home situation. The end result is that Margaret, by focusing on her own situation, comes to a decision on what to do next; this is client-centred work (see p. 90).

- *Supportive interventions.* A mother with two bedwetting children brings up an idea as to what else she might do to help her children. The health visitor empathetically encourages her solutions ('supportive' is a word frequently used in health visiting but there is a difference between facile approval and empathic understanding).

EGAN'S (1986) THREE–STAGE COUNSELLING MODEL

This is a structured approach to counselling that involves three stages in the helping process and can, therefore, be modified for health visiting intervention in problem solving. The three stages are:

- *Stage 1: Problem clarification.* This is a collaborative working relationship in which the

health visitor 'attends and responds' (Egan 1982, p. 51). The health visitor listens actively to what the client is saying, helps the client to focus on the pivotal aspects of all the problem areas and during the whole process, communicates empathetic unconditional positive regard.

- *Stage 2: Goal setting.* Within this developing helping relationship, the health visitor enables the client to develop new perspectives on the problems identified and the players in the situation, and helps them to establish new goals.

- *Stage 3: Action.* The means of achieving these goals is the focus of this stage, and the health visitor may challenge the client on steps they propose as the way forward. At the end of this process the client, through this intervention method, gains confidence in their own ability to take control in response to problem situations.

STRATEGIES FOR PROBLEM–FOCUSED AND EMOTION–FOCUSED COPING

Sarafino (1994) uses the work of various psychologists to explore two approaches to coping with stress: strategies to deal with the problem and strategies to deal with the emotions that result from it.

Strategies to deal with the problem include *direct action*, when the client is helped to carry out an activity that may distract them from the problem, e.g. going away, negotiating, consulting. By *seeking information* the client acquires knowledge about how to proceed, e.g. seeking legal advice or approaching alternative accommodation providers. *Turning to others* involves seeking social support from friends and family, applying for a loan or some other means by which other people can help towards solving the stress-creating problem.

In emotion-focused coping the health visitor may help the client in several ways, e.g. helping them to come to terms with the problem – *resigned acceptance*: 'it will not go away, so how can it be accepted in my life?' Another focus is *emotional discharge*; here the client is helped to express their feelings or reduce the tension in such ways as by screaming when angry, crying or using jokes. A third way of emotion-focused coping is to use strategies to re-examine or change the client's view of the stressful situation. A health visitor might encourage the client to talk or write about their problems and negative feelings, which may reduce their stress and benefit their health. Pennebaker (1990) suggests that to write things down enables the person to organize, consider and assimilate his or her thoughts and feelings more carefully than talking. A comparison of therapeutic approaches is discussed by Cody (1999) and this is complemented by using health psychology to reach the same conclusions, i.e. being with and questioning a person, helping a client to develop personal insight and knowledge.

ROGERS'S (1951) CLIENT–CENTRED APPROACH

This is a model of counselling that is used selectively by health visitors. As with most health visitor interventions, this model involves the client seeking a solution to their own problems. However, when used by health visitors in its original format, one of the main requirements is that there is sufficient time for the client to work through their own situation. It is therefore more likely that health visitors will use it with individuals who have issues in their personal life. Rogers's model concentrates on the process of the relationship between client and counsellor, involving warmth, genuineness and positive regard for the client, leading to a gradual understanding of the client's problems, unfolded at the client's own pace. It is particularly valid in a helping relationship such as support visits in response to an identified need, over a planned length of time.

WORKING WITH INDIVIDUALS AND FAMILIES IN THE HOME

The following health visiting skills and intervention strategies are used when working at the individual/family end of the horizontal axis of the model (Fig. 4.2) These skills and intervention strategies will range along the vertical axis of proactive–reactive approaches.

PARTNERSHIP IN HEALTH VISITING (A PROACTIVE ACTIVITY, Fig. 4.2)

Health visitor education has embraced the introduction of advocacy, enablement and empowerment into client interaction and these lend themselves well to reflection on intervention outcomes. The traditional paternalistic approach to health visiting precluded any use of partnership because health visitors were ill equipped to working with confident, questioning clients, choosing to leave them to manage alone because they clearly needed no direction. Partnership requires professional and client to be on the same level; when health visitors chose to undertake home visits unannounced this puts the client/family at a disadvantage – an imbalance in the power relationship between the professional and the client.

The effective way of initiating partnerships is for health visitors to make appointments to visit clients in the home. This really emerged as the result of *Working for Patients* (Department of Health 1989d), the *Patient's Charter* (Department of Health 1991) and, to a lesser extent, the *Children Act 1989* (HMSO 1989). It has since been reinforced in *Liberating the Talents* (Department of Health 2002b) and the *NHS Improvement Plan* (Department of Health 2004b). Visiting by appointment not only puts the health visitor into a position of seeking client invitation, but also allows the client time to prepare by thinking about what is wanted from the health visitor, whether objectives set from previous visits are effective and appropriate, and how these should be developed. Health visitors have their own agenda of objectives based on child health and child development needs, and these are introduced if and when appropriate. The true partnership approach, however, involves the client setting the agenda on the basis of an understanding of the health visitor's role. This is established at an introductory visit, described by Chalmers (1992) as giving and receiving of information, when the health visitor explains her/himself as a resource for the client and the client gives whatever background personal information they wish. Empirical evidence shows that health visiting is ineffective if the role is not clearly understood either by clients or by other professionals, for example, GPs.

Thus a partnership begins on the sound footing of clearly established professional and client information exchanges. The transaction is entirely non-judgemental and allows communication to flow uninhibited between health visitor and client. Once unconditional regard is established then true partnership can function, with the client bringing their own unique personal situation and the health visitor bringing knowledge based on education and experience. The knowledge is offered in response to client need, when prompted by the agenda, with the client in the position of making an informed choice as a result of the discussion raised. Health visitors may select knowledge from experience but their professionalism is in being able to recognize the client's perspective and offer information or knowledge appropriate to client perspective. Clients may reject the practical knowledge/know-how that the health visitor is suggesting but it should be offered with information about the research underpinning its effectiveness and presented in a meaningful way. If there are conflicts between modern and traditional practices, the partnership aspect is to acknowledge traditional practices and their value, but then to show the differences that new research and methods can make to healthcare issues.

Partnership also embraces the concept of mutual esteem, which is determined by unconditional regard. To ascertain whether the information/knowledge offered is acceptable from the client's perspective, the health visitor will check this out by questioning. This puts the health visitor in the position of possible rejection by the client and this can be uncomfortable unless they have developed the type of relationship in which mutual respect plays a prominent role. Similarly, clients may have to be challenged by health visitors about an apparently dangerous practice in relation to the

health or safety of a family member. Challenge is not necessarily aggressive or even assertive but requires an ability to speak plainly without offence in order to modify behaviour – on the basis of research evidence.

Partnership is also based on client and health visitor using the same record tool, as shown in Chapter 15. This system resulted from national concerns about the freedom of information in relation to databases held by the NHS. Charles (Ch. 15) discusses the value of client-held records from several perspectives, but one of its prime uses is to serve as an agenda for each home visit while remaining the property of the Trust; this difference between client access and Trust ownership makes the partnership approach questionable. It is acknowledged that the red book is only a record of the child. Any records on other family members are kept on supplementary records, of which the client should have a copy; their content should be based on a family health plan mutually agreed by client and professional.

A family health plan is defined as a core tool for enabling a family to think about their health and parenting needs. The *Health Visitor Practice Development Resource Pack* (Department of Health 2001e) suggests that the plan should identify:

- the family's needs as they see them
- how they wish to address these needs
- an action plan for the family, including support to be provided by the health visitor and others
- what has been achieved.

A challenge to the concept of partnership can arise in relation to parents and their children's development. Health visitors are educated in normal and abnormal child development, and first-time parents in particular may have little knowledge or experience about child growth or care. Many parents themselves come from small nuclear families and have not gained the experience of sibling rearing that was the rule in large, early-20th-century families. The *Child Development Programme* (Barker 1984) offered parents the opportunity to focus on the continued developmental achievements of their children and other health factors such as diet, and to develop their own ideas for care and stimulation. This gave health visitors a flexible approach, based on parental knowledge and observation, where an idea for anticipatory safety guidance, for example, is fostered through an analysis of developmental progress. The health visitor may say, 'Belinda is beginning to move so fast now that she will probably be crawling before long. How do you think that will affect the way you look after her?' This allows the parent to suggest stair gates or fireguards without the need for 'telling' by the health visitor. In everyday life our own ideas are more productive than other people's.

First-time mothers may be overwhelmed by advice from well-meaning family members that they find difficult to challenge. Discussion with a health visitor bringing research-based information allows the client to balance this new knowledge against traditional advice and make a truly informed decision about her child health care. To retain good relationships with influential family members is important in reducing the stress experienced by mothers in this vulnerable position. The Marcé Society (1994) has shown in published articles that this need to retain a harmonious balance between the knowledge she would like to take up and the knowledge forced on her can frequently lead a mother into a downward spiral of depression over child health care management. Gogna and Hari (2000) identify the same dilemma in first-time Asian mothers, where care may be delivered by the mother-in-law and the new mother has knowledge that she would like to use if traditional practices did not prevent her.

CARE THROUGH PRACTICAL ADVICE (A REACTIVE ACTIVITY, Fig. 4.2)

One of the charges formerly levelled at health visitors is that they never ceased to give advice and that on many occasions it was unsolicited. The development of the public health role of the original sanitary nurses from which health visiting grew was to advise and teach in homes on health and hygiene relating to babies and young children. The point of this is to emphasize

the word 'advise' and to examine it in the context of modern health visiting within the arena of a far better educated public. Originally, the advice given by health visitors was paternalistic, assuming complete ignorance of the basic tenets of child health and hygiene, and in the majority of situations the health visitor was working only with working-class people. Today's health visitor is working in a knowledgeable society, which central government considers to be classless and whose hopes and aspirations are based on material acquisitions. Both these statements could be criticized for their generality but are included to show the changes apparent in the society in which the health visitor of today is working. Clearly, the skills of the earlier health visitors were based on a didactic approach, albeit with kindly intentions. Those skills would be challenged today and found to be unacceptable by their recipients.

> A young family has a 4–year-old daughter with a carcinoma of the kidney with bone secondaries. She was treated by surgery and chemotherapy but sadly a recurrence of the bone metastases took place several months later. The family 'used the Internet' and discovered a drug used in America for this particular recurrence. They informed the paediatric consultant and requested this treatment.

The vignette is included to illustrate the depth and breadth of information available to clients, which clearly means that health visiting has to approach from a totally different stance than in the early part of the 20th century.

The practical advice that may be sought from health visitors falls into three main areas:

- social and environmental problems
- problems of child rearing
- family health problems.

SOCIAL AND ENVIRONMENTAL PROBLEMS

Care must be taken when discussing such problems not to assume that the health visitor is working in a socially deprived area. Social problems in families living in more affluent circumstances can be as severe and different from those of families living in material poverty.

The practical advice offered depends, of course, on how important the problem is to the client. Clients living in damp and run-down property need urgent advice on how best to solve this problem, and this is one of the most frustrating areas of the health visitor's work. It is easy to empathize with families in these situations and it is also not difficult to recognize the problems of housing departments with dwindling stock and rising lists of needy clients – coupled with a greater tendency on the part of clients to seek litigation against local authority housing departments.

Health visitors may attempt to help clients by writing to housing departments on their behalf or encouraging them to enlist the help of local councillors in their fights for rehousing (influencing policy). Many families are in despair over their situation and one of the skills of the health visitor is to encourage clients to take positive action to enhance their demands by, for example:

- documenting the instances of nuisance
- taking photographs of damp or other unhealthy situations
- drawing other tenants together in an effort to collectively influence the housing department
- documenting health problems experienced by children which may lead to school non-attendance.

The type of advice discussed in the list above is designed to develop people's confidence and motivation to do something themselves to alter and improve their situations, and requires the health visitor to have a wide knowledge of the whole system of housing in both the public and private sector. Often, this gives the health visitor a better chance of developing good links with clients and the 'giving and receiving' concept proposed by Chalmers (1992) is a clear result of advice over the initial problem. In this concept, Chalmers argues that each party 'gives' and 'receives' in order to manage health

visitor–client encounters. The health visitor gives the focus of 'routine' (thus not making it intrusive) and 'client centred' in the entry phase. This is followed by information, teaching and support in a health promotion phase and finally a negotiated or non-negotiated termination phase. The client 'gives back' information and interest and 'gives' positive reception that the help has been well received. It is important that the entry work is successfully established before attempting to move onto subsequent phases.

It is difficult for a health visitor to empower families or individuals in isolation. This is where the health visitor should work in collaboration with health, education and environmental health to combat social exclusion. Collaborative working (see Ch. 5, p. 110) with school nurses, social services, the local GP and environmental health departments can provide a powerful force to enable empowerment for influence and change. It is also useful if the health visitor has good links with the housing department in order to gain support and sympathy for some situations. Being a single parent with two small children in a second-floor flat with elderly people both above and below calls for real understanding of the difficulties in keeping peace and harmony.

Isolation is a problem in urban areas with large detached houses. Some professional women with small babies have high expectations of their own mothering abilities and cannot run nextdoor to seek help without appearing to concede personal failure. The health visitor making a planned visit may be consulted on a presenting problem, e.g. infant colic, which may have little to do with the real problem of isolation. The perceptive health visitor can see the real problem but has to allow the client to take agenda leadership over the secondary problem, working to find an appropriate management strategy for the colic until the real problem becomes apparent to the client. Again, Chalmers' work on giving and receiving becomes the underlying theoretical perspective within care and advice in health visiting. Provided the health visitor and client have satisfactorily achieved a solution to the colic then it may be possible to open up the debate on isolation. However, if the colic is not satisfactorily resolved, will the client allow the health visitor to challenge the situation by suggesting that isolation may be the principal problem?

The skill of perception in health visiting is essential to satisfactorily identify the root cause of problems. Clients are very close to their own difficulties and ascribe reasons for problems from a narrow selection of choices. Health visitors coming with wider perspectives can work with the client in partnership by offering alternative coping strategies.

PROBLEMS OF CHILD REARING

The care and advice given in this area is endless and is the recognized focus of health visiting work. Advice can be as detailed as guidance relating to feeding or dealing with infant constipation, or fundamentally broad ranging in relation to child development and behavioural management. Child protection also draws on every aspect of the health visitor's knowledge in relation to the law, research on at-risk situations, material evidence of abuse or neglect, and family dyadic relationships.

The skills of care and advice in health visiting duplicate those of nursing in response to practical guidance, e.g. on infant feeding practices or home safety. Health visiting skills used must be in partnership with clients because authoritarian approaches compromise future working relationships. The approach 'Have you tried …?' is often more acceptable than 'You must …'.

Where there are issues of possible risk to, or neglect of children, approaches determined by Trust guidelines must be employed. Here health visitors must be vigilant about potential risk factors, honest with clients if there is a doubt over an explanation given about, for example, an injury, and confident enough to record openly in the client-held records the concerns identified. Advice given must be immediate and the situation must be observed regularly and frequently. Clearly, formal policies must be adhered to by health visitors but the fundamental work in the initial stages has translated 'advice' into 'instruction'.

The trap that health visitors can fall into is that they are so concerned about maintaining working relationships with carers that they may minimize the potential risk to the child.

FAMILY HEALTH PROBLEMS

Health visitors are often drawn into family discussions on the best way of solving health problems. This is often a fruitful partnership approach in which the client can discuss their own health solutions and the options open to them until they reach an appropriate and satisfactory outcome. In this scenario the family tests its own knowledge against that of the health visitor to see whether compromises or alternative strategies are needed. Other situations that can develop are when a client is unaware that there is a problem, e.g. in an area of child development where the client sees no problem but the health visitor recognizes abnormality or delay. An example here might be a speech delay identified by the health visitor that has been accepted as normal by the parent.

However, it is also important to recognize that the health visitor needs to sensitively challenge the parents' view that there is no problem with the child's speech, and referral for a hearing test and to a speech therapist for a second opinion could be encouraged. It is also important that the means whereby a health visitor may judge delay is also culturally sensitive, for example, the use of building bricks as a test when a child has never seen bricks before and refuses to build a tower. If it is possible, group developmental checks can be useful to allow children to copy and mimic to demonstrate their own abilities.

Advice on family health must be tailored to family circumstances and this may mean the health visitor compromising and negotiating acceptable advice. The beginning of the process is about determining the problem in relation to the family knowledge level and then building upon this knowledge level. This may mean that the same problem from one family to another elicits an entirely different response from the health visitor – depending on family circumstances.

EMPOWERMENT IN HEALTH VISITING (A PROACTIVE ACTIVITY, Fig. 4.2)

Empowerment is a term overused in health visiting practice and yet it has an important place in the health visitor–client relationship. In health visiting practice, empowerment means giving clients the means of exerting their own authority over the circumstances in which they find themselves. Authority is based on confidence and knowledge: knowledge is gained in partnership, as discussed above; confidence giving is another skill of health visiting. It begins by using processes to improve clients' self-esteem. In Chapter 3, Carnwell discusses the use of Twinn's (1991) model of supporting roles and paradigms in health visiting and this is an important link in recognizing self-esteem as a fundamental need.

A criticism of empowerment in health visiting is that there has been insufficient exploration of the psychological perspectives underpinning the process. Tones (1991) takes a psychological perspective whereas other writers (Blaxter 1990, Blackburn 1991, Gibson 1991, Twinn et al 1996) all consider the socio-political perspective to be the root cause of lowered self-esteem and advocate empowerment and education as a solution. Education has an important part to play in reversing a loss of self-esteem but it is by no means the only answer. Taking a psychological perspective requires investigation and an understanding of theoretical concepts. Several may be helpful and relevant but the most useful are locus of control and self-efficacy.

LOCUS OF CONTROL WITH RELATION TO HEALTH

Rotter (1977) particularly focused on enabling people to understand whether they had an internal or an external locus of control. He described people who believe they have control over their own successes or failures as having an internal locus of control, whereas people who believe that their lives are controlled by forces outside themselves – e.g. fate – have an

external locus of control. For example, in the health field, patients who prefer doctors and specialists to make decisions about their treatment and don't want to know the details – 'just tell me what to do' – could be seen as having an external locus of control. Patients who want to know exactly what their condition is and what treatments are available before they make decisions as to which they want have an internal locus of control. Some commentators (Blackburn 1991) have argued that personal circumstances such as lack of education and social deprivation override this notion of locus of control. However, health visitors have noted that although clients appear to have the same set of reduced sociological circumstances, some appear to be more able to cope and rise above their difficulties, and it is argued here that this is due to their having an internal locus of control. Health visitors who are aware of this theoretical perspective can fairly easily identify whether their clients have an internal or an external locus of control. This gives the health visitor more insight into the way the client can be empowered. If the client has an internal locus of control, the more education and information they have the more they are enabled (empowered) to use their internal locus. Clients with an external locus can also use education and information but to a far lesser extent and need support primarily through advice and encouragement.

A family has an autistic child of about 5. The mother had a minimum education and left school at 16. None of the specialists to whom the child was referred was able to give a diagnosis of his behaviour. It was only when the mother saw a television programme on autism that she realized that that was her child's problem and subsequently persuaded the professionals of the diagnosis. She has constantly asked for her child to be statemented but the Education Authority in the borough in which she lives refuses to comply. The mother has asked questions and explored the situation, discovering that the Education Authority in the next borough is willing to statement her child, who as far as they are concerned lives at an address in their borough. To all intents and purposes the family now live in the next borough. The father of the family became very depressed by the whole situation and was unable to see any way forward. He was so stressed by the circumstances and the battle they were having that he ultimately lost his job and the family now live on income support.

This vignette is useful in exemplifying the difference in the parents – the mother has an internal locus of control; the father has an external locus of control. The mother responded to education via a television programme and sought as much information as she could from her health visitor; the father has required antidepressants to be able to cope with the stress the situation has created within him. Interestingly, the mother later confided to the health visitor that when her husband began to feel better he stopped taking his medication. His wife knew that he should continue until he became more stable, so she crushed the daily dose up and, unbeknown to him, mixed it into his breakfast cereal! A good discussion point.

The locus of control theory highlights a dilemma in health visiting – the control element. If a health visitor recognizes that their client has an external locus of control then they may offer their services from a benevolent motive that may be interpreted by others as a means of taking control. Mayall & Foster (1989) use the following interpretation (p. 146):

It is particularly where the work is interventionist that [this] conflict comes to the fore. For instance, when a health visitor visits with the benevolent intention of supporting and educating a mother, her visit on private territory can be perceived both by herself and the mother as a move towards assuming some power over activities in the home. This will be especially so if she takes the initiative in proposing and developing topics of conversation. Doctors in the preventive child health services avoid the problems because they offer a responsive rather than an interventionist service.

The interpretation above is part of a discussion on the possible powerlessness that professionals can feel when practising interventionist work, particularly in home health visiting. The dimension of a theoretical perspective of health locus of control can be an explanation of why health visitors feel powerless. They recognize an external locus of control in the client and thus wish to satisfy client need; indeed the client may push the health visitor into an advising or apparently control-taking position. In a sense, the client who has an external locus of control, if unable to take control of their lives, can drift into the condition that Seligman (1975) called learned helplessness – which he described as a principal characteristic of depression.

It can be easier for health visitors to work with a client with an internal locus of control. They appear to respond better to information and rarely ask for advice. The fact that in a fairly brief encounter health visitors may have insufficient time to gauge locus of control in the client may be the reason for clients criticizing their approach – information giving or advising – as inappropriate for that particular client.

The apparent anomaly in responses to personal control can be explained by an alternative theory: that of self-efficacy.

SELF–EFFICACY

Bandura (1977b) suggested that self-efficacy is the belief that we can succeed at something we want to do. People gauge their chances of success and failure by their observation or knowledge of the success or otherwise of others in the same circumstances. Bandura showed that people would attempt to do something if they thought that they could succeed or that the circumstances were favourable enough for them to do so. Bandura et al (1985) showed that people with a strong sense of self-efficacy experienced less psychological and physiological strain in response to stressors than those with a weak sense of efficacy.

This could explain why clients who make even small improvements in their personal circumstances despite negative situations cope more effectively. Bandura (1977a) suggested that self-efficacy came about through social learning theory, i.e. we learn from observing the behaviour of others. In early development the significant others are members of the family, who serve as models of behaviour and standards for comparison. Parents who are caring, encouraging and consistent in their standards of behaviour tend to have children with an internal locus of control and a strong sense of efficacy (Harter 1983). Health visitors, particularly in the home setting where there is more time to focus on client ability, will recognize that those parents who have reached adulthood with poor intellectual and social skills and many self-doubts tend to find life events and parenthood stressful.

Health visitors recognize that knowledge is not the only need that many clients have: their circumstances play an important part not only in how they see themselves but also in their self-efficacy.

> Jane is aged 16 and pregnant and is working with Annette, her health visitor. Jane is tearful at the antenatal visit. Her mother is present and is very disappointed in her daughter, whom she sees as shameful and deceitful. She is angry with the baby's father, whom she knows, and embarrassed by the shame brought upon her and her husband, Jane's father. She had such high hopes and expectations of her daughter's life, which she now sees as shattered. Jane says nothing at all. Annette listens to Jane's mother and after a while things quieten down. At this point, Annette asks Jane how she feels about the situation and acts as a mediator to give her an equal right of reply. Giving Jane permission to hold centre-stage in the same way as her mother helps her to begin the long haul back to self-esteem.

This vignette above is a mere skeleton of the knowledge that Annette has about why educationally underachieving 16-year-olds become pregnant, repeat the same patterns that Annette knows their mothers went through, living in council-owned property in a deprived area of the city and never achieving their hopes and ambitions. Health visiting work here is long term, based on a comprehensive knowledge

of the socio-economic influences on bio-psychological development of the individual. To enable Jane, her mother and ultimately the baby to achieve their potential calls for a subtle use of empowerment through support and education. Again, in this situation, collaborative working with education and housing as well as the school nurse will help to develop a support network which will help to empower both Jane and her mother. For Jane it will help to boost her independence as a new mother-to-be; for Jane's mother it will help her to recognize the positive influence she can have on her daughter, despite the undesired situation. It is also important that health visitors in this situation do not make assumptions: this is a set of circumstances that many will recognize but while it may seem classic it is still unique.

Empowerment is also about helping people to reflect on ways to change their circumstances, by enabling them to recognize their own potential and achieve their aims. This is carried out at the client's own pace: for example, the health visitor may be in a position to give the client information on how to communicate with community leaders or agencies. Client confidence is boosted by positive support that is non-patronizing and based on enabling clients to recognize their own achievements, encouraging them to unravel the process and reflect on their own abilities within it. Clients often fail to see that where an outcome is only partially achieved, they have nevertheless gained immense confidence and can use this to greater effect later in similar circumstances. Reflection is not just a professional practice tool but can be used in partnership with the client to achieve positive outcomes. Guided reflection in this case does not require tools but does require equal partnership with the client to explore situations, circumstances and feelings of self-worth. It is important that reflection is a continuum of action and that the client is helped to explore the process according to their own beliefs and values. It is equally important for the client to recognize that the guided reflection approach is both non-patronizing and also non-judgemental.

Empowerment is shown by Naidoo & Wills (2000) as an approach to health promotion, helping people to identify their own concerns and health issues and giving them the skills and confidence to deal with them. Naidoo & Wills (1994) suggest that there are two main mechanisms: self-empowerment based on non-directive client-centred counselling; and community empowerment through enabling them to challenge and change aspects of their environment.

Locus of control and self efficacy are aspects of health behaviour that are present in both client and health visitor and are used particularly in empowerment – the skill of the health visitor is to enable the client to understand and use these skills. However, the next section on assessment lies particularly with the health visitor.

ASSESSMENT OF HEALTH NEEDS AND BEHAVIOURS (A PROACTIVE ACTIVITY, Fig. 4.2)

The wider debate over health needs assessment has been covered in Chapter 2. In this chapter we are more concerned with basic health visiting skills in relation to families and individuals, and health visitors need to be skilled in health needs analysis in relation to both the current and long-term situation.

A number of tools are available to health visitors to structure their assessment of health needs. Traditionally, health visitors have annually analysed their caseloads and the information that this revealed was enormously important, giving a clear view of how their work was progressing. Unfortunately, the evidence produced from these caseload analyses was, as mentioned previously, never acted upon. The ways in which they viewed their work were restricted by the overwhelming need to ensure that the 'box of records', for which they felt acutely responsible, was worked. Interestingly, if challenged on the number of families they were really working with, most health visitors would identify some 30–50, and the remainder were visited regularly because it was 'routine', whether the client wished it or not.

Despite the criticisms above, the annual caseload evaluation does provide health visitors with two essential pieces of information and we would argue it is important to continue this practice. Firstly, the results can reveal a true evaluation of the health visiting practised on that caseload, e.g. details of infant feeding patterns, child behaviour problems, maternal depression, family disorganization problems, and many other factors. All of these should be used as a basis to examine how health visiting input has influenced any recorded changes. Perhaps an emphasis on antenatal classes in relation to infant feeding can be measured against an emphasis in the following year on individual discussions with pregnant women in their own homes. This would allow a clear analysis of which has been more effective – group work or individual work. Balanced against this must be cost-effectiveness, in terms of time and effort, in achieving improvements in infant health. Previously, health visitors have ignored this opportunity to undertake 'real' evaluation, for the reasons outlined above. It is also very important that this annual caseload analysis is not viewed in isolation but must be in comparison with the local public health report and other local data. These should then be considered within the context of government targets such as National Service Frameworks (NSFs). The health visitor should look for gaps or differences between their own caseload analysis and the other data and the meaning of these. For instance, if there is a low level of violence identified in the caseload analysis, does this mean a problem with the health visitor caseload? Does it mean that there have not been needs expressed or identified?

Secondly, caseload evaluation should be used in conjunction with a regular community health needs assessment (Department of Health 2001e) to determine the focus of health visiting practice. This may lead to a shift from the prime focus on mothers and under-fives to another age group in need – for example, a rise in breast cancer rates in the area for women aged 44–60. It could be argued that working with the under-fives allows the health visitor to undertake an assessment of the health needs of all the family. However, a criticism of this argument is that often the assessment of health needs of all the family is not undertaken in relation to the wider perspective of the epidemiological and social factors of the area. Good caseload evaluation should be undertaken annually to acknowledge the use of these two important factors.

As a result of the evaluation of health visiting interventions outlined above it is possible to recognize that outcomes of health visiting practice are essential to satisfy the health needs of the individual, the community and the purchasers. Health visitors must also recognize that successful health visiting interventions may be perceived by both client and purchaser to be the result of their own work, not that of the health visitor. It is therefore important that health visitors clearly identify what they have done and measure this against clearly defined outcomes related to accurate evaluations of health needs. It should be borne in mind that identified health needs are peculiar to each individual client or family and that these will be part of the family health plan. It is they who identify their own needs in conjunction with the health visitor, and it is important for health visitors to document where they have raised awareness of health needs towards which they and the family are working, as well as working with the client's own agenda. Good examples of this are seen in relation to smoking and similar health behaviours.

Many Primary Care Trusts have developed tools for use by health visitors on initial-contact health-needs assessment. These are based on a scoring system for risk factors in a similar way to the public health scoring systems such as the Jarman index (Jarman 1983), although on a more personal basis. Some health visitors find these useful for giving a baseline of family need and they are known to have been used by purchasers to establish resource allocation. Many other health visitors challenge the whole basis of risk scores on the premise that these can change so rapidly that they become meaningless as a tool to influence intervention and are out of date the minute they have been completed (Lightfoot 1994, Hudson 1997). There is also the criticism that families are being labelled by their score and indeed, who is making the assessment: the health visitor or the family? These tools do,

however, have a value in providing a checklist so that in moments of concern about overriding problems a brief response can be inserted for use at a more convenient time. Risk scores can also be useful for identifying patterns or trends at a population level.

The skills of dialogue between client and health visitor to establish health needs are essential and in many ways will override any tool designed for the purpose.

> During an antenatal visit, a health visitor discusses, with the client, general family support systems and the influence of significant family members in her life. All the time the health visitor is alert to other health needs. The physical needs are very evident and have been dealt with by the midwife. However, discussion on the wider family brings to the fore a realization that the client hasn't thought through sibling rivalry and has not yet prepared the toddler for her loss of unique child position. There will be a host of other factors but this one identified item is used to illustrate preparation for the psychological health needs of the toddler.

MANAGEMENT OF CARE PATHWAYS AS IDENTIFIED BY THE CLIENT (BOTH PROACTIVE AND REACTIVE ACTIVITIES)

There are no clearly defined management programmes for this area of health visiting skills. Few nursing models are appropriate in these situations and it is far more likely that health visitors will borrow health psychology models based on Bandura's self-efficacy model (1977b) or Becker's health belief model (1974). In most situations these necessarily require adaptation to the client's needs but the value of flexible models is shown in Chapter 3. Here, the skills of health visiting are twofold: first, being able to identify and use the most appropriate model; and second, enabling the client to solve the problem using the health visitor in client-listening sessions. In this second aspect the health visitor is probably using a variant of

Rogers' (1967) person-centred approach, discussed at the beginning of this chapter.

Many client problems are long term and health visiting skills are mobilized towards helping the client to set short-term goals that are achievable. Positive reinforcement of what clients have already achieved is essential in raising self-esteem and this is done without any aspect of paternalism on the part of the health visitor. It means that the health visitor takes time to listen to the client story, to help them unpack the complexities of the situation, and for the client to recognize their own strengths in the process.

The health visitor can help the client to record what they are doing, to keep a diary of the problem, e.g. where there are toddler sleeping problems and it is necessary to see how regular the problem really is. Other ways in which clients may be encouraged to keep a record may include a food diary (see Ch. 9), a diary of moods and feelings in relation to postnatal depression, management of infant crying or temper tantrums and so forth. The management skills of the health visitor are to enable discussion and analysis of diary contents, determine the severity or otherwise of the problem, pick out themes and patterns and negotiate a planned programme of change suitable for the client's agenda.

Present-day life circumstances (stress, pace, pressure, change) require health visitors to enable individuals to find a way around the difficulties they face, and this means a focus on changing the situations in which people live rather than concentrating solely on individual behaviour and knowledge. Helping clients to change their focus calls for health visitors' ability to promote discussion, challenge their belief system where appropriate and offer alternative frames of reference. For example, modern family behaviour has, in many cases, lost the rhythm of regular mealtimes. Young children do not respond to erratic patterns in their lives and thus do not settle into established eating behaviours. Helping mothers to recognize the benefit of their own childhood patterns and rhythms in establishing beneficial eating behaviours may mean establishing better rhythms within the family, encouraging family conversation and relaxing harmony. The circadian rhythms identified in relation to sleep (Kerr et al 1997) apply equally well to eating behaviours in young children. If carers have not experienced regular patterns and rhythms in their own young lives then health visiting skills of suggestion and education would be of value here.

PLANNED ACTIVITY MANAGEMENT (BOTH PROACTIVE AND REACTIVE ACTIVITIES)

This skill of health visiting differs from the clinical nursing skill of preparation and planning for care on discharge in that it is client driven in health visiting rather than being carried out in consultation with the patient and other care organizations, as in nursing.

Activity management can cover topics such as working with families with disabled children, working with children with behaviour problems, working with families with chronic illness in one of the parents, and working with families with dependent elderly relatives.

> Mr and Mrs B are both teachers with seven children ranging from 17 down to 6 years, and at her last and eighth pregnancy Mrs B gave birth to a baby with Down's syndrome. There was good support from the outset, with neonatal nurses, midwives, paediatrician and GP all combining to help in the care. The health visitor was also involved from the beginning but recognized that in this case the greatest need was support of the family rather than the new infant, who was supported by other professionals.

This brief vignette shows the need for perception in the health visitor to recognize where within the family is the greatest need for support. The initial focus of activity meant that all concerned were included in planning and work with the new baby. Often, having made the initial introduction to the family (and, of course, knowing them from past contact), the health visitor steps back and appears to have a limited input into what is going on. However, the health visitor and the mother have agreed a home visiting programme, which is revised regularly. It is critically important to recognize that the health visitor skills here are to maintain contact with the other professionals in order to keep abreast of the situation, and possibly to remain in the background until the situation is normalized. The health visitor realizes that the family supports each other but visits or makes periodic contact to monitor family dynamics and minimize any breakdown. What is vital about this type of scenario is that the health visitor is more effective when observing from the outside than when working from within. There are other professionals dealing with the day-to-day matters, but knowledge of family dynamics means that the health visitor is working to identify any changes that may lead to long-term difficulties. A common situation is that when the health visitor is discussing the needs of the family the mother remembers that, when she picked the second-youngest child up from school earlier in the week, the teacher had mentioned that he was becoming more disruptive in class. Because the mother's attention is focused on the needs of the baby she has not recognized the needs of this other child. The opportunity to look at the whole family that has arisen from the health visitor's visit means that together the health visitor and the mother can discuss the situation and plan how she can perhaps focus more attention on that child, whose behaviour is possibly demonstrating lack of his mother's attention.

Dependent older relatives can influence family dynamics by disrupting normal family home life, if brought into the family home, or by creating pressures and drawing a parent from the family home in order to attend to their needs. The skills of the health visitor centre on dialogue with both the older relative and the family to ascertain the needs of each, linking in with other agencies to provide alternative support. The health visitor plans with the family and the relative a programme of activity that meets the needs of each, reduces the older relative's feeling of dependency and helps the family to function with less guilt and pressure. A very useful model that can be used in this situation is that of Procaska & Diclemente's (1984) stages of change model, which is discussed by Carnwell in Chapter 3.

OTHER HOME VISITS

Health visitors and older people in the family unit

The bulk of health visitor intervention is undertaken with older people who are living on their own. Perceptions and attitudes in health visitors who work with older people are a major factor in determining how best to intervene in potentially deteriorating situations. Health visitors working in these areas of practice should have developed the skills of reflection and should practise these regularly, as well as having a knowledge of systems and policies. It is also important to understand how we develop attitudes towards older people and what creates bias within cultures. The types of intervention using the Heron (1986) analysis (see earlier in this chapter) are likely to be skewed towards the authoritative categories, in particular prescriptive interventions, e.g. in encouraging improved nutrition or minimizing danger in the home.

Health visitors working with older people and their carers may offer practical support in material terms, obtaining finance or equipment such as a continence service or a laundry facility, respite care in an alternative situation for both the older person and their carer, or a sitting service. Therapeutic interventions require an education approach and the opportunity to see an endpoint, otherwise they may well be considered of little value. They may include strategies such as helping the carer to understand the difference between protection and personal liberty and how to introduce these. Other education approaches include advice and information on a wide range of issues, which may include medical information about health/illness, housing or financial benefit advice, or ways in which the carer can continue in employment. Another major benefit can be gained from multi-agency support but this is fraught with difficulties where there is no key worker who can act as coordinator to ensure a smooth service.

Visiting older people in their homes can be instigated in the following ways:

- referral from the GP
- referral by another agency
- referral from a colleague from another discipline
- referral by relatives or neighbours
- self-referral as the result of an initial visit.

The skills are very similar to the visit outlined above, again requiring the health visitor to arrange the visit by letter or telephone. Either way, this is a planned visit and again requires skills of entry and agenda setting, as outlined above. Skills of health visiting require listening closely to the presenting problem, bearing in mind the possibility that it may not be the real issue. The nursing models of Roy (1975) and Orem (1991) are very useful when working with this age group because it is the activities of daily living that the client and the health visitor are negotiating.

If there is a carer in the home, the health visitor has another agenda with the carer alongside and yet separate from that of the older person. In these situations the alert health visitor often seeks to avoid any secret agendas and ensure that all concerns are fully explored. Chapter 10 discusses abuse of older people, and sensitivity to this possible situation must be maintained.

Robinson's (1998) work on effectiveness of health visiting in the homes of older people found that it reduced carers' coping stress, enhanced their quality of life, reduced mortality among older people and reduced hospital admissions. In addition, work on the effectiveness of reminiscence therapy is also relevant – the very dialogue that health visitors have with older clients is likely to include reminiscence.

CONCLUSION

The range of activities that are carried out by health visitors in the home calls for comprehensive observation, communication and application of knowledge skills. Although home visiting is often considered by managers and other professional disciplines to be very time consuming, nevertheless feedback from clients and research undertaken (Robinson 1998), shows that it is greatly effective. There are many instances when health visitors can effectively use group work with individuals and families, and indeed do so. However, the opportunity for a parent to be able to access professional advice and support in the ambience of the family home, and the effectiveness of this work, should never be underestimated.

The skills required for effective intervention are widely recognized and it is important that health visitors do not underestimate their value to families and individuals in the home. Recording of the contents of a home visit should also include a brief analysis of the interventionist skills used.

Chapter **5**

Skills in specialist community public health nursing–health visiting: working with social groups and communities

Anne Robotham

INTRODUCTION

Health visitors have traditionally always worked with social groups and in communities. However, up until the last decade of the last century the tendencies have been for the social groups to be focused around common core activities: for example, groups of mothers in the postnatal period, groups of young children in schools and nurseries, groups of people seeking similar health support, such as smoking cessation groups, or older people in singing, exercise and reminiscence groups. In working with communities the evidence was that the communities tended to be specialized, such as working with travellers or particular ethnic groups, or in deprived areas mainly made up of people living on certain council estates. This work has called for the use of a wide range of skills within the health visitor portfolio. However, before these skills are examined it seems appropriate to consider how health visiting has been affected by government legislation and policy at the beginning of the 21st century.

THE EFFECT OF GOVERNMENT POLICY ON HEALTH VISITOR SKILL DEVELOPMENT

Porter (Ch. 2) has traced the development of public health alongside health visiting from the

Box 5.1   Skills related to the competencies of working with social groups and communities

- Interagency working
- Working with groups
- Population health needs assessment
- Family health needs assessment
- Multidisciplinary team working
- Addressing health inequalities
- Health protection programmes
- Community involvement and development
- Priority parent education
- Population-based health promotion
  (Health visitor practice development resource pack, Department of Health 2001)

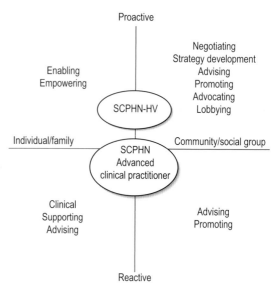

Figure 5.1 The new model of health care for the third part of the register – Robotham and Frost (based loosely on Twinn's 1991 adaptation of Beattie 1996)

19th century until the present day, and has shown how the adoption of the public health role requires new skills in assessing the health needs of populations and using the data generated. She cites the many recent government reports that have had, and will have, an impact on health visiting. The Department of Health (2001e) identifies sets of skills related to the competencies of working with social groups and communities in a public health role. These are shown in Box 5.1.

If these competencies are examined against Figure 4.2, repeated here as Figure 5.1 for ease of access, it can be seen how they all belong to the upper right-hand quadrant of the figure, which is based loosely on Twinn's (1991) adaptation of Beattie's (1991) model discussed by Carnwell in Chapter 3. The skills of strategy, proactive advice, promotion in relation to health and advocacy for enablement are the major facets of a health visitor's armoury in this focus of practice.

Carr et al (2003) undertook a study in the north-east of England to explore the possible differences between public health nursing and health visiting. Their results suggested that there were differences between the two roles, but the comments identified from individual and group interviews suggest that it was in the organization of their work that the

main differences lay. The models of practice, i.e. the skills of working with groups and communities, differed in one major aspect; this was that health visitors maintain caseloads from their individuals/family work, which they cannot let go of when it comes to their public health work. In addition there seemed to be few records of the work that health visitors did with social groups and communities. Following on, and independently, from these results, Forester (2004) showed that there is little in the literature about the organization of health visiting services to support community development. The tension of combining caseload responsibilities with community development has been identified in practice examples.

Forester (2004) found that there are conflicting views from health visitors concerning caseloads and community development:

individual caseload work would always detract from the developmental approach of community based work

caseload work allowed for legitimate entry into communities and helped in making initial contacts and learning community networks

caseload work created a tension in the different philosophical approaches to clients with regards to agendas and partnership

the advantage of not having a caseload was that it enabled more work at strategic level and gave the role a clearer position within multi-agency arenas.

(Forester 2004, p. 143)

However, despite the recent impact on health visiting practice that has evolved from government reports and policy advice, there were earlier examples of health visitors working both with families/individuals and communities/groups, but they did require teams of health visitors working with or without caseloads. In 1990 in Stockport a decision was made to create a tripartite approach to health visiting organization consisting of these different components:

- a generic primary care health visiting service based on GP attachment
- a first parent visitor programme providing a dedicated service to first-time parents in deprived communities
- a health visitor-led team of community development workers located in the most deprived areas of Stockport, none of whom holds a client caseload.

In assessing the effectiveness of this tripartite model, Swann & Brocklehurst (2004) considered that there were several organizational aspects that were important:

1. continuity of effective leadership
2. a commitment to design services to reduce health inequalities
3. pragmatic decision making
4. willingness to take calculated risks
5. true partnership-working.

In addition, Swann & Brocklehurst pointed out that it was important that health visitors developed skills appropriate for the particular aspect of practice in which they were involved.

The following health visiting skills are examples of proactive work with social groups or communities. They involve a wider dimension of anticipation and strategic planning, which nevertheless may be based on the individual or family group.

COMMUNITY DEVELOPMENT

Social exclusion is the modern term applied to estates throughout the UK characterized by large families, single parenthood, low income, poor physical and mental health, an antisocial environment and poor access to health services. A high number of the population are under 35, and are at a time when their only vision for the future is an ever-increasing spiral to the bottom of the heap. It was the publication of the Black Report (1980) that first really brought to the fore the social and health inequalities that were evident in the Victorian era but had surely disappeared by 1980. Since then there have been a number of studies exploring methods in which communities could start to develop themselves. In the next section, DeVille-Almond describes one way in which she enabled some members of a socially excluded community to develop themselves. Daniel (1999a, 1999b) reported on an initiative in the Ore Valley in Sussex, in which the community worker/health visitor co-ordinated and enabled the agencies – housing association, local continuing education centre (part of the local university), residents' association, playlink scheme and representatives from the local health and social services and local residents – into a community project. In enabling by empowering through knowledge, listening and negotiating, the project team decided its own requirements and action approaches in consultation with local residents at every step on the way. A community centre was developed in a flat owned by the Housing Association and dedicated to the welfare of the residents. In time this has been used by so many different groups that further flats were added to make a multi-agency resource centre including health support services, social support services, training and education facilities, office space and a support and information service.

This was a successful initiative which has gone on to become one of the trail-blazers for Sure Start, and the most important factor is that the whole project has been undertaken in the community by the community, with health professionals/social service professionals acting as co-ordinators, listeners and supporters. Various reports on community initiatives over the years emphasize the need for the community to be the main workers in the project for it to succeed. Due to management policies less support has been given to health visitors to develop this aspect of their work. This may be historical in the way that public health practice was seen as belonging to health promotion departments or lay community workers (see Ch. 2: Building capacity and capability).

In the next section health visitors as partners with the community will be discussed.

PARTNERSHIP WITH COMMUNITIES

Partnership has been discussed in relation to home visiting but it also involves working with communities. Twinn (1991) uses Drennan's (1985) and Hennessy's (1985) earlier work to show health visitors sharing their knowledge and expertise openly with community groups to create emancipatory care (not subject to official authority or control), which they consider fundamental to working practice. It is also argued, on this basis, that emancipatory care belongs as much to home health visiting as to community work. The outcome is freedom of choice to a client liberated from traditional practices.

Fagan (1997) looked at a partnership approach to child health surveillance as recommended in the Hall Report (Hall 1991, Hall & Elliman 2003), using a pre-Child Health Surveillance questionnaire sent out prior to each session at 9 months, 18 months and 3 years. This showed that clients responded to requests to undertake their own surveillance linked to the major areas of child development discussed in the parent-held child health record. This small-scale study suggested that there was an improved attendance at child health surveillance sessions and that, even if they did not attend, parents completed the questionnaire, indicating their interest in the process. It also gave the health visitor a chance to applaud parents on their vigilance and care about child development and maintain the positive regard between professional and carer.

In Chapter 2, Porter discusses a model of health needs assessment which has three main approaches: an epidemiological approach, a health economist approach and the rapid appraisal approach. Porter covers the epidemiological approach and Powell in Chapter 16 looks particularly at the health economist approach. In the section below DeVille describes a modification of the rapid appraisal approach. Ong (1986) identified the key informant groups in the community to be:

- people who work within the community, e.g. school teachers, police, health visitors
- people who are recognized leaders, e.g. councillors, church leaders, chairs of self-help groups
- people who are important within informal networks e.g. corner-shop owners, bookies, lollipop persons.

Informal interviews with a semi-structured questionnaire will soon provide data that can be used to ascertain a hierarchy of information such as that shown in Box 5.2.

It must be remembered that some members of the community see themselves as the 'community voice', who are the more vocal members. It is the marginalized and inarticulate members that the professional, i.e. health visitor or specialist community public health nurse, needs to seek out and advocate on their behalf.

Initiating a community development

In setting out to work in partnership it is important that health visitors recognize that they cannot approach this using a middle-class frame of reference. In writing about a community project development, Friend (1999) cited the example of a health visitor and project leader who were aiming to reduce the incidence of coronary heart disease in a community. 'It soon

Box 5.2   The uses of data

Data gained	Can be used with other data to inform
Policy and local strategies	Health policy
Service provision	Health and environmental services; Social services
Socio-ecological environment	Physical environment improvement; Socio-economic environment, e.g. Housing; Disease and disability provisions
Demography	Community composition; Community organization and structure; Community capacity

became apparent that the residents were well aware of the cocktail of ingredients that make up an unhealthy lifestyle, but they were too busy surviving to make any adjustments. The community was in agreement and declared to the project team that public health enemy number one was stress.' (p. 81).

It is vital in setting out to develop partnership work in a community that the health visitor identifies with the community. DeVille-Almond (2000, p. 47) makes these comments on her approach into community:

> To truly get the feel of a community I felt it was important to integrate with and more importantly to be accepted by the community. However, before being able to do this I had to ask the question: 'What is a community, and should we expect everyone to take us on board?' Communities are very hard to define – just because there is a natural boundary in terms of either houses or area the people inside those boundaries do not automatically see themselves as part of the community. I found there to be a very definite divide between the older people and the young, the youth and the 'grown ups' and the

men and women. However, if the older people had grandchildren and great-grandchildren in the community it gave them a link with the young. There was also a 'class structure' within the community, which at times became quite complex. This appeared to be defined by several factors, including:

- which road you lived in
- how long you had lived in the area
- whether you were married or were single with a child
- whether your family was a long established name that had dominated the community for many years or whether you were new to the area
- whether you or your partner was presently in work.

There were several other factors that defined a community, but trying to work within these complex rules often caused friction between others and myself.

An example of this became apparent when I first set up a keep-fit class: many of the younger mothers came, which put some of the older residents off attending. There were also a few local notorious members of the community who had dominated other sections of it for many years. Once these people became involved in any new initiative it put many others off. It became quite a task to decide whether to exclude the dominant people, thus making room for many others, or to try to integrate them with the other members of the community without frightening the others off. After working within the community for a while it became apparent that it would have to be a mixture of both. There were also barriers created by working from a church-owned building. Some people felt that the fact that events were run in the Community Centre, which was owned by the church, would put a large number of local residents off attending. I had to try and make sure this did not happen.

Partnership in community as object

For larger and more heterogeneous communities, however, one of the striking features can be conflict, possibly stemming from a variety of divisions such as race, age or class. Hawtin et al (1994) quote Haggstrom's (1970) concept of the two appearances of community: community as object and acting community. The first is the network of interest groups, political parties, bureaucratic organizations and so forth that is acted upon. The second identifies its own needs and problems, participating in the decision making and engaging in collective action.

An example of community as object (acted-upon community) was seen when, on behalf of a charitable organization, a researcher was profiling child care needs in a community in a deprived area. From going round and speaking to all the leaders and organizers it became clear that they were very enthusiastic about their own particular project. Potentially, there was enormous energy and some excellent work was being done in many aspects of community support, from children's holiday play schemes, through groups for young mothers run by an older citizen in order to discuss problems of parenting, to classes in the local community school for the unemployed to learn computer skills. However, each of these groups was beavering away independently of the others. When one worker was asked why he thought this was, his response was: 'You are all doing to us.' Reflection on this helped the researcher to understand that this community area, although deprived, had had quite a lot of money invested in it for a number of projects, all of which had been quite successful. However, what this worker was saying was: 'We cannot work together because we are not encouraged to take responsibility for the distribution and effective use of the money invested in us – give us the money to use and we will make it effective.' He was clearly right and thus the recommendation to the organization who wished to donate money to set up a scheme was: 'Just give them the money and they will use it effectively – don't put in any other project organizers.' Sadly, the donating organization felt unable to let their money go without retaining control themselves and so a further small project started up, running alongside and overlapping with others, and the community came no closer together.

Partnership in acting community

DeVille-Almond (2000, p. 48) considered one way of getting a community to come together was by increasing communication through the production of a newspaper. At the same time she emphasizes that it is vital to listen to the community as they define their own needs.

I was asked by the Trust to address women's and children's needs, in accordance with the Health of the Nation (Department of Health 1992b) targets, and to progress from there.
My main aim was to ensure that I worked collaboratively with all the people in the area: this included social services, the local council, local churches, local schools, the local community association, local health professionals, local voluntary bodies and, most importantly, local residents. I soon discovered that there was an immediate need for many health provisions and as a starter I decided to address two that I could rectify almost immediately. The women who lived locally expressed concern over there being no adequate baby clinic in the area and also they felt that some sort of keep-fit class would be good. There had been a Weight Watchers group in the area for a while and, although there was a great need for such a service, it had closed down as many found it far too expensive.

I needed to find a suitable building to run the clinics in and I was unable to use the GP's surgery. However, the local health authority had given some funding towards the building of a community centre owned by the church. These funds were given on the understanding that the local authority could have free room space for 10 years for all health activities. The community centre was in the heart of Moxley and made an excellent venue. My only concern was that the fact that it was a church building which might be a bit of a stumbling block with some of the local residents.

I asked local schoolchildren to help design posters to promote the forthcoming clinics and asked local businesses to donate prizes for these. I awarded eight prizes for the best posters and well over 100 local people attended the awards ceremony. I announced to all when the two new clinics would be starting. This all happened within 6 weeks of taking up my job.

One of the first comments I had from local residents was that people often spoke about what was needed but then nothing ever got done! They also expressed concern that no one ever consulted them on issues such as what day and time would be best for the clinics. I therefore had a panel of local residents to help me with these issues. I felt that it was important for people to see that things were being done. Within weeks both these clinics got off the ground.

We started a baby clinic in the Community Centre, which we ran on a much more informal basis than is commonly done. We provided a crèche facility for older children, had complimentary light refreshments, and encouraged mothers to discuss issues not only with health visitors in group sessions but also between themselves. Many of the mothers now help with the running of this clinic. The demand has been so great that we now have a Child Medical Officer on a monthly basis and a second clinic has been started for new babies only. Here two of the local health visitors encourage the mothers to set up support groups and run discussions on the specific health needs of newborns and their mothers.

On Tuesdays we have a 'weigh-in' clinic, two keep-fit sessions (the local community association pays for the instructor), a blood pressure clinic, a reflexology clinic and invite speakers on a whole range of topics – talks for which we provide crèche facilities. I also run 6-week cooking courses where cheap, low-calorie meals are prepared within half an hour and everyone gets a taste. At the end of the 6 weeks each person is issued with the recipes and a breakdown of cost and calorie content. Women in the audience help me to buy and prepare the food and also supply me with recipes. We make a small charge for the keep-fit classes and 'weigh-in' clinic and this money goes towards monthly prizes for achievement by participants, food for the cooking courses and the complimentary refreshments. Every 6 months, for extra-special effort, I offer the opportunity for two women to attend a health farm for the day. At least six of the local women have lost 35 kg or more in weight.

Many of the women said that they would like to attempt other sports but felt they were not the type to join a tennis club or go to the gym. The keep-fit instructor and I decided to work together with the local sports and leisure services and get tennis coaching, swimming lessons and other activities organized at a knock-down price. Many of the women took advantage of this and I also used some of the award money to fund these events. Over 40 women completed tennis courses that were offered and some have continued playing. We will hopefully run similar events this year.

I was given an initial £500 by the Trust and opened an account in the name of Moxley Community Clinics. Any money raised from the charges for the 'weigh-in' clinic and keep-fit classes and any other funds I receive are paid into this account. This then enables us to run these clinics at a relatively low cost to the Trust. Much of my equipment is provided by sponsorship from outside the NHS, by fund-raising by the local community or by applying for research-based money.

I have instigated the setting up of a chiropody clinic in the Community Centre on the same day as around 55 pensioners meet for bingo, making the clinic more accessible for the users. This was started at the request of the local pensioners and the Trust provided a session every 2 weeks. It soon became apparent that the need was for more than this and the service is now provided on a weekly basis. Very few appointments are missed as many of the attendees are on site on this day anyway.

I have also worked with a community arts team to get local young people involved in a theatre workshop looking at health issues.

It became apparent that I had truly started to empower the local residents when I mentioned recently that I would have to close down some of the classes for a week because the nursery nurses and myself would not be there.

'You can't do that,' was the reply. 'We don't need you lot here. We can run this on our own.'

It is often difficult as a health professional to let go and it was at this point of the project that I realized that I had stopped being the instigator of better health in this community and the community had started to take over. I was simply a player in the team. Changing attitudes is possibly the most difficult task one has to encounter in the public health field and it takes more than a few years. However, once the seed has been set it will soon start to spread and hopefully in years to come it will be possible for this community to truly reap the benefits of better health for all.

DeVille-Almond shows, in the vignette above, that her health visiting skills contributed very much towards her public health nurse role and she was very proactive in her approach to partnership development with the community in which she found herself. It could be argued that she was equally *reactive* in her work because she based her two initial community needs on her health visiting knowledge. Firstly, of the need for education and support in infant and child rearing and, secondly, of the self-esteem and health needs of women living in educationally and materially deprived circumstances. The development of Sure Start programmes (see Ch. 8) has now taken over much of this type of work.

COLLABORATION AND PARTNERSHIPS IN THE COMMUNITY

Although the word 'collaboration' can be used interchangeably with that of 'partnership', as has been shown by El Ansari et al (2001), nevertheless it is quite possible to make a distinction in terms of health visiting skills. The Universal Dictionary suggests that to collaborate is to work together especially in an intellectual or artistic manner, whereas partnership suggests working together with others in some common interest. Where health and well-being are the main focus then partnership is probably appropriate. However, there are several situations where health visitors may experience finding various groups

in the community which have been set up and actively involved in, for example, learning English classes, learning IT skills, and learning creative skills such as card making and decorating. These groups have usually been set up by the local further education college and have been specifically designed for a certain age group of people who are not working, because they are usually held during the day.

A health visitor or public health nurse can then capitalize on these group situations once a relationship has been made with the college tutors. The sessions could possibly be extended to include health teaching, exercise classes or social well-being discussions. Where these are successful the word is spread and the group classes grow, to the benefit of the college and health professional alike. Funding can often be gained from city partnership sources or charitable organization sources. The health visitor will have used a data collection technique which will have shown where small sources of funding are available in the area (see Ong, Box 5.2, above).

In exploring outcome evidence of the effectiveness of collaborative partnerships, El Ansari et al (2001) make the point that 'collaboration is complex and enquiries into its effectiveness by different parties will be on the basis of different agendas with contrasting criteria and potentially conflicting perceptions'. El Ansari et al recommend an outcomes model that takes into account the different perspectives (e.g. Barr et al 1999). This enables measurement of a range of outcomes, from the learners' reactions to the intervention to the impact this has had on the community and organization.

Clearly the use of collaborative partnerships is not just about an easy opportunity to find a group. In the new NHS the need for accurate targets is important as a means of demonstrating the value of public health work by collaboration.

ADVOCACY IN PARTNERSHIP AND EMPOWERMENT

Advocacy by health visitors on clients' behalf can be viewed as part of empowerment and may be regarded as the beginning of the process. It is not necessarily inhibiting to client development for health visitors to make initial representations on their behalf, and does not reflect the traditional role of the health visitor, putting the client into a passive role. Advocacy is particularly appropriate when health visitors are working with clients from ethnic minority groups who have little or no spoken English and do not understand the health care system in general and health visiting in particular.

Mayall & Foster's (1989) research showed that health visitors intervened in the private sphere of the family as advocate for the child and to represent the child on the behalf of society. Discussion with health visitors made it clear that they saw their work as not only protecting the child from abuse but also ensuring that the child was given every opportunity to fulfil its potential. It is interesting that in the study health visitors considered this to justify any amount and type of intervention they thought necessary but saw it as benevolent rather than controlling work because it was for the protection of children. This highlights the need for health visitors to be aware that their work is susceptible to varying interpretations depending on the values and beliefs of the person making the interpretation.

There is evidence from an east London project (Harding & Pandya 1995) that health advocates are used not only as translators, working alongside health visitors, but also for independent home visits. This system was also used in Sparkbrook in Birmingham by Weaver (1996). Comments from health visitors involved in the project to use health advocates as part of health visiting teams were positive and there were clear guidelines on preparation for home visits by the advocates, visiting following an initial joint visit with the health visitor, and subsequent debriefing sessions.

Advocacy is not just about health visitors representing clients' views but, as in the project above, enabling clients to make best use of the health service as well as promoting flexibility in the delivery of health visiting which serves to suit different cultures. Gogna & Hari (2000) make the very clear point that effective health visitors with ethnic client groups must be prepared to listen and learn. The assumption that the Asian family is all-protective and supportive is far from the truth.

ANTICIPATION OF PHYSICAL, SOCIAL AND PSYCHOLOGICAL NEEDS IN SOCIAL GROUP WORK

Anticipation in the acute nursing care field is designed to prevent the occurrence of further physical problems in relation to the immediate illness, and to prepare patients for interventions to minimize adverse psychological responses. In a sense the anticipation is clearly relevant and immediate.

Anticipation in public health–health visiting enables clients to identify the possible impact of wider issues. This includes both short-term and long-term responses to client situations. For example, health visitors working with mothers of growing infants draw on and extend the mother's knowledge of infant development, encouraging aspects of safety such as ensuring that the rolling infant is not placed on an unsecured surface above floor level. In addition, situations that may not yet have occurred are identified and discussed by health visitors. Examples include dangers in relation to equipment that has become apparently necessary for infant growth, such as baby walkers, but in reality has no part to play in child development. Health visitors help mothers to challenge some of the traditional practices of child rearing that have been found by research to be unsafe, e.g. placing a young baby to sleep in the prone position.

Anticipation of social needs is more difficult to conceptualize and yet there are many ways in which health visitors can enhance mothers' social situations. Examples here include introducing new mothers to other mothers in similar circumstances to establish peer group support networks. Helping women to understand their social circumstances is also included in the anticipatory work of health visitors, particularly women who are trapped in unhappy marriages and who need to realize that there are ways out. This theme is further explored in Chapter 10 on violence and health.

Social needs of older people are anticipated by health visitors and frequently these involve networking and liaison with other agencies to access group activities or social support visits. Often, health visitors listen to the reminiscences of older people and are criticized for apparently social visits. However, current work on reminiscence therapy has shown that these are vital for social health and as such are important aspects of health visitor anticipation.

Research (Browne et al 1988, Cox & Holden 1994) has shown that health visitors are well equipped to anticipate psychological needs and health breakdown. Listening to women and allowing them to express their concerns is one well-used method, as is knowing the vulnerability of women with particular personal histories. Examples include the knowledge that women who lost their own mothers before the age of 11 are more at risk of postnatal depression, or that parents who had harsh childhoods themselves are more likely to deal harshly with their own children. These exemplify the very real need for health visitors to listen to families and seek for possible at-risk factors during the early getting-to-know-the-community period. It is critical that health visitors do not gain information through question-and-answer sessions; rather, they use skills to draw parents out and discuss with them the relevance of information about past situations to current or future situations. This is discussed further in Chapter 11.

When it comes to working with other age-groups, some health visitors are in a position to target adolescents and have set up clinics particularly to provide support, again in the form of listening sessions to enable adolescents to work through problems of emotional development. Often these are of relation to family-planning advice and counselling and the adolescent is encouraged to anticipate their own needs and health behaviour.

SPECIAL SOCIAL GROUPS – CHILDREN WITH SPECIAL NEEDS

Although the health visitor will have visited the family in the home, yet there are several examples around the country where health visitors work with parents and children with special needs in social groups outside the home.

There appear to be two basic models of organizational practice in health visiting work with children with special needs. In the first model, specialist health visitors are appointed on an outreach scheme and receive referrals from the family health visitor to provide more intensive support and counselling about practical aspects of parental handling of the child with special needs. The second model is where a child has multiple special need problems and is looked after at home by a multidisciplinary team of physiotherapists, speech therapists, possibly the community children's nurse in the case of nursing needs, and available portage helper schemes. In this latter case the family health visitor may act as a coordinator for the professionals involved with the special needs child, as well as possibly working with other family members, especially other siblings.

The health visiting team is likely to include nursery nurses and community assistants who can provide regular practical help such as helping the mother to carry out, for example, portage tasks or catheterization in the manner in which she has been taught by the hospital. The individual helpers and professionals involved will depend on the organizational policies of the particular Community Trust and whether the paediatric unit has a community outreach scheme. If there is an outreach scheme that helps mothers with clinical care then the special needs health visitor has a supportive and planning responsibility to ensure that the overall care pathway is contingent on the family requirements. For example, concentration of services on one child can have negative effects on other children within the family and the special needs health visitor will need to be ever-vigilant in monitoring the developmental progress of the other children. Robinson (1998) shows that health visitor effectiveness particularly involves improving the psychological functioning of families with a child with special needs.

Where the family health visitor is working in the dual role as a special needs health visitor then her/his situation is likely to be more of a coordinator of the other professionals involved as mentioned above. In many ways the health visitor may need to concentrate on supporting the parents: mother, who may be almost overwhelmed with the number of supporting carers that her child needs, and father, who may have to work long hours to bring in money for the extras that the family requires. There is empirical evidence from health visitors that many mothers find it hard to cope with all the attention being focused on the child while their own needs lie buried. These needs may involve feelings of guilt, anxiety, lack of ability to be a 'normal' parent and so forth.

SPECIAL SOCIAL GROUPS – FATHERS IN THE FAMILY UNIT

Health visitors' interactions with fathers vary with the level of employment in the area. Mack & Trew (1991) quoted research showing that fathers often have different tolerances and attitudes towards child behaviour from those of mothers, both within a normal community and in the event of referral to a psychologist because of behaviour problems. Repeated research studies in breast-feeding have shown clearly that where fathers are supportive, mothers breast-feed more effectively and for a longer period of time. The pilot perinatal study (Sheldrake et al 1997) also showed that fathers could become postnatally depressed alongside their wives. Indeed, one mother asked the health visitor for a scale for her husband and brought the results back to the health visitor; between them, she and the health visitor worked to support the father through his difficult period.

Traditionally health visitors found it difficult to work with fathers, but in recent years attitudes have changed towards men in the parenting role and in many cases, particularly in employment troughs, there have been role reversals, with women working and men staying at home to look after the family. Health visitors need to examine their skills in working with men and recognize that many men have intimate knowledge of child care and development. Intervention categories remain the same as when working with women: authoritative and facilitative approaches are used in context.

Barna (1995), focusing on work with young fathers, suggested that one of her main aims was to challenge sexist attitudes and values, ensuring that in so doing she did not compound stereotypical male images but allowed issues of masculinity to be addressed in the context of parenting. Clearly, this type of work relates more to group work in clinics; nevertheless, health visitors may have to challenge men on their sexist attitudes and, if the mother is there, to make sure that this is done in such a way that the father does not feel that 'women are ganging up on him'.

Some Sure Start programmes have shown that group meetings of fathers, with or without their offspring, have been effectively used by the health visitor and father as discussion, information, education and fun sessions for all concerned.

HEALTH PROMOTION ON A HOLISTIC HEALTH BASIS

Bunton & Macdonald (1992) suggest that health promotion combines aspects of the disciplines of psychology, education, epidemiology and sociology; it also embraces other disciplines such as social policy, communications theory, marketing, economics and philosophy. Health education is a means whereby recipients have health promotion communicated to them. In a sense it is the didactic sharing of health promotion, and is less frequently seen as part of health visiting because it cannot be presented in partnership with the client. Catford (2001) described 10 components of health promotion:

1. Understanding and responding to people's needs
2. Building on sound theoretical principles and understanding
3. Demonstrating coherence
4. Collecting, analysing and using information
5. Reorienting key decision makers
6. Connecting with all sectors
7. Using complementary approaches at both individual and environmental levels

8. Encouraging participation and ownership
9. Providing technical and managerial training
10. Undertaking specific programmes – avoiding 'analysis paralysis'.

This list, in effect, encapsulates all the domains for the specialist community public health practitioner but professionals from different discipline backgrounds will bring different skills which contribute toward proficiency in public health domains.

Health visiting skills in health promotion range from working with individuals through working with groups to working with communities. In many ways, promoting health in communities is about bringing people together and encouraging them to work for the health and safety of the community. Examples of this include the student health visitor who worked with a group of mothers in North Staffordshire. They were particularly concerned that their children had to cross a busy main road to reach school. By bringing the mothers together and helping them to realize that they shared the same concerns, the student encouraged them to make representations to the local council and police department; the upshot was that a pelican-controlled crossing was installed. This might be criticized as not being health promotion because there is a preconceived idea that health promotion is targeted at the individual, albeit possibly using a group methodology. However, the skill in health visiting is about being able to mobilize communities to promote the health of their more vulnerable members.

Neighbourhood Watch schemes have often been set up as a result of health visitors raising awareness of the anxieties of local people about burglary and theft. The pulling together of the community has not only reduced the threat to its more vulnerable members but has also enabled other members to become actively involved in its organization, giving them a clear application for their skills and the satisfaction of having a worthwhile part to play.

Health visitors promoting health to families often build on concerns expressed by women discussing their families. A classic example of this is the mother of a family of growing children who is concerned about their predilection for junk food. With the support and encouragement of the health visitor she is able to confidently make changes to the meals that are offered and discuss with her family the reasons why such changes have been made. Work by Mayall & Foster (1989) has shown that mothers often have a wide knowledge of what their families ought to eat but financial constraints force them to forego more expensive nutritious foods in favour of more filling ones. Health promotion in these circumstances means that health visitors encourage and support women in their concerns and discuss with them ways of making cheaper food equally as nutritious as more expensive items. This particular example of family feeding has been discussed in the vignette (DeVille-Almond, above).

SKILLS IN INTER-AGENCY WORK

In her discussion on health visiting with the homeless, Marian Jones (see Chapter 6) is praised by the research evaluators for the success of her inter-agency group. Marian is at pains to point out that this group was in existence before she moved into the post; however, she has maintained and fed this group through effective continuity of meetings. The results are a much closer understanding of health staff and local teachers and others about their own roles and the community which they are serving. DeVille-Almond (2000, p. 51), in her discussion of community development, says the following:

Local officials, businesses and voluntary groups were useful sources of information but the most valuable source was discovering the knowledgeable members of the community and working closely with them. Once people started to approach me with health issues within my area and put forward agendas of their own I realized that I was on my way to a successful partnership.

DeVille-Almond (2000, p. 51) also has an important point to make in relation to the need to communicate well, and also that this type of work does require time resources and the need for flexible working:

> *It would be arrogant of me to suggest that there have not been problems in working with the local community and other agencies, and there have of course been failures as well as successes. Some of the failures were brought about by lack of communication between myself and other community members and some by personality clashes. However when working in the public heath arena one has to remember that upsetting one person can often have a knock-on effect to 50 others, especially where the community contains very close knit groups. I had a great deal of difficulty in delegating work. This was mainly because there was no one to delegate it to. However, once I became involved with the community, many people were willing to commit themselves to helping in the setting up and running of projects. I also had a great deal of difficulty persuading other professionals within the Trust about the value and priority of the role. I feel, however, that for the project to work successfully it is important to learn from the failures and build on the successes. This type of work takes lots of commitment and a 9-to-5 approach would be out of the question. I have often worked evenings and weekends to truly involve myself with the community and feel that now, more than 3 years into the project, this hard work has started to pay off. (p. 51)*

There is nothing new about inter-agency work through common-cause meetings. In the mid 1970s an inter-agency group of health professionals, local teachers, social workers, educational welfare officers and community police met on a regular basis in a particularly deprived area in Wolverhampton. The meetings were very effective in enabling professional members to understand their desired outcomes and to recognize the differences between themselves and other meeting members. The main difference between that type of meeting and now is that at that time it was community acted on unlike public health work today, which is community in action.

Working with mixed groups of health professionals and users Buggins (2000) suggested asking the membership to complete a statement such as 'Being a health professional is …' and 'Being a user representative is …' She suggests that the exercise underlines many commonalities between users and health professionals – both groups find their role both tough and satisfying – but the perceptions of where the power and control lie provide a lot of discussion. Health professionals often don't feel powerful and in control, but users perceive them to be amazingly so.

Buggins (2000) also raises a point made earlier by DeVille-Almond (2000), that people are often tired of consultation without results and this breeds frustration and apathy. Managers and organizations need to connect front-line work together and embed it into the organizational decision-making process. This means that specialist community public health practitioners need to be in a position to act upon the expressed needs of the community and ensure this reaches policy makers.

HEALTH VISITING IN THE HEALTH CENTRE/GP SURGERY

The health visitor working in the health centre, and to a lesser extent the GP surgery, is very much part of a team. However, in larger health centres health visitors may be a team in themselves working within the wider team of paramedical staff. This approach is not the intention of the philosophy of integrated teams because among the professionals there is in effect still only the concept of 'working alongside' rather than working in a truly integrated manner. Integrated teamwork is slowly being introduced into GP/community care but the models used differ widely across Health Authorities and Trusts. It is recognized that not all primary care trusts subscribe to the same model of integration, because of the diverse nature of the communities they serve and the human and material resources available.

Various examples of integrated teams have been evaluated. Lawton (1996) was an early commentator on an integrated team approach introduced into a Welsh general practice. In this model the main focus was on the inclusion of all practice professionals in a team with regular meetings and joint discussion on responsibilities; for example, each discipline was responsible for running certain clinics within the practice. The team was managed by a member of one of the professional disciplines (at the time of writing, the health visitor). Future objectives were to use audit and undertake PREP requirements, staff appraisal and practice profiling. In addition, the team was looking at shared records, practice guidelines and treatment protocols, monitoring continuity of care, developing health promotion initiatives and setting up library facilities within the practice.

The CPHVA (1997) issued a professional briefing paper that included full references and bibliography on various models available. They included a useful definition of integration: 'A team of community based nurses from different disciplines, working together within a primary care setting, pooling their skills, knowledge and abilities in order to provide the most effective care for the practice population and community it covers' (p. 229).

The CPHVA particularly commented on the often-raised concern that the concept of integrated teams would lead to a generic community nurse. They recommended that it was important that professional disciplines worked together not to compete but to recognize each other's philosophies, values, roles and responsibilities and to promote both differences and areas of commonality to GPs. There was also the concern that within integrated teams the public health remit might be lost in overriding concern for 'care' of the individual rather than the needs of the wider community. 'The wider community' may also come to mean the GP practice catchment area only, and thus practice concerns may override the social concerns of the community.

It is most likely that this competitive element has disappeared with the loss of general practice fund-holding and its divisive effects, and the establishment of Primary Care Trusts. The very composition of the new Primary Care Trusts ensures an equal balance between social and health care needs. The most appropriate model of integration should ensure, among other things, that the whole primary health care team produces an annual plan of action, building on the community nursing profile and identifying specific public health issues.

In many ways the organization of health visiting within general practice is secondary to the different skills necessary to practise in centres and surgeries, and within or outside teams. The siting of health centres in the heart of the community acts as a central focus for clients seeking the health visitor, and the knowledge that the health visitor is to be found in the health centre means that clients have easy access without the need for appointments. In some areas health visiting teams who work closely together have organized themselves to allow for someone always to be available in the centre during opening hours. Criticism of the cost-effectiveness of this system was avoided by the fact that the health visitor is thus readily available and may well be running clinics or groups during this time, or catching up on the volume of paperwork that seems necessary to today's practice. A survey undertaken in one centre in the West Midlands (Windsor 1990) to evaluate the number of callers for the health visitor during a week showed that the number of client contacts easily surpassed those made by all health visitors away from the centre except at the beginning and end of the day. Clearly, this method is only effective where there is a health visiting team working together. It does not replace planned home visits but it does give clients the possibility of immediate access.

Where there is one health visitor in a GP surgery, or smaller teams in health centres, a combination of fixed health centre times and home visiting remains the more cost-effective method. Cost-effectiveness in this sense is not about contact numbers but about the immediacy of access to a health visitor that some clients in deprived areas have found so useful. This system can also operate in rural areas provided there is a sufficiently large team of health visitors to be able to organize it. Marley (1995) describes the need that was identified for a 'duty drop-in rota' of health visitors within the Strelley nursing development unit project. Because of resource issues in the GP practice it proved impossible to continue this. Analysis of one week's client-initiated contacts showed 62 as against 46 planned contacts and clearly demonstrated a need that in this instance was, unfortunately, not possible to meet.

There is a major difference between the client visiting the health visitor in the health centre, on 'independent' territory, and visiting at home on the client's territory. Thus the environment of the health centre has to be welcoming and give the client what they want. If the client is coming to attend a group, then the organization of that group should be such that clients have control over what they want from it. They may organize the group themselves or want to be sure that it is not too large or too small, with the attendant difficulties of being overwhelmed or exposed. Clients come to health centres, whether for individual discussion or group activities, with their own agendas. Thus it is easier for the health visitor to concentrate on their needs and what is being said. Despite this, alert health visitors will be aware that occasionally the problem is secondary to another unspoken difficulty. What is necessary here is for health visitors to have the astuteness to identify those health care concerns that can be safely tackled within a group setting and those that merit one-to-one conversation.

Another factor that must be considered by health visitors is time management, which may particularly be addressed by attendance at clinics or group sessions. Too much time spent with one client means someone else waiting and it may be necessary to suggest a home visit, after ensuring that the urgency of the problem is not affected by delay. The important skill in working with clients in clinics is the ability to recognize immediacy and to help clients themselves to give priority to health visiting time.

Skills in a group setting rely on the education of health visitors to work with groups, understanding their dynamics and characteristics. Tuckman's (1965) model of group behaviour is a useful knowledge base for group interaction, as is Belbin's (1993) model of team roles at work. The two models mentioned are most

useful because they clearly aid the organization of groups in the initial stages by health visitors, and then later give health visitors an understanding of how to withdraw successfully, enabling the group to continue functioning productively. In addition, health visitors' group skills and knowledge encourage group attendance and participation by shy attendees, allowing them to feel secure and comfortable in the group situation. Similarly, the same skills enable more controlling members of the group to use their skills without detriment to the shy ones. It is a skilled health visitor who enables the first-time mother to feel confident enough to sit alongside the experienced mothers, who also do not feel held back by the novices.

WORKING WITH PERINATAL WOMEN IN THE HEALTH CENTRE/GP SURGERY

The first introduction of health visiting to the family unit may be in the home during the antenatal period. It is also likely that where pregnant women attend the GP surgery for antenatal care and attend parentcraft classes they will also meet the health visitor outside the home. Health visitors work with women in the antenatal period to establish a relationship, introduce the perspective of health visiting and, if possible, identify any factors in the pregnancy or family history that might create vulnerability in the family. Green & Murray (1994) surveyed the literature to assess the extent to which women were found to have depression during pregnancy and from the studies found that the prevalence of rates of depression in pregnancy were comparable with those found after delivery. They went on to use the Edinburgh Postnatal Depression Scale to record scores of women in the antenatal period and found a close link between these and the postnatal score. Further pilot studies (Sheldrake et al 1997) have confirmed the increasingly common finding of depression in antenatal women.

Clement (1995) reported on the use of 'listening visits' in the antenatal period, highlighting their value both in helping women to identify early depressive feelings and in ensuring continuity into the postnatal weeks. This

Mother's name: ....

Today's date:..

Baby's date of birth: ....

Health Visitor: ....

I would like to know how you are feeling now **underline**, a few weeks after your baby's birth. Please the answer which comes closest to how you have felt **in the past week**, not just how you feel today. It has been found that responses are more accurate if they are not discussed with other people, so it is advisable to fill in the form on your own when you have a few spare minutes. Please complete ALL items.

Here is an example, already completed.

I have felt happy:
> Yes, all of the time
> Yes, most of the time
> No, not very often
> No, not at all

This would mean: 'I have felt happy most of the time' during the past week.

Please complete the other questions in the same way.

In the past week:

1. **I have been able to laugh and see the funny side of things:**
   As much as I always could
   Not quite so much now
   Definitely not so much now
   Not at all

2. **I have looked forward with enjoyment to things:**
   As much as I ever did
   Rather less than I used to
   Definitely less than I used to
   Hardly at all

3. **I have blamed myself unnecessarily when things went wrong:**
   Yes, most of the time
   Yes, some of the time
   Not very often
   No, never

4. **I have been anxious or worried for no good reason:**
   No, not at all
   Hardly ever
   Yes, sometimes
   Yes, very often

5. **I have felt scared or panicky for no good reason:**
   Yes, quite a lot
   Yes, sometimes
   No, not much
   No, not at all

6. **Things have been getting on top of me:**
   Yes, most of the time I haven't been able to cope at all
   Yes, sometimes I haven't been coping as well as usual
   No, most of the time I have coped quite well
   No, I have been coping as well as ever

7. **I have been so unhappy that I have had difficulty sleeping:**
   Yes, most of the time
   Yes, sometimes
   Not very often
   No, not at all

8. **I have felt sad or miserable:**
   Yes, most of the time
   Yes, sometimes
   Not very often
   No, not at all

9. **I have been so unhappy that I have been crying:**
   Yes, most of the time
   Yes, quite often
   Only occasionally
   No, never

10. **The thought of harming myself has occurred to me:**
    Yes, quite often
    Sometimes
    Hardly ever
    Never

Figure 5.2 The Moods and Feelings Questionnaire (Copyright 1987 British Journal of Psychiatry; from Cox JL, Holden JM, Sagovsky R 1987 Detection of postnatal depression: development of the 10-item Edinburgh Postnatal Depression Scale. Br J Psychiat 150:782–786)

is a counselling process under Heron's (1986) facilitative category and can embrace all three interventions under that category: cathartic, catalytic and supportive. The particular counselling structure used would be along the Rogerian lines of client-centred discussion.

The introduction of the Edinburgh Postnatal Depression Scale (Cox et al 1987) has created a means whereby health visitors can identify depression in women and gauge the effectiveness of their interventions. The tool has been readily taken up by health visitors in various parts of the UK and may be used in different ways. In the Southern Birmingham Primary Care Trust the tool was originally modified by a change of title only and is used in both the antenatal and postnatal periods (Fig. 5.2).

The title 'Moods and Feelings Questionnaire' was felt to be less clinical and therefore I did not perpetuate an idea that depression belongs to the perinatal period. The tool was to become integrated into home visits aimed at an antenatal period between 22 and 28 weeks and three postnatal periods: 1 month, 3 months and 6 months after delivery (following Holden 1994). The tool could, of course, be used at other times when the health visitor and mother wanted to check progress or effectiveness of particular interventions.

The tool is used primarily to give women permission to talk about their negative feelings and to identify low moods. There is also evidence that some women are able to conceal depressive moods and that in others it helps to prevent the spiral of depression (Cox & Holden 1994). The tool is first introduced to the woman and the underlying research is explained; they are given the option to fill it in or not. Women are given space to complete the questionnaire and are encouraged to do it on their own, but it is important that they have a chance to discuss the reasons for their responses with the health visitor or a close confidante. Often underlying issues emerge that have little to do directly with the pregnancy or birth. Evidence (Green & Murray 1994) shows that there is a relationship between low moods and feelings (from any cause) in the antenatal period and postnatal depression. It is not necessarily the scoring

system that is important but the ensuing dialogue, which clearly belongs among the cathartic and supportive interventions in Heron's (1986) facilitative category. There is a division of opinion as to where the tool should be offered to women: in the home or the clinic. The pilot project mentioned above (Sheldrake et al 1997) indicated that women preferred to use the tool at home with the health visitor.

Despite the effectiveness of this tool it is being used less because it is no longer recommended in Hall and Elliman (2003). However, it must be recognized that although it is not seen as part of a developmental check system, nevertheless many health visitors and their clients have had need to be grateful for the way in which it has helped to identify and support perinatal depression in both men and women. It continues to be used in many parts of the UK.

HEALTH VISITING IN COMMUNITY-BASED CENTRES

This area of practice has usually only been open to those health visitors who have the opportunity to undertake project work in communities. It must also be made clear that there is a difference between this and health visitors who have used community centres as a base to work from in the absence of physical space in a GP surgery or health authority clinic. These latter situations call for skills similar to those identified in the previous section. They call for vision on the part of a Trust or Health Authority to recognize that health visitors have the special skills to enable them to undertake community work, and it also calls for a special type of health visitor to carry it out.

One of the earliest workers in the community was Drennan (personal communication, 1984), who set up and developed health promotion initiatives in Paddington and Kensington Health District communities. She worked against considerable difficulties in finding centres to use for group discussions and activities, ascertaining residents' health needs and requirements and encouraging and motivating colleagues to help. It is largely as a result of the knowledge and experience that she gained from this work that other centres have been set up.

Clearly, one of the major skills is networking – with other professionals, non-health agencies, community leaders and vocational and charitable organization workers. This particularly calls for patience, ignoring frustrations resulting from other workers' differing agendas and recognizing that it is often difficult to create interest in the community for the enthusiasms of the few who are motivated. There have been well-documented reports of difficulties of communicating with communities and, increasingly, community development workers attached to social services find that an early task is to motivate a small group of community leaders to take responsibility for the organization of a newsletter. This may call for a round of discussions with local businesses and organizations to seek support to cover production costs – possibly by charging for the opportunity for local advertising.

Both DeVille-Almond (2000) and Gilbert (Gilbert & Banks 1997) have shown the need for health visitors to develop community projects to provide information to funding bodies about:

- the aims, objectives and achievements of the project to date
- the work that needs to be achieved at periodic reviews
- the work at risk of not being achieved
- options on the possible way forward, with returns on investment.

The objectives of Gilbert's work are included here to show the potential value of health visiting in the community in developing the public health role for the benefit of the population of a particular area:

- to work with mainstream services to develop a health-related focus in the community
- to work with children and their families to:
  - increase their level of social and financial support
  - increase the developmental opportunities for young children

- to create structures for health action by tenants and services
- to improve the resettlement of new tenants by the provision of new information about a wide range of services
- to develop a model by which health gain can be achieved at the level of the GP practice population.

Possibly one of the most important skills attached to working in the community, with the community, is enthusiasm. Closely following this is an ability to be creative, to be able to work in any ambience, and an infectious, challenging manner. It also calls for a resilience that outweighs despondency when one of the best ideas 'bites the dust' because of lack of resources.

HEALTH VISITING SKILLS IN HOMELESS ACCOMMODATION OR WOMEN'S REFUGE HOSTELS

Health visitors work in hostels or homes on two organizational bases: either because they are working as specialist visitors or because the home or hostel is part of the general practice caseload.

Health visitors working as specialist practitioners often cover the whole catchment area of the health authority and thus become the specialist expert for their colleagues, receiving referrals and linking with colleagues when clients are moved on. The skills of health visiting in the specialist approach are a knowledge of all aspects of homeless law, knowledge of alternative options to bed and breakfast accommodation, and skills of negotiation for and on behalf of the client. The work of the specialist health visitor service for homeless families has been expanded on by Jones in Chapter 6.

Health visiting in single-parent hostels calls for yet another group of skills from the health visitor. Personal selling is particularly relevant to this aspect of promoting the service (de la Cuesta 1994). Adjusting the approach through physical appearance and language to appear trendily acceptable is a means of gaining a client's confidence. Many young mothers in single-parent hostels are deeply suspicious of possible paternalism and resent any suggestion of criticism of their child-rearing practices. Often they have been in the care of the social services themselves during part of their lives, lack experiences of positive parenting and are fearful that their children may be taken away because of their present circumstances.

The skills of the health visitor in these circumstances lie in breaking down barriers, trying to create trust and confidence in the young mothers and at the same time promoting parenting and teaching child care and maternal health. Group work is often a way forward, particularly if a young member of the team takes this on, but the contents of sessions for discussion have to be determined by the group and the skill here is in introducing areas of health or child care that have not initially been seen by the group as relevant. Often, young women are under considerable pressures from their families, the baby's father and other friends, and in many cases resent the herding together of people all with the same difficulties into one hostel. Added to this they may be separated from their extended family because of lack of space in the family home, the breakdown of relationships or merely the absence of accommodation nearby.

A major concern of young single mothers invited to group sessions is that they will be subjected to a school approach; in many cases they have not completed their schooling or failed to gain any qualifications and thus have a negative conception of education.

PROFESSIONALS AND NON–PROFESSIONALS IN THE COMMUNITY

Health visitors were the original non-professionals in home visiting until the time of their registration and qualification. This has meant that for a period of over 50 years child care in the UK has been the domain of mothers and families and professional health visitors. It was only in 1983 that a scheme was set up in Dublin as part of the Child Development Programme pilot study. Because of lack of resources the intervention programme hitherto

run by health visitors could not continue. Experienced volunteer mothers in disadvantaged areas were recruited to implement the programme instead of health visitors and underwent 4 weeks of training. They aimed to support 5–15 first-time mothers each under the guidance of the child development programme advisor. Later, a random controlled trial (Johnson et al 1993) was set up to examine the effectiveness of these volunteer community mothers against a control group of general health visiting (public health nursing). The trial concluded that the child development programme could be delivered effectively by non-professionals, but effectiveness was not compared with health visitors working in the Child Development Programme.

Jackson (1992) discussed two projects pioneering community mothers in England, each with a slightly different focus. One project trained community mothers to visit families with more than one child who, although not experiencing serious difficulties, would in the view of their health visitor benefit from ongoing support. If further problems arose during the community mother's work with a family then this would be reported back to the health visitor, and there were guidelines over what community mothers should report on without losing their credibility with client and health visitor. One of the comments about the effectiveness of community mothers in this project was that the support they offered often helped to defuse family crises before they exploded. The second project reported on by Jackson was a programme that aimed to offer a community mother to all mothers in the city's Asian community for whom English was not their first language. It began because the routine health visiting service was failing to meet the needs of Asian women, largely because of the language and cultural divide.

Since these pilot projects in the early 1990s there have been further developments in other parts of the UK. Friend (1999) also showed the value of a community mothers programme in North Tyneside run to help first-time mothers and those who needed support. The training enabled the community mothers to set goals together with the first-time mother. The visits were semi-structured and they were not giving advice, the whole idea being to increase the new mother's self-confidence and self-esteem.

The original notion of community mothers arose, as has been mentioned, from shortfalls in the health visiting service. However, more recent projects have been set up for the more esoteric reason of avoiding the language and cultural divide and addressing the higher rates of perinatal mortality and low birthweight that occur in Asian babies. Criticism has been levelled at the potential for breaking of confidentiality and relationship difficulties when mother and community mother meet outside the home. However, with a good selection and training process and with fairly average rates of pay, it is likely that the 'right' women are employed in this position. Well-structured ground rules and good working relationships between health visitors and community mothers ensure that the beneficiaries are the families and children.

Suppiah (1994) uses evidence from one such research-based community mother programme to show benefits in three areas:

- facilitating empowerment
- bridging the client/professional gap
- costs and benefits.

In the first area the training encouraged community mothers to discuss with families a range of options to enable them to find solutions to their own problems, enabling parents to raise their self-esteem and avoid dependency on the community mother because they could make their own choices. In the second area, community mothers were able to bridge the gap between professional and client, being seen as 'street-credible' because of similarities in background and experience. In the third area,

although some health visitors found community mothers a threat to the notion of professional expertise, others described a sense of shared endeavour and increased job satisfaction. As one community mother wrote in *Health Visitor* in 1992, 'one of my mums said, "I like you, Donna, 'cause you're just like me – dead common."'

The non-professional position of community mothers employed by the NHS differs little from the position of nursing assistants employed in community units or acute units. They are given minimum training and are part of a team, whether a district nursing, ward or health visiting team. It is therefore difficult to understand why some health visitors (Jackson 1992) are so threatened by community mothers. In the same way, skill mix in health visiting was initially seen as equally threatening. The major question thus arises of whether health visitors are so inflexible or didactic in their work that they cannot see that partnership and support is the main benefit of any home visiting.

CONCLUSION

Each group of specialist community public health practitioners will focus on their specialism, which is drawn from different knowledge sources, to concentrate on an aspect of public health care. Using the model of public health care (see Fig. 5.1) this chapter has considered several intervention strategies for working with social groups and communities at the right-hand end of the horizontal axis. Other chapters within this book also look at working with particular individuals or groups and the reader should use this chapter to consider what intervention or psychological skills are best suited in these different situations.

Chapter **6**

Working with socially excluded groups

Joanne Davis, Helen Hoult, Marian Jones, Marian Evans and Anne Higgs

INTRODUCTION

The United Kingdom is a multicultural society which is working at ensuring equality for all cultures. Despite the fact that racial harmony can become fragmented on rare occasions, nevertheless health, social and educational benefits are available to all in equal measure. That is the theory. In practice there are certain groups who are socially excluded in society today and have limited access to health services, social services and occasionally education. Davis and Hoult have worked extensively with Travellers and Gypsies for a number of years, providing a health visiting service as effectively as possible. Jones has set up a good first point of contact system for the homeless in a hostel – people who have limited access to health primary care services because of their no fixed abode status. Evans and Higgs work on the fringes of the primary care service in providing a first point of contact to primary health care services for asylum seekers whose apparently necessary transient lifestyle creates very real inequality even on a humanitarian scale.

WORKING WITH TRAVELLERS AND GYPSIES

Joanne Davis and Helen Hoult

DEFINITION OF TRAVELLERS/GYPSIES

The definition of 'Travellers', under the 1968 Caravan Sites Act, is: 'Persons of nomadic habit or lifestyle, whatever their race or origins'. The recent Criminal Justice and Public Order Act 1994 that replaced the 1968 Caravan Sites Act adds the concept of: 'purposeful travel for economic independence and to a degree a tradition of travelling'. Okely (1983) described Travellers as: 'a self-reproducing ethnic group based on a principle of descent, with an ideology of travelling, a preference for self-employment and a wide range of economic activities'.

The Travelling community see themselves and are regarded by others as a separate ethnic group by virtue of the following characteristics:

- A long shared history, which, even though largely unresearched, can be traced back for many centuries.
- A shared set of values, customs, lifestyle and traditions associated with nomadism.
- A shared language.
- Endogamy (marrying within the group). Travellers come from a small number of ancestors. Different families are associated with different parts of the country. One becomes a Traveller not by choice but by birth.
- Self-ascription as Travellers (Irish College of General Practitioners 1995).

Travellers and Gypsies see themselves as two distinct groups in society; however, to the outsider it can be hard to distinguish them. Travellers are Irish in origin and have come to live in the UK over the centuries, mainly for personal economic improvement. They are often wrongly called 'tinkers', which, apart from being derogatory to them, is in fact a highly skilled trade and not a descriptive label of a group of people. Gypsies are English and Welsh in origin and some of the families acknowledge Romany ancestors. These Romany Gypsies can ascribe their roots directly to nomadic tribes deriving from the Indian sub-continent. However some of the English and Welsh Gypsies one meets have also become nomadic for usually economic reasons and have intermarried with Romany Gypsy families. Over the past few years it has become commonplace too for English/Welsh and Irish to marry, thus blurring the boundaries further.

HISTORICAL OVERVIEW OF TRAVELLERS' AND GYPSIES' CULTURE AND BELIEFS

There are documented records of Gypsies living and working in Britain since the 15th century. However, the Travelling population is a very complex one and to consider Gypsies as a single group of people is wrong. Today's Traveller may be descended from one of a variety of groups once important to the UK's economy. Their former vital economic role protected them to an extent from the discrimination they now face.

Despite this economic importance, during the reign of Henry VIII and subsequently, the Gypsies' nomadic lifestyle has been viewed with suspicion by the settled population. Gypsies were seen to use local resources such as land and food without the responsibility of local taxation and duties. This has a familiar ring to it, as it is this non-payment of tax that is commonly used in accusations of criminality today. Legislation under Henry VIII banished them under pain of death, thus confirming local suspicion.

This persecution, when it has suited the settled population, has continued through the centuries. In the 20th century, under the Nazis in Germany, 300 000 Gypsies were killed in concentration camps and the plight of Eastern European Gypsies is in the news today. In this country, although supposedly protected by the 1976 Race Relations Act, it was not until 1988 (Commission for Racial Equality v Dutton) that it was clarified that Travellers were not to be discriminated against either directly or indirectly. Despite these judgements, prejudice is inherent in our society.

Gypsies see this discrimination as part of everyday life. This resignation, alongside poor education, allows the media – particularly newspapers – to publish and broadcast offensive and discriminatory views. This covert and insidious discrimination is all the more dangerous because it is constantly reinforced by the state's criminalization of Traveller lifestyle and work opportunities, thus serving to convince the general population that their views are justified.

The Traveller population of Britain is impossible to assess accurately, but it is thought that there are at least 12 000 caravans inhabited by about 60 000 people. Families in Britain tend to be either Irish Travellers or English and Welsh Gypsies. Although these two groups have some cultural similarities, they also have fundamental differences and share a mutual antagonism; these occur through perceived attitudes to

each other's racial grouping. As already stated, English and Welsh Gypsies can trace their heritage back to Indian nomadic tribes and will indicate that their traditions of travelling are descended from centuries of nomadism. They criticize Irish Travellers as having less of a tradition of travelling and also as being less economically self-sufficient and often dependent on state benefits.

Naturally it goes without saying that these beliefs and antagonisms are usually founded in misunderstanding and unreliable information, and as a consequence Travellers do not have a common voice and are not a united community. As society has marginalized and now criminalized their lifestyle, they suffer discrimination and prejudice at the hands of most statutory services and so have unequal access to everything we take for granted.

The recent legislation (the Criminal Justice and Public Order Act 1994) withdrew the statutory duty of local authorities to provide site facilities for them (although they still can if they want to) and allows for eviction of camps every 24 hours, with powers to enter and remove vehicles from land. Penalties can be imposed of up to £1000 if Travellers do not leave land as soon as possible, or reoccupy it in less than 3 months. Under this legislation, penalties, if found guilty of an offence, can be a fine of up to £2500.

TRAVELLER AND GYPSY CULTURE

It is said that you cannot become a Traveller, you have to be born one. A culture is essentially a series of beliefs that are shared by a group of people and give those people a sense of belonging. A culture also distinguishes those members who share it from others. As with all cultures, there are the old-fashioned ways and beliefs held by older members of society, while young people may have different attitudes. Naturally, with television and video Travellers are not immune to the changes in our society and some of these have become adopted into theirs.

Much has been written about the Gypsies' hygiene and pollution beliefs (Okely 1975, 1983, Miller 1975, Sutherland 1987), and this is an area of academic dispute. These beliefs are based on a view held by Gypsies of there being an inner self denoting cleanliness and the secret ethnic self, and the outer self, which is *public* and the one presented to the outsider or *gauga*. These beliefs are held to be the basis of the rules about separate bowls for washing people, clothes and food. This is an area where it is easy to fall foul as a health professional: inadvertently using the wrong bowl to wash hands can cause great offence. Most families adhere to the use of different bowls for different uses. When this is discussed with them, they all say it is for preventing germs spreading or to 'be clean', are amazed to be asked and even more amazed that these rules do not apply within the settled population. None has ever mentioned views about the outer world being polluted and polluting them, and certainly none has mentioned this as being a reason for refusing immunization. It is probable that the use of different bowls is a pragmatic response to a lack of clean water and of there being many people in a small space.

The more elaborate concepts of hygiene proposed by Okely, among others, have been used to explain poor uptake of childhood immunization among Travellers. Travellers are said to see the immunization of a child as polluting the inner self with something from the outer world. In our experience, the most frequently voiced reason for refusing immunization is a commonly held, but mistaken, belief that the whooping cough vaccine causes brain damage. This is a view shared by a significant minority of the settled community. Travellers also have a marked reluctance to 'hurt' their child with the needle.

Family life is the mainstay of their culture, children being the centre of their world. The rearing of Traveller children is a curious combination of extreme indulgence in the form of material things like sweets, clothes, money, gold jewellery and lack of discipline, coupled with an acceptance of the responsibility of young children for jobs around the site, e.g. working with their father (boys) and care of and responsibility for their younger siblings (girls). It is not uncommon for girls as young as 6 or 7 to look after the baby, being responsible for feeding, clothing and changing and also playing with and comforting the child. Such types of responsibility, along with cleaning the trailer and making men and boys meals and drinks, make many child care specialists and professionals from outside the community uncomfortable, feeling that the children's own childhood is being denied. What they fail to see is the difference between Traveller/Gypsy culture and their own. The expectation of Traveller parents of their children is firmly set in the gender rules by which they themselves have been reared and accept, i.e. that boys particularly are adults by 11–12 years old and, as such, can contribute to the family economy. They thus reject education beyond that age in favour of learning their 'trade', be it tarmacking, garden labouring, tree-felling, scrap, stripping old cars or hawking. Most now accept, however, that their complete illiteracy is a handicap to modern life and want their children to be able to read and write a little. For girls their 'trade' is to be able to look after a home, cook, clean and look after children.

Much academic discussion has focused on these strongly defined gender roles (Acton 1974, Okely 1983) within the community, where the taboos about acknowledging and voicing issues of sexuality, sex education and associated issues are often talked of by health professionals as vital to both understanding and working with the community. The discussion centres on issues of social control (Acton 1994). This gender role of differentiation has been linked with the hygiene taboos previously discussed as an attempt to keep women suppressed and not a threat to men. Thus anthropological studies (Thompson 1929) talked of the 'uncleanness of women' while discussing the pollution of childbirth and menstruation. These views are probably not widely held now. It is more likely that this gender differentiation, avoidance of sexuality and the maintenance of the 'private nature of female sexuality' (Pahl & Vaile 1986) is to do with the very close and un-private nature of their lifestyle and the diminished economic role for the women outside the home. Work for Traveller men has declined on the whole with the advent of industrialization, recycling and our disposable, throw-away society, so a strengthening of the home role for women is the probable result (Okely 1983). However, both Okely and Acton indicate that this preservation of gender roles is essentially cultural and almost reinforces Gypsy culture.

This clear boundary of men's work and women's work is broadly adhered to among the community, but as with all populations there are greater and lesser degrees. We have seen trailers where 'baby' dolls have nappies firmly sellotaped to their nappy area to prevent the boys of the family seeing the doll naked, through trailers where pregnancy and childbirth have been openly discussed in front of adolescent girls, to a young couple where the father was present at the birth of his second child.

REVIEW OF THE LITERATURE

There is little published research about Traveller/Gypsies, especially with regard to their health and health care. The literature available on the subject is divided into four main areas: culture and folklore, accounts of intervention by health service personnel and epidemiological studies, reports of activity by pressure groups and charities, and discussions about the problems of undertaking research with Travellers.

There are many books about traditional Gypsy life (Sampson 1930, Kendrick & Bakewell 1995). These explore traditional Gypsy culture and the folklore that surrounds it. The majority of published literature comprises descriptive accounts written by health visitors and associated health personnel. They usually give evidence of methods and actions taken to offer health care and service access to Travellers. The accounts give details of custom and practice among Travellers with regard to health issues.

There is little epidemiological research evidence available. The best-known study is by Pahl & Vaile (1986), who looked at a group of Kent Gypsies. The study dealt mainly with women's and children's health and concluded that prenatal mortality, stillbirth and infant mortality were considerably higher than in the general population and the incidence of low-birthweight babies was also higher. The study looked at child and adult health and morbidity and concluded that the health status

of Travellers is worse than that of social class V (Registrar General's classification). The causes identified were:

- poor sites and environmental conditions
- enforced nomadism
- poor access to primary health care services and preventive health measures.

Other studies have looked at the impact of mobility on health (Durward 1990). Further studies have tried to look at child health in particular but all suffer from a lack of reliable collected data, e.g. immunization uptake (Simpson & Stockford 1979) and growth (Carroll et al 1974, Creedon et al 1975). Also, the studies are small scale and it is difficult to draw reliable conclusions from them. The same problems occur for studies of adult Travellers' health – some have looked at lifestyle factors (Wilson 1987, Crout 1988) and others at chronic disease (Thomas 1985, Thomas et al 1987). However, again these are small studies that draw few reliable or widely applicable conclusions.

Reasons for the problems with research about Travellers – which makes up a large body of literature by itself (Feder 1990) – include the fact that the population is highly mobile and is not an ideal research population. The absence of medical records and poor memory recall of illness render retrospective studies of health inaccurate and impossible to check for reliability. This makes it difficult to formally reference views about Travellers and their health and so most of the evidence given to support argument is experiential or anecdotal.

Finally, there exists a large amount of literature in the form of reports, mission statements and conference proceedings. These explore issues of relevance to Travellers' health (e.g. service provision, site conditions and provision) and make local and national recommendations about conditions that affect Traveller health.

SETTING THE SCENE

Traveller/Gypsies live in Britain in a variety of settings – on local-authority-provided sites and on privately owned sites, on both of which payment is made for rent and utilities. Others live on unauthorized encampments in fields, by roadsides, in parks and on derelict land, where they are subject to regular eviction under the terms of the Criminal Justice and Public Order Act 1994. Others live in houses, both privately owned and rented, where they maintain the culture and lifestyle of being Travellers.

Generalizations have had to be made in this section because the experience of both authors has in the main been of mobile Travellers who resort to urban areas to live. We are aware of differences in culture among urban groups and also that Travellers who live in settled rural communities and the health workers who work with them may have different experiences of health care provision.

THE RANGE OF HEALTH VISITING WITH TRAVELLERS

All generic health visitors possess and use a range of skills that enable them to successfully achieve their remit within their client group. For a health visitor working with Travellers these skills must be further complemented, refined and their presentation made appropriate so that the community is able to uptake services successfully.

NETWORKS

The overriding difficulty of working with Traveller/Gypsies is the one from which their name derives – they travel. This nomadism poses many problems for the health visitor (and this is true not only of permanently mobile families but also of those who are sited or live in houses, most of whom spend some part of the year in other areas of the country where they have connections). Firstly, it becomes an impossible task to successfully profile the caseload, although individual families can be profiled. However, it is not possible to accurately state which families are resident in the specialist's area on any particular day. Actual caseload numbers can fluctuate enormously, particularly when large groups – sometimes of over

100 trailers – move into an area for a short time, increasing the specialist's workload dramatically.

These problems are further compounded by the difficulty of rigid health authority boundaries. Unknown to themselves, Travellers cross these boundaries daily and often have no idea which local authority's jurisdiction they are in until an eviction officer arrives. Health visitors are in general unable routinely to cross boundaries. When working with the Traveller community, particularly if neighbouring authorities have no provision for health visiting Travellers, it may be necessary to cross boundaries for follow-up care.

Other difficulties faced when families cross from one health authority to another is that the authority they have left has no obligation to continue supplying services. For potentially lengthy service input such as speech therapy or physiotherapy the transfer of care to another authority would be inappropriate, families usually having moved on before further input could be arranged. This bureaucratic nightmare makes it necessary for the health visitor to be somewhat vague when asked about the actual location of the client's trailer. Individuals are usually happy to travel many miles to an appointment with a practitioner they know rather than recommence treatment elsewhere where their reception may be less positive.

Many families have no contact address and, for those that have, the address may be used by up to 100 individuals or more. The likelihood of one individual receiving their post is minimal, given that a large percentage of the community are illiterate or have very poor literacy skills, and have very similar names. It is common within Traveller culture to name children after relatives; therefore large numbers of family members of varying ages often have identical names. It is particularly important when visiting Travellers that both parents' forenames and dates of birth, if possible, are taken to avoid confusion.

With mobile Travellers not having a postal address, many use the health worker's address for the receipt of medical appointments. It is a particular quality of specialist working to acquire knowledge about family networks, and so the worker will know mobile phone numbers or relatives' contact points through which messages can be passed.

Using the specialist's address has another advantage. Travellers do not generally have tools such as diaries and calendars that are used by literate society. They have to rely upon their memories to remember forthcoming events such as appointments. If these appointments are far in advance, without any further prompt it is highly likely that they will forget to attend. Most specialists keep a record of forthcoming appointments for families and remind them, using a variety of methods, nearer to the time. It is worth noting here that some families genuinely have little idea of months of the year and sometimes even days of the week. It is not uncommon to be asked 'Which month comes before September, love?' and they almost always refer to December as Christmas month. Older individuals often do not know their own date of birth and many forget to celebrate their children's birthdays or their own – their mental calendar is very different from ours.

HEALTH CARE

Families' expectations of health care is generally low as often their positive experiences have been few. They are often refused access to services the general public take for granted such as GP services and the preventive services allied to them. Travellers tend to be led by curative rather than preventive medicine. They would not see, without input, the importance of preventive clinics but would attend for medical treatment once ill and experiencing symptoms. They very quickly attend, particularly to the Accident and Emergency department (A&E), if children are unwell or suffer accidents. Travellers tend to prefer the 'drop in' nature of A&E care as they are never refused treatment and seem to believe that hospital doctors and hospital premises, with their banks of machinery and facilities for various investigations, are much more thorough than any GP. Travellers often use A&E inappropriately for illnesses that would generally be treated by a GP, but because of registration difficulties they are often unable to access GP services, particularly in the evening or at weekends.

OUTCOMES

Audit and outcomes are phrases routinely used in many aspects of primary care, but in preventive work quantifiable outcomes are difficult to determine.

Immunization rates are the most commonly recorded outcome for health visiting activity. Health visitors with Travellers give many home immunizations; however, mobile families often move on before immunization courses can be completed – it is therefore unknown whether a child has completed the course elsewhere or not. This inaccuracy results in poor immunization statistics for Travellers, but experience shows that many families who decide to have immunizations ensure that their children receive the full course wherever they happen to be staying.

Parent-held records have become invaluable for health visitors working with this community as many Travellers are very poor historians and often, in common with many members of the settled community, have no idea what previous injections any of their offspring have received or when or where the last one was given.

A study undertaken in Glasgow in 1985 by Riding found that of 109 Travellers aged 5–61 years, who had no previous recollection of ever being immunized, over 80% had antibodies to polio and diphtheria and over 50% had antibodies to tetanus.

PARENT–HELD RECORDS

Travellers in the Black Country region have had purpose-produced parent-held records since 1990 and for new births Travellers are now given the national record. This up-to-date information allows health visitors to immunize children on first contact and complete the record appropriately for any injection or developmental assessment undertaken. The record also allows accurate chronological information to pass between professionals as many families ensure that they take the record with them to all hospital or GP appointments. Further information can also be gained easily if necessary from professionals who have previously seen an individual, using the contact numbers in the book.

ADVOCACY

Health visitors in this field need also to be knowledgeable regarding housing and benefits. Travellers are often discriminated against by staff in these departments and health visitors acting as an advocate for the client often find themselves in the same situation, at times being dealt with with cynicism and rudeness.

Travellers often find themselves in a 'trap' with regard to housing. In most areas it is local authority policy that persons applying for housing must have been resident within the borough while their application is being processed and until accommodation is offered. Mobile Travellers are constantly evicted by the local authority, who try to ensure that families move out of their borough at each eviction. Therefore Travellers who need to stay within the borough to qualify for housing with the local authority are being moved on by a branch of the very organization that insists they must reside there to qualify. Many therefore apply but fail to remain long enough to be successfully housed.

Another common problem arises when local authority housing departments cannot decide through which channel Travellers should apply for housing. Some insist Travellers apply via homeless services, others that they apply via the standard route as they are not literally homeless. However, in a letter to all chief planning officers in England (Ref: PDC 34/2/7 dated May 1998) Richard Jones, Head of the Developmental Control Policy Division of the Department of Environment, Transport and the Regions, stated that 'a person is regarded as being homeless if he or she has a caravan but no place where they may legally put it and reside in it'. This may go some way in ensuring that Travellers no longer fall into such gaps in housing policy.

The health visitor's role with Travellers is very varied. Travellers are a demanding group to work with, whose culture must constantly be considered prior to every contact.

HEALTH NEEDS OF TRAVELLERS

This section will look at the health needs of Travellers both in a private sense and in the area of public health. It will give details of some of the problems and barriers faced by Travellers concerning their health and try to show why health visitors are well placed to work with this group of people. One of the fundamental roles of health visitors is to seek out health needs and address them. To do this they must be able to use and give information and secondly to empower people to use this knowledge in their own situation in a constructive way.

Travellers as a group, with some notable exceptions, are disadvantaged in today's society. Socially they are marginalized and criminalized by legislation. Their culture reinforces this in that their first loyalty is to their family, and so Travellers are not a cohesive cooperative group and therefore are not organized to work together to improve their social standing within the wider society.

Economically they are also disadvantaged. Many traditional occupations for men have disappeared or become less financially viable (e.g. scrap dealing, labouring on railways and road systems) and many Travellers now are dependent on benefit at least for part of the year.

Educationally Travellers are disadvantaged. The vast majority of Travellers have patchy educational careers and are thus illiterate. As a group they place little reliance on written information, preferring to rely on passing information around verbally. However, illiteracy poses many problems for them when they come into contact with the settled society, where documents are regarded as evidence of existence and forms are used to access many different services.

Having demonstrated that Travellers are a disadvantaged group we can turn our attention to their health needs. Fundamentally they have the same health needs as everyone else in society. As with other groups, young families and the elderly are high consumers of health care and Travellers are no exception; however, unlike the settled community, which has an ageing population, the Traveller community is dominated by the young. Services needed range from the care of the healthy (e.g. contraception and pregnancy) through preventive health care measures (e.g. immunization and health screening) and the needs of the ill (e.g. care of minor illness in children) to the care of the chronically sick. Other commentators have attempted to quantify their needs in terms of morbidity but statistical evidence is very limited. It is thought that Travellers suffer from raised levels of morbidity related to lifestyle and inherited factors as a result of consanguineous marriages and have a significantly shorter life expectancy than the settled population. If asked about their health needs Travellers almost universally respond that their main health need is not based on what medical task needs completing but about how access to health care is achieved. This leads us on to a discussion of the public health needs of Travellers.

PUBLIC HEALTH ISSUES

The most important need Travellers have is somewhere to live. This for many would be a small permanent site where they could live with members of their extended family. Many would choose only to move off for a few weeks of each year – for work, for family reasons or just for a change of scene.

Many would not like to settle at all but pursue a mobile way of life. This involves living for short periods of time in one place while looking for work or dealing with family matters and then moving on. The most suitable accommodation for these families are transit sites or short-term stopping places.

The advantages of sites to Travellers are that they are legitimate places to camp so that:

- they are not continually evicted
- they have a permanent address from which to gain access to services
- they have access to proper sanitation facilities and clean water.

Sites also reduce the amount of discrimination and abuse suffered by Travellers from the general public when they stop in unauthorized areas. Naturally, on the other hand they reduce

the nuisance experienced by the local population. Temporary roadside sites have neither of these and so pose a health risk to Travellers and the settled population alike. For professionals working with Travellers, site facilities mean that relationships can be built up with local service providers, e.g. health centres, schools, play facilities and DSS/social services. Cooperation and communication can be improved and cross-cultural training can be given to improve understanding on both sides. It also allows resources to be targeted and used effectively. Campaigning to increase the number of sites is part of the political role taken on by specialist health visitors.

Activity is usually undertaken in three ways. Firstly, there is the development of inter-agency groups working together at a local level. These usually comprise representatives from public health, local council officers responsible for eviction, education for Travellers, health (usually the health visitor) and housing. Sometimes representatives from police and social services attend. The group seeks to influence policy changes within the local council with regard to site provision and planning.

Secondly, health visitors play a significant role in raising the awareness of individuals from many organizations with which Travellers often need to liaise. Many individuals working with statutory organizations discriminate against people whose lifestyle they judge as meaningless and it is the role of those who work with and know the community to challenge this behaviour and attempt to resolve it. Thirdly, there is a National Association for Health Workers with Travellers (NAHWT), which seeks to influence national policy towards Travellers, particularly with regard to discriminatory legislation concerning lifestyle, and planning and site provision. This group acts as a consultative body commenting on any new policy documents concerning Traveller issues.

From a public health perspective sites for Travellers would allow campaigns such as home, road and play safety to have a focus and also ensure that campaigns targeted at the wider literate population could be directed at Travellers, e.g. folic acid, meningitis awareness.

Finally, with regard to benefits, contrary to popular belief Travellers often do not receive benefits to which they are entitled, such as child tax credits, carer's allowance and disability living allowance. Many benefits to which families are entitled can be sent only to a private address, i.e. not a post office or PO box, and post is not delivered to mobile unauthorized stopping places. Some families use the address of a relative to receive post, but for some it may be necessary to use the health visitor base as a secure address through which to receive mail.

Problems with benefits are usually concerned with verification of people's identity and postal addresses; sites that have correct postal addresses would go some way to solve these problems.

BARRIERS TO HEALTH CARE

ACCESS

Having discussed the health needs of Travellers in depth, what are the problems that create barriers to health? Access to health care is regularly denied to Travellers on the grounds of having no permanent address. Primary health care is organized (usually) on the basis of GP practices covering geographical addresses and remuneration is received per head of population. After this, remuneration is given on items of service. Although temporary registration is available this may also depend on postal address. Commonly Travellers are denied access on these grounds alone. However, our experience is that there is a commonly held belief that Travellers do not accept preventive health measures such as immunization and health screening; this mistaken view discourages GPs from registering Travellers even on a temporary basis, as they believe that this will prevent them meeting targets and consequently affect their remuneration.

These difficulties with registration lead the health visitor to be frequently in contact with the local primary care trust or shared services agency requesting GP allocation forms and completing these on the client's behalf. However, when clients are allocated in this way GPs are obliged only to offer care for a minimum of 3 months, in the same way as temporary registration, and can then remove them from their list. The whole procedure then begins again.

It may be difficult for health visitors to influence this situation greatly. It is possible to visit GPs local to the newly arrived site and discuss the situation, and this can often be useful for both Travellers and GP practice alike. However, Travellers often find GPs who are sympathetic to their situation and where they receive a positive experience. They will then contact them again, as will their families and other members of their community. This usually only involves one or two practices. Consequently the health visitor is able to liaise closely and ensure that relationships are maintained and any intervention considered necessary by the GP is properly communicated to the Travellers. It is possible to maintain quite a high level of care in this way.

The major problem for many Travellers with regard to health care is their inability to register permanently with a GP. People with no permanent address are unable to register permanently with a GP, and if an individual has no permanent GP they are not issued with a medical card. Many Travellers do not realize that without a medical card they still have a right to be seen by a GP (in Ireland this is not the case, which often leads to confusion).

Mobile Travellers are generally registered temporarily with GPs for a period not exceeding 3 months. This type of registration leads to difficulties for the client as many GPs are unwilling to refer temporarily registered patients for consultant appointments and many preventive services such as cervical cytology and breast screening are regulated via the health authority, whose listings are of permanently registered patients only, thereby further denying access to services.

Travellers/Gypsies are often viewed by GPs and society in general as demanding and difficult. Practices become concerned that if Travellers are accepted on to their caseload permanently, immunization and health screening targets will not be achieved, thus affecting the practice budgets, although in our experience if

Travellers can gain access to these services the uptake rate is good.

It is too early yet to give any opinion on whether Primary Care Trusts will go some way to change this problem of difficulty of access for Travellers.

CULTURE

Within the primary care relationship, culture plays a great part and where cultures meet misunderstandings and discrimination can occur on both sides. Work with Travellers is defined by their own agenda and there are both positive and negative aspects of their cultural attitude to health. It is here that health visitors try to bridge the gap. A health visitor is the most common response by primary care trusts or shared services agencies to work with Travellers. Some work specifically with Travellers and others have some dedicated time for Travellers alongside the demands of their own caseload. What all health visitors for Travellers deal with is that they are from an outside culture working within another. It is vitally important not to lose sight of the positive aspects of Traveller culture when trying to help them access health care designed for a different culture – and in circumstances in which Traveller culture is not viewed positively by wider society.

Positive aspects of Traveller culture are based on their many strong family relationships. Most families help support each other with care of children, the elderly and the ill and would not expect statutory services to take over that role. Also, family life is the mainstay of their lives, with children being regarded as central to this. Children are thus cared for and protected by the whole community, with all members taking responsibility. Occasionally the NHS culture clashes when Travellers are not aware of the structure and functioning of health services, e.g. specific appointment times and appointments that only cater for one person, not the whole family.

Travellers also have high expectations of what primary care can offer or achieve and so are regarded as demanding of services. Health visitors are fundamental in advising Travellers of the limitations of what is possible or available and have to try to work in partnership with them concerning their health.

PARTNERSHIP AND EMPOWERMENT

These two areas of a health visitor's work – to empower clients to act independently and make their own choices about health and also to work in partnership with clients – are not easy to achieve with Travellers. Their lack of knowledge and the barriers to services that exist preclude them from exercising choices at the moment, although with continuous health visiting intervention future generations will hopefully develop these skills.

Specialist health visitors for Travellers form relationships with all members of large extended families and often find themselves working with clients in different parts of the country, especially where there is no health visitor provision. In this way influence filters through several generations and they in turn learn how to use health services appropriately and for their benefit.

As for working in partnership together, this is difficult where clients have limited skills and where the structure of services and society generally seeks to prevent it. Generic health visitors can only create limited partnerships because their contact with Travellers is usually only brief, while the camp is in their area. In this situation the health visitor usually has to deal immediately with any needs the Travellers may express.

As a specialist covering a wider area the health visitor will probably have contact with a group over a longer period. In this situation it is easier to facilitate Travellers to deal with their own health needs by giving them the information they need, paving the way with relationships and prompting them to act. As Travellers learn to function independently they carry this information and skills with them as they travel to different places.

Already discussed have been rules and regulations surrounding access to GP care, and problems when clients cross primary care trust boundaries when they move camp – particularly when being referred to secondary or paramedical care. These issues have both organizational and financial implications for shared services agencies and primary care trusts.

ETHICAL ISSUES

Finally, health visitors will face some ethical dilemmas when working with Traveller families. Certainly, many members of society would say that if Travellers settled on sites or in housing their difficulties with access to services would cease. Certainly with some families with multiple needs and difficulties health visitors would agree. This can create dilemmas when needs are apparent and cannot be met simply because of the mobile nature of their lifestyle. In this situation solutions are found by working flexibly across all agencies and also, with regard to health, across community and acute health trusts. Individual solutions are tailored to each different situation. However, only by educating other professionals across the country to respect the family's choice of lifestyle and seeking to work with them to confront these difficulties can any progress be made.

Other issues that can be equally problematic are the interrupted education of children due to mobility and the very limited play opportunities for pre-school children. Many Travellers now acknowledge that education is of benefit to their children but it is unusual, though not unknown, for children to attend school after the age of 11–12 years. Travellers tend to see the benefit of literacy rather than education in its wider sense, and Travellers alerted by visual media fear that if their offspring attend secondary education they may become involved in substance abuse, sexual abuse and other reported problems, which they view as inherent in general society. Traveller children, however, are educated for life and work from a very early age, and their knowledge of what would be deemed adult skills such as extended child care (girls) and the value and subsequent selling of scrap metal (boys) are far in advance of the average non-Traveller house-dwelling child. By nature of the limited space available in caravans and the poor environmental conditions outside, many toddlers spend considerable amounts of time confined in caravans or strapped into car seats. As a health visitor it is difficult not to acknowledge parental concerns of safety and a pragmatic approach to protecting their children but also difficult to see the curbing of a toddler's natural desire to learn by investigating his environment.

These issues of a safe place to play are hard to address. However, many permanent sites, particularly small, privately owned family ones, do make play areas available. On temporary roadside sites the situation is impossible to alter, as it would only be by the provision of transit sites for mobile Travellers where safe play facilities could be provided that any difference could be made.

SPECIALIST HEALTH VISITORS WITH TRAVELLER FAMILIES

Health visitors working solely with Traveller families are not an extravagance: it has been found that they represent value for money, for the following reasons:

- They are knowledgeable about Traveller lifestyle and culture and therefore will not offend families by asking unacceptable questions or giving inappropriate responses; in short they give appropriate care acceptable to Traveller culture.

- They become known to families, who often have had very negative experience of authority, including health care workers – they become known to be trustworthy and stand or fall by their reputation among large extended family networks.

- They act as a resource for peer groups and other professions within and outside the health service.

- They are able to carry out cross-boundary work to encourage continuity of care – they often act as a link between services that may otherwise find it difficult to locate families.

- They have national knowledge and connections with other health visitors for Travellers around the country, enabling networking and further continuity of care.

- There is evidence that if it were not for health visitors' work, Travellers would not receive preventive care such as immunization, family planning and antenatal care.
- The health visitor's role can ensure investigation and follow-up for families with specific difficulties.
- The community is receptive to health promotional ideas and again health visitors are at the forefront in disseminating this information.
- The advocacy role of health visitors is another success and applies equally to dealing with other agencies such as the Department of Social Security and housing departments, as discussed in previous sections.

At a local level health visitors take a major role in ensuring that health needs are considered before eviction of camps, particularly with regard to the access of women about to give birth to hospitals and follow-on midwifery care. Circular 18/94, Gypsy Sites Policy and Unauthorized Camping (Department of the Environment 1994), reminded local authorities of their obligations to Traveller families under other legislation such as the Children Act 1989, the Housing Act 1985 and various circulars from the Department of Education. Circular 18/94 suggests that, prior to eviction of unlawful encampments, local authority officers should liaise with other relevant statutory agencies who may be involved in these families' welfare, prior to a decision being made regarding eviction.

However, it should be noted that at the time of writing the Office of the Deputy Prime Minister is reviewing this circular (18/94) with reference to the proposals contained within the forthcoming Planning and Compulsory Purchase Bill. It is hoped that this review in consultation with representatives of the Gypsy/Traveller community and associated policy pressure groups will go some way to support better site provision for Gypsy Travellers. More

details about this process are contained within the section entitled National Policy Change.

An example of how health visitors are involved in welfare considerations prior to evictions is where families who have a newly delivered woman among them should not be evicted until such time as the statutory services have fulfilled their obligations. In practice, local authorities may request information from professionals involved with the families' care but then evict all the families in trailers other than the trailer in which the newly delivered woman is living – it is highly unlikely that this action would result in the woman staying: as the local authority is aware, she will move off to be with the rest of her extended family. This 'consideration' of health needs also applies to families with a member suffering from severe illness or in hospital or requiring other community health services, e.g. district nursing.

There are many successes at a local level that are due to health visitor intervention. Two points need to be made. Firstly, successes are local and due to personal activity; change in national policy is far harder to achieve and this will be discussed more fully in the next section. Secondly, and contributory to this lack of national success, health visitors are not well placed or supported to collect data or evaluate their activity to provide any statistical or proven evidence of the effects of their interventions nor of the health needs they encounter. Although the number of families/individuals may be fewer than those seen by the generic health visitor the actual input per capita is much higher, resulting in little quantitative data, only qualitative. This makes it difficult to present the case of Travellers as a supported argument rather than as a statement of what workers know to be true.

NATIONAL POLICY CHANGE

NEW INITIATIVES

There has been no national policy change to improve the position of Travellers in society. Indeed, current legislation in the form of the 1994 Criminal Justice and Public Order Act serves to criminalize their lifestyle further and allows harsher penalties. Legislation combined with discrimination and the cultural inability of Travellers to organize into cohesive pressure groups has prevented social change from occurring despite activity by those who work with them and seek to represent them.

Politically, mobile Travellers have no voice in that they have no vote and Traveller issues are regarded as vote losers for local councillors seeking to represent residents. It is also appropriate to mention that Travellers are not included in the national census. There is thus no information available to highlight government policy changes that may be necessary.

The above paragraphs were written in 2000. In this updated edition it is good to be able to report that things have begun slowly to change. The intervening years have seen the development of an important pressure group for national policy change for Travellers called the Traveller Law Reform Coalition (TLRC). This body comprises a number of groups who seek to challenge government policy concerning Traveller/Gypsies. Very importantly, the coalition has several representatives from the Traveller community working with it in partnership which has given it a more powerful voice, in that it clearly does represent the views of the community and goes some way to include them in the democratic process. The National Association of Health Workers with Travellers has been part of this consultation. Briefly this coalition has had several key achievements.

As mentioned in the previous section the government is reviewing Circular 18/94 with reference to the Planning and Compulsory Purchase Bill. This calls for a change in the guidance given to Gypsy/Travellers to help them identify appropriate sites for development. It calls for local authorities to identify specific pieces of land for Travellers to live on, rather than purely setting criteria for locations for Gypsy sites.

It also includes changes to planning laws, so that Gypsy/Traveller site and accommodation needs would have to be included into Regional Housing Strategy, which would then be reflected in local planning authorities' 'regional planning strategies'. These would identify the number of and location of sites in each local area. These would be the responsibility of local planning authorities in their local development documents. It is possible that this legislative change will be sufficient to persuade local authorities to allocate sufficient land for Traveller/Gypsy identified site needs.

This change in policy has been directly influenced by the TLRC and Institute for Public Policy Research publication in 2004, of a significant document, *Moving Forward*. This reported on Gypsy/Traveller accommodation. It stated that the government should urgently review the shortage of authorized sites and address the issue in terms of equality and Gypsy/Traveller human rights rather than within the criminal justice system such as antisocial behaviour and public order.

Secondly, the TLRC has sought to amend the Housing Bill to ensure that local authorities have a clear duty to provide and facilitate sites and use housing corporation money to fund them. They have joined with Shelter, the Children's Society and the Commission for Racial Equality (CRE) in order to influence this, although it is not clear whether the government will accept these amendments.

Thirdly, in support of the previous two points regarding potential legislation, 100 MPs have signed up to an Early Day Motion in the House of Commons calling on the government to create more sites for Gypsy/Travellers.

Fourthly, the Office of the Deputy Prime Minister (2003) has produced a document entitled *Guidance on Managing Unauthorized Camping*, which clearly states that all public authorities must take account of 'humanitarian considerations' before considering eviction, which must include some sort of welfare inquiry. This means that all public bodies must comply with this, for example the Department of Transport, Ministry of Defence, Forestry Commission.

In addition to these changes pushed forward by the TLRC, the CRE has published their own strategy for working with Gypsies and Travellers produced after lengthy consultation with Gypsy/Travellers and other bodies including NAHWT. Briefly it prioritizes better site provision and also promises to:

- support for the above proposed legislative changes to become law
- campaign for a fairer planning system in order to reduce the discrimination experienced by Gypsy/Travellers in trying to develop their own sites
- work to get a category for Gypsy/Travellers in the Census
- challenge legal and media discrimination of Gypsy/Travellers
- campaign on health and welfare issues.

It is impossible to predict what the outcomes of these proposed policy changes will be. However, it is clear that the issue of Gypsy/Traveller exclusion within our society is both on the government agenda and becoming part of the mainstream debate about equality.

OTHER ISSUES

The position of GPs and primary care has already been discussed, as has the value of specialist health visitors to work with Travellers. Policy makers should be made aware of the way reform of the NHS has increased the inflexibility of services, thus preventing access to secondary care by marginalized groups with no named GP. It is now difficult to achieve direct access to maternity units and other services because of financial barriers. This has removed one of the major ways in which health visitors worked to allow Travellers increased access to care, with the result that much time is wasted finding a GP who is willing to refer people to hospital.

It is clear that health visitors are the main deliverers of services to Travellers. Notwithstanding the previous discussions of how national policy towards Travellers needs to be altered in order to offer them equality of access to health care and meet their health needs, it is worth considering how health visitors alone can improve their service to Travellers.

Over the years a common response has been to take the service to them, i.e. to use mobile facilities. Although the advantage of this is that once on a site the Travellers are able to seek a service spontaneously and do not have to travel anywhere else, the disadvantages are that a full range of services cannot be offered and as a result Travellers are again not treated equally. It is not usual for these services to have a GP with them and so problems with access to primary care still exist. The other disadvantage is that often funding is removed from these facilities, particularly if there is a wide fluctuation in uptake, which naturally occurs with mobile groups.

Other changes that would improve the situation greatly would be the development of salaried GP/primary health care teams specifically employed to work with 'difficult' inner city populations. These may of course be nurse led with the advent of advanced practitioners and nurse prescribing. However, it may be that these teams/sessions are also intended for use by the homeless, mentally ill and substance dependent. It is difficult to envisage how appropriate this setting would be for Travellers, whose health needs have already been described as the needs experienced by young families with children.

Health visitor services are already improved for the highly mobile by the use of parent-held records for child health activity, and women also carry their own antenatal records. It would be ideal if Travellers could carry their own primary care records, particularly those members of the community who suffer from chronic conditions requiring follow-up and regular medication.

WIDEN THE SCOPE OF HEALTH VISITOR PRACTICE

The extended role of the health visitor to include advanced practitioner roles has already been mentioned in this chapter. Within the health visitor for Travellers network this is seen as probably the most likely practical way to improve Traveller health in the short term, notwithstanding the need to keep up political pressure for policy change. Although most health visitors have other practical skills, e.g. midwifery and family planning, it is in the area of diagnosis and treatment of minor illness that an extended role would be so useful with Travellers. Nurse prescribing has gone some way to improving their situation as diagnosis and prescribing for some minor problems, e.g. head lice, eczema, fever, is now part of everyday health visitor activity. Previous issues about funding have generally been resolved.

Advanced nurse prescribing is in its early stages and despite the obvious benefits to Travellers who do not have access to GPs there are major issues for practitioners in terms of supervision and support for their diagnosis, treatment plans and monitoring of the patients' condition.

CONCLUSIONS

Much has been written about the effectiveness of health visitors and how that effectiveness can be measured. It is extremely difficult to assess the impact of the intervention of a health visitor on parenting. As described in the section on partnership and empowerment, it is possible to be positive about the impact of health visiting on Travellers' lives and its influence across generations, with regard to health. As Travellers have more contact with health visitors influence can be brought to bear on their cultural patterns of child rearing.

In the wider population, evidence can be shown of the health visitor's impact on public health, e.g. the nutritional requirements of babies, children and their mothers, hygiene and sanitation issues, the use of family planning to space children and reduce the size of families, and more recently the campaign to reduce cot deaths. Health visitors may not have been the instigators of these campaigns and may well have not done the research but it is they who carry these messages day after day into people's homes.

It may be possible to audit a health visitor's day-to-day work with Travellers by looking at issues raised by Travellers and assessing the amount of time spent by the health visitor in dealing with problems raised by her clients. Although not designed to evaluate the

effectiveness of the role, it will demonstrate the breadth of needs met by the health visitor and highlight those issues where the health visitor is not in a position to help. It is hoped that this will show how the service is used by Travellers and what if any extra resources would improve it.

Services could further be monitored using the already existing data collection models based on ethnicity. Certainly this would demonstrate birth rates, death rates and use of secondary care services. However, Travellers are well aware of the settled population's dislike of them as a group and would understandably be reluctant to describe themselves as Traveller/Gypsy on official forms or to figures in authority. It would be unwise to expect those who complete forms with clients to decide a person's ethnicity merely on appearance or accent. In Birmingham consideration has been given to using a particular post code (e.g. B99) or even to using one nationally to encompass anyone giving a caravan site address (whether official or unauthorized), but this would exclude all those Traveller/Gypsies who use a relative's or spurious address when asked in an attempt to make services more accessible for themselves.

As previously mentioned, the CRE has made the inclusion of Gypsy/Travellers in the Census an aim.

Among public health strategists there is a debate, at present, about including ethnicity on birth registration documents. Whether this will become policy is unclear. However, the justification for this is that it could attempt to quantify the birth rate among Traveller/Gypsies and see at what rate the population is increasing. This in turn could begin to inform service planning, in particular future site accommodation, to meet their needs. As stated previously the issue of who decides the correct ethnic category at registration has not been resolved.

It is clear that health visiting practice, as with all professional practice, should be evidence based and grounded in research. It is not always possible to research or prove as fact all aspects of health visiting. As already indicated earlier in these conclusions, the impact on health and parenting of health visiting is hard to assess but should not be underestimated.

Research with Travellers has many practical problems to overcome. Briefly these are a lack of verifiable records due to problems with accurate names and dates of birth, and little opportunity for longitudinal data collection due to Travellers' high mobility. This is combined with generally poor history/life events recall by Travellers. Because of the use of family names within extended families, the possibilities for duplication of data are endless. Lastly, Traveller illiteracy at such a high rate does not allow any questionnaire-style surveys.

It should be noted here that as Gypsy/Traveller involvement with the political process (with the TLRC) has developed, there has been some criticism of how research is done 'to' Travellers, not 'with' them. It is to this end that the Inequalities Programme of the Department of Health has commissioned a large scale epidemiological study using valid and standardized measures of health status. The study also explores inequalities in health service access through service use questions followed by in-depth interviews with a subsample.

The results of this large study have provided the first valid and reliable estimate of the health needs of Travellers in England. In brief the findings have demonstrated that there are marked inequalities in health between the Gypsy/Traveller population studied in comparison with other ethnic minorities and social deprived and excluded groups. Gypsies/Travellers reported between two and five times more health problems than the other groups, particularly in relation to chest pain, respiratory problems and arthritis. The authors noted a high reported rate of miscarriages, stillbirths and premature deaths of children. Gypsies/Travellers reported very high rates of anxiety and depression, relating this to the many difficulties they face in day to day life, particularly concerning accommodation.

The report found that despite Gypsy/Travellers' evident increased health needs, they had a significantly lower use of health services; it was noted that barriers to access reported were

refusal of some GP practices to register them and also widespread communication difficulties between themselves and health workers. The report contains specific recommendations for improving the health of the Gypsy/Traveller community and mentions specific implications for both policy and health provision. The report is being considered by the Department of Health and the authors are planning publication in the medical and nursing press.

In addition to this completed study there is another being conducted by the Maternity Alliance, an independent national charity, which will report in 2005. This is looking at Gypsy/Traveller women's experiences of care during pregnancy, birth and after birth. This study has arisen following the publication of the 1997–2001 Confidential Enquiry into Maternal Deaths entitled *Why Mothers Die*. This highlighted the fact that of all ethnic minority groups Gypsy/Traveller women had the highest death rate due to pregnancy and birth-related events and that this was as a result of substandard care and discriminative attitudes towards them.

These studies will inform policy makers and service providers about the Travelling community and its health and for the first time will enable them to make evidence-based provision to meet their needs.

It is hoped that the studies will also demonstrate a community view of health and health-related topics which will also better inform those who work with them to provide appropriate high-quality health care.

WORKING WITH HOMELESS PEOPLE: FIRST–CONTACT CARE

Marian Jones

THE SITUATION OF THE HOMELESS

People become homeless for two obvious reasons: because they have lost their previous home due to refugee or financial reasons, or because they are running away from an intolerable situation. The latter applies mainly to young people leaving home because of unhappiness/abuse, or to women running from domestic violence, or to refugees who have been signed off by the formal NASS system and were free to settle anywhere in the country. The former may be those asylum seekers who have been moved on from a dispersal unit due to permission to stay in the UK, or people who simply cannot afford rent or mortgage. The charity Crisis estimates there are 400 000 single, hidden homeless people in England. This includes those staying in hostels, bed and breakfast accommodation, squats and on friends' floors (Crisis 2003).

Crisis (2003) also estimate that 600 people sleep outside in England on any one night. The government's Social Exclusion Unit estimates that around 25% of rough sleepers are aged 18–25, and 6% are aged 60 or over; 90% of rough sleepers are male.

It is interesting that most of the statistical information available is linked to the roofless homeless and there is little research available in relation to homeless people who are living with friends, sleeping on floors of bedsits and squatting in empty buildings.

Hostels for the homeless are run by local councils, who by law are required to provide temporary accommodation for people without homes; or by charitable organizations who seek to provide support and counselling for those in poverty or have drug addiction problems. Official figures suggest that there are 85 500 households living in temporary accommodation; around 5600 families with children living in bed and breakfast hotels; and 9600 families living in hostel accommodation (with shared amenities). Of homeless people, 69% are classified as white, 11% Afro-Caribbean, 8% South Asian, 8% other ethnic origin, and 6% unknown (ODPM, 2002).

Until recently the only access to health care that was available to homeless people was by attendance at the local Accident and Emergency department. As stated elsewhere (Working with Asylum Seekers, next sub-chapter), most GPs are reluctant to take the homeless onto their lists because of the transient nature of their residence and because there is usually no access to previous medical history. No previous medical history also means that a GP is reluctant to refer a homeless person on for specialist or secondary care.

HEALTH ISSUES IN HOMELESSNESS

Many homeless people have extremely high health needs, ranging from minor infectious illnesses to serious organic problems arising from substance abuse or sexually transmitted disease. Women and children fleeing from domestic violence may have contusions, abrasions or fractures. Women refugees may be suffering from sexual disease or rape trauma, or from cultural practices such as female genital mutilation. People who have been homeless for some time may have become part of the drug addiction scene or have become alcoholics. Refugees may be suffering from the effects of physical trauma, amputation or blindness. Many will have mental health needs arising from past experiences.

Research evidence (ODPM 2004a) points significantly to a rise in respiratory diseases in the overcrowding present in hostels, but this must be associated with other factors such as smoking and household income.

STRATEGIES FOR DELIVERING HEALTH CARE TO HOMELESS PEOPLE

Under a scheme for creating sustainable communities, the Office of the Deputy Prime Minister coordinates information concerning homelessness and health services. The following extract is taken from such an information sheet:

Homeless people can face great inequalities in accessing health services, yet their health often suffers from being homeless or living in poor accommodation. Moreover, poor health – physical, mental or both – can cause a person to become homeless in the first place. Homeless people may often leave health problems untreated until they reach a crisis point and then rely on treatment at A&E or will present at other primary health services with multiple and entrenched problems. If we are to tackle health inequalities and homelessness, local authorities and health services must work together, through homelessness strategies and the Priorities Planning Framework, to provide services that are appropriate and accessible. Personal Medical Services (PMS) schemes are locally negotiated alternatives to General Medical Services (GMS). They offer opportunities to provide new services to groups experiencing difficulty in accessing GMS. PMS is implemented through contractual arrangements with Primary care trusts to provide core primary care medical services to locally agreed priority groups, such as homeless people.

(ODPM 2004a)

According to information (ODPM 2004a), there are now 86 PMS schemes around the country which focus on homelessness, and successfully provide primary medical services for this group.

THE NURSE PRACTITIONER ROLE RELATED TO A HOSTEL FOR THE HOMELESS

A homelessness centre was opened in Birmingham without prior consultation or planning with service providers, and the problems of this homeless population soon became apparent to the nearby GP practice. This was a small practice of two GPs and two practice nurses. They were sympathetic to the plight of the homeless and were soon inundated with requests from a needy population in terms of health care and high social need. The practice applied for PMS funding for a full-time nurse practitioner to be based in the homeless centre. The health authority would only provide funding for a half-time practitioner. Subsequently, the volume and success of the work enabled the

practitioner to apply successfully for another 50% funding from the Birmingham City Council (Supporting People programme). The current nurse practitioner is both a trained district nurse and a health visitor.

The hostel where the nurse practitioner is based will accommodate up to 100 adults and children at any one time, and between 500 and 1000 individuals will have been resident in the centre over a 12-month period. The period of residency varies from overnight to 12 months. The average length of stay appears to be increasing due to a shortage of local authority housing.

During a 3-year appointment the nurse practitioner, in setting up her clinic, found that a high percentage of the residents presented with symptoms such as fever, headache, cold/flu, vomiting, sore throat and so forth. In addition there are other compounding issues such as alcohol and drug misuse, mental health issues, physical and learning disabilities, domestic violence and many other problems.

It is clear that to operate effectively the nurse practitioner should possess a qualification of advanced clinical skills, so that the issues of minor illness diagnosis and management can be treated without further referral. Much of the nurse practitioner's time is in offering advice, treatment, referral and support for social as well as health problems. Seventy-eight per cent of the hostel residents have taken the opportunity to register with the GP and only about 10% actually need to see the GP.

The nurse practitioner, sensitive to the many forms of questioning that residents have to endure before admission to the hostel for the homeless, does not see clients until they request the services of a GP. Once a GP is requested the nurse practitioner will see the client and begin an assessment of their identified need. However, if the client is admitted to the hostel and has already disclosed health problems then the nurse practitioner can begin to support them from the outset. In an analysis of the nurse practitioner role (Frodsham & Jones 2004), it is already clear that the identification of, and support towards these needs have had a very positive impact on several other services. Every resident is given a printout of their relevant medical information to give to their new GP when they leave the hostel, and the nurse practitioner gives them contact details of the nearest GP practice to their new address.

The nurse practitioner developed the previously set up weekly inter-agency meetings at the hostel to promote the exchange of up-to-date and comprehensive information. These meetings are attended by the nurse practitioner, housing staff, educational social worker, head teacher or deputy at the local infant and junior school, CAMHS representative, child development worker and (very infrequently) social services. Some of the comments from agency members include:

From a midwife: *She gets a complete history and the excellent information provided saves us an awful lot of time otherwise spent on the phone chasing up information. Because she has done such a thorough job we no longer come 'cold' to a client. When you are there on site on a full-time basis you get to know people much better; she has got a much more holistic picture of the residents. It has certainly helped us very much as midwives.*

From a midwife: *There is much better coordination and referral to other agencies since M took up the post. We have very restricted time with people and don't get to know the whole picture. She is very good at coordinating what happens next and planning to meet their future needs when they move on. It's very easy for people to get lost in the system and some people want to get lost in the system and away from social workers and the police. M is very good at preventing this and passing information on.*

From CAMHS: *I see M as the anchor person at the Homeless Centre, to bring everyone together. She's done a lot of networking with other agencies. She played a big part in developing the steering group for tackling female genital mutilation. At the time there were a lot of Somali families and this was an issue. M took it on and networked with other agencies to develop educational approaches with Somali mothers.*

SOCIAL WELL-BEING WORK – CHILD PROTECTION ISSUES

There is evidence (Amina Mama 1996, ODPM 2004c), that children are at risk when fleeing with their mothers from domestic violence situations. The risks that lead to high degree of child protection work by the first-contact care worker for homelessness, range from fear and anxiety in the child, through to respiratory infections from overcrowding in hostels, to adverse effects on growth and development in the child. The nurse practitioner will be notified of any homelessness involving children and has to ensure that a full history of circumstances is acquired as soon as possible. This will mean intensive work making contacts with those professionals previously involved, with the full knowledge of the mother. Any legal proceedings that have been instigated must be obtained from social workers involved and continuity of support ensured by collaborating with the local social services department.

The other important issue in child protection is that of education, and the link that the nurse practitioner is involved with in the inter-agency meetings which include local teachers is invaluable. In their report Frodsham & Jones (2004) cited the following comments from education staff:

For inter-agency working M's post is brilliant. We can point people in the right direction – building up a fuller picture of each child's needs.

We are duty bound to pass on information about children. The problem is that records don't come from the previous school because they have only been there short term. It's very difficult to track children. In particular it's hard to track Somali children because their name changes frequently. The nurse practitioner helps in the tracking process because she alerts the medical authorities in the area where the child is going or has gone.

Where there appear to be growth or development problems then the ease of referral to the GP practice ensures that, as far as possible, the child is followed up, under the suggestions of the Hall Report (2003).

FUTURE DEVELOPMENTS IN WORKING AS FIRST POINT OF CONTACT WITH HOMELESS PEOPLE

The current nurse practitioner at this hostel for the homeless in Birmingham has become very familiar with the problems she meets when working with different organizations. Most health visitors working with the homeless are involved in influencing policy in their local areas. Their public health approach enables them to be at the interface between relevant services, such as housing, environmental health and the voluntary sector, and they can be proactive in raising awareness of the difficulties experienced by homeless people in accessing both mainstream and specialist services. In terms of working with personnel in the various agencies, it is relatively easy to implement change where staff are able to work independently (in a decentralized way) of the organization. It is when any funding is involved that there is an immediate bottleneck because the decision-making process reverts to centralized control with its slow bureaucratic process. Clearly one of the important skills required is good knowledge of IT processes and immediate access to a computer which preferably can be linked with the associated GP practice.

One factor that is important in this type of role is that of support and supervision for the practitioner. The post is very isolated in the sense that the practitioner is not working in a team and has little opportunity to offload the stress that comes with working in isolation. In many cases there is so little link with the local health services that the first point of contact practitioner doesn't know which manager is responsible for her, or to whom she/he can turn to for support. Clearly under clinical leadership this is a priority in the maintenance and support this post requires.

There are a variety of different ways in which working with homeless people schemes are being run throughout the country. In some,

where the project is large enough, there will be a combination of professionals working as a team which is devoted entirely to the project. This will allow, for example, a team consisting of a worker for mental health, outreach and support workers, a nurse practitioner/health visitor, possibly a GP, a drugs worker and other combinations. This is a clear example of the use of professionals skills as advocated in *Liberating the Talents* (Department of Health 2002b).

WORKING WITH ASYLUM SEEKERS: SPECIALIST HEALTH VISITING

Marian Evans and Anne Higgs

SETTING THE SCENE

People seeking asylum arrive in the UK from different parts of the world and with very different histories and experiences. They bring with them a diverse understanding of health and health care expectation according to individual and cultural background. An asylum seeker is someone who is trying to achieve refugee status through claiming 'a well-founded fear' of persecution for reason of race, religion, nationality, membership of a social or political group (1951 UN Convention). A refugee has been granted leave to stay in the UK and has the same rights as a UK citizen, i.e. benefits, health care, education, work, etc. The asylum process is very confusing and frustrating, and both client and professional have limited control and influence.

Woodhead (2000) states that:

- Most asylum seekers and refugees arrive well and in apparent good health. They expect to find security. Asylum seekers and refugees arrive very confident and 'upbeat' and come to the UK ready to contribute to society in the hope of securing better lives for themselves and their families.

- An important minority of asylum seekers arrive in considerable distress. Some are victims of torture, seeking safety and security for their families in the aftermath of conflict or war. They may have a number of complex physical and mental health needs (e.g. amputation, bullet wounds, trauma or depression).

- Health might not be the number one priority upon arrival – housing, asylum, security, food and warmth are more likely to be needed. However, serious ill health is likely to appear as a pressing concern later on.

Home Office policy towards asylum seekers has evolved as the numbers have increased, particularly after the conflict in Afghanistan. All asylum seekers must apply for asylum immediately on entry into the UK, although in certain parts of West Africa applications from U.N. refugee camps are being encouraged. Once in the UK, the National Asylum Support Service (NASS) has contracted accommodation into which asylum seekers are dispersed around the country. The policy is to try to place asylum seekers in language clusters to enable the development of efficient language support services. Not all asylum seekers are supported by NASS: some are supported by friends or family and may find it more difficult to access some of the benefits available to them.

ENTITLEMENT FOR HEALTH CARE SERVICES

All people who have formally applied for asylum are entitled to NHS treatment without charge as long as their application (including appeals) is under consideration. NASS will issue HC2 certificates when they are being dispersed; this entitles them to free prescriptions, dental and eye examinations and other health costs. Prior to being dispersed, or if living with friends or family, they need to apply for an HC2 by submitting an HC1 form so that they can get immediate help with health costs. Since asylum seekers are entitled to free NHS treatment, they can apply to a GP to register as a patient. Asylum seekers are exempt from charges for NHS hospital treatment. It is likely that in the event of a failure to gain asylum

(including failed appeals) asylum seekers will be charged for health care as though they are private patients. For information on local provision of healthcare see references.

EXPERIENCE OF ASYLUM ON ENTERING THE UK

Studies (Woodhead 2000, Johnson 2003) have shown that asylum seekers lose control of their lives in being dispersed around the country not knowing where they will end up. Dispersal often means that the asylum seeker is forced to move away from relatives and friends who may already have settled – probably in London. Currently, on entering the UK, asylum seekers are placed in emergency accommodation or induction centres, which predominantly consist of large hostels/hotels or multi occupancy accommodation. Much of the E/A is of poor quality being overcrowded, damp and inadequate heating. Children's needs are unmet with no provision of play activities. Food provided is unsuitable to the needs of babies and young children and many are ignorant and suspicious of western foods. Hostel accommodation is probably more acceptable to UK citizens who have grown up with youth hostels and higher education hostel living. Dispersed accommodation is of generally better quality and allows the individual to purchase their own food.

Another problem arises when an asylum seeker has received a decision from the Home Office that they can stay in the UK. They have then to move out of their dispersed accommodation within 28 days and are then effectively homeless, resulting in the need to rely on homeless accommodation until such time as they can attempt to climb the housing ladder. Again, refugees find themselves sharing accommodation with friends or families, resulting in overcrowded conditions until social housing is available. There is a lack of suitable housing in Birmingham because much of it has been bought up by NASS-contracted housing agencies.

Asylum seekers are not entitled to work and welfare benefits but are supported through erratic NASS provision. (Financial support frequently fails to arrive.) In emergency accommodation, basic needs such as food, accommodation and toiletries should be provided by the hostel owner (women often have to ask for sanitary towels from male workers) but they have no money. In dispersed accommodation they receive NASS support, which is equivalent to 70% of welfare benefits.

Despite the Home Office policy of trying to keep asylum seekers in language clusters, this has become increasingly more difficult due to lack of accommodation. Communication is difficult and the quality of interpreting varies according to availability of interpreters. Some interpreters are very good, but some are young and inexperienced and lack the vocabulary to describe minor ailments, e.g. measles. Some GPs find the struggle with interpretation increasingly difficult (BMA 2004). Some practices have tried to gain access to the Language Line telephone interpreting service with concerns about the quality and cost (Johnson 2003).

HEALTH CARE NEEDS ON ENTRY

Many asylum seekers are relatively healthy on entry into the UK, although others may have experienced problems following long traumatic journeys or experienced imprisonment or abuse/torture in their home country. The average babies seem fairly healthy and are of good weight as the majority are breast-fed. Children generally appear well apart from normal childhood ailments.

Physical health issues amongst adults include amputation, abdominal pain, headache, musculoskeletal/joint pain, pregnancy (frequently as a victim of rape), sexual disease and various minor illnesses. Many have also existing diagnosed conditions and may have been without medication for some time.

Accessing services is a major barrier to asylum seekers due to communication difficulties and lack of awareness of health provision. Many are unaware of how to self-care for minor illnesses and have a different perception of illness; for example, a Somali mother was extremely anxious when her baby vomited: 'In

Somalia, he might die.' They have no facility or knowledge to purchase over-the-counter) remedies and rely on A&E for free medication.

Knowledge of sexual health issues varies according to each individual and country of origin. Most countries have limited health education, especially sexual health, and many are ignorant of safe sex practices. People from the Middle East appear to be ignorant of HIV and AIDS because it was not prevalent in their own countries. If they are aware, they think it possible to buy antibiotics over the counter, as is common in their home country, and so they think sexual infection is not a problem. People from sub-Saharan Africa are afraid that they may have HIV and either want to be tested or are wary, as they assume that it would affect their asylum claim.

The most difficult problem to deal with is mental health, as there are few mental health teams who are interested/willing to take on this type of client. Much of this is due to lack of trained interpreters and to the complex needs and extent of their problems, in addition to lack of resources The asylum process itself causes stress and anxiety and this, compounded by a history of trauma and loss, leads to further mental health problems.

Many asylum seekers cannot sleep due to flashback nightmares of their traumatic experiences. One young African man had been made to lie in a pit with dead bodies for about a week – he didn't know exactly how long because he became delirious, but 6 months later he cannot get the smell of the bodies out of his nostrils.

Finding a service to help him to deal with that is not easy.

Individuals may have been tortured through beatings, electrocution, rape or emotionally damaged by threats of harm to family, or publicly shamed. Initially, there are often no mental health concerns; problems arise when the client has settled and has the time and perhaps feel secure enough to revisit the past.

Mothers can be vague as to an infant's immunization history. For example, with asylum seekers from Africa a mother may say, 'Save the Children were doing a clinic one month so

I went there and next month I saw Oxfam doing a clinic and so I went there and we had another immunization.' Some are wary of immunizations as they were linked to abusive government campaigns.

Research (Woodhead 2000) has shown that many asylum seekers are better nourished on entry than 6 months later. This deterioration in nourishment is linked to poverty that occurs once they are in the UK and the fact that on the whole they are not global travellers and are thus unused to different foodstuffs. Western people are now global travellers but those from Africa are not aware of food types in other countries and are suspicious of trying new foods. They want comfort food, as we all do when under stress.

One mother fed her weaned child on ten packets of crisps a day because she noticed that adolescents are always eating crisps and thought this was the right kind of food.

This demonstrates a level of ignorance as one problem and a level of availability as another problem. If you are living in a hostel you have no choice in the food fed to you. The food quality may not be good, the hostel buying cheap fruit and vegetables. There are currently no food standards imposed on hostels, only the normal health and safety issues.

Many women arrive in various stages of pregnancy. They are referred directly to a midwife. They have little or no resources. Some want termination; many have had to flee homes leaving their children behind. There are also young unaccompanied minors aged 14–18 years, pregnant following rape and needing a lot of support, i.e. antenatal care, emotional and mental health support.

DELIVERY OF HEALTH SERVICES IN BIRMINGHAM

Coventry, Birmingham and Leicester are the main locations for asylum seekers in the Midlands and were the focus of a series of scoping studies commissioned by the Home Office to examine the provision of health care services for asylum seekers (Johnson 2003). Birmingham has 600 council places which are used as emergency accommodation and 3000–4000 dispersed accommodation places. The lack of racial tension makes Birmingham an acceptable city. Many other towns in the West Midlands now have a designated health care professional who is responsible for responding to the needs of asylum seekers, but there are often very different levels of response facilities available.

Primary Care Trusts have set up their own methods of handling the refugee situation. In the Heart of Birmingham there are two specialist health visitors who work with asylum seekers. They get referrals from NASS which are very inaccurate (reflected in the Woodhead 2000 report), or directly from the hostel providers and managers. The health visitors then try to see all referrals with an interpreter to sort out the issues. In Birmingham, most asylum seekers are housed in the poorer, deprived areas, where there is a lack of health care resources. Many GPs are single handed and are very reluctant to take on refugees because of lack of interpreters and the time-consuming needs of the asylum seeker. The high mobility of asylum seekers due to NASS constant movement requirements also makes it difficult to give consistent service. The health visitors work closely with statutory agencies such as NASS, Birmingham City Council, education providers (ESOL classes), the not-for-profit agencies, e.g. Refugee Council, Refugee Action, various voluntary agencies, the Red Cross, church voluntary groups, and with a broad spectrum of health care workers from genitourinary clinics to rehabilitation centres.

Following introduction of themselves and their role (usually through an interpreter) the health visitor discusses with the client their health and triages their needs. Currently in use is a medical assessment form that is available in many languages, but the Department of Health is piloting a personal health care record in some areas that is similar to the child health record. One copy is sent to the GP, one is kept by the team as a record and a third copy is given to the asylum seeker as their own permanent record. The health worker seeks information on the client's current health problems, prioritizes their needs and refers accordingly. Once the specialist health visitor has found a GP who will take them, families with children under 5 years are referred to the practice health visitor. The team often provides continuing support to asylum seekers with ongoing problems, such as physical disability, mental health problems, housing and other social problems.

CONCLUSION

Specialist health visiting work with asylum seekers is both rewarding and frustrating. Frustrations are often due to the failure of the NASS system, as already identified (Woodhead 2000, Johnson 2003, BMA 2004). The system fails everyone, individuals get lost in it, as do professionals who work alongside it, because of asylum seekers constantly being moved and therefore untraceable. This makes duty of care very difficult. It is frustrating because asylum seekers have huge needs and there are limited resources, e.g. mental health. Frustration is felt because of legislative boundaries that we have no control over.

Rewards come from being able to change or influence even a small part of their lives, meeting basic human needs – food, clothes, warmth – before we can think of other public health issues.

The skills to work amongst the asylum and refugee population entail developing a high cultural awareness based on an understanding of our own values and practices. Knowledge of culture may influence delivery of health care and the practitioner has to be adapt to meet the need. People and advocacy skills are required, as are networking skills. We need a great knowledge of service provision and how to access it. Knowledge or awareness of world and national politics and legislation is essential.

The new practitioner should be able to look at strategy as well as the holistic needs of the individual in their current environment. Working with asylum seekers demands 'going the extra mile' on their behalf, recognizing that there are some things that cannot be changed at local level.

Chapter **7**

Quality improvement through leading and managing change

Marion Frost

MODERNIZING THE NHS

The past few years have seen the introduction of many changes in the way the National Health Service (NHS) is organized. Strategic health authorities have replaced health authorities, leading to the ongoing organization and delivery of services at the Primary Care Trust (PCT) level. The Department of Health (2001f) specifically requires PCTs to develop health improvement plans based on the needs of the local community with the aim of improving health and health care for individuals and communities. The vast majority of client contact with services takes place in the primary care setting, providing both a challenge and an opportunity for health visitors and community nurses to lead and manage the changing agenda. The Health Minister, John Hutton, stated at the Chief Nursing Officers' conference in November 2002 that nurses, midwives and health visitors needed more effective leadership to enable change to happen (Hutton 2002).

In order to improve the quality of care received by clients, the government expects high national standards and a system of clear accountability as part of the clinical governance framework (Department of Health 2002b). Client and public expectations are also changing in relation to the delivery of health care. Clients are demanding accessible services based on meeting their individual identified needs, while the public expects to have a greater say in planning changes in current service provision and the development of new services. Health visitors and nurses working in the community will therefore be required to undertake a wider range of duties. For health visitors this provides the opportunity to innovate and develop the leadership and public health aspect of their role, working at the population level (Department of Health 2003b) which, for some, has been stifled by GP attachment and fund-holding. For all practitioners working in primary health care there will be an opportunity to extend current roles and, where appropriate, take on work previously seen to be the remit of doctors as the new General Medical Services contracts are negotiated.

Within the changing agenda, three core functions have been identified by the Department of Health (2002b) to form the basis for planning services across primary and community care:

- first contact assessment and appropriate interventions
- continuing care, rehabilitation and chronic disease management
- public health/health protection programmes.

While this appears to provide the opportunity for health visitors to extend their public health and leadership role, for many health visitors there will be an uneasy tension between the *Chief Nursing Officer's 10 Key Roles for Nurses* (Department of Health 2002b) (see Box 1.1, p. 11), as the emphasis is placed on the assessment and management of conditions rather than the promotion of health and the prevention of ill health.

Prior to this, the White Paper *Saving Lives: Our Healthier Nation* (Department of Health 1999c) set out the Labour Government's plans for improving health and tackling health inequalities. Nurses, midwives and health visitors were viewed as central to the public health strategy proposed as part of the modernization programme. It was recognized that implementation of the plan depended on a skilled workforce that would be able to meet the challenge of managing strategic change through acting as leaders and champions of public health, working collaboratively with all parties involved and using evidence-based practice where available.

Health visitors as public health practitioners were encouraged to work with individuals, groups and communities in their role as leaders of public health practice.

Furthermore, *Making a Difference: Strengthening the Nursing, Midwifery and Health Visiting Contribution to Health and Health Care* (Department of Health 1999a) recognizes that the changes involved in modernizing the health service require effective leadership at all levels. Specifically, professionals are needed who can inspire, motivate and empower their colleagues to achieve improvements in the quality of service delivery. This theme is further reiterated within the *Health Visitor Practice Development Resource Pack* (Department of Health 2001e), with leadership being viewed as the key to changing practice and enabling the delivery of the public health agenda. Health visitors must therefore harness this opportunity to take on a leadership role and be proactive in leading change to improve the quality of service provision and the health of those with the greatest needs. The current training of health visitors endorses this leadership role with the Nursing and Midwifery Council (NMC 2002c) requirement for pre-registration health visitor programmes, including a domain 'lead individual practitioners in improving health and social well-being'.

LEADERSHIP

In order to promote leadership development as part of the modernization agenda, the government set up the NHS Leadership Centre in April 2001 with the aim of developing high-quality leadership at all levels of the service. As well as supporting the development of leaders from both clinical and non-clinical backgrounds the centre aimed to contribute to policy development and research on leadership issues. Effective leadership was seen as being central to managing and delivering the modernization programme for the NHS.

The NHS Leadership Centre commissioned research to identify the qualities of effective leaders at the chief executive and director levels of the service. Participants were asked to focus on the future challenges facing the service, rather than identifying leadership patterns of the past. Patients and carers were also consulted about their views of what leaders do to make improvements in service provision. Over 200 people from the Department of Health, Regional Offices, Health Authorities, Acute, Combined, Mental Health, Ambulance and Primary Care Trusts were involved in contributing towards the development of the NHS Leadership Qualities Framework (www.NHS LeadershipQualites.nhs.uk). The model developed reflects the core values and principles of a leadership approach that:

- focus on patients
- create a culture of inclusion and involvement – of patients and the wider community
- empower patients and staff
- allow collaborative working – with patients, advocacy/voluntary groups and partners
- are supportive of taking calculated risks, i.e. not risk averse
- recognize that making mistakes or misjudgements is an essential part of learning.

NHS LEADERSHIP QUALITIES FRAMEWORK

This evidence-based framework describes 15 qualities to which leaders should aspire and sets standards for leadership in the NHS as part of the *NHS Plan* (Department of Health 2000c) and *Shifting the Balance of Power* (Department of Health 2001f). It provides a basis for individual and organizational assessment in a changing care environment and includes benchmarking against identified standards. Central to the leadership role is the need for political awareness, the development of a vision for the future and the ability to work across sectors in order to improve service delivery. Effective leadership is therefore considered to be central to the government's modernization programme for improving health service delivery and achieving health gain. The assumption appears to be

that leadership is a skill that can be learnt rather than an innate characteristic.

CLINICAL LEADERSHIP

Leadership is a dynamic process whereby the leader influences others in order to achieve a desired goal. Heider (1992) suggests that leadership includes learning to lead in a nourishing manner, learning to lead without being possessive, learning to be helpful without taking the credit and learning to lead without coercion. The skills required for leadership are similar to those previously identified for health visiting in Chapters 4 and 5. In essence, the main skills are:

- the ability to develop a vision
- two-way communication: the ability to talk and to be understood, and to listen
- to give encouragement to people who need it, to make them feel that their contribution is wanted and valued, thus developing a trusting relationship
- being able to build on one's strengths and compensate for areas that require improving.

Girvin (1998) explores leadership through three key interpretations: as a personal quality, as a behavioural style, as a contingency approach. Handy (1999) suggests that although each of these approaches contributes towards a greater understanding of the nature of leadership, they fail to explain the difference between effective and ineffective leadership and may be of limited practical use unless other factors are considered. He recognizes the complexity of the role and advises that how these theories are used to inform practice is more important than adopting one approach to match all circumstances.

LEADERSHIP AS A PERSONAL QUALITY

Girvin suggests that the characteristics of integrity, lateral thinking, intelligence, enthusiasm, ability to make decisions and self-confidence are often present in the individual leader but on their own do not necessarily mean that an individual possessing them is a leader.

not because of their characteristics or personalities but because of situational factors and interactions between the leader and group members. Fiedler believed that leadership behaviour is fixed and that the right style needed to be matched to the right situation. Effectiveness could only be improved by restructuring the task or changing the amount of power position of the leader. More recently, contingency theorists have concluded that leadership is a complex process and involves the relationship between the leader and the follower and the importance of needs of the followers. Bass (1990), using path–goal theory, suggests that the job of the leader is to assist followers in achieving goals and to ensure the goals are compatible with those of the organization, which fits well with the current government ethos of continuing professional development to be discussed later. The leader facilitates, coaches and rewards effective performance helping to clarify the path and acting as a source of motivation and expressing concern for employees' needs.

LEADERSHIP AND GROUP/RELATIONSHIPS THEORY

Girvin adds to above interpretations by suggesting that the relationships formed by a leader at all levels of the organization also influence the relationships with the team. Complex organizations such as Primary Care Trusts will often have a number of differing cultures and the skill of the leader will lie in the manner in which these are negotiated, particularly when change is being managed. Leaders therefore need a good knowledge of organizational structures and cultures in order to understand the values, philosophies and objectives of the working environment and to ensure credibility with the team. As new working patterns emerge within the NHS, the increase in part-time working and flexible contracts of employment may effect the team relationship and require differing responses from leaders.

Having considered these four theories, Girvin proposes the notion of choosing a leadership style once the leader has considered several factors. These include the nature of the decision

to be made, the personal characteristics of the group members, the environment in which they are working (including the organizational culture) and the understanding that leadership is about relationships and working together. Girvin then adds to the picture by suggesting that styles cannot exist without a portfolio of skills from which to draw, including:

1. having and achieving goals
2. initiating and implementing change
3. having and using influence
4. having and using power
5. taking responsibility for the growth of self and others
6. mentoring
7. having and articulating a vision
8. forging and sustaining relationships.

Clinical leadership may have interpretations such as those outlined above, but to these should be added other dimensions such as educational, political and strategic/managerial skills and the power or position of a leader supported by appropriate resources.

TRANSFORMATIONAL LEADERSHIP

According to Girvin, the concept of transformational leadership, attributed to James MacDonald Burns (1978), is gaining increasing popularity within the world of nursing. Rather than relying on rewards and transactions to generate results, the transformational leader is able to articulate a realistic and credible vision for the organization, motivating and inspiring colleagues to use their knowledge and abilities to achieve a desired goal. The relationship developed with the workforce is meaningful and stimulating, resulting in higher levels of risk taking and entrepreneurial activity which embraces a culture of change (Duckett & MacFarlane 2003). Individuals are valued and trusted and problem solving is encouraged. There is a need for the leader to understand themselves and others and to adapt their behaviour to the context in which they are leading change. However, in being adaptable, the clinical leader needs to recognize the danger of being viewed as inconsistent and insincere (Bennett

1997) and use approaches suitable for the situation, moving fluently in and out of these as the situation demands.

MANAGING CHANGE

Delivering improvements in primary care is at the heart of current government policy. For the NHS, organizational change is frequently triggered by the need to respond to challenges in the external environment. A recent major force for change has come from the government's modernization agenda with its increased demand for improving health and health care for clients and communities (Department of Health 2002b). Practitioners may experience change at a professional level, with changes in the registration process leading to new roles and competencies, at an organizational level with the development of Children's Trusts, and at the individual level by implementing and enabling change as a health promoter. Change is inevitable; the problem for practitioners is how to use change for the benefit of clients, staff and the organization. Effective management of change is challenging and requires knowledge and understanding of the dynamics of the process, including a shared vision that the benefits outweigh the costs.

THE DYNAMICS OF CHANGE – FORCE FIELD ANALYSIS

A useful model for professional practice was developed by Lewin (1951) and involved the identification and analysis of 'driving forces' which sought to promote change, and 'inhibitors' which led staff to resist change. He further suggested that the manner in which people responded to change depended on the relative strength of the 'driving forces' and the 'inhibitors'. Applying this model to leadership issues, a 'driving force' for change could be a transformational leader with a vision that motivates staff such as enabling the development of the public health role of the health visitor through consultation and the support of a skill mix workforce. Conversely, an authoritarian management style could be an 'inhibitor' when trying to change health visiting practice if skill mix working is imposed on a health visiting workforce that is concerned about accountability issues and the loss of health visiting posts.

Hyett (2003) reports on some of the factors that block health visitors from taking on a leadership role, including limited resources, high vacancy rates, working independently and crisis management. She suggests that health visitors need to move away from working independently and work in teams which share the vision and goals of the PCT. However, the goals of the PCT may be based on a medical model of health which conflicts with the preventive philosophy of health visiting practice.

RESISTANCE TO CHANGE

Change is often resisted at the individual and the organizational level for many reasons, in spite of potential benefits for clients, carers and health service staff (Bennett 1997, Mullins 1999). For health visitors this may include:

- Feelings of insecurity generated by the proposed change.
- Disruption of the existing status quo.
- Threats to individual status such as the loss of professional titles, with a new emphasis on a flexible team approach to meet the needs of clients.
- Disruption of familiar work patterns such as the introduction of skill mix, with support workers, health care assistants and registered nurses being part of the health visiting team.
- Loss of competence, loss of self-esteem, having to learn new skills such as nurse prescribing.
- Group norms that oppose change and perpetuate traditional practice that may not be evidence based, such as routine developmental checks.
- Resentment over lack of consultation.
- New ways of working may mean old ways become redundant. Organizing workloads on a corporate basis may replace individual caseload management by health visitors. This

may lead to a sense of loss as the concept of 'my clients' is challenged as work is delegated on a priority basis.

Lewin (1951) proposed that three phases needed to occur as part of the process of overcoming resistance to change:

- *Unfreezing*. Reducing the behaviour and factors that inhibit change, and strengthening the drivers.
- *Movement*. Develop new attitudes and implement change.
- *Refreezing*. Establish and stabilize new norms and practices.

While this model acknowledges the dynamic nature of the planned change, factors such as the cost of the process and whether the change is a worthwhile undertaking also need to be considered. Hyett (2003) views empowerment as central to the process, enabling health visitors to believe in their ability to instigate and manage change. A transformational style of leadership is proposed which recognizes the servant–leadership model of working, whereby staff move between being leaders and active followers to meet the demands of the task.

An important priority is to create an environment of trust and shared commitment through encouraging staff to participate actively in the decision-making process. Staff are more likely to feel valued and respected if their ideas, innovations and relevant experiences are used to plan and drive the change process. It is therefore essential to consult with those affected by the change before it happens, however time consuming this may be. People need to understand the benefits of the proposed change and take ownership for its implementation. Benefits must be seen to outweigh the costs. In order to motivate those involved with the change, there needs to be a clear and shared purpose with feedback systems to monitor and evaluate the consequences of the change.

MOTIVATION

Encouraging and motivating practitioners to change the manner in which a service is delivered to clients or embracing new ways of working can seem to be an enormous and complex task. Herzberg (1966) suggests that there are motivating factors which may lead to greater job satisfaction and involve such factors as recognition and responsibility, and hygiene factors such as pay and working conditions which, if lacking, can lead to dissatisfaction. An increase in the strength of motivating factors is thought to significantly improve performance. The value of this theory is that it reminds the leader that enabling workers to influence and direct change is more likely to lead to job satisfaction and end in a successful outcome. Handy (1999) also suggests that it is important for the leader to understand how individuals perceive themselves within the work environment and the direction in which they want to progress. Many of the changes within the NHS, such as clinical governance, have been imposed from above and there is a danger that people get left behind.

STAGES IN IMPLEMENTING A CHANGE IN CURRENT SERVICE PROVISION TO CLIENTS

In considering the priorities for change, the Department of Health (1998a) made the following statement: 'It will be important not to let change overwhelm us. The philosophy will be to take it one step at a time: plan the pace of change and prioritize and understand that the aim is evolution not revolution.' A SWOT analysis can be a useful tool for identifying attitudes, motivations and spheres of influence (Swage 2000). Strengths and weaknesses are identified in relation to both the current and desired ways of working, and the opportunities and threats are considered which are likely to influence the change process. Useful questions to ask include:

1. What are the main issues to be addressed?
2. What needs to be done to achieve the change in practice?
3. What are the strengths of the current service provision that can be built upon?
4. What are the weaknesses that need to be tackled and changed?

5. What opportunities are there to support and develop?
6. What threats must be counteracted or minimized?

Firstly individual and community needs should be identified and the availability and effectiveness of resources assessed. Professionals working at the front line need to question whether their knowledge and skills are being used appropriately and whether the service provided is effective in promoting the health of the local population.

Consultation with, and involvement of, service users is central to current government policy (Department of Health 2002b, 2003b). Users and carers as well as front-line workers should identify gaps in local service provision. Leaders need to ensure that all staff are trained and supported in working effectively with the public. Working closely with such organizations as Patient Advice and Liaison Services (PALS), Volunteer Service Managers (VSM), patient/client forums and lay members of PCT boards is an essential part of the change process. A shared vision should be developed that takes into account the local health issues identified by professionals and actual, and potential, service users, and considers how health inequalities could be reduced in line with government targets and PCT policy.

Once key stakeholders agree the vision, factors that will aid the implementation of the change must be identified and strengthened and obstacles minimized. Changes need to be managed in stages with careful evaluation and adjustments. An essential part of the process is to develop effective communication channels to keep people informed of progress. The impact of the proposed changes on the local community and staff should be carefully analysed. The aim is to achieve a 'win–win' situation with benefits for all parties. Change is often a stressful process and it is therefore important to be realistic and keep changes at a manageable level.

Finally, when the change is established it is essential to maintain support from clients, the community, other agencies and sectors, the PCT and other interested parties. Results of the evaluations need to be responded to and practice improved accordingly, with progress reports being disseminated to all concerned.

PROJECT DEVELOPMENT AND MANAGEMENT

As well as managing a change in current service provision, leadership skills will also be required to develop and manage specific projects that ultimately result in health gain and tackle inequalities in health. Projects are frequently time limited and resources allocated accordingly. There is a pressing need for project work in relation to health needs assessment, collaborative working, human resource management, setting quality standards for practice and implementing research studies, as well as developing the use of information technology. The writing of a project proposal follows similar guidelines to a research proposal. It is important that proposals are characterized by succinct and unambiguous writing to give the sponsors, stakeholders and team members a clear picture of what is to be achieved. Roberts & Ludvigsen (1998) have put together a useful and simple text containing tools and case study examples for carrying out project management in health care, and this is recommended to readers.

The six stages of setting up a project are:

- *Stage 1*. Developing a project idea
- *Stage 2*. Bringing together an appropriate team to implement the project
- *Stage 3*. Planning the project
- *Stage 4*. Implementing the project
- *Stage 5*. Completing the project
- *Stage 6*. Evaluating the project.

STAGE 1: DEVELOPING THE PROJECT

Most projects will be based on some evidence of need or as the result of a feasibility study or strategic planning meeting. It is important that as much data or literature evidence is gathered as is possible and that this is closely examined to judge its reliability and validity. As in research proposals the clarity of the research question is all important, so in project development the clarity of the aims is critical. In the early stages the project team may be small but as the project develops it may be necessary to bring in particular expertise and collaborate more widely across different sectors and with a variety of agencies.

The position of stakeholders, particularly clients and carers, needs to be carefully considered in order to prevent failure at a later stage. For example, if they are clients or the local community, they will need to be involved at the development stage. If they are providing funding, then early identification of the resources required and inclusion in the key stages will be essential. Similarly, if the project involves changes in work patterns or responsibilities, then the staff affected will need to be involved from the outset.

STAGE 2: BRINGING TOGETHER THE TEAM

- The project leader must have credibility through adequate seniority within the organization, and have the support of management.
- The sponsor who is funding the project may, for example, have put the project out to tender, or the project team may have applied for funding from various sources.
- The stakeholders may be staff, service users/carers or other interested parties, or suppliers of materials or technology.
- Partners, e.g. the PCT or a charitable organization, might be contributing funding, expertise or resources.

Team members are usually selected for their skills, enthusiasm, motivation and drive, and possibly for their technical expertise. The team should have identified roles and responsibilities and there needs to be good communication channels. The project team may have a steering committee that is able to approve decisions and progress the work of the team.

STAGE 3: PLANNING THE PROJECT

In-depth sharing of ideas may be facilitated by an 'away-day' to encourage focusing on the task in hand and allow team members to get to know each other. The project aims, objectives and outcomes should be determined at an early stage and a time-scale set. Tasks should be identified and allocated in the early planning stages, taking into account staffing issues and possible training requirements.

Costs and resources must be identified at this stage, as will the need to ensure quality of the project design and its strategy for evaluation. It is essential that all stages of the planning and implementation of the project are clearly documented and that team members and key personnel have access to reports. Feedback from team members is an essential element of the process and this must be clearly documented and scrutinized for appropriateness in relation to the original aims and objectives.

Another important aspect to consider at the planning stage is dissemination of the results of the project. This may occur at regular intervals, by means of a newsletter for example, or at a more formal event such as a conference or workshop. The aim is to share good practice and prevent duplication of work and consequent waste of resources.

STAGE 4: IMPLEMENTING THE PROJECT

The better the planning the more likely it is that the implementation stage of the process will run smoothly. The leader must have good control of the process and be able to see the whole picture, comparing this with the original plan and checking for any discrepancies. If problems arise, action needs to be taken as soon as possible and the relevant people consulted if any changes are required.

Control of a project involves time management, resource and cost management, quality management and human resource management. Contingency planning is also important in terms of what to do if something goes wrong, e.g. if materials requested do not arrive on time or if someone withdraws from the project team.

A good project leader recognizes that there will be fluctuations in the speed of implementation of the project. Communication skills are essential to keep the team involved, motivated and supported. The project leader must be mindful of the stress that change can bring and needs to monitor team members. In addition, project leaders need to have a highly developed sense of self-awareness, recognizing their own personal traits and the effect that these may have on other people. People management may also mean conflict management and this is essential to good project leadership. Above all, the ability to listen to people involved in the project, be they stakeholders or team members, and hold an unconditional positive regard for each individual will help to carry the work forward.

STAGE 5: COMPLETING THE PROJECT

This involves pulling together all the information, ensuring that the aims and objectives have been met and that the planned outcomes have been delivered on time. All documentation must be up to date so that an evaluation can be made and also that standards and quality can be shown to have been met. The process of dissemination should be planned into the programme at the relevant stages of the project.

STAGE 6: EVALUATING THE PROJECT

Many projects have evaluation built into the implementation process. The evaluations can be drawn together to form a summary report. The team may wish to put together a report on the process of the project and their roles within it. Stakeholders, including service users and their carers, should be canvassed for opinions using questionnaires, interview schedules or focus groups.

A useful framework, originally developed by Donabedian and adapted by Maxwell (1984), can be used as an evaluation tool:

- *Relevance*. What was the rationale for developing the project?
- *Accessibility*. Was the project accessible for the target population in terms of location, timing, staffing, culture, language etc.?
- *Effectiveness*. Did the project achieve health gain for the target population in the short and long term?
- *Acceptability*. Were the expectations of the target population met?
- *Efficiency*. Were the benefits acceptable in relation to the costs incurred?
- *Equity*. Was there a fair share for all of the target population?

Evaluating practice is an essential part of the learning process for the project leader and team and is the key to developing and improving services, ensuring that they are accessible and acceptable to the public. Project management and change management occur within a culture of clinical governance that places the responsibility for the quality of care within the NHS at both the individual and organizational level.

LEADING AND IMPROVING QUALITY IN PRIMARY AND COMMUNITY HEALTH CARE

CLINICAL GOVERNANCE

A key aspect that needs to be considered by leaders and all concerned in the management of change in the NHS is the ultimate aim of improving the quality of client care. Central to the government's vision of modernizing the NHS is a framework of clinical governance to improve quality and safeguard high standards of care. Evidence of significant variations in client care, including a postcode lottery, medical and nursing errors and poor standards of care, have led to the need for a culture change that transforms the way in which clinical care is provided (RCN 1998).

Clinical governance is defined as 'a framework through which NHS organizations are accountable for continuously improving the quality of their services and safeguarding high standards of care by creating an environment in which excellence in clinical care will flourish' (Department of Health 1998a).

The principles of clinical governance apply to all those who provide or manage client care services in the NHS, both in the hospital and community.

The requirements of clinical governance are backed by the new statutory duty of quality which is placed on NHS trusts and PCTs. In essence, the three aspects of clinical governance are:

- setting of clear standards
- delivering of these standards locally
- monitoring the standards.

As part of the arrangements for clinical governance, chief executives of PCTs are legally responsible for clinical quality and the various components that come together under the governance umbrella. The government requires all professionals involved in health care organizations to work together in multidisciplinary teams and across organizational boundaries to improve clinical effectiveness in a client-focused manner. The emphasis is on partnership working, with clients being viewed as central to the process of clinical decision making and service planning. The use of evidence-based practice where available is central to the process. There is a requirement to develop local information and organization information systems to aid standard-setting and to collect data to demonstrate improvements in the quality of care and services (see Chapter 15). Clear policies must be put in place to manage and reduce risk where appropriate, recognizing that 'risk taking' is often an essential part of the change process. Poor performance must be addressed within a 'no-blame' culture which enables practitioners to learn from mistakes and encourages continuing professional development. While the role of the leader/manager is to provide a supportive environment which embraces the new culture, the responsibility of practitioners is to be accountable for their own practice and participate in continuing professional development.

Two statutory bodies have been set up to support the clinical governance agenda. Firstly, the National Institute for Clinical Excellence (NICE), which came into existence in April 1999, has the responsibility of developing standards for a National Service Framework (NSF) to specify the manner in which particular services are to be provided. The first framework in place was for coronary heart disease (CHD), which was originally brought to public attention when Townsend et al (1988) demonstrated the

inequality of service provision between the north and south of England. Estimates at that time were made of the potential for complete recovery from coronary thrombosis for sufferers in the south as against the north, including such variables as: economic equality; dietary equality; emergency care, including ambulance service response; and subsequent clinical care and aftercare. It was clear as a result of these estimates that there was a marked inequality in delivery and care, and epidemiological studies of non-infectious disease show clearly that coronary heart disease is one of the most preventable and treatable diseases. To date, NSFs have also been developed for cancer, paediatric intensive care, mental health, the older person and diabetes, medical and children, young people and maternity services.

The expectation of NICE is to draw up and issue scientifically based guidelines to doctors and other health professionals, setting out the best treatment options for patients using the best available evidence. This whole concept is a massive undertaking and culture change. Indeed, although quality assurance mechanisms and health care quality standards have been in place for many years, imposing the legal responsibility on NHS trust chief executives requires the setting up and maintenance of effective systems and standards of care management and measurement. When setting standards there are always concerns about their underlying basis and the motives of those setting them. Economic constraints have been cited as reasons for deliberately setting standards that are easily achievable, and this should be minimized by ensuring that all interested parties, professional and consumer, have a voice to ensure that appropriate targets are set and met.

The second statutory body, the Commission for Health Improvement (CHI) (now the Healthcare Commission), was set up during the period 1999–2000, and has conducted a rolling programme of visits to each organization in the NHS to check that the systems for ensuring quality are in place. CHI has been responsible for monitoring the implementation of standards such as the NSFs. Each health care organization has been required to produce an annual clinical governance report. As with other government measurement mechanisms, the Department of Health has used these to publish 'league tables' for different aspects of care quality. The main problem is that they tend to focus on short-term successes and, as the health visiting profession is well aware, most of the value of preventive work is long term. This points to the need for health visiting to explain and demonstrate the effectiveness of long-term preventive health care and to be party to devising its own standards and measures/indicators of quality.

The new Healthcare Commission (Commission for Healthcare Audit and Inspection) covers both the NHS and the private and voluntary sectors, taking over the duties of CHI, the health care part of the National Care Standards Commission work, and the NHS national value for money aspects of the Audit Commission's remit. It aims to improve care for all patients and will inspect services, review performance and publish the results. Sir Ian Kennedy, Chair (2004) stated, 'when care is good, we get out of the way, but when we have concerns, we can address them quickly and effectively. We will work alongside others who share our purpose – to promote improvements in health care – so that we can pool our knowledge, coordinate our reviews and reduce the burden of regulation on staff who actually care for patients.' How effective it will be remains to be seen.

CLINICAL EFFECTIVENESS

The NHS Executive defines clinical effectiveness as 'the extent to which specific clinical interventions, when deployed in the field for a particular patient or population, do what they are intended to do, that is, maintain and improve health and secure the greatest possible health gain from the available resources' (NHS Executive 1996). In nursing disciplines the most commonly quoted definition of clinical effectiveness is that of Kitson: 'Clinical effectiveness is about doing the right thing in the right way and at the right time for the right patient' (RCN 1996). To the above definition can be added 'at the right price'. All health service professionals are aware of the negative results of rationing of

health care although the reality is that resources are constrained by finite budgets. As part of clinically effective practice, health visitors and their leaders should influence policy decision making to ensure that service provision and resource planning are based on best evidence of need.

Clinical effectiveness has three main approaches:

- *Inform* describes the sources of information available and what is being planned for the future to make information more readily accessible.
- *Change* describes and suggests ways in which changes to services can be encouraged, based on well-founded information about effectiveness.
- *Monitor* describes ways in which changes to services can be assessed to show that change results in improvement.

If evidence-based health care is to dominate then it has to combine evidence for intervention with client preferences and clinical/practitioner expertise. Evidence for intervention may come from a variety of sources, including research publications and guidelines of protocols. Good-quality guidelines, recommendations and policy for good practice should all indicate the source of the evidence on which they are based and who agreed it. Client preferences can stem from a variety of experiences and influences in context and are the least controllable of the three factors. Clinical and practitioner expertise comes from best-practice information and experience but skilfully modified to the context.

Clinical audit may identify areas where practice needs to be altered to improve clinical effectiveness and the original practice can then act as a baseline against which change is made. If areas of practice require examination then the issue becomes a researchable question and action research in practice becomes the reality. This reality is then a clinical effectiveness cycle (Fig. 7.1).

Dissemination of good practice is also an essential part of clinical effectiveness and should be encouraged and supported by leaders. Health

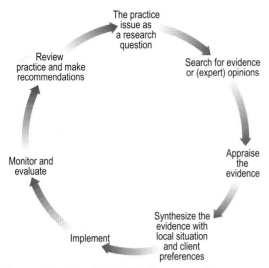

The practice issue as a research question

Search for evidence or (expert) opinions

Review practice and make recommendations

Appraise the evidence

Monitor and evaluate

Synthesize the evidence with local situation and client preferences

Implement

Figure 7.1   The clinical effectiveness cycle

visitors are becoming increasingly involved in innovative outreach programmes and activities that are clinically effective and fairly easily evaluated. It is essential for health visitors to recognize that they have a responsibility under clinical governance to disseminate their results. Many leaders/managers value and support the good practice and innovations carried out by their staff, recognizing how it reflects on the organization and that job vacancies may be fewer where staff are encouraged to develop such skills. The development of information technology through electronic means should be recognized as an important mechanism whereby dissemination of evidence-based effective practice can take place. The development of websites such as http://www.innovate.hda-online.org.uk have done much to help disseminate new ways of working, enabling practitioners to learn from each other. As well as this national resource, many PCTs are recognizing that by developing and using their own website they are in a position to act as role models for others, thus saving time and preventing 'reinvention of the wheel'. All health visitors should have access to a well-resourced, accessible library with electronic searching facilities for staff and student use, in order to:

- keep up to date with journal articles and new texts, particularly electronic journals

- access important sources of material such as nursing databases, PubMed or the Cochrane database
- access Department of Health command papers, health service circulars, health service guidelines and local authority circulars.

The availability of information is crucial for the implementation of clinically effective practice. Leaders and managers must influence organizations to develop cultures that support learning and inquiry in order to improve the quality of care for clients.

EVIDENCE-BASED PRACTICE

Changing the way care is delivered has become an increasingly important part of the clinical governance agenda and a challenge for all leaders and managers. Evidence-based practice is based on the notion of rational decision making and involves 'finding, appraising and applying scientific evidence to the treatment and management of health care' (Hamer & Collinson 1999). The implications for the leader are to ensure that evidence-based practice is used where available, to act as a role model to motivate staff and to ensure that staff are appraised and updated on current changes in practice. The setting up of the National Institute for Clinical Effectiveness (NICE) to give a strong lead in clinical and cost-effectiveness by drawing up guidelines has created a momentum within all the professional disciplines working in the NHS. In ensuring consistent access to services and quality of care right across the country, the aim of the National Service Frameworks is to bring together the best evidence of clinical and cost-effectiveness, with the views of service users, to determine the best ways of providing particular services.

The work of Sackett et al (1997) has raised awareness of the importance of recognizing different levels of medical evidence and Table 7.1 provides a useful guide for professionals. While randomized control trials (RCTs) are viewed as the 'gold standard', Le May (1999) warns that it is important not to ignore other sources of evidence used to inform practice and, in reality, affect decision making. These include:

- evidence from research, both published and unpublished
- evidence based on experience from reflection-on-practice
- evidence based on theory that is not research based
- evidence gathered from clients and carers
- evidence passed on by experts, including Delphi surveys
- evidence based on policy directives.

Evidence-based practice is important for the NHS in that it should enable greater consistency in decision making, reduce variation in service delivery, promote cost-effectiveness and accountability to the public for the service provided.

In a summary of a systematic review of health visiting (discussed in Chapter 4) Robinson (1998) consistently found weaknesses in studies available for meta-analysis using RCTs. This was mainly due to the small size of the studies, giving them insufficient research power, poorly documented randomization, insufficient reported detail to allow meta-analysis, and non-blinded assessment of outcomes. Controlled trial research deals only with outcomes, whereas much of health visiting work is associated with processes and this results in many studies being inappropriate as evidence unless they are more rigorously constructed and better documented.

Table 7.1 displays the obvious medical underpinning for graded evidence and the science of the medical research approach is clearly acknowledged. However, as level III shows, well-designed studies rooted more in the field of sociology are also important additions to research evidence. Health visitor students typify much of the nursing profession approach by using, or developing proposals that use, survey methods to collect attitudinal, biographical and demographic information and the tools are usually questionnaires, interviews or observation. Qualitative methodology is of great value provided that the sampling techniques are rigorous. There is little problem in accepting surveys as a methodology. It is essential that

Table 7.1   Definition of levels of evidence

Level	Descriptor
Level Ia	From a meta-analysis of randomized controlled trials (RCTs)
Level Ib	From at least one RCT
Level IIa	From at least one well-designed controlled study without randomization
Level IIb	From at least one other type of well-designed quasi-experimental study
Level III	From well-designed non-experimental descriptive studies, e.g. comparative studies, correlation studies, case–control studies
Level IV	From expert committee reports or opinions and/or clinical experience of authorities
Level V	From a meta-analysis of observational studies (an observational study is classified as level III but where the research question is best addressed by a cohort study then systematic reviews of valid, relevant cohort studies match level I evidence)

the aims are clear from the outset and that the study design is focused in every stage of the methodology, including decisions about sampling, size, the techniques by which subjects will be allocated to a group, how the intervention will be introduced, statistical applications required and the methods for evaluating the outcomes of the study. Any limitations must be critically discussed.

Clinical trials in medicine almost always embrace a drug or equipment trial but there is no reason why clinical trials in health visiting should not embrace a supportive or educational procedure. An example of this is a health visitor who offers intervention to a group of fathers who have postnatal mood-lowered partners and compares the EPDS scores against a control group of similar postnatal mothers whose partners have not elected for/been offered health visitor support. It is not necessary for any of these studies to include very large sample sizes because the use of meta-analysis can combine the populations and findings of many trials, provided that the design and documentation have been meticulous.

Nursing, midwifery and health visiting professionals aspire to deliver research-based knowledge, information and advice to patients and clients as required by the NMC Code of professional conduct (NMC 2002a). In the past, many nursing and health visiting practices were based on experience, tradition, intuition, common sense and untested theories (Burrows & McLeish 1995, Hunt 1996, Kitson et al 1996). French (1999) argues that evidence-based practice needs to be evaluated and validated in the practitioner's own context whenever possible, therefore undertaking 'small-scale' rigorous research projects in the practice setting.

Upton (1999) considers it difficult to achieve evidence-based practice if there is a theory–practice gap in nursing, but French (1999) suggests that a significant attribute of the concept of evidence-based practice is the focus on the practitioner's own experience and the practice context, and that this is important in minimizing the theory–practice gap. In essence, he says, the 'evidence-based practice' approach to research is determined by the practitioner researcher's personal judgement regarding the aims, relevance, feasibility, constraints and significant variables associated with the particular research issue. Much of the blame for the difficulty that nursing has in using evidence-based practice Upton (1999) places firmly at the door of education programmes.

Action research has become more commonly used in nursing and health visiting research and has its theoretical basis in experimental design, in that the practitioner undertaking the research makes a change and then sees what occurs. Much of this happens in direct work with clients when the health visitor and the client work in partnership by making a change and observing the results. This particularly occurs in behaviour modification of a young child, when various approaches are tried using a quasi-controlled approach to find which one is the most effective. As with any partnership, the recording of changes is of great importance, both from the viewpoint of communication and also

as an essential feature of action research. Action research involves working closely and actively with groups to identify problems, implement solutions and evaluate their effectiveness as part of a cyclical process. It must include negative as well as positive outcomes.

Changing to evidence-based practice is critical for improving the care of clients. Promoting a change in culture from traditional practice to one in which the philosophy of evidence-based practice is accepted and promoted continues to raise concerns for practitioners. A current example is the Hall Report (Hall & Elliman 2003), which has challenged the evidence base for some of the child development surveillance programmes carried out nationally by health visiting teams. Critical appraisal of the report and support in changing practice are required in order to ensure clinical effectiveness in practice.

CLINICAL AUDIT

Audit is a means of identifying whether clinically effective service provision is taking place and seeks to improve the quality and outcome of client care. It is a necessary part of evidence-based practice as it measures whether set standards are being met. The results may confirm the consistent use of best practice or identify poor-quality care. There should be three continuing objectives:

- to continually improve overall standards of clinical care
- to reduce unacceptable variations in clinical practice
- to ensure the best use of services so that patients receive the greatest benefit

and care provided should be

- appropriate – to people's needs
- effective – drawing on the best clinical evidence
- efficient and economic – to maximize health gain for the population.

Quality mechanisms and total quality management have been part of the NHS for several years. Kogan & Redfern (1995) draw together some of the aspects of the early work of

Donabedian (1980) in analysing health care quality, as follows:

- Goodness of technical care, which refers to the effectiveness of health care, its ability to achieve the greatest improvement in health status possible within the conventional wisdom of medicine, i.e. of science, technology and clinical skills.

- Goodness of interpersonal relationships among those involved in health care, in particular the relationship between the service user and the provider (therapist, nurse, doctor, other health care professional); thus an important aspect of high-quality care is that patients are treated with respect and their autonomy and interests are safeguarded.

- Goodness of amenities, which refers to creature comforts and aesthetic attributes of the health care setting. These can be difficult to distinguish from interpersonal care because privacy, courtesy, acceptability, comfort, promptness and so on are relevant to amenities as well as to interpersonal relationships.

Donabedian emphasizes the inextricable intertwining of these components, thus demonstrating his appreciation of quality as a whole entity.

A SIMPLE QUALITY AUDIT IN HEALTH VISITING

In its simplest form, clinical audit is about assessment, planning, implementing and evaluating (APIE), and most health visitors will recognize that this was the basis on which the nursing process was first premised. Indeed, readers of the record-keeping section in Chapter 15 will note the quality process in the SOAPIER mnemonic that Charles uses in her record-keeping standards. The nursing process was originally devised as a problem-solving cycle but in addition lends itself to an audit process, as in Figure 7.2.

This is insufficiently rigorous to act as an audit tool as it stands because there are no standards identified and it assumes an ability to

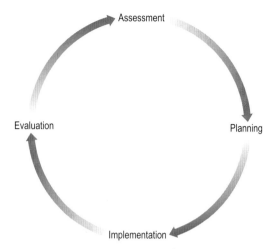

Figure 7.2   The nursing process/care plan

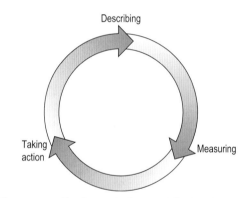

Figure 7.3   The Dynamic Standard Setting System

identify a problem, so that it is not possible to measure any quality performance.

To set quality standards many health visitors have been involved in a process called quality circles, which has the following basic steps:

- select a topic of relevance
- select indicators of quality for the care
- develop criteria and a level of acceptable performance
- identify standards for each criterion.

In 1990 the RCN published the Dynamic Standard Setting System (DySSSy) which is a cycle consisting of three elements (Fig. 7.3). However, the process is not as simple as Figure 7.3 suggests because each of the elements has

Table 7.2   Components in a quality cycle (RCN 1990)

Element	Component
Describing	Select a topic for quality improvement
	Identify a care group
	Identify criteria in relation to Donabedian's structure, process and outcomes definition
	Agree the standard
Measuring	Refine the criteria
	Select or design an audit tool
	Collect data
	Evaluate the data
Taking action	Consider action to be taken
	Plan the action
	Implement the plan
	Audit

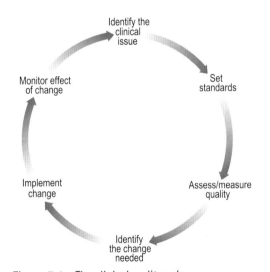

Figure 7.4   The clinical audit cycle

several components that must be achieved before an element can be completed (Table 7.2).

Audit is a critical element of the quality cycle and is the catalyst for changing practice. It is essential that planning for improvement, taking action and evaluating the results of that action must follow the audit process (Fig. 7.4).

> A trust in the West Midlands was required as part of its purchaser/provider contract with the health authority to set breast-feeding rates as an impact measure of health visiting (i.e., a clinical audit of the effectiveness of health visiting in relation to breast-feeding advice and support). The authority required quarterly information on the percentage of babies breast-fed at the time of the primary visit and 6 weeks after birth. The baseline measure set was for the last 6 months of 1996 when the breast-feeding rates were 44% at the primary visit and 33% at a 6-week check. Breast-feeding rates have since been collected quarterly and include all breast-feeding even if mixed feeding has been introduced. Since the commencement of the audit little change has been seen in the rates at the primary visit but the breast-feeding rates at the 6-week visit have improved slowly from the initial 33% to a current 40.5%. In real terms this represents 95 more babies benefiting from breast-feeding and their mothers decreasing their risk of pre-menopausal breast cancer.

Since 1996, alongside the increased awareness among the staff of breast-feeding rates by case-load, clinic locality and trust, many other activities have taken place. A significant number of staff have undertaken nationally recognized breast-feeding training. The trust is currently a pilot site for the UNICEF Baby Friendly Initiative in the Community.

AUDIT TOOLS

It is not the intention of this chapter to critically analyse the wide range of audit tools available to management, but mention of one or two of the more common tools that are more suited to health visiting audit is felt to be useful here.

The *Rush Medicus Nursing Process Quality Monitoring Instrument* was developed in the USA and is probably the instrument most widely used to measure the quality of nursing care. Like many of the nursing quality audits it is based on the 'nursing process' and has six main objectives of care:

● The plan of nursing care is formulated.
● The physical needs of the patient are attended.

- The psychological, emotional, mental, social needs of the patient are attended.
- Achievement of nursing care objectives is evaluated.
- Procedures are followed for the protection of all patients.
- The delivery of nursing care is facilitated by administration and managerial services.

Each of the objectives has a subset that links across the initial range and also takes into account medical care. Observers are experienced nurses not directly involved in the ward/department, who work with the nursing staff to feed the results into a computer package that generates a set of criteria questions directly relevant to the patient information input. The system is used randomly across a sample of 10% of 1 month's admissions, but has not found real support in the UK because it is seen as a top-down management tool rather than a local professional quality tool.

Monitor was developed in the UK (Goldstone et al 1983) and is a modification of the Rush Medicus tool. It was originally designed for acute care nursing but subsequently modified for a wide range of special care groups, including health visiting. It was championed in health visiting by Barker (1988), who developed it to run alongside the early childhood health and development programme, and it became the Early Health and Development Monitor (EHD). The objective for EHD was to assess the effectiveness of health visiting as a support service focused on prevention and development goals for the parents of 0- to 4-year-old children. The tool consists of detailed questions relating to the health and development of the child and views these against the socio-educational environment of the family. It is used at 1 month, 6 months, 12 months, 24 months, 36 months and 48 months and should take 15–20 minutes to complete. Barker (1991) considered it the most effective tool to measure outcomes of health visiting interventions, but critics have considered that the number of visits calculated for a 400-family caseload (500 visits in any one year/approximately 11 visits per week in a 45-week year) to be too time consuming to be cost effective. Nevertheless, pilot studies in two West Midlands community health care trusts provided a wealth of evidence over many fields: epidemiological, socio-educational, maternal and child health, nutrition and developmental progress. As with most audit tools, the commitment of the professionals using the tool must be 100% and good electronic systems should be readily available for the information to be quickly downloaded and easily accessed for future consideration.

The *Edinburgh Postnatal Depression Scale* (EPDS), in its original design, identified the presence of postnatal depression in women and used a scoring system to measure the intensity of depressed moods and feelings. A study undertaken in the West Midlands has shown that it is possible to use the EPDS tool to measure the effectiveness of different types of health visiting and other clinical interventions by scoring women after a period during which the client-determined intervention has taken place. The development of this study into using the EPDS tool both as a focus for identifying level of mood and feeling and to audit the effectiveness of a variety of interventions is currently being explored.

The majority of audit tools are designed to elicit quality information in connection with planned client-centred interventions. In health visiting, some of the more common audit tools are effective when exploring, for example, breast-feeding or immunization uptake rates and quality control mechanisms. It is for the profession to challenge auditors to use mechanisms whereby the quality of the intervention is set in context against the long-term effects of support and working in partnership with clients.

CLINICAL RISK MANAGEMENT

Part of the underpinning values of the Leadership Qualities model is to be supportive of taking calculated risks. Health visitors should be aware of the tools for risk identification within their PCT and have a responsibility for ensuring that the procedures are followed accurately and professionally. Indicators that ensure a good clinical risk programme is in place include the following:

- use of incident reports, including reports for near misses
- criteria for clinical audit, effectiveness or quality control
- reports and minutes available for any planning meetings held
- a speedy system for dealing with client complaints
- adherence to the appropriate service agreement charter in relation to visiting times and schedules
- policies and procedures for all aspects of care and surveillance
- client-held records, supplementary records, computer data entry systems
- channels of communication, especially to the child protection advisor.

It is important not only that these systems are in place but also that they work effectively; where there seems to be substandard quality in any of these areas it is the responsibility of each health visitor to make representations to the appropriate person, both verbally and in writing.

Risk in its simplest clinical definition is 'the potential for unwanted outcome' and is the reason for complaints of suffering, delay, lack of communication and many other concerns that may be experienced by patients and their relatives. Clinical risk modification provides the best service for patients and clients by the establishment of multidisciplinary standards of care and best practice guidelines to enhance professional development of nursing, medicine and other therapy professions. The changes in health care delivery, with much higher expectations from patients, greater clarity of roles and responsibilities of clinicians and the emphasis on devolving decision making as close to the patient as possible, are meant to affect the entire performance of health care delivery. The focus of health care risk management is on the systems and practices that affect patient care in order to proactively manage overall cost and appropriateness of care delivered. The NMC Code of Professional Conduct (2002a) states that 'as a registered nurse or midwife, you must act to identify and minimize the risk to patients and clients'.

Wilson & Tingle (1999) usefully propose that risk management is the systematic identification, assessment and reduction of risks to patients and staff:

- through providing appropriate, effective and efficient levels of patient care
- by prevention and avoidance of untoward incidents and events
- by learning lessons and changing behaviour/ practices as a result of near misses, incidents and adverse outcomes and
- through communication and documentation of care in a comprehensive, objective, consistent and accurate way.

The risks that apply to health visiting differ in many ways from those of acute nursing and midwifery. Communication and documentation is one of the categories of practice where risk may occur. Decision making by the client can be difficult in the light of limited knowledge, and an immensely important aspect of health visiting practice is in ensuring that clients have all the knowledge they wish. However, as Rose points out in Chapter 12, how much knowledge can a client be reasonably expected to cope with and how does the client know the legitimacy of that knowledge?

The health visitor, Jasmine, is discussing with Jane the impending immunization session to which her daughter Lizzy has been invited. Jasmine makes the following record in the parent–held personal child health record:

- Date and time of immunization plus signature.
- Immunization discussed and reference made to the immunization leaflet that Jasmine has given to Jane. Any concerns regarding Lizzy's health at the time of immunization to be notified to the health visitor present at the time or the doctor giving the injection.

Jasmine also reminds Jane verbally to bring the child health record to the immunization clinic so that a correct record can be made.

This is where documentation is all-important because clear recording of what has been said will ensure that, should there be a question in the client's mind, scrutiny of the records should prompt memory. Equally, should there be a complaint against the health visitor for the advice given, records should show the principle of what was discussed. It is vital not only to record but also to tell clients what is being recorded and why. It is also important to have previously checked that the parent can read or that there is someone who can read records to them.

Clearly, recording detail of discussions would be time consuming and result in cumbersome records; nevertheless it is important that notes include such statements as in the vignette above. This type of detail does mean that should there be an untoward complaint about possible lack of information from health visitor to client, the record can give a clear outline of the original discussion content.

REDUCING CLINICAL RISK

Incidents tend to be related to clients on health centre or GP practice premises or to health visitors while out on home visits or in public places. There should be clear guidelines and protocols to follow should an accident occur to a patient or client. The transfer of many child health clinics to GP surgeries sometimes means that they are being held in a less than appropriate setting, where rooms are not purpose built. A parent/carer attending the clinic with a small baby and an inquisitive toddler is an accident waiting to happen. There are two major issues:

1. The well baby is being brought to a building in which there are people with communicable diseases, because the health visitor is running a well baby clinic at the same time as the GP has a normal surgery.

2. The only room available is a treatment room. The surgeries are being used, the practice nurse has her own office and so the health visitor is using a room with many movable pieces of equipment and an uncovered floor.

General practitioner surgeries are still primary care centres and as such should be safe for all primary care clients to attend. Health visitors involved in working in general practice where such situations are common have a responsibility under their professional code of conduct, and health and safety legislation, to promote health care environments that are safe (NMC 2002a). Child health clinics held in GP surgeries should be held at a time when ill patients are not attending. The rooms which parents/carers, young children and toddlers are using must be fit for the purpose or alternative arrangements made. If the situation is not resolved, a senior person with sufficient authority should be informed in writing of the concerns.

There are situations in practice where the health visitor is likely to be working alone and at as much risk of an accident as any other member of the general public. There are also certain situations where health visitors may find themselves in potentially violent circumstances and these mean that they must ensure their own safety as well as the safety of any particularly vulnerable person present at the time. While it is not possible to provide guidelines for every set of circumstances, there are general safety strategies that should be used by every health visitor. These include:

- If the client or partner/family has a history of violent behaviour then find out, if possible, the circumstances in which such episodes have occurred.

- If the client or partner/family has a history of violent behaviour or has been abusive in the past, a health visitor should always visit with a colleague who either comes into the house with them or waits in the car for a predetermined length of time.

- Health visitors should be aware of the fact that in most violent circumstances it has been a move on the part of the victim that has precipitated a violent response. Such moves may be:
  - the use of assertive language or behaviour
  - moving too close to the perpetrator – invasion of space

- appearing to threaten the perpetrator by representing 'officialdom'
- appearing frightened or failing to maintain eye contact.

- Health visitors should ensure that they do not unwittingly, for example, pass the perpetrator a weapon such as a pen.

- A health visitor should always tell colleagues or the clinic receptionist when they are going to visit a client about whom they are concerned.

- When visiting clients health visitors should always go back to their base at the end of the day or ensure that the base receptionist or a colleague knows they are safe as per PCT guidelines.

> Barbara, a health visitor, is notified that a family has moved into her area. She checks to find that only the mother and two children have registered with the practice and writes to make an appointment to visit. On arrival at the house Barbara introduces herself to the mother and children but the man present ignores her. Conversation about the family and the children ensues and gradually the man gets drawn into the discussion. It eventually emerges that he is the father of the two children and because of his violent behaviour towards GP receptionists he cannot find a local GP who will accept him on the practice list. As he explains, he does not like to be kept waiting in an appointment system.

This type of situation is not uncommon. Information can be very slow in catching up with mobile families and therefore there are times when health visitors or members of the team may come unwittingly into potentially dangerous circumstances.

MANAGING COMPLAINTS MADE BY CLIENTS

In the past, health visitors had few complaints from clients about clinical tasks. However, this appears to be changing as a result of public litigation awareness and advertising by law firms. It is possible that health visitors could be sued for failure to screen for a hearing defect, a mobility problem thought originally to be late walking, missing developmental delays and so forth. There is also the possibility of complaints from clients where the health visitor is intervening in potential cases of child neglect or abuse, particularly if the health visitor has not worked openly in partnership with a family where there are suspicious circumstances. The most important factor to be remembered is that accurate and contemporaneous recording is essential in these situations. It is also important that the health visitor does not appear to be defensive when a complaint is made but has a clear explanation as the result of careful listening to the client's concerns.

> An incident occurred because a father telephoned the health visitor to seek advice over how much formula milk his 2-month-old daughter should be taking. The health visitor was surprised that the baby was on formula milk because she had recently seen the baby at home with its mother, who was breast-feeding the baby. Apparently the father, who was separated from his wife, had found the child left on its own the day before, and had since taken parental responsibility for the baby. The health visitor could not answer the question because she had to find out from the mother what the feeding arrangements now were. The father objected to this last response and made a formal complaint to the health visitor's manager saying that she was unhelpful and would not give him the advice he sought.

In this vignette the health visitor had taken the telephone call at a time when she happened to be alone in the office. She immediately logged the content of the call so that when she was summoned to explain to the manager there was a clear record of what had happened and her subsequent actions between the phone call and her meeting with the manager.

MANAGING POOR CLINICAL PERFORMANCE

It is a requirement for all practising professionals to ensure that their registration with their professional organization is current. Primarily, this requirement is aimed at protecting the client and all recognized professions have their appropriate regulatory committee to whom representations can be made where professional conduct or performance is below the level of acceptability. Standards for nurses, midwives and health visitors have been set in relation to professional practice in documents such as the Code of Professional Conduct (NMC 2002a). It is the duty of any professional to act to identify and minimize risk to patients and clients.

Registration with the professional body also ensures that the required amount of professional updating and development is undertaken within a prescribed period of time: a minimum of 5 days' study every 3 years. A culture of lifelong learning supported by continuing professional development (Department of Health 1998a, 2001f, NMC 2002a) is central to the government's clinical governance agenda.

> Four health visitors share an office. Two of them, Doris and Ann, work with the same practice; the other two each work for a different GP team. The office acts as a good forum for sharing work-based experiences and ideas and generally supporting one another. Gradually over a period of time, Doris becomes more withdrawn, less sociable and ceases to join in office discussions. She still attends in-service training days but there is no noticeable improvement in her practice. Questions directed to her elicit monosyllabic responses. This situation slowly develops over about 3 years. Ann, from the same practice, becomes increasingly concerned because not only do the GPs seek her out in preference to her colleague but clients are also asking for Ann rather than Doris. Periodically the three health visitors quietly discuss what they can do to help Doris, but find it increasingly difficult even to get her to come to any social occasions

they are involved in. Some 18 months from the beginning of this period the advice of the manager is sought but no changes are made. Managers come and go, some with health visitor qualification, some without, but the situation continues to deteriorate until finally a GP in the practice writes a letter to the current manager, detailing his concerns and itemizing instances where he feels Doris has been practising particularly ineffectually. Doris is seen by her manager and it is decided that she should take sick leave and seek help from her family doctor.

> The situation took a long time to develop and no one closely connected with Doris in her workplace felt in a position to act. Management felt trapped: there was little direct evidence of dangerous practice but clearly it was ineffective. Most of the managers approached by the three health visitors asked for a statement in writing but none of the three felt that she had sufficient evidence to make any accurate or detailed statement. Even if client records were subject to an audit procedure poor practice might only become evident if an entry made by a colleague on behalf of Doris proved to have a substantially different content. Educational courses that Doris was asked to attend were completed but this did not contribute to a change in practice. All the health visitors felt guilty, but disabled; they knew that something should have been done much earlier; they felt sorry for Doris, who lived in difficult circumstances, but they lacked the mechanisms to allow them to intervene.

This type of situation is probably best coped with through clinical supervision, although there is a fine line between ineffective practice and dangerous practice. It can be argued that if a health visitor gives inappropriate advice a client need not take up that advice and thus client choice may act as damage limitation. If a health visitor fails to notice developmental delay or an obvious physical defect in a baby, is this dangerous or merely unfortunate? The profession has perhaps an even greater need to ensure that systems are in place to prevent or deal with poor clinical performance. The main mechanisms open to health visitors that could anticipate this occurrence, particularly when there is an insidious onset, are regular use of a reflective journal, clinical supervision and appraisal.

CLINICAL SUPERVISION

A crucial role of the leader/manager is to ensure that clients receive safe, effective care delivery and that staff are supported and developed through the process of clinical supervision. Clinical supervision is defined by Butterworth & Faugier (1992) as 'an exchange between practising professionals to enable the development of professional skills'. Bond & Holland (1998) suggest that there are 'core' elements to the clinical supervision process and these are listed as:

- modification and empowerment of skills
- critical debate about practice authority through reflective processes
- protection towards independent and accountable practice
- clinical supervision education should commence after qualification as part of professional development
- clinical supervision must be seen as 'active' time and energy on the part of the developer.

Clinical supervision has been in place in midwifery for some considerable time but with a disciplinary element attached to the process. The comparison with the models used in mental health nursing, clinical psychology, social work and counselling shows these to be developmental for staff concerned. Quality in midwifery practice is statutorily linked to the supervision process in that where poor practice is identified the midwife is not allowed to practise alone until a professional standard is re-established.

However, if clinical supervision is used as intended in the nursing and health visiting professions, it serves to enrich practice and becomes a tool for professional growth and development. Primarily, clinical supervision is where two practising professionals meet regularly to discuss the effectiveness of their practice. The clinical supervisor should be an experienced practitioner and the most favourable scenario is likely to be where the supervisee has chosen the supervisor and an informal contract is drawn up by them to clearly identify their roles, the purpose and ground rules.

The Open University (1998) suggest that the clinical supervisor should have skills covering the following:

- To develop and maintain the relationship
  - by practising empathy
  - by attending and active listening
  - by reflecting back and paraphrasing
  - by self-disclosure.

Situations where a health visitor is concerned about any aspect of work with a client are explored through challenge and support. The more these skills are used at the beginning of the supervisory relationship the more fruitful such a relationship will become.

- To manage the process
  - by monitoring
  - by managing time
  - by using intuition
  - by reviewing and evaluating
  - by summarizing and integrating
  - by decision making and action planning.

Monitoring, in clinical supervision, refers to monitoring those aspects of practice that are explored within the session rather than actual health visiting work. An experienced health visitor supervisor possesses the ability to use intuition as an extension of the skill practised in working with clients. Within the supervisory relationship, familiarity with the complexities and contexts of health visiting will allow thoughtful reflection on the totality of practice in relation to the individual practitioner's perceptions and self-awareness. It is also important that the ground rules related to the timing of each session do not allow it to overrun, enabling both practitioners to remain focused. The most effective sessions are those when, at the end, the supervisee comes away with a clear idea of their own capabilities (restorative), support for the practice under discussion (normative) and an enthusiasm for exploring alternative strategies (formative) for similar working circumstances.

- To carry out the supervision processes
  - by questioning
  - by focusing
  - by using silence
  - by giving constructive feedback
  - by informing
  - by confronting.

Chapter 4, discussing the skills of health visiting, showed the value of Heron's six-category intervention model in health visiting practice. The use of the same model in the clinical supervision process allows for both the authoritative and facilitative aspects to be used within the supervisory process. Clinical supervision is about using intervention strategies to promote discussion, reflection on and analysis of practice, and the Heron model facilitates this as well as promoting positivism and support within and for the supervised practitioner. Implicit within this is the capacity for effective reflective skills in both supervisor and supervisee.

Clinical supervision places an emphasis on personal and interpersonal aspects of supervision and encourages self-actualization. In health visiting it encourages practice feedback at times when the isolation and autonomy of the role make this otherwise difficult. Clinical supervision encourages interpersonal regard and the development of trust, caring and interdependence between practitioners. Properly organized and set up it manages tension between practitioners and helps the supervisee deal with uncertainties, fostering clinical autonomy. Clinical supervision facilitates the recognition of practice boundaries and limitations in skill and competence. When carried out in a positive environment it enhances morale in order to inspire and motivate towards excellence. Supervisees are helped to recognize the service delivery functions of their role in relation to the ethical and moral values of the profession. Furthermore, it supports the development of the leadership role in health visiting, in that good morale and motivation are essential qualities for facilitating and managing change.

The West Midlands Clinical Supervision Learning Set led to a network being established that has produced a guide to clinical supervision. This is based on the experience of implementing clinical supervision in various trusts, with a view to identifying good practice, particularly in audit and evaluation. The combination of the learning set pack with the Open University (1998) and the Royal College of Nursing's pack (RCN 1998) gives a comprehensive overview of the methodology and implementation of clinical supervision, which is still in its infancy in many areas. The Learning Set Guide (Brocklehurst 1998) has a useful section on case studies of implementation within several trusts in the West Midlands. Box 7.1 lists pointers to success, recommendations and what to avoid, and are extracted from each trust case study.

A pilot project in clinical supervision set up in a West Midlands community health care trust in 1998 yielded the following response. Of the 16 respondents, 14 said that clinical supervision significantly improved job satisfaction and 15 said they would be influenced in applying for a new post if it provided access to clinical supervision. When asked if they had benefited from their clinical supervision sessions 15 respondents had benefited but one was uncertain; 14 respondents had made changes to their practice as a result of receiving clinical supervision. One supervisor felt that with the development of primary care groups they needed clinical supervision more than ever and another felt that the process was vital for ongoing development. In discussing the question of whether supervision should be from someone from the same discipline or another discipline, eight respondents had same–discipline supervisors and eight had supervisors from a different discipline. Comments from supervisees with a supervisor from the same discipline were: the person is more important than the discipline; she/he understands the problems; it's wonderful/ most appropriate. Comments from supervisees with a supervisor from a different discipline were: discipline not significant; 'with me it's better, I have more freedom to talk and have to be more objective'; a positive decision that worked well; advantages and disadvantages – helpful to have a different perspective; difficult to discuss certain issues, they need explaining rather than reflecting.

Box 7.1   Pointers to success in setting up a clinical supervision system

Recommendations for success

- Involve the practitioners in the planning stage as early as possible
- Allow a long time for planning, consultation and marketing
- Arrange the best training that can be afforded for supervisors or group leaders
- Allow clinical supervision to be practitioner led and confine managerial input to support only
- Plan the project carefully in line with current issues within the organization
- Carry out a comprehensive evaluation
- Set ground rules in all clinical supervision settings, including confidentiality
- Make sure that there is management/stakeholder support at all stages of the development and implementation of clinical supervision

What to avoid

- Avoid excluding management when trying to encourage a practitioner-led approach to the development of clinical supervision
- Do not overemphasize the mandatory nature of clinical supervision
- Do not assume that once people are trained they will necessarily start providing supervision without encouragement
- Avoid making claims for clinical supervision that are hard to substantiate or fulfil
- Avoid planning the detail before practitioners have had a chance to influence the development
- Do not begin with a group of practitioners who do not appear motivated to try clinical supervision

---

The education of effective supervisors requires a non-threatening setting where potential supervisors come with a desire to be educated. The basics of supervisor education hinge on an ability to further develop personal self-awareness and to work on the Heron (1986) six-category intervention skills. A contract between the participants in the supervisory relationship and clear guidelines of responsibility for supervisor and supervisee are essential tools for a purposeful relationship. Written records are kept about issues discussed during supervision, their confidentiality being part of the contract. Clinical supervision should help to identify gaps in knowledge and skills which need to be addressed through continuing professional development.

CONTINUING PROFESSIONAL DEVELOPMENT (CPD)

The Department of Health publication *Working Together, Learning Together* (Department of Health 2001i) set a framework for learning and development based on a vision of client-centred care. CPD is advocated for all professionals working in the NHS to enable them to keep up to date and realize their potential through gaining new knowledge and skills. Under the statutory requirements for periodic re-registration with the NMC, nurses, midwives and health visitors are required to show that they have undertaken a minimum of 5 days' study since their last registration, and must produce a current portfolio of their professional development. The Department of Health (2000d) advises that every nurse, midwife or health visitor needs to match personal and professional aspirations for continuing professional development with the needs of the NHS organization. Personal development plans are viewed as central to this process with accreditation for learning.

The current emphasis on work-based learning supports the notion of lifelong learning and requires universities and NHS organizations to work closely together to provide quality learning environments in the workplace. There are many ways in which learning opportunities may take place: through distance learning, the use of learning sets, self-directed learning through journal learning articles, reflection, project work and so forth.

> A locality action forum in a multicultural area of the West Midlands had been concerned for some time about the amount of adult violence occurring in the area. Key workers decided that a day conference might be helpful to raise awareness of concerns and bring together many of the agencies working in the area. Funding was provided by the social services department and invitations were sent to police, social workers, health care workers (health visitors, practice nurses, district nurses), health coordinators, local religious leaders and community development workers. The community health council sent a representative. The local university provided a keynote speaker from the public health degree course. The entire day was spent exploring the problem and learning about the underlying theoretical causes for adult violence.

This type of education initiative is very much in the spirit of clinical governance, in that it is focused on the problem, and all the disciplines involved gain education and information in a problem-based learning approach. It means that key workers can understand the thrust and perspectives of the other workers and recognize the reasons for varying approaches. As discussed in Chapter 10, research (Bennett et al 1997) shows that social workers perceive psychological abuse and neglect as more common than physical abuse; police, lawyers and mental health workers perceive verbal abuse as more common than physical abuse. Community mental health nurses report more physical abuse whereas social services staff report more financial abuse. As a result of these factors the studies found that in approaching intervention social workers sought to change the situation or behaviour, police sought to detect or prevent crime and nurses attended to health needs. Problem-based learning allows for understanding and consolidation of the different approaches, particularly in consultation with the local community leaders. This approach to education crosses old boundaries between disciplines and will clearly be a more effective use of funding to the benefit of the community.

CONCLUSION

Organizations must put in place structures and resources that enable leaders to develop innovative practice, and support front-line practitioners in the provision of high-quality client-centred care. Practitioners need to embrace change, working together in multidisciplinary teams to deliver services that meet clients' needs and reflecting on practice to improve the client experience. Good practice based on research evidence should be used as the basis for interventions, while variations in the process, outcome and access to health care must be actively addressed. Risks and hazards need to be reduced to as low a level as possible, creating a safety culture for all. Strong leadership and commitment are central to the process of driving forward the changes that enhance the quality of care for clients. Leadership stems from the practice and knowledge base of health visiting, which enables the provision of a flexible, responsive practice in line with the health needs assessment of the population. Current government policy supports strong leadership, and health visitors need to take the opportunity to influence and lead developments in community and primary care to ensure clinically effective practice for clients based on sound evidence.

Chapter **8**

Contemporary influences in safeguarding children

Jane McKears, Margaret Reynolds, Sarah Forester and Jane Middleton

INTRODUCTION

The early years of the 21st century have, as never before, seen a significant emphasis placed on raising the profile of child protection. Demand has come both from government and from society as a whole. The Laming Report (2003) has acted as a catalyst in this respect. McKears and Reynolds consider the major influences on child protection from two main influences: central government and the professional and voluntary sector.

Forester gives an overview of Sure Start and its aims to support families with young children. The place of local programmes within the larger Sure Start agenda will be discussed against the background of Sure Start principles. The bulk of the section will discuss how these principles are being put into practice in one Sure Start local programme in south London. This will focus in particular on the challenges of putting the user perspective central to service development. The health visiting team within this local programme will be described and some principles identified which have relevance to health visiting both within and without Sure Start programmes.

Middleton describes the information currently available concerning Children's Trusts, and explores the potential implications for health visitors. She considers the role of health visiting in relation to children's centres and extended schools, including integrated team working and leadership.

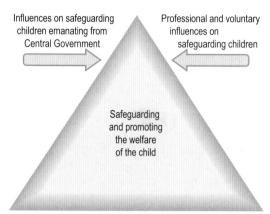

Figure 8.1 Diagram indicating contemporary influences on child protection

CONTEMPORARY INFLUENCES IN CHILD PROTECTION

Jane McKears and Margaret Reynolds

Contemporary influences on child protection will be considered under the two main areas as indicated in Figure 8.1.

INFLUENCES ON SAFEGUARDING CHILDREN EMANATING FROM CENTRAL GOVERNMENT

WORKING TOGETHER: A GUIDE TO INTERAGENCY WORKING TO SAFEGUARD AND PROMOTE THE WELFARE OF CHILDREN (DEPARTMENT OF HEALTH 1999d)

Working Together places an even greater emphasis on professionals working together to protect children from harm as well as carrying out their other professional duties with children and families to enable children to achieve their potential.

Working Together (1999) encourages quality assurance and recommends basic skills and knowledge levels required of trainers delivering training for child protection. There is also a recommendation that training is evaluated and learning outcomes inform future training.

McKears (unpublished research 1994) found wide variations in the level of skills and knowledge of the trainers across five different towns in Britain. She found that some trainers had undergone in-depth training to undertake their work and also had high levels of personal professional knowledge about the issues involved. Other trainers had had little or no training to become trainers and had widely differing levels of knowledge and experience, which led to inequity of training provision across the country. By reviewing the evaluation of training and baseline standards for trainers these issues will be addressed.

The key outcome, described as 'appreciation of own role and that of others', reflects many public inquiries into the deaths of children as a result of abuse. However, in her research, McKears found that the multi-agency training did not always achieve this outcome.

Attendees at Area Child Protection Committee (ACPC) training events did not always reflect the diverse range of staff involved in working with children, which limited the opportunity to understand their role. In addition she found that even when there were representatives from a wide range of professional groups at the training events this in itself did not mean that greater understanding of one another's roles was achieved. It is essential when planning training that exercises are designed which are targeted with this aim in view.

Working Together also places emphasis on group development of trainers, which would enhance the process of inter-agency understanding of roles. Perhaps a serendipitous outcome of group development would be emotional support and understanding between the trainers, which would equip them to deal with the ongoing demanding nature of their work with families.

AREA CHILD PROTECTION COMMITTEES (ACPCs)

ACPCs came into being following the inquiry into the death of Maria Colwell in 1974. Their role is to coordinate agencies responsible for protecting children at risk, which the report showed was seriously lacking within child protection services (http://www.guardian.co.uk/print/0,3858,4521410-108861.00.html). Each local authority is required to ensure there is an ACPC covering their area. Problems may arise where local authority boundaries are not coterminous with other agencies, for example health and police, or where one ACPC covers more than one local authority. This can mean some professionals having to work to different protocols according to the area involved.

Working Together (Department of Health 1999d) further details the role and responsibilities of ACPCs. These include a duty to ensure that agencies within their area cooperate in effectively protecting children, formulation of local policies and procedures for inter-agency work to protect children that accords with the guidance set out in *Working Together*, training in child protection and to produce an annual business plan. They are required to undertake serious case reviews in instances where a child has died or suffered serious injury as a result of actual or suspected non-accidental injury, and ensure that lessons are learned from these cases so that improved ways to protect children are implemented in the working practice of each agency involved.

Membership includes senior members from the main statutory agencies, including, besides social services, education, police, housing and probation service, as well as voluntary organizations. Membership from health includes the designated doctor and nurse for child protection.

Although much has been achieved through the work of ACPCs, safeguarding children will be further improved through establishment of Local Safeguarding Children's Boards as statutory successors to the non-statutory ACPCs, as required by the Children Bill 2004. The latter puts in place legislative arrangements for implementing the proposals in the 2003 Green Paper *Every Child Matters* (DH 2003a), placing working together on a statutory footing for both the statutory and voluntary agencies and the community. It also puts into effect the recommendations from the Laming Report regarding protecting children through creating a Director of Children's Services, a lead council member for children and a Children's Commissioner, to be a children's champion ensuring that children's views and interests are kept at the heart of policy making (Department for Education and Skills 2004b).

Although the Children Bill will not create Children's Trusts it will facilitate their development while acknowledging that different areas may want to tailor their structure to meet local need. The primary purpose of Children's Trusts will be to ensure integrated commissioning of services for children and young people with pooling of budgets from education, social services, connections and some health services. They may also commission services on behalf of the Local Safeguarding Children Board (the statutory successor of the ACPC).

As the planned transition from ACPCs to Safeguarding Children's Boards gets underway, together with other requirements of the Children Bill over the next few years it clearly shows the increasing seriousness with which government views protecting children and their desire to get things right.

THE LAMING REPORT INTO THE DEATH OF VICTORIA CLIMBIÉ

The Laming Report (2003), resulting from the inquiry into the death of Victoria Climbié as a result of numerous horrific injuries inflicted by her great-aunt and her boyfriend, in February 2001, contains key proposals for safeguarding children. These include national standards for safeguarding children, more training for all staff in all agencies, in particular those working directly with children, in recognizing and dealing with deliberate harm to children, and a proposed national agency for families and children reporting to a children and families board chaired by a cabinet minister. Recommendations at local level include Safeguarding Children's Boards to be the statutory successors of ACPCs.

The report contains 108 recommendations: 17 general ones aimed at central government or local authorities, 46 recommendations for social care, 27 recommendations for health and 18 recommendations for police. All are required to be implemented across the country within the time limits set against each recommendation, either 3 months, 6 months or 2 years from the time of the report's publication.

In dedicating the report to Victoria's memory, Lord Laming said 'The report is intended to have an impact on practice now – not some time in the future. Its recommendations cannot be deferred to some bright tomorrow.'

The report found that simple, basic good practice was found wanting to a significant degree by many of the professionals involved with Victoria's case, from the time of her arrival in the UK until her death a brief 9 months later. Not only was the practice of front-line staff not acceptable, but senior managers failed in their duty to ensure services to children and their families were properly staffed and financed, together with effective staff supervision to deliver quality care. Victoria and her great-aunt were known to a number of agencies right from the time of their arrival in England. This was not a case that was hidden away, and there were a number of opportunities during the last months of her life when Victoria could have been saved.

- Key messages from the report are a need to:
  - work together to safeguard and promote the welfare of children
  - learn the lessons from the past in order to improve practice and management in the future
  - identify significant shortfalls in resources within children's services and seek ways to address them.
- Issues for health include:
  - better record keeping, including observations, conversations and discussion, and a single set of records for each child in a given area.
- Within the hospital setting:
  - being clear about who has responsibility for child protection concerns
  - clear admission, discharge and follow-up arrangements
  - ensuring hospital nurses' care plans take into account concerns about child abuse
  - involving the child in compiling a case history
  - all designated and named doctors in child protection, and all consultant paediatricians, must be revalidated in the diagnosis and treatment of deliberate

harm to children, and in the multi-agency aspects of child protection.
- Within the community recommendations include:
  - ensuring primary care staff know who to contact if they have child protection concerns
  - appropriate training for all staff in child protection.
- Particular issues for GP practices are:
  - ensuring all GPs and their practice staff receive training in recognition of deliberate harm to children and in the multi-agency aspects of child protection investigations
  - new registrations of child patients with a GP practice to include wider social and developmental issues.

The GMS Contract (NHS Confederation 2003) clearly states the responsibilities that GPs have in respect of child protection and the need for relevant training. This is facilitating improvements in many areas in implementing training programmes for GPs and practice staff in child protection.

This is a particularly important development in safeguarding children from harm when considering that GPs and their staff are often the first professionals to encounter cases of possible child abuse.

A significant response to the Laming Report, published in September 2003, is *Keeping Children Safe: The Government's Response to the Victoria Climbié Inquiry Report and Joint Chief Inspector's Report Safeguarding Children* (Department for Education and Skills 2003). This response considers what is wrong with the present system for safeguarding children, what is needed in a system for safeguarding children for the 21st century and what the government is doing about it. In considering the last point, the document considers each of the recommendations from the Laming Report as well as how the government proposes to ensure the system is improving through the Commission for Health Audit and Inspection (CHAI).

It is to be hoped that ongoing monitoring of the Laming Report recommendations through

Commissioning for Health Improvement (CHI), metamorphosing to CHAI, the strategic health authorities and implementation of the Children Bill will ensure an improved standard of practice in safeguarding children. Above all it is not about major organizational changes, but about basic good practice.

NATIONAL AUDIT OF CHILD PROTECTION ARRANGEMENTS

Following the death of Victoria Climbié, Lord Laming published the Inquiry Report in 2003. Of the 108 recommendations, many were related to accountability for child protection and some were concerned with basic good practice. Self-assessment check-lists were sent to all NHS organizations, councils with social service responsibilities in England and all police forces in England and Wales. The results were audited by CHI, HM Inspectorate of Constabulary (HMIC) and the Social Services Inspectorate (SSI). What is unusual in this is that despite having published inquiries into the deaths by abuse of children for over 20 years, this was the first large scale audit of child protection arrangements (CHI 2004).

While the audit found areas of good practice within all sections of the report, there were significant areas of concern. Of particular relevance to PCTs and health visitors are the following:

- Although joint working is essential, some NHS staff felt unable to influence working in other agencies despite a clear edict for collaborative working.

- Strategic health authorities and PCTs lacked clarity in their responsibilities for performance management in child protection.

- PCTs needed to increase their understanding of the responsibilities of independent contractors. For instance, it was found that GPs were sometimes unwilling to share information about adult family members. They were also reluctant to take up PCT-led training in relation to child protection. However, not all NHS boards appeared to have sufficient awareness of the issues.

- Variations found in service provision within the NHS were believed to put children at risk.

- There were noted difficulties with training of agency staff, variations in take-up of training by key staff and exclusion from training of some staff, e.g. ambulance personnel.

- Some NHS staff have only limited access to child protection registers and previous case notes. Access to ACPC procedures varies between PCTs and audit regarding staff compliance with these policies is not equitable.

- Cross-border arrangements for children in hospital outside of the area caused concern. Not all NHS organizations have designated or named doctors, nurses or midwives for child protection.

- Criminal Records Bureau (CRB) checks were inconsistent and especially likely to be lacking with agency staff.

- Record keeping within the NHS was criticized regarding timelines, quality and lack of monitoring.

- While the report found many areas of good practice there were serious concerns in some areas.

- Where the CHI, SSI, HMCIC (Her Majesty's Chief Inspector of Constabulary) report is very positive, is in its commitment to ongoing audit and inspection to bring about continuous improvement.

From April 2004 CHI became CHAI (Commission Health Audit and Inspection) and this work will continue. What remains clear is that audit and reporting can provide the information but the Primary Care Trusts will have the responsibility for implementing the changes.

GUIDANCE TO PRIMARY CARE TRUSTS REGARDING THEIR RESPONSIBILITY FOR CHILD PROTECTION

Child protection is a public health responsibility for Primary Care Trusts (PCTs). Guidance (DOH 28 January 2002) to PCTs clearly indicates that it is essential to maintain an effective focus on child protection as power is devolved down from the old local health authorities to PCTs in line with *Shifting the Balance of Power within the NHS: Securing Delivery* (Department of Health 2001f). The start of this transfer took place against the background of the Victoria Climbié inquiry, undoubtedly emphasizing the gravity of the responsibility they were taking on for many trusts and the devastating consequences if they got things wrong.

Child protection forms part of the public health responsibility that PCTs have for the whole population which they serve. In exercising that responsibility, as commissioners of services, they have a key duty to ensure the health and well-being of children in need as identified under the Children Act 1989 within their area, working together with social services and other local authority agencies including education, to provide coordinated services across agencies, with relevant sharing of information. They will have a clear duty for regularly reviewing local health arrangements for child protection, ensuring they are in accordance with *Working Together* (Department of Health 1999d), and *the Framework for the Assessment of Children in Need and their Families* (Department of Health 2000b), and with local Area Child Protection Procedures (ACPC).

PCTs have a duty to ensure all health professionals have the opportunity to attend child protection training. This will include GPs and their practice staff. PCTs must ensure that child protection training is available to those in organizations within the trust area whose work means they are in regular contact with children. This can be achieved through the local ACPC, which has a responsibility for arranging multi-agency training.

The responsibilities of the designated professionals, nurse and doctor, are outlined in the guidance and accord with that in *Working Together* (Department of Health 1999d). These professionals may cover more than one PCT depending on the size of the trust, and must establish effective links with the named professionals in each trust.

The designated doctor is required to be a senior paediatrician and the designated nurse a senior nurse with a health visiting qualification. Their role is to take a professional lead in all aspects of the health contribution to safeguarding children, to provide professional advice on child protection to other professionals and to social services. Additionally they have a key role in influencing training and professional development in child protection processes in line with ACPC protocols, and to participate in case reviews. They should also be part of the health service representation on the ACPC.

It is recommended that each NHS trust, including PCTs, should identify a named doctor and nurse or midwife to take a professional lead on child protection matters within the trust. These professionals are required to have expertise in child health and development, as well as child maltreatment, and comprehensive knowledge of local arrangements for safeguarding children. They will provide expert advice and support to fellow professionals and other agencies, and be responsible for promoting good professional practice in safeguarding children within the trust. They will also have responsibility in conducting the trust's internal case reviews unless they personally have been substantially involved in the case. In these circumstances the designated professional will take on that responsibility.

Assuming responsibility for safeguarding children as part of their public health role began on 1 April 2002, but many PCTs have still to complete the relevant arrangements. Although CHI inspections, which have focused on progress in local trusts' development of arrangements for child protection, is a driver to ensure effective development in this field, financial restraints, with no extra funding being provided by central government to develop the service, remains a significant issue. Yet this is an opportunity for PCTs to meet the challenge within their public health role by promoting children's health and well-being, particularly in the early years, by investing in and implementing an effective child protection system.

THE ROLE OF PRIMARY CARE IN THE PROTECTION OF CHILDREN FROM ABUSE AND NEGLECT (ROYAL COLLEGE OF GENERAL PRACTITIONERS 2003)

Published against the background of the Laming Report, the position statement is endorsed by the Royal College of Paediatrics and Child Health, the Faculty of Public Health Medicine, the National Society for the Prevention of Cruelty to Children, the British Association of Medical Managers, and the NHS Confederation. It is the first position statement concerning the protection of children from abuse and neglect in primary care published by the Royal College of General Practitioners.

Acknowledging that child abuse and neglect remain prevalent in our society, it emphasizes the role that members of the Primary Health Care Teams (PHCTs) have in identification of those at risk of abuse and neglect, and in subsequent work with children and families. It is interesting to note that Sinclair & Bullock (2002), in reviewing serious case reviews, identified health professionals, and health visitors in particular, as being more likely to have been involved with the children, 12 of the 40 children in the review being unknown to social services.

Barriers identified in GPs' participation in child protection work included anxiety, concern over damage to their relationship with families, legal implications, disbelief and disgust, and lack of awareness due to inadequate training.

Proposals for a way forward focus on acknowledging that the rights of the child are paramount, and that policies and procedures are in place, in line with the local Area Child Protection Committee (ACPC). It emphasizes the importance of basic training in child protection for GPs and 3-yearly updates, and that child protection training should be part of the vocational and continuing professional development, commencing with SHOs (Senior House Officers), whether they go on to become paediatricians or GPs, or want to make child protection an area of expertise. Mention is also made of the need to develop a strategy between ACPCs and those responsible for GP training.

The GMS Contract, published at the same time as the position statement, is concerned with patient protection and the need to participate in guidelines and procedures to effect this, for both children and vulnerable adults.

Although primarily aimed at GPs, the position statement emphasizes the role of primary care, including all members of PHCTs in child protection work. It identifies the need for ongoing training in this field, for GPs and their staff, an issue neglected in many areas, but identified in the Laming Report as a crucial recommendation, and the importance of working together to safeguard children.

WHAT TO DO IF YOU'RE WORRIED A CHILD IS BEING ABUSED (DEPARTMENT OF HEALTH 2003e)

This clearly states that safeguarding children is the responsibility of everyone who comes into contact with children and families in their everyday work, irrespective of whether or not they have a specific role in relation to child protection. It sets out what everyone should do if they have concerns about a child's welfare, which includes being familiar with their own organization's procedures and protocols for safeguarding children in their area. It also indicates how social workers and their managers should respond to a referral, and what police officers should do when they become involved with a child about whom they have welfare concerns.

It offers useful guidance on information sharing with other agencies in cases where there are child protection concerns and what the main restrictions of disclosure of information are. These are common duty of confidence, the Human Rights Act 1998 and the Data Protection Act 1998. In the NHS, discussion with the Caldicott Guardian may be helpful in reaching a decision as to whether it is lawful to share particular information.

Flow charts summarizing action to be taken when a practitioner has concerns about a child's welfare have in many cases been incorporated into local child protection policies and procedures.

While the guidelines in *What to Do if You're Worried a Child is being Abused* are clear, it remains the responsibility of all practitioners not only to follow them, but also to maintain a culture of vigilance in order to identify and afford help to vulnerable children at an early stage.

EVERY CHILD MATTERS (CM 5860) AND EVERY CHILD MATTERS: NEXT STEPS

Published in September 2003, *Every Child Matters* is described by Lord Laming as a statement of vision, and by the Director of the NSPCC as the most significant opportunity for children since the Children Act 1989. The Education Secretary described it as a turning point in the way children are nurtured, protected and supported. It is government's response to the Laming Report and puts forward a range of proposals to reform and improve child care. For the first time it requires local authorities to bring together in one place, under one person, services for children, requiring social services, education, health and police to work together.

Proposals are aimed at reducing the number of children who suffer ill health, educational failure, or become involved in offending and antisocial behaviour. It puts the role of parents first in improving outcomes for children, then links this to challenges that are faced when families are poor. Policy challenges are:

- better prevention
- a stronger focus on parenting and families
- earlier intervention.

In order to bring about these reforms, it is crucial to address weak accountability and poor integration, and workforce reform.

The five key outcomes for every child and young person are:

- being healthy – good physical and mental health and healthy lifestyle and growing up to care
- staying safe – protection from harm and neglect for themselves
- enjoying and achieving – getting the most out of life
- making a positive contribution
- economic well-being.

Four key areas for action are:

- supporting parents and carers
- early intervention and effective protection
- accountability and integration locally, regionally and nationally
- workforce reform.

The Green Paper affirms government's support for effective intervention and effective protection. It proposes removal of barriers to information sharing. Using a shared assessment system is particularly important when many professionals are involved with one child. It proposes a lead professional acting as a gate-keeper for information-sharing systems, developing a common assessment framework, with work at an advanced stage in the *Integrated Children's System* (2002). There are proposals for an accountability framework at local and national level which will include a Children's Director at local level, and services brought together into Children's Trusts. It should be noted that the Children Bill 2004 has put back the establishment of Children's Trusts until 2008. The Green Paper identifies the need for more foster parents and proposes the appointment of a Children's Commissioner who will act as a 'champion' for children.

The Green Paper goes on to affirm government's commitment to tackling child poverty and ensuring children have the best possible start in life by extending the Sure Start principles and network of centres in disadvantaged areas, and improved access to antenatal and postnatal care. This last is being done increasingly with midwives attached to Sure Start centres. It also proposes extending free education for all 3-year-olds and improved support for disabled children in the early years. Further proposals include improving access to primary health care and specialist health services, tackling antisocial and offending behaviour, tackling bullying and supporting children entering the country, particularly those entering as unaccompanied asylum seekers.

Multidisciplinary teams are seen as the way forward, working in places accessible to children and families, for example around schools, primary care and Sure Start centres. Proposals for workforce reform in respect of those working with children include raising of educational standards, and developing a pay and workforce strategy with the aim of improving both the attractiveness and status of working with children, while at the same time improving workforce skills and collaborative working.

The consultation period on proposals in the Green Paper ended at the beginning of December 2003. It clearly shows that government accepted the recommendations in the Laming Report, with proposals to address them clearly defined, with set time limits for this to be achieved. As such it is a significant step towards more effective safeguarding of children.

The Children Bill 2004, which received Royal assent in November 2004, will put into effect proposals contained in the Green Paper. *Every Child Matters: Next Steps* (Department for Education and Skills 2004b) sets out the timetable of developments as well as discussing the response to consultation on *Every Child Matters*. While this is to be welcomed, it has been criticized by some who feel it does not go far enough in affording children effective protection.

FRAMEWORK FOR THE ASSESSMENT OF CHILDREN IN NEED AND THEIR FAMILIES (DEPARTMENT OF HEALTH 2000b)

The *Framework* draws on requirements of the Children Act 1989 to provide care and protection of children, as well as reflecting the principles in the United Nations Convention on the Rights of the Child, which were ratified by the UK government in 1991.

Protecting children from all forms of harm and ensuring all aspects of need are met is a primary aim of government. Locally, social services and other local authority departments, together with health, has a duty to work together to identify children in need in their area. They are required to provide such services as are necessary to promote their welfare and satisfy their developmental needs within the family setting wherever possible.

The *Framework* provides guidance for use by professionals and other staff involved in undertaking assessment of children in need and their families. Its use provides a clear understanding of what is happening to the child within the family and the wider context of the community in which they live. This allows for the making of professional judgements as to whether the child being assessed is suffering from, or likely

to suffer from, significant harm, what actions must be taken and which services will best meet the needs of this particular child and family.

Assessment focuses on three main areas: firstly the child's developmental needs, including health, education, emotional and behavioural development and social skills; secondly the parenting capacity of the child's parents, which includes basic care, ensuring safety, emotional warmth, stability, stimulation, guidance and boundaries; the third area, family and environmental factors, includes issues around community resources, family history and functioning, housing, income, employment and the family's social functioning. Protocols have been developed in a number of areas to give practical step-by-step guidance in implementing the *Framework* in addition to those developed nationally.

GETTING THE RIGHT START: NATIONAL SERVICE FRAMEWORK (NSF) FOR CHILDREN, YOUNG PEOPLE AND MATERNITY SERVICES

The NSF, published in late 2004, sets standards for health and social care services involved in working with children, as well as considering how these link with other services, particularly education. It covers children from pre-birth up until their 19th birthday.

The first of the eleven parts, covering children's hospital care, was launched in April 2003, with implementation planned over a 10-year period. Topics include play, use of medicines and planning for discharge from hospital, the latter overlapping with recommendations from the Laming Report. Of particular relevance to safeguarding children are dedicated A&E departments, already implemented in some hospitals, together with child protection available on a 24-hour basis.

This part of the framework is relevant not only to hospital staff involved in caring for children, but also to health visitors and school nurses, as they seek to work collaboratively with hospital staff as the child moves from hospital to community. Many areas have a children's liaison nurse, who acts as a vital link in relevant information sharing concerning child care and protection between hospital and community.

PROMOTING THE HEALTH OF LOOKED AFTER CHILDREN (DEPARTMENT OF HEALTH 2002c)

Promoting the Health of Looked After Children is a comprehensive guidance for the delivery of services from health and social services, the aim being more effective promotion of health and well-being of children and young people in the care system.

The framework is informed by the Children Act 1989 and by revision of the legal framework within which it operates in the Children Act (Miscellaneous Amendments) (England) Regulations 2002. The NSF, now developed, sets new national standards for service delivery.

Most children looked after by the local authority have been identified as children in need, many having been in need of protection. Many have significantly increased health needs when compared with other children and young people in similar socio-economic backgrounds. They have poorer access to services, for example routine child health surveillance and health promotion, owing to language or cultural barriers. They do less well at school, meaning fewer go on to further and higher education, and their job opportunities, economic status and quality of life are less good than those of their peers living with their parents.

The holistic model of health in the new guidance uses the domains of the *Framework for the Assessment of Children in Need and their Families* (Department of Health 2000b). This has now been merged with the Looking After Children system to create the Integrated Children's System (Department of Health 2002c), which will provide a common framework for assessment, intervention and planning for all children in need, including 'looked after' children.

In respect of health care, a designated doctor and nurse are required to be appointed to enable PCTs to fulfil their responsibilities in commissioning services to improve the health of 'looked after' children. The designated doctor will be a senior paediatrician, clinically active in community paediatrics, with extensive experience in the health needs of these children. The designated nurse will be a senior nurse or midwife, with considerable experience pertaining to children and young people.

Duties will not only include regular health assessments as detailed in the guidance, but also a monitoring role concerning the effectiveness of delivery of health care services to these children and evaluation of the extent to which young people and children's views are taken into account in the design and delivery of health services for them.

Other services must include health promotion and access to child and mental health services. The latter is particularly important as 'looked after' children, owing to their life experiences and vulnerability at particular points in their life, for example leaving care, may benefit from this service in terms of support and help in instances of mental health disorders, and in prevention of mental problems.

Many areas have already appointed the designated professionals for 'looked after' children. Some have incorporated them into the team for child protection, while in others the two teams are separate. The rationale for the first model is that many 'looked after' children enter the system through the child protection route, and both groups of children are children in need. Close working between team members facilitates the sharing of relevant information quickly and effectively. It can also facilitate joint working where necessary, to provide cover for leave for the designated nurse for 'looked after' children, ensuring continuity of care, and can be more cost effective in terms of sharing resources, including clerical support. The second model can mean more emphasis placed on the needs of each group of children and more autonomy for professionals, but less opportunity for information sharing and joint working, and greater difficulty in obtaining cover for leave, a particular issue at present when taking into account the shortfall in staff resources, as discussed later in this chapter.

Whichever model is decided upon, it must be seen to be working effectively in improving the health and well-being of 'looked after' children in the area.

CHILDREN IN WHOM ILLNESS IS FABRICATED OR INDUCED: SUPPLEMENTARY GUIDANCE TO WORKING TOGETHER TO SAFEGUARD CHILDREN (DEPARTMENT OF HEALTH 2002d)

This supplementary guidance is particularly relevant to safeguarding children as the outcome for a child can be death or long-term health problems and impairment of psychological and emotional development. Following publication of the research framework in North Staffordshire Hospital NHS Trust (Department of Health 2000), the Department of Health responded to the report's recommendations to develop guidelines to identify children in whom illness had been fabricated or induced by their carer. It has been formulated within the framework of *Working Together to Safeguard Children* (Department of Health 1999d) and the *Framework for the Assessment of Children in Need and their Families* (Department of Health 2000b).

While there has been much debate in describing the fabrication or induction of illness in a child, including Munchausen's syndrome by proxy, illness induction syndrome, fabricated illness by proxy and factitious illness, the guidance does not use any particular term, but refers to the 'fabrication or induction of illness in a child'. What is important is the impact of fabricated or induced illness on the health and development of the child and how to safeguard their welfare rather than which term to use. This is emphasized in the work of Professor Roy Meadow. In spite of the current controversy over expert witnesses, in the past this has safeguarded the lives of many children.

There are three main ways in which a carer fabricates or induces illness in a child. These are: fabrication of signs and symptoms which can include fabrication of past medical history; falsification of hospital charts and records, letters and documents and specimens of body fluids; and induction of illness by a variety of means. Additionally there is the situation where a child has to undergo unnecessary or invasive treatment based on symptoms that have been deliberately falsely described or manufactured by the carer.

Fundamental to the guidelines are the principles of the United Nations Convention on the Rights of the Child and the Human Rights Act 1998. The latter provides a framework for the care and protection of children. Additionally there is a shared responsibility for all professionals in all agencies as well as the wider community to safeguard children from harm and to promote their welfare.

The guidance details arrangements where there is reasonable cause to suspect a child is suffering or is likely to suffer significant harm. This includes a strategy meeting, or more than one if the child's circumstances are complex, at which representatives of the relevant agencies will be present. This will include the GP, health visitor, school nurse, senior ward sister if the child is a hospital inpatient, and the local authority legal advisor.

If a decision is made to initiate Section 47 inquiries, the strategy discussion will have to make a number of decisions, including whether the child needs constant professional observation, designation of a medical clinician to oversee and coordinate medical treatment for the child, and the needs of siblings and other children with whom the alleged abuser has contact, collation of medical records of all family members, including children who are either deceased or no longer living with the family, and the needs of parents. At all times there is a need for the utmost care concerning confidentiality and the securing of records.

A decision will also be made about the nature of police investigations, including analysis of samples and covert video surveillance. Where the latter is used, it is police led and coordinated, and forms part of the criminal investigations.

Most children in these circumstances are too young to be interviewed as part of the criminal investigation, but where it is decided they are of sufficient age and understanding, the interview will take place following the guidance in *Achieving Best Evidence* (Home Office 2002). The outcome of the inquiries may indicate that concerns are not confirmed, or that action to protect the child from significant harm is required, where an initial child protection case conference will be held and recommendations made regarding the child's welfare.

In spite of the guidance on children who may be suffering from illness that is fabricated or induced, taking into account research and experience in this particular area, and lessons learned recently, there has been much controversy over the diagnosis, casting doubt on the efficacy of medical experts in this field. While controversy will no doubt continue about the rights of the parent/carer and whether investigations into this form of abuse, including the use of covert video surveillance, infringes those rights, the focus on the rights of the child must remain the central point. It must be remembered that most of these children are too young to speak for themselves or to understand what is being done to them.

It has been acknowledged that although there is always the possibility of human error, the child's welfare must remain paramount. If professionals fail to keep this concept central in their thoughts and actions in these circumstances, they may well lose the child.

THE RESPONSIBILITIES OF EMPLOYERS IN PREVENTING UNSUITABLE PEOPLE FROM WORKING WITH CHILDREN AND YOUNG PEOPLE

The employer's responsibility in this respect is becoming an increasingly important issue, following publicity around recent cases of Schedule 1 offenders working with children or those where concerns have previously been raised. Working with children includes work which is paid or unpaid. This can be in the statutory, voluntary or private sector; it may or may not be under a contract or apprenticeship, and includes all 'regulated positions'.

Employers need to be aware of the law, acts and reports relating to who may or may not be employed in working with children and young people. These include the Warner Report (1992), Utting Report (1997), the Children Act List (1999) and the Police Reform Act (1998), which set up the Criminal Records Bureau (CRB), operational

from the spring of 2002. All new posts in the NHS where post holders will be working with children are subject to satisfactory CRB check, but it does not as yet cover existing employees, nor does it include periodic rechecking. At best it will give a snapshot of a person at a moment in time, but will not cover future offences against children unless a system of rechecking is put in place.

The list of Schedule 1 offences has its limitations as it does not include a number of new offences, for example pornography. It is also concerning that, without a conviction, the 'offender' cannot be regarded as a Schedule 1 offender. It should also be remembered that where a disqualification order has been issued by a senior court, if the individual attempts to breach that order it is a criminal offence for both the individual and the employer.

New offences include 'abuse of a position of trust'. Where a complaint is made against someone employed to work with children by the child, and that complaint is upheld, an employer who knowingly employs that individual against whom the complaint was upheld, or obtains work for them knowing they are barred, that is an offence for both the employer and the employee. It also has to be remembered that the Rehabilitation of Offenders Act does not apply to 'regulated' positions. This means that where work with children is concerned, convictions are never spent. Within the health service, 'regulated positions' include health visitors, school nurses, nursery nurses, midwives and nurses working with children in hospital.

What can employers do in practice to safeguard children? In choosing the right people to work in posts directly or indirectly involved with working with children, they should not rely on a single method of checking, but should maintain a level of ongoing vigilance, creating a sufficiently high barrier to act as a deterrent to committed abusers from seeking employment in working with children.

As part of that ongoing vigilance, consideration should be given to undertaking CRB checks for existing employees, some of whom have been in post for many years, as well as periodic rechecking for all staff whose post is subject to a satisfactory CRB check.

Mindful of the Bichard Inquiry (House of Commons 2004) following the Soham murders, employers need to balance the cost of increased CRB checks and any other checking methods deemed appropriate, and the rights of the prospective employee and the rights of the child, against the lifelong cost to a child, or even loss of life, by allowing just one person to slip through the employment net.

PROFESSIONAL AND VOLUNTARY SECTOR INFLUENCES ON SAFEGUARDING CHILDREN

CHILD PROTECTION AND PUBLIC HEALTH

Within Walsall Sure Start centres, a pilot based on parent empowerment with regard to child protection is being undertaken. Its aim, over a 4-week period, is to bring to life the concept that protecting children really is everyone's business.

Parents are engaged in a training course where child protection principles are imparted in an interactive and safe environment. The emphasis is on promoting the safety of children while enhancing the knowledge and skills of parents and carers within the Sure Start area.

Identification of individual feelings, controlling stress levels and using supportive networks together with person responsibility for the children within their care introduce the course. By the second session, parents are observing role-play between facilitators which provokes discussion about what actually constitutes abuse. Behavioural indicators of abuse are considered, as well as how we can make people feel safe.

In later sessions, the concept of 'trust' is analysed – both how it relates to them personally and also to a child. 'Safe secrets' and the importance of listening to and observing children are highlighted. Developing confidence in children follows on from an exercise with parents relating to the development of their own self-confidence.

The course is conducted within an environment which respects individuals and takes account of some participants' inability to read and others where their first language is not English. A nurturing emphasis for parents includes storytelling and games.

This programme is a good initiative in that it places responsibility for child protection closest to the source – with the parents.

THE SOLIHULL APPROACH

The Solihull Approach (SA) is a health visitor intervention which can be used where identified behaviour problems are causing parental concern. Behaviour problems can lead to over-chastisement, physical abuse and emotional abuse. Where parents find their children's behaviour difficult to manage it can lead to deteriorating parent–child relationships and weaken bonding.

The SA was developed in Solihull by health visitors and psychologists but was so successful that the training has now been extended to many PCTs across the UK and also in Australia.

The approach, which is based on containment of the parent's or carer's anxieties, reciprocity between parent and child and behaviour management, has been shown to have better outcomes for parents and children. This has led to reduced Child and Adolescent Mental Health Service (CAMHS) waiting lists, meaning a shorter wait for those children who need the service. To successfully implement the SA, it is essential that health visitors and CAMHS workers train and work in partnership. Paediatricians and Sure Start workers also benefit from this training, which ensures a collaborative approach.

CHILD PROTECTION AND THE EDINBURGH POSTNATAL DEPRESSION SCALE

The Edinburgh Postnatal Depression Scoring (EPDS) is a tool which is used in conjunction with professional judgement, by health visitors, to identify the possibility of the need for intervention. If the scoring is high, then health visitors can introduce 'listening visits', which have been shown to reduce the likelihood of the condition worsening. Referrals to GPs or community psychiatric nurses (CPNs) would be made where appropriate.

In Walsall, a pilot is being undertaken to address the needs of women whose first language is not English. A survey had shown that these clients were not accessing EPDS as it was not appropriate to do so via an interpreter.

Using pictorial booklets, whose message is also reinforced on each page in the relevant language, e.g. Urdu or Punjabi, the health visitor can now use the tool to provide an equitable service across the PCT.

The pilot is being led by the psychology department, who are working in collaboration with the health visiting service and the local Sure Start centres.

Postnatal depression can be associated with child neglect. By identifying and addressing issues regarding postnatal depression, the likelihood of child neglect can be reduced, and the enhanced enjoyment of her child which a mother may subsequently feel might also prevent potential emotional abuse.

PROFILING

Profiling of families to assess their vulnerabilities when they are not within the child protection system includes using a list of factors which are sometimes associated with child abuse. Profiling families for child protection is different from community profiling, which tends to be more quantitative. For instance, if 50% of the community smokes this is a hard fact supported by statistics showing a relationship between smoking and lung cancer and heart disease. However, child protection profiling is related to 'stop and think' factors which prompt a health visitor to provide an individual care plan and to consider mobilizing other resources There is not necessarily a cause-and-effect relationship, however.

Many public inquiries into the deaths of children as a result of abuse show that the families were isolated. This might prompt health visitors to encourage families to attend parent and toddler groups or other community activities. However, many isolated families never need child protection input and satisfactorily care for their children. Boxes 8.1, 8.2 and 8.3 suggest factors which may impact on parents' ability to safely care for their children and have been recognized by researchers (e.g. Browne et al 1988, Parton 1990) as being important in the profiles of abusers and abused children.

Box 8.1   Factors which may make parents abusers

- Parents abused previous children
- Parents themselves abused as children
- Parent has severe mental health problems
- Parent has severe physical health problems
- Parent has drug-related problems
- Parent has alcohol-related problems
- Domestic violence
- Parent has learning disabilities
- Parent has low stress threshold
- Parent has unrealistic expectations of children
- Parent has no support network
- Parents are isolated

Box 8.2   Factors which might make children more vulnerable to abuse

- Short gaps between birth of children – can result in mother becoming physically depleted with little 'recovery time' and also has several highly dependent children to care for at once
- Low-birthweight children who may require more frequent feeding and where parents may experience greater anxiety
- Children with feeding difficulties
- Child has disabilities
- Child is 'wrong sex'
- Child reported as crying a lot – may be a negative perception or could accurately reflect the extra tension experienced by parents whose enjoyment of the child may then be reduced

---

Box 8.3   Social factors which may precipitate child abuse

- Poor housing
- Overcrowding
- Homelessness
- Racial harassment
- Financial problems
- Poor provision of community facilities

Where there are several factors present a child may be considered vulnerable. However, a single factor in a serious form would also warrant greater support, for example, if a parent had a serious drug problem which impacted badly on the family. When using such a profile, health visitors assess the impact of the factors on the family. There is usually a complex interaction between the factors that result in abuse. Of course many families suffer from some of the above factors, while raising happy and confident children. A large percentage of children in the UK are raised in poverty without, as far as we are aware, being abused.

Profiling is not universally accepted as being useful. Appleton (1994) described how health visitors expressed concern at the lack of definition of vulnerability, which led to disparity in identification of such families due to different perceptions. Her study acknowledges the sometimes transient nature of vulnerability but showed that health visitors had difficulty removing children from the 'vulnerable status' once they were so identified . Others (Dingwall 1989) have highlighted pitfalls in identifying families as vulnerable: staff overreacted in some situations but failed to react in others due to the families' 'vulnerability status'. It may be possible that someone seeing a bruise on a child whose name is on the Child Protection Register might be more likely to be responded to as though it was abuse than if the child's vulnerability status was low. Roberts (1988), shows that there are some influences frequently associated with violent or neglectful parents, but it is essential to remember that it is ultimately the individual's response to the stress which leads to abuse. Having identified vulnerable families, the health visitor will provide an individually tailored, evidence-based package of care to support the child and family.

HALL REPORT AND CHILD PROTECTION

Professor David Hall, in his recently published *Health for all Children* (Hall & Elliman 2003) states:

> *the evidence base for … parent education and health-promoting schools … is more robust than the evidence for some screening tests.*

As a result of this, his recommendations for child health screening include six contacts pre-school age, with three more during school life. Further contacts for support should be agreed between the parent and health visitor, including the nature of the contact, e.g. telephone call.

While there have been concerns expressed by health visitors that reducing the number of contacts could mean vulnerable children being missed, it is clear that such children will have their individually planned programme of care. Children where names are on the Child Protection Register will receive the health visiting service agreed within the Child Protection Plan.

With the ensuing time freed up from performing routine health surveillance of dubious value, health visitors will be empowered to extend their public health role, with its many advantages, including the potential for the reduction in child abuse.

By working in collaboration with community groups, Sure Start projects, children's centres, mother and toddler groups and various women's groups, health visitors can tackle some of the root causes of child abuse.

Over-chastisement of children can result from unrealistic expectations of their development. Child development workshops could address these issues while reducing the isolation, which is often a contributory factor.

Parent-friendly child assessment folders can be a fun way for parents to access their own children and highlight any concerns, while emphasizing the wide variations in normal development, which can be very reassuring.

Assertiveness skills, which may help women remove their children from dangerous relationships, can be fostered in group climates of mutual support.

In considering education regarding the potential for sexual abuse within community settings, health visitors need to enhance their skills and work in multi-agency and multi-disciplinary settings. Parents and carers must be genuinely engaged in the process with the child at the heart of the process.

By engaging the recommendations of Professor Hall, the child's health requirements are met while facilitating the move of the Health

Visiting Service towards making a real difference in lives of children.

There are ten principles involved in implementing the plan. Universality of availability is an ongoing principle but Hall emphasizes the need to include the socially excluded, vulnerable and those not registered with a GP.

While there are no explicit standards of primary care for children at present, the NSF for children will have a specific heading for vulnerable children. This will regulate care across the country, and should drive up standards and reduce inequalities. Information is emphasized, both in its provision to parents and its use in monitoring outcomes for professionals by audit.

With the resulting change in health visiting service provision the audit results regarding child protection will be awaited with optimism.

STOP IT NOW, UK AND IRELAND

Originating in the USA in 1993, 'Stop It Now' has charitable status and has had funding from the Home Office, although local projects are encouraged to bid for funds locally. It has a number of projects up and running in England, namely Surrey, Derby and Derbyshire, and Thames Valley. Others are at the early planning stage, including that in Dudley, where the aim is to cover the whole of the West Midlands area.

As a national and local public health campaign, its aim is to stop child sexual abuse by offering help to abusers and potential abusers. According to information from the organization, indicative prevalence in the UK is that one in six child sexual abusers is under the age of 18 years – young people who could potentially be lifelong abusers.

The main thrust of the work is primary prevention aimed at adults through education to enable them to change behaviour by identifying risk signs in themselves and what they can do about it. The work covers not only those who have previously abused, but also those who feel that they may abuse. Work includes a free confidential phone line follow-up support for a limited number of phone line contacts,

and training for professionals. Besides raising awareness, the aim is to change people's attitudes so that they are more willing to talk about child sexual abuse and to listen to both adults and children when they raise the issue. Although research as to its effectiveness is limited, indications are that this approach is valuable in preventing child sexual abuse and the potentially lifelong effect on victims.

Attitudes to abusers, or potential abusers, will no doubt continue to differ as to whether they deserve to be offered help. Yet it has to be remembered that statistics indicate sex offenders do reoffend in spite of monitoring through the sex offenders' register. Add to this the young age of many offenders, it makes sense to focus on prevention.

It is of paramount importance to focus on the rights of children to safeguard them from this form of abuse. The approach taken by 'Stop It Now' indicates that it can and does work, and as a public health initiative is an effective way of helping to safeguard children.

GOOD ENOUGH PARENTING AS A MEANS OF PROTECTING CHILDREN AND PROMOTING THEIR WELFARE, AND CHANGES IN THE LAW REGARDING UNMARRIED FATHERS OBTAINING PARENTAL RESPONSIBILITY

Parenting is possibly the most important public health issue that our society faces today, a deficit in this area having been linked to a wide range of factors including childhood illness, teenage pregnancy, school disruption, child abuse, juvenile crime and mental illness (Hoghughi & Speight 1998). These inevitably have implications for adulthood and the next generation.

The current public health agenda is committed to improving the health of all, while at the same time narrowing the gap between advantaged and disadvantaged people in society (Department of Health 1999c). The Sure Start programme, which continues to expand to different areas of the country, offers good social experiences from pre-conception to school age, and is directly aimed at disadvantaged or socially excluded groups, with particular emphasis on teaching parenting skills in order to enhance all aspects of children's lives (Government Green Paper Supporting Families 1998). A number of health visitors are already involved in Sure Start projects using their particular skills to advantage, working alongside other agencies and professionals. Others continue to incorporate teaching of parenting skills in their everyday work with families on their caseload.

Much has been said about parenting skills, but what are they? Why is it more appropriate to talk about 'good enough parenting' rather than 'good parenting' and why is this such an important topic? Winnicott (1965) argued that it was unrealistic to and unhelpful to expect parents to be perfect. He argued that the term 'good enough parent', i.e. good enough to meet their child's needs, was more realistic.

The concept of parenting refers to a relationship, a group of activities and a process. Although generally undertaken by biological parents, it can involve anyone concerned with the care of a child, including grandparents, teachers, nurses and others fulfilling parenting tasks with the child (Long 1996). It has three components, the first being love, care and commitment, which protects children from harm and promotes emotional as well as physical health. The second is control/consistent limit setting, which involves setting and enforcing boundaries to ensure children's and others' safety. The third, the facilitation of development, is concerned with both optimizing children's potential and opportunities for using it (Hoghughi 1998).

Why is 'good enough parenting' so important particularly in the early years of a child's life? Children's needs are at their greatest in the first 5 years of life in terms of physical and emotional care and protection from harm by their parents. This is the time when consistent love, care and commitment are essential for a child to develop secure attachment, a sense of security, to learn and explore within the boundaries of a safe environment if they are to grow into well-adjusted, confident, stable adults.

Bowlby (1953) highlighted the importance of secure attachment to a parent/parent figure in a child's development in the first 5 years of life. This is reiterated by Tizzard (1977), who stressed that in his studies of older adopted children the duration of this period could be longer.

Although many families today in which there are children are made up of parents not married to each other, fathers – unlike mothers – do not have an automatic right to parental responsibility. This has made it difficult to be actively involved in parenting their children and taking responsibility for decisions made regarding their welfare. Following the amendment of the Children Act 1989 into the Adoption and Children Act 2002, 1 December 2003 was the appointed day for bringing into force section 111 (parental responsibility of unmarried fathers). This has made it easier for unmarried fathers to obtain parental responsibility. The law now states that if unmarried parents register the birth of their baby together the father gets equal parental responsibility.

Research evidence supporting the change in the law suggests that where fathers devote time to their sons, there is an increased chance of them growing up to be confident adults and early involvement protects against delinquency in later life. Fathers' involvement with their children of both sexes encourages a positive attitude to school; and fathers' involvement with their children's education at age 7 is predictive of higher educational attainment by the age of 20 (http://www.fnf.org.uk/usefuld.htm).

It is acknowledged that there are many factors both in the parent and child that can affect the parent–child relationship, including physical and mental health and social factors, and the absence of one parent. According to Green (1999), if a child is reared by one stable parent he or she is likely to do better than if there are two warring parents remaining together.

The importance of a child receiving 'good enough' parenting from one or ideally both parents to enable them to optimize their abilities is a significant factor in their maturing into stable adults – the building blocks of a healthy and stable society of the future. This is an important area in which health visitors working together with other professionals in the early years can have a positive effect on children's lives by working with all parents, particularly those from disadvantaged backgrounds, to develop 'good enough' parenting skills and to effectively safeguard children from abuse.

DOMESTIC VIOLENCE

Messages from Research (1995) presents a challenge in which the emphasis is on prevention of child abuse and identification of children in need. Where there is domestic violence in a family children may be at risk of physical abuse due to 'cross-fire' injury. They may also suffer physical injury when trying to protect a parent (usually the mother).

The government's response to this – *Safety and Justice* (2003) – shows that one in five men think it acceptable to assault their partners, for example, if there has been sexual infidelity. In addition, research shows that some women choose violent partners even after an unhappy experience of violence.

Interestingly, the government then funded projects to fill the acknowledged gap in knowledge regarding how best to change young people's attitudes towards domestic violence. Before the evaluations were produced and made available to inform such work, the government had already started work in schools to address young people's attitudes.

Using an information pack, teachers were encouraged to stimulate discussion about domestic violence and conflict resolution. This has also been introduced into the citizenship agenda of young offenders institutions and the core curriculum in prisons.

Raising the profile of domestic violence amongst the general public has been approached by the issuing of the leaflet *Loves Me Not*. Womankind, a voluntary agency, also coordinated a white ribbon day aimed at ending violence against women.

Evidence suggests that 32% of perpetrators of domestic violence had been drinking and 8% had been using drugs. As part of the National Drug Strategy the government has commissioned research into these links (Home Office 1999). As 30% of domestic violence starts during pregnancy (Mezey 1997) it is clear that an awareness programme for young people is essential to forewarn them of potential problems.

As part of the government's proposals it is intended that prosecution and sentencing become a deterrent and that any child contact arrangements would ensure the safety of all parties. For further discussion on violence see Chapter 10.

IMPLICATION OF STAFF SHORTAGES FOR SAFEGUARDING CHILDREN

The age distribution of all nurses, midwives and health visitors qualified to practice shows an increasingly ageing workforce, with over half of those registered as being under the age of 40 years 10 years ago, compared with the 2003 figures, which show that over half are over the age of 40 years, and one in four is over 50 years. This also reflects the changing pattern of students entering nursing, of which health visiting is a part, and midwifery, as an increasing number are mature students rather than school leavers (http//www.nmc-uk.org).

When relating this workforce age trend to health visiting, in September 2003 the total number of health visitors practising was 12 984, of which 53% were aged 45 years and over, and 33% were over the age of 50 years. The numbers entering the profession on completion of training shows figures between 638 in 1994–95 to 709 in 1999–2000. As can be seen, the percentage of those entering the profession is smaller than the percentage of those of retirement age who have been active practitioners and those leaving for other reasons, including ill health (http// www.publications.doh.gov.uk/public/ nonmedicalcensus2003).

In practical terms mature students entering training in the profession can be advantageous as they bring with them the benefit of life experiences as well as experience in other fields of nursing or other occupations. However, it also means that they will have fewer years to practise in health visiting than if they had entered the profession in their twenties following qualification in a branch of nursing.

Of further concern is that if the number of those leaving the profession due to retirement, ill health or other reasons continues to be greater than the number of new registrants, the result will be a continuing shrinkage of the workforce. The effects of this are already being felt as nationally it is becoming increasingly difficult to recruit to health visiting, meaning that caseloads are left vacant and existing staff are required to oversee vacant caseloads as well as their own.

Implications for safeguarding children include less time to devote to individual work with children and families where children are on the Child Protection Register, increase in staff stress and sickness levels, and an increase in the possibility of failure in detecting cases of suspected child abuse.

It is in the pre-school years that children are most vulnerable. Without sufficient health visitors working with these young children and their families, offering advice and support in an enabling, non-judgemental and non-stigmatizing way, there is a real risk that vulnerable children will not be identified and the relevant help and support given in order to safeguard them from harm. This is particularly concerning when linked to the national shortage in social workers, although the two services should be working together and not the one compensating for the shortfalls in the other.

Further work needs to be done to increase the number of students entering the profession, consideration being given to direct entry and alternative methods of training. Retention of staff once qualified, and attractive remuneration compared with other professions outside the NHS, also need to be considered if children are to be adequately safeguarded.

THE IMPACT OF CHANGES WITHIN SOCIAL SERVICES ON HEALTH VISITING

The interface between and the collaborative working with social workers are vital to health visitors and the families with whom they work. Until the turn of the century, most health visitors could involve social workers with families who were not coping and, while there were no actual child protection concerns, it was clear that unless considerable support was given the situation would deteriorate dangerously.

In recent years there has been a national shortage of qualified social workers, reflecting the position in teaching and health visiting. Across the board, public services have enhanced skill mix. Family support workers now assist social workers, e.g. for contact visits, nursery nurses take on some of the child health surveillance and classroom assistants hear children reading. This skill mix has enabled qualified staff to target areas of work where a higher skill and knowledge base is required.

For many social services departments this has meant social workers targeting identified child protection cases and 'looked after' children. The knock-on effect for health visitors has been that the previously perceived safety net for vulnerable children has not been there.

In some areas, the family centres which previously supported any vulnerable children are often now offering targeted services. In Solihull, for instance, the family centres now work with families where parents are struggling with drug and alcohol problems or where there is domestic violence.

The government is trying to address these workforce issues across agencies by attempting to make working with children a more rewarding and attractive career. With the new Children Bill now law (2004) there will be greater integration of departments within children's services. The common assessment framework spreads responsibility across all agencies to develop a preventive strategy. Health visitors will collaborate with social workers, Sure Start and schools as well as neighbourhood services. Each patch will assess and respond to a local needs transforming children's services plan and will provide financial assistance for recruitment and retention of social workers to enable this to become a reality.

Every public inquiry into the death of a child as a result of abuse has highlighted the need for inter-agency collaborative working. If the future plans materialize, this will eventually happen.

ASYLUM SEEKER CHILDREN

These children have the same universal rights as all people, and as with all children their needs are best met within the context of the family. This means providing support to refugee families to enable them to meet their children's needs.

Children's needs relating to development should be considered by the professionals involved and resources made available to them and their families if they are to make progress physically and psychologically, and be able to cope with the trauma of the circumstances leading to their arrival in Britain. These can include language barriers and cultural differences, as well as accommodation, benefits and education.

Where the health professional has possible concerns, for example if the child is with someone other than their natural parent and may be subject to exploitation or the standard of care is deemed inadequate, referral to social services is in the child's best interests to give the family the relevant help needed. As in other areas, the West and East Midlands social care regions have a protocol for dealing with safeguarding children from abroad, but this has to operate within the context of immigration law (Dudley Area Child Protection Committee 2004). For further discussion see Chapter 6.

CONCLUSION

Following the publication of the Laming Report in particular, increasing recognition has been given to the importance of safeguarding children. Audit through CHI has highlighted deficits in the service nationally. The plethora of publications, including *What to Do if You're Worried a Child is being Abused, Every Child Matters* and the Children Bill, and the proposed formation of local Safeguarding Children's Boards, Children's Centres and Children's Trusts, in such a short space of time indicates how seriously the government is treating this issue.

No system will ever be foolproof, but the onus is on professionals from all agencies who work with children to make working together a reality, remembering that child protection is everyone's responsibility.

SURE START

Sarah Forester

BACKGROUND

The first Sure Start local programmes were set up in 1999, as the result of a 1998 Comprehensive Spending Review (HM Treasury 1998). This review of services for young children reflected a recognition of equalities in health and a concern that the provision of services for young children appeared to be failing those in greatest need. In addition, there was evidence from programmes like Head Start and the Perry Pre-School programme in the USA, as well as experimental programmes in the UK, that comprehensive early years' programmes could make a difference to children's lives (Glass 1998). These programmes worked by bringing together early education, child care, health and family support for the benefit of young children living in disadvantaged areas and their parents.

The review established that while there was no single blueprint for the ideal set of effective early interventions, they should share the following characteristics:

- involve parents as well as children
- be non-stigmatizing: avoid labelling 'problem families'
- multifaceted: target a number of factors, not just, for example, education or health or 'parenting'
- persistent: last long enough to make a real difference
- locally driven: based on consultation and involvement of parents and local communities
- culturally appropriate and sensitive to the needs of children and parents.

These points then became enshrined into the guiding principles of the Sure Start unit and local programmes. The first programmes began in 1998/9 with a commitment of 10 years of funding and cross-party agreement to ensure their continued development across time and potential governmental change.

THE SURE START UNIT

Since these early beginnings, the Sure Start Unit has developed a larger remit and encompasses a range of interventions designed to improve the early health and well-being of children under 4, their families and communities. While some services are targeted on the 20% most disadvantaged wards across the UK, other services are universal. Funding has been provided by central government to local authorities to provide:

- Early education for all: free part-time nursery education available to all 3- and 4-year-olds. There is also guidance for an early years curriculum, the *Foundation Stage*, which aims to promote quality education provided by qualified nursery teachers.

- More and better child care; extending the opportunity for parents to return to work and get out of poverty, through such programmes as the neighbourhood nursery initiative (NNIs), increased childminder support and the development of after-school places.

- Making child care better quality – working with Ofsted to inspect and approve early education and child care, recruiting and training people to work with children. This also includes the provision of guidance such as *Birth to Three Matters* as a guide for early-years carers.

- Children Information Services (CIS). Every local authority is required to have a CIS where parents and carers can expect up-to-date information on local child care services. In addition, these services are expected to monitor whether provision within their areas is adequate with respect to demand and plan for expansion of appropriate child care places.

- Linking employment advice to information on child care through work done by Job Centre Plus child care advisors.

- Extended schools – ensuring that school resources are at the centre of community initiatives and can be used flexibly by other agencies to meet the needs of families more effectively.

Local Sure Start initiatives are targeted and include both the development of children's centres in the 20% most deprived wards (Sure Start Unit 2003a) and Sure Start local programmes, of which there are now 524 across England, Wales and Northern Ireland. In Scotland money available for local programmes has been put into all areas of the country and a different model has been adopted (see the Sure Start website for details).

SURE START LOCAL PROGRAMMES

Sure Start Local Programmes (SSLPs; Department for Education and Employment 1999b) became the cornerstone of the 1997 Labour Government's campaign to tackle child poverty and social exclusion. From the initial 'trailblazers' these programmes have developed in a series of rounds, with the final Round 6 programmes being agreed by March 2004. Each programme has to work within an agreed set of Sure Start principles (see Box 8.4).

Each SSLP has a defined geographical area that is identified at the planning stage and has to be approved by the Sure Start Unit. Factors such as demographics, especially numbers of children under 4, employment status of families and other measures of deprivation are considered at this stage as well as natural boundaries of communities. The original intention was to ensure all Sure Start services would be available to families within 'pram-pushing' distance of their homes. Plans submitted for

> **Box 8.4   Principles of Sure Start local programmes**
>
> - Community driven and professionally coordinated
> - Working with parents and children
> - Services for everyone but not the same services for everyone
> - Flexible at point of delivery
> - Starting very early
> - Respectful and transparent
> - Outcome driven

approval also had to ensure consultation with a wide group of local families about local services and that the result of this consultation was integral to the Sure Start plan (Sure Start Unit 2003b).

Plans also have to identify a budget for both capital and revenue expenditure, with detailed plans for how this money will be spent in each area of the Sure Start programme. This includes ensuring that services address the following areas:

- outreach and home visiting
- support for families and parents
- primary and community health care
- play, learning and child care
- building community involvement
- special needs support
- improvements to parents employability
- management and evaluation.

SURE START OBJECTIVES AND TARGETS

SSLPs have to identify how the services they are delivering are meeting the four key Sure Start objectives (Box 8.5). Within each objective the SSLP agrees to a number of Public Service Agreement (PSA) targets and Service Delivery Agreement (SDA) targets. Performance against these targets is monitored for each SSLP either on a quarterly, yearly or three-yearly basis depending on the target. For a full account of the complexity of these targets and monitoring requirements see Houston (2003) and the SureStart website.

This is a complex and wide-ranging set of expectations, which means delivering services at individual, family and community levels.

While these principles and targets are national expectations, each local programme has to identify how they will be met on the ground. Thus local strengths in services and communities can be built upon, while at the same time gaps in services are identified. A key part of this process is to bring all service providers together into a Sure Start partnership or management board. This must include all statutory agencies, voluntary agencies as relevant locally, and local parents and community representatives. The

---

> **Box 8.5   Sure Start objectives with SDA targets**
>
> **Objective 1: Improving social and emotional health**
>
> - Support for women suffering postnatal depression
> - 100% contact by programmes to families within first 2 months of baby's life
>
> **Objective 2: Improving health**
>
> - Reduction in smoking amongst pregnant women
> - Increased support for breast-feeding
> - 10% decrease in admissions to hospital for gastroenteritis, respiratory infections and severe injury
>
> **Objective 3: Improving children's ability to learn**
>
> - Access to high-quality play and learning support
> - Increased use of libraries
> - Reduction in number of children requiring speech and language intervention
> - Improved Foundation Stage assessment scores
>
> **Objective 4: Strengthening families and communities**
>
> - Families report improved levels of support
> - Local parents are represented on Sure Start boards
> - Reduction in non-working households and improvements to parents' employability

---

success of SSLPs in delivering this complex agenda depends on the ability of all these partners to work together. Each local programme has a lead agency accountable to the Sure Start Unit both financially and for delivering the PSA targets. However, it is clear that not one agency can deliver this agenda in isolation. The need to develop good working partnerships both at strategic and operational levels is crucial but this is a process that takes time and commitment (NESS 2002).

PARENT PARTNERSHIP AND INVOLVEMENT IN SURE START

One of the key differences and strengths of Sure Start to previous initiatives for families is the key role of parents within local programmes. This is based on the belief that parents and carers are in the best place to identify and suggest solutions to the difficulties faced by families in their area. In this respect Sure Start embodies some of the key principles of a community development approach to service development. Many programmes use community development approaches as a key tool in engaging with communities, especially those groups that have been traditionally 'hard to reach'. Integral to both community development and Sure Start principles is the emphasis that the process of working with parents and communities is as important as the outcomes. The engagement of parents as equal partners in the development of programmes is viewed as an end in itself and as such is inherently empowering.

COMMUNITY DEVELOPMENT AND HEALTH

Community development as a strategy for health has been supported by the literature in health promotion (Alma Ata declaration, World Health Organization 1978, Health 21, World Health Organization 1999) and increasingly by policies which seek to increase user participation in health services (NHS Executive 1998). The background to community development comes from radical social movements and in particular the work of Friere (1972). It is an inherently political process which seeks to move marginalized groups from exclusion to inclusion in decision-making processes (Dalziel 2002). Mackereth (1999) provides a useful overview of the principles of community development (see Box 8.6).

These principles are easily transferred to a Sure Start programme with its emphasis on empowerment, community capacity building and promoting health and well-being of children and families. However, some critiques of community development suggest that a truly bottom-up community-led agenda is impossible

> **Box 8.6 Principles of community development (from Mackereth 1999)**
>
> - Adopts a social model of health
> - Challenges and seeks to influence public policy
> - Derives its mandate from users, not providers
> - Uses a collective approach with groups normally excluded from resources and service planning
> - Places emphasis on confidence building and defining own needs
> - Is free from bureaucratic structures and professional constraints
> - Aims to reduce inequalities in health that derive from socio-economic factors and unequal access to services

to achieve within statutory-led services. Beattie (1991), for example, suggests that community development can be a strategic option to get official health agendas to 'hard-to-reach groups'. For health visitors with experience of working in this way this is not a new issue. Both Craig (1998) and Forester (2002) found that health visitors working in community development often mediated between community and health service agendas in order to develop services that were acceptable to communities. For those of us working within Sure Start, these tensions do exist. An obvious example is the target around smoking reduction, which is rarely raised as a priority for parents. However, within such a wide-ranging project as Sure Start, and given a realistic time-scale to achieve outcomes, the two apparently contradictory perspectives can be accommodated.

SURE START ROEHAMPTON

This section will describe how some of the Sure Start aims and principles are being implemented in one Sure Start local programme. This is only one example. The Sure Start website provides a wealth of information about projects across the country as well as contact details for all local programmes.

Roehampton is an area at the boundary of Inner London consisting of four distinct estates set within the London Borough of Wandsworth. On three sides the area is bounded by the green common land of Richmond and Wimbledon Parks and Putney Heath. The fourth boundary is mostly an affluent part of Putney. Within this area there are approximately 1000 children under 4, of whom a third live in one-parent families and a half in households where no adult is employed. Roehampton has the highest concentration of teenage pregnancy in the borough. The community is 80% white with a huge number of different ethnic groups making up the other 20%. At least eight main languages are spoken within this ethnic mix, although one local primary school reports at least 30 mother tongues amongst its children. Although the area is very green, the housing is characterized by high-rise blocks with very few of the dwellings having access to gardens or safe play spaces. Shops in the estates are small, expensive and offer limited choice. There is no specific place to buy fresh fruit and vegetables, for example, and no provision for ethnic dietary requirements. There are many bus routes going through the area but generally access to transport is poor. Less than 50% of households have a car. In these respects Sure Start Roehampton is probably like many other estates of concentrated deprivation surrounded by relative affluence.

Within a community development approach, it is important to look for resources within a community from which to build. In theoretical perspectives this is referred to as salutogenesis (see, for example, Cowley & Billings 1999) Professionals often only focus on problems within an area. For people living within these communities there are often many positive aspects and resources, both personal and communal. Within Roehampton, as in other Sure Starts, the challenge is to harness the health and social capital within the community and facilitate its growth and development. The positive aspects within Roehampton are:

- A mixed community with many different languages and cultural practices.

- Highly committed parents who give energy and drive to the programme.

- Enthusiastic workers in a number of services, such as 1 o'clock centres, library, churches, youth service, health visitor team, voluntary sector, nursery schools, adult education, Job Centre Plus etc., who are keen to work better together and 'join up' provision on the ground.

- Space and environment – a lot of potential green space and a leafy environment. Roehampton is possibly the only Sure Start with flocks of wild parakeets regularly flying around!

- Regeneration initiatives – a number of projects are being initiated looking at shopping, housing, transport and bringing more employment into the area.

The Sure Start local programme is a Round 6 programme and was given approval in July 2003. It is the second SSLP within the borough, the other being a Round 3 programme. The lead agency is the London Borough of Wandsworth through the Early Years Section of the Education Department. The advantage of being a sixth-wave programme is that planning the programme has been based on lessons learned nationally from other Sure Start programmes (NESS 2002) and from the partnerships forged locally from the other Round 3 programme in the borough. In addition, further guidance from the Sure Start unit (Sure Start 2003b) and that related to Children's Centres (Sure Start Unit 2003a) has and will inform the development of the programme. Sure Start Roehampton will be developing in tandem with the Children's Centre in the area. Also, the emphasis on mainstreaming services has been integral to the thinking from the beginning of the programme.

The overall aim of Sure Start Roehampton is to:

- 'make Roehampton a place people want to move to rather than away from' (London Borough of Wandsworth 2002)
- improve the ability of all children in the area to make the most of their opportunities
- create more opportunities for the families of Roehampton
- ensure equity and quality in all we do.

SURE START ROEHAMPTON CORE SERVICES

There are five core services within the Roehampton programme and a number of other services that are developing to meet identified needs as the programme progresses. Each service is provided by separate providers contracted by Sure Start Roehampton. This model of service provision has been adopted as a step towards early mainstreaming plans and to ensure the engagement of different services within the Sure Start partnership.

Sure Start Roehampton core services are:

1. An enhanced health visiting team, employed by Wandsworth PCT (see next section for details of this team).
2. A crèche and child care service employed by Wandsworth Preschool Playgroup Alliance. This will provide crèche facilities, quality initiatives across all child care provision in the area, a toy library and a low-cost home safety equipment scheme.
3. A group work programme running a range of fun and therapeutic groups.
4. Family support service employed by the Family Welfare Association, providing practical and emotional help to families in their homes and running a volunteer programme.
5. Social worker – joint appointment with local social services children and families team.

In addition the Children's Centre initiative provides the programme with a part-time nursery teacher employed by a local nursery school. There are Sure Start-funded activities delivered by the local library, the Further Education College and Contact a Family. The Sure Start base will also have on site an employment advice project, Citizens Advice Bureau and Job Centre Plus sessions.

These different teams each have a team leader or coordinator who, with the programme coordinator, form a core team for Sure Start Roehampton. The role of this team is to ensure that services work together providing a seamless service to families, that policies and procedures are consistent across services and that parental involvement in service delivery and planning is prioritized.

Box 8.7 identifies how Sure Start Roehampton services map to Sure Start objectives.

Box 8.7 Objectives for Sure Start Roehampton

Objective 1: Support for families and children

- Child care services, crèche, quality initiative across all providers in the area
- Enhanced health visiting team provides outreach and enhanced health visiting service
- Family support service
- Social worker
- Group work programme
- Activities and outings for families

Objective 2: Improving health

- Health visiting team with lead health visitor for specific targets
- Low-cost home safety equipment scheme
- Breast-feeding mentors
- Midwife
- Antenatal groups
- Cooking groups
- Exercise groups

(Continued)

Box 8.7 *(Continued)*

Objective 3: Improving ability to learn

- 'Chatterbox' and 'babblebox' sessions, 2-year tea parties with speech therapist
- Crèche and quality schemes for all child care settings in area
- Book of the month reading scheme at library
- Playgrounds improved and increased outdoor play a priority in crèche
- Group for parents and children together (e.g. PEEP music and exercise)
- Toy library
- Activities and outings
- Family learning
- Support for 'English for speakers of other languages' courses

Objective 4: Strengthening families and communities

- Parents' participation in Sure Start through forum and management groups
- Job Centres advice service
- Neighbourhood nursery, childminding support
- Parent survey forms basis for plan and evaluation
- Education opportunities and taster courses
- Collaborating with HEART (regeneration and employment project)
- Creating employment and training opportunities within services
- Community cafe

THE ENHANCED HEALTH VISITING TEAM

Drawing on the experiences of earlier rounds of Sure Start and with the vision and drive of local health visitors, the Sure Start Roehampton plan developed a model that puts the health visiting team central to the programme. This 'enhanced health team' provides the first contact between families and Sure Start and for referrals into Sure Start. The team is responsible for delivering the reach targets, the targets related to Objectives 1 and 2 of the programme (improving social and emotional development, and improving health) and contributes to supporting families. In this respect the health team is totally integral to Sure Start.

This model was adopted for a number of reasons:

- The health visiting service is a universal community-based service working with families to promote health and well-being, so is the natural home for Sure Start aims and objectives.

- There is some evidence that in other Sure Start programmes the health service has been marginalized or has been seen as the work of a single health visitor.

- In some Sure Start programmes the home visiting function has been duplicated by another service.

- Integrating the service from the beginning will allow for better mainstreaming when Sure Start funding diminishes.

- One of the principles of Sure Start is to change existing services and this was seen as an opportunity to reshape the health visiting service in the area and to promote the public health role of health visitors.

HOW DOES THE ENHANCED TEAM WORK?

Sure Start Roehampton has contracted with Wandsworth Primary Care Trust to deliver an enhanced service for which a service specification has been drawn up. In effect Sure Start pays for two health visitors, one nursery nurse and a midwife over and above the existing establishment. Additional funding has increased speech therapy hours by two sessions a week.

In return the PCT has designated all workers in the area, Sure Start workers, and are developing a team approach to working with families with children under 5. The total team consists of seven health visitors (one a team leader), three nursery nurses, a midwife and a full-time administrator. The team leader is a member of the Sure Start core team and is responsible for developing the team and ensuring both PCT and Sure Start expectations and targets are met.

The team is expected to deliver services related to the Sure Start objectives which are detailed within the specification. This will mean more intensive home visiting, more group work, and better information tracking to help inform, develop and manage the programme.

The team has decided to work geographically while retaining a named link with local general practices. Each staff member is also the named link to a local child care provision: playgroup, 1 o'clock centre, nursery school, etc. This facilitates a public health role approach to health promotion. For example, in dental care every setting has signed up to the same healthy snacks policy.

Each member of the team is developing a speciality role such as teenage parents, promoting breast-feeding, postnatal depression, special needs, accident prevention and baby massage, which relate to both the objectives and local needs. For this health issue, they will become a resource to both the health team and the wider Sure Start team. For example, the health visitor working with teenage parents initiative, represents Sure Start on the locality teenage parents multi-agency group and the health visitor and nursery nurse working in special needs are working with the portage service to improve and reinstate regular inter-agency reviews.

In addition, training needs of this team and the other Sure Start teams are identified together. The aim is to provide consistency in response to parents and carers about issues wherever that family choose to access services or advice. Therefore training about domestic violence, managing debt, challenging behaviour and

other common issues is undertaken across teams. In some areas, for example the promotion of breast-feeding, the health team will take the lead in developing consistent information to enable all Sure Start services to be updated and informed.

At the time of writing this team is at the early stages of development; however, there are already examples of how this team integrates with the rest of the Sure Start programme:

- One health visitor co-facilitates the parents' forum.
- A family health group and a multicultural parenting group are being run by two health visitors with the group worker.
- One nursery nurse runs music sessions at the outreach events.
- Two health visitors sit on the Sure Start management board and subgroups.
- All events and groups are coordinated through the Sure Start core team.
- The health team is an important source of information and encouragement to parents to attend trips and events. The team will accompany parents to such events and work with them in order to be a 'friendly face' for parents.
- An audit of health visitors records cross-referenced to GP records provides sound baseline data for planning how services develop.

Information gathering and exchange is being constantly reviewed to ensure that health systems are compatible with Sure Start systems. This remains a major challenge both in terms of compatibility of IT systems but also the ethical issues it raises. The aim is to get systems that enable not only the recording of monitoring data for both PCT and Sure Start but also will provide accessible data for practitioners to monitor, evaluate and develop their own work.

HARD-TO-REACH STRATEGY

A major concern within Sure Start programmes is that those families most in need are able to access and influence the services that are on offer. Within monitoring procedures each programme has to ensure that new families are continually being involved and engaged with services. This means not only having an actively implemented equal opportunities policy but also identifying hard-to-reach groups within the local community and ensuring resources are used to meet their needs. To ensure equal outcomes for children there need to be different inputs for some families. Each programme is therefore required to develop a hard-to-reach strategy that identifies particular groups within its community and outline actions for engaging these groups within the programme.

In Roehampton the following groups have been identified:

- those families who have little or no spoken English
- families with chaotic lifestyles who do not currently use services
- teenage parents
- families with children or adults with special needs
- fathers.

In order to achieve equal outcomes for these groups additional resources are required to ensure that the programme engages with these groups in a way that facilitates their involvement. Examples of how Roehampton Sure Start has started this process include:

- paying child care costs for people attending 'English for speakers of other languages' (ESOL) courses
- holding specific events for fathers (see Sure Start 2003c)
- participating in a multi-agency teenage pregnancy locality group and supporting the current Young Mums groups
- working with Contact a Family to survey services for families with special needs and consult with families in a fun day
- ensuring through an increased home visiting service that isolated families have their needs identified and met.

In this project extra resources have gone into the team but the methodology for looking at service provision anew is not specific to Sure Start. Ways of working developed within Sure Start projects are transferable to non-Sure Start health settings. Information about community development in health visiting can be obtained from the CPHVA special interest group for community development and websites listed below. The Sure Start website and publications give examples of many projects that could be transferred to other settings.

USER INVOLVEMENT

As described above, parent participation within the Sure Start programme is an essential component and one which Sure Start Roehampton is committed to as it develops. User participation within health service planning has often been paid lip service and rarely been moved much beyond user satisfaction surveys (Poulton 1999). In the past, this may have been due to professional protectionism (Ashton & Seymour 1988) but a review by the Health Development Agency (2000) suggests that issues of power still have to be addressed if community participation in planning services is to become a reality.

Parents are the best ambassadors for services, and if parents who have been involved feel that they have been taken seriously and their opinions valued they are likely to bring others along. In Roehampton, the commitment to addressing these issues has meant really challenging both staff and provider organizations to look at what barriers might exist to ensuring local parents can be equal partners. This requires:

- developing a culture of user involvement in all aspects of the programme at both strategic and delivery levels
- ensuring parents' concerns are central to how the programme develops by a continual process of consultation with parents and carers
- identifying and removing barriers, both practical and attitudinal, to parental involvement
- promoting reflective practice in relation to user participation in all core services.

The following describes some of the ways that Sure Start Roehampton ensures these principles happen.

MANAGEMENT COMMITTEE AND SUBGROUPS

In order to facilitate parents' full participation in these the following practices have been adopted:

- The constitution requires that parents are the majority group on the management board with six seats. Three parents have to be present for any decisions to be made.
- If parents have to leave, for example to pick up children, then the meeting stops even if the agenda has not been finished.
- The parents' report is a standing agenda item at the beginning of the meeting to ensure their concerns are given due consideration.
- In the running of the meeting parents are often asked their opinion first before more powerful professionals to ensure their views are not influenced or diminished.
- All meetings are held at a place and time to suit parents and have a free crèche available.
- Papers are written in comic sans font, which is more easily read by people with low literacy skills in English.
- Our subgroups each have at least two parents on them, so parents do not feel isolated.
- Wherever possible a smaller meeting of parents is held the day before the management committee to go through the agenda (which can be very lengthy), to ensure everyone understands what issues need decisions and for them to discuss together who will say what.
- The finance officer and Chair are working on making the finance report more easily understood, which will help both parents and professionals alike.
- Items are regularly passed back to the parents' forum for discussion before decisions are made.

PARENTS' FORUM

The parents' forum is viewed as a central component of the development of Sure Start Roehampton. It meets weekly with a usual attendance of between 12 and 15 parents out of a regular pool of about 24 parents. It is open to anyone and regularly readvertised. This discusses any aspect of Sure Start, with some items coming from parents and some from workers or the management committee. Again 'pressing issues' from parents are dealt with at the beginning of the meeting. At the parents' request, meetings are facilitated by workers. Ground rules are regularly revised and systems for decision making discussed. A crèche and lunch are provided.

INTERVIEWING FOR ALL WORKERS

Parents have been involved in interviewing every worker for Sure Start services. This includes the coordinator, administrator, health staff, crèche staff and social worker. They have participated in shortlisting and interviewing alongside professionals. Some training has been given but not all parents who have participated in interviews have had this and it is not a requirement. This has been a learning experience for workers and parents alike. Parents have developed some very clear and insightful questions to ask potential employees and given reasoned assessments of workers' abilities and qualities that would make them suitable to work in the area. Initial concerns from some professionals with this process have not been borne out in practice and the added value to recruitment is now accepted as the norm. Parents feel ownership of the appointments.

CONSULTATION ON SPECIFIC SERVICES

Parents have been involved from the beginning in developing both the wider plan and specific briefs for all services. Particular views have been sought for particular services; for example, childminders were asked to a meeting looking at services for them and a consultation fun day was held for families with children with special needs. Other services have been discussed in the parents' forum. For example, 'What do you want from a midwifery service?' was a discussion that was fed in, in writing, to the midwifery provider and informed the job description of the midwife. On another occasion the local librarian attended the parents' forum and as a result the times of 'baby rhyme time' were changed. This has resulted in increased uptake of that service.

ORGANIZING ACTIVITIES AND EVENTS

Parents have been involved in organizing events and activities to attract other families into Sure Start and to provide social fun times for families. There is no doubt that the events that have been parent driven have been the most successful. Small groups of parents have met with one worker to organize each event and have worked within a budget. Criteria for trips have been developed in the parents' forum, which is where ideas for events are agreed. Care has been taken to make events open and accessible to all. Discussions around inclusion for all members of the community have developed from both planning and evaluating events.

NEWSLETTER, OUTREACH AND PUBLICITY

Parents have designed and written newsletters and publicity material, and have helped at outreach and publicity events. Within the parents' forum, people have volunteered to translate material into six of the eight languages required locally. To produce the newsletter one parent has use of a laptop bought by Sure Start, and parents can use the facilities of the office to make telephone calls or photocopy and write letters. In addition, mobile telephone top-up cards have been bought from petty cash for parents arranging events. Financial issues have arisen when parents may wish, for example, to do shopping for an event but do not have spare cash. Money 'upfront' from petty cash facilitates parental involvement and provides a marker of mutual trust and respect. Staff aim to treat parents using the office as valued members of the team and give priority to their needs.

GENERAL PRACTICAL ISSUES

Child care is the single biggest barrier to full participation. Workers may be welcoming of children but parents have repeatedly said that they cannot concentrate or feel fully involved in meetings if their children are present. This can be resolved by using a crèche, childminders or other child care provision such as play workers or nursery nurses. Experience shows that this provision has to feel safe, secure and of good quality for both parents and children, in order for parents to feel able to participate fully.

Attention needs to be paid to using simple jargon-free language in all verbal and non-verbal communications to parents, with translation into other languages and visual images or other media used as much as possible. Explanations of how services work, how decisions are made and important terminology are given repeatedly so that all parents can feel properly informed.

HOW TO MAKE PARENT INVOLVEMENT HAPPEN

This level of parent involvement will only happen with the commitment of all staff and services. As a first step a basic principle of community development is to go to where the community is. This means meeting people in 1 o'clock centres, schools, shopping centres, post offices, chemists, GP surgeries – anywhere people with young children go and meeting them with an open agenda, and being prepared to listen. The second step is to take people's concerns seriously. If people feel they are being listened to they are more likely to want to engage with the service. Through the parent forum, workers have realized that parents' concerns have to be dealt with first before being able to discuss workers' agendas. This happens in individual meetings but there is a wider point to be made. Often staff are pressurized to get something achieved but working *with* parents takes time and patience to develop. Meetings and activities need to be at convenient times and places. The simplest way to achieve this is to ask parents and not assume that parents are comfortable with venues or arrangements set by workers.

TENSIONS IN DEVELOPING PARENT PARTICIPATION

There is no doubt that developing real user involvement takes time and energy and at times can be challenging. The community is not necessarily a homogeneous group and different factions may have very different views. Some groups may be more powerful than others within a consultative body, for example. Many heated discussions have taken place in our parent forum around issues of inclusion. These have ranged from dealing with parents and children's behaviour at Sure Start events to accusations of racism amongst parents. These discussions reflect the real concerns of the community within which Sure Start operates. These conflicts have been managed in a number of ways:

- Ensuring, at the parents' request, that the parents' forum is facilitated by two experienced group workers.
- Regularly reviewing and developing ground rules.
- Regularly reviewing the Sure Start objectives and principles with parents.
- The implementation of the hard-to-reach strategy. Within this there have been many discussions regarding separate versus inclusive development for different groups. Sure Start Roehampton is currently taking a staged approach whereby, for example, we run a separate Somali parents' group with the long-term aim of ensuring their inclusion in all services.

For Sure Start Roehampton workers, parent involvement is a culture that we wish to foster. This is an ongoing challenge. It is often easier to do something oneself but much better in the long run to involve others in the process.

CONCLUSION

This sub-chapter has given an overview of Sure Start and described just one local programme. It has aimed to raise some of the issues that Sure Start Roehampton has addressed in the early stages of its development, in particular a real commitment to user participation. Every project of this kind will transform over time and develop as new needs are identified. It is important to retain that developmental aspect and be continually responsive to local communities.

The Sure Start principles provide an excellent framework for working with families and communities and can be transferred to any setting where workers are keen to make a difference to outcomes for children and families and address inequalities in a positive way.

USEFUL WEB SITES

Sure Start: www.surestart.gov.uk
National Evaluation of Sure Start: www.ness.bbk.ac.uk
Community Development Exchange: www.cdx.org.uk
    (formerly the Standing Conference for Community
    Development)
Health Development Agency: www.hda-online.org.uk
HDA evidence-based home page:
    www.hda.nhs.uk/evidence/
The Kings Fund: www.kingsfund.org.uk

WHAT WILL CHILDREN'S TRUSTS MEAN FOR HEALTH VISITING?

Jane Middleton

This section will describe the information currently available concerning Children's Trusts, and explore the potential implications for health visitors. It will consider the role of health visiting in relation to Children's Centres and extended schools, including integrated team working and leadership.

POLICY BACKGROUND

Children's Trusts were described in the government paper *Every Child Matters* (Department of Health 2003a), and further detailed in *Every Child Matters: Next Steps* (Department for Education and Skills 2004b). The legal framework for their existence is being introduced in the Children Bill 2004, and most recently they were described again in the *Five Year Strategy for Children and Learners* (Department for Education and Skills 2004a). Here, it was made clear that 'Children's Trusts are not new statutory bodies – they are partnership bodies that give effect to the new duties to cooperate in promoting the well-being of all children.' While Children's Trusts do not have to be in place until 2008, most will be operational by 2006. They relate to all children aged 0–19.

Local authorities have been given the duty to ensure that these trusts come into being, and this has led to scepticism on the part of many that health partners will be enabled or be willing to take part. The key documents concerning children that health bodies will regard as their planning tools are the Children's National Service Frameworks. These are still awaited, and it is imperative that the theme of integration is also contained in these frameworks, and that government works closely between the DOH and DFES, in order to demonstrate that this must also happen at local level. Early indications are positive in this respect.

The main components of a Children's Trust described in *Every Child Matters* are that it should have all the functions of the local education authority (but not school management, as LMS remains), children's social services and potentially the following health services: community paediatrics; services commissioned by drug action teams; teenage pregnancy coordination; locally commissioned and provided CAMHS; speech and language therapy; health visiting; and occupational therapy services concerned with children and families, and services which PCTs have decided to delegate to the Children's Trust with funds they have provided.

To give some early leadership and shape to future local developments, in 2004 the Local Government Association (LGA) and a range of national partner organizations including the NHS Confederation produced a document called *From Vision to Reality: Transforming Outcomes for Children and Families*. They have nominated a model of integration of services which does not depend on structural change, but on shared outcomes, delivered from service hubs, and have 37 pilot areas nationally where this is happening. The potential providers are from health, social care, education and the voluntary sector.

Additionally, there are 35 Pathfinder Children's Trusts in the country that have been in existence since September 2003 which do involve structural change. They vary in size and purpose: some are commissioning trusts, some

service provider trusts, and some do both. Some apply to one area of children's services, e.g. early years, and some to all. Most, but not all, involve health partners as full participants. It is too soon for any meaningful evaluation of these trusts to have taken place.

The main theme of all of this work has been the better integration of planning and delivery of services for children and families, particularly in areas of deprivation and where individual children are at risk. This is one of the platforms of the Labour Government's reforms for children, based on an intention to reduce or eradicate child poverty. The policy is outcome driven, but also arises from reviews of existing services, and a view that they are not being delivered in the most effective way for families and children. The policy places equal importance on protection and prevention, and expects services to be commissioned and delivered to this ethos.

Additionally, the Laming Report into the death of Victoria Climbié highlighted again what happens to children when service providers do not work together, and emphasized the view that it was time for a radical change. (Not radical enough for some, who would have liked a Children's Trust to herald the beginning of a new legal structure for the planning, commissioning, funding and delivery of children's services.)

CHILDREN'S CENTRES AND EXTENDED SCHOOLS: WHAT ARE THEY, WHAT ARE THEY TRYING TO ACHIEVE AND WHY? WHAT DO THEY DO?

The key delivery mechanisms for the required joint or integrated working of a Children's Trust are Children's Centres and extended schools. These centres are the manifestation of the government's view that families should be able to access, or to be signposted to, seamless support for themselves and their children through one centre in their community. Services should join up around the child and the family, not vice versa. They should provide universal and preventive services as well as catering for families with greater needs. They should operate within an overarching context of protecting children.

Children's Centres will all provide child care and early education for 0- to 5-year-olds (known as 'educare'), and will also provide family support, health services, employment advice and specialist support. 'Ante- and postnatal care will be linked to Children's Centres, and each family will be supported by a team of midwives and health visitors linked to the Centre' (Department for Education and Skills 5-year strategy for children and families). Additionally, Children's Centres will provide outreach work to families unable or unwilling to access the main centre. Additionally, many centres have developed a hub and satellite approach, and will provide outreach services via local satellites that are at venues acceptable to local families. There will be a Children's Centre in most of the top 20% most deprived wards in the country by 2006, and there is an aim that by 2008 all poor children should have access to such a resource.

Children's Centres present something of a dilemma for the future of health visiting. Currently, health visiting is a generic service, while the move to Children's Trusts is requiring a proportion of the service to be dedicated to the care of children aged 0–5 and their families. Also, while Children's Trusts are for all children, Children's Centres require a preventive approach, which for health visiting pulls the resource towards the public health role. While this fits the ideological perspective of many, it does bring questions in terms of resource allocation for child health surveillance and child protection matters. Ironically, it is in the inner cities where this dilemma will have the most acute impact, for it is here that there will be the most Children's Centres, and here that the most intensive child protection work with families is required.

Of course, if the preventive work bears its expected fruits, the number of families requiring intensive specialist child protection input from qualified professionals will reduce. However, research has demonstrated that there is generally an increase in the number of child protection cases when preventive services move into

an area before there is a subsequent decrease. Also, the inner cities have high levels of mobility, so the continuity of work with families is lost. A possible consequence of Children's Centres is therefore that PCTs will have to rationalize their resources to areas of most need, and the opportunity for preventive work in more affluent areas will be diminished. This is already happening in many cities as a result of the demographic age profile of health visiting, and the consequent lack of available staff. However, it is an unintended consequence of the development of Children's Centres which would need to be addressed by the Children's Trust when it is looking at its funding policies regarding health visiting for children and families on a whole population level.

Extended schools are those that offer services other than education to the school population and neighbourhood. They can be based on a primary or a secondary school. They have more of an impact on the role of school nurses than health visitors, but contribute to the pressure on PCTs to consider geographical rather than GP-attached allocation of community-based nursing. Extended schools can be attached to Children's Centres, thus creating an opportunity for care and support for the whole family.

LEADERSHIP AND DELIVERY ETHOS

Children's Trusts will either directly employ staff or operate on secondments on a 'dotted-line' accountability path, as in Youth Offending Teams, thus enabling clinical governance to be offered by PCTs (Integrated Care Network 2004).

What is clear is that for children's services post Climbié there is a determination to create multi-agency, multi-skilled teams, where staff receive training together which draws on the skills and expertise of each discipline. It is also highly likely that a new form of generic children's worker will arise from the process of joint working, who will need a new form of training, qualification, support and management. These staff are sometimes referred to as 'paraprofessionals'.

They would offer support to parents which provided information on local services, offered direct advice on parenting, and drew on the knowledge and skills of professionals in the team in relation to play, education, child development, child and family health, diet and nutrition, breast-feeding, stopping smoking, child behaviour and more. They would offer home visits, outreach services and group work. This would leave the specialist professional staff free to offer extra and more skilled support to families at times of crisis in their lives, or where there were concerns.

There is an enormous opportunity for health visitors to become leaders in the field of training, and to be the supporters and supervisors of teams of paraprofessionals. Health visitors have, throughout their history, had a holistic and generic approach to their work. Experience from Sure Start local programmes shows that, with training in management skills, health visitors make extremely effective leaders of generic teams. Health visitors have been enthusiastic about the Sure Start programme, and have often led the local partnership working required to make these programmes a success. Skills in fostering and maintaining partnership working are key to the success of Children's Centres, and, at strategic level, Children's Trusts.

The Department for Education and Skills is currently developing a leadership programme for staff working in Children's Centres, and it is likely that health visitors will be offered the opportunity to join this programme once it is complete. It is not difficult to conclude, therefore, that health visiting could be in the forefront of the change processes required to take forward the development of Children's Trusts.

CONCLUSION

The plethora of influences on strategy towards child protection illustrates the concerns that government, professionals and the voluntary sector place on safeguarding children. The major government documents following the Laming Report all have a potential influence on the work of specialist community public health workers who are concerned in the duty of care towards children. Sure Start programmes that have successfully developed show the benefits of that government initiative, and local PCT and Health Trust organization of Children's Trusts will further strengthen safeguarding of children. The following chapter looks at practical issues in relation to safe care and development of children.

Chapter 9

Safeguarding children – issues and dilemmas

Margaret Reynolds, Janice Frost, Joan Leach and Jean Glynn

Traditionally health visitor education has had a major focus on the development of the individual and, in particular, children. Modern thinking suggests that a general overview of the child's growth and progress is sufficient to identify problems that may occur. A dilemma is that if a health visitor is legally challenged in a court of law over professional concerns about developmental delay, a general overview is not scientific evidence. Reynolds argues coherently for a combination of the use of a Schedule of Growing Skills linked to a carer's assessment of their own parenting skills and self-esteem can form a good basis for safeguarding the child from ill care, neglect or abuse. Health visitors frequently are asked advice concerning child development problems and Frost offers some practical intervention suggestions. Leach offers advice on safeguarding children from accidents and Glynn is particularly concerned with health inequalities that can inhibit the promotion of good sexual health.

SAFEGUARDING CHILDREN BY DEVELOPMENTAL SCREENING

Margaret Reynolds

INTRODUCTION

The 21st century has seen significantly increased importance placed on safeguarding children and raising the profile of this area of work. This research project is of potential, particular relevance to health visitors working in this field in enabling them to evaluate their work with children and their families and to share information with other relevant agencies and professionals, as well as promoting the partnership approach between the family and the professional.

There is a shift in thinking away from the term 'child protection' to the more proactive, all-encompassing term 'safeguarding children'. This concept originated from concerns about children and young people in the care system ('looked after' children), to include protecting all children from harm. Although it has no

definition in law or in government guidance, the report, *Safeguarding Children* (Department of Health 2002d) defines it as:

- 'all agencies working with children, young people and their families take all reasonable measures to ensure that the risks of harm to children's welfare are minimized'; and
- 'where there are concerns about children and young people's welfare, all agencies take all appropriate actions to address those concerns, working to agreed local policies and procedures in full partnership with other local agencies'.

The main elements of the project, which is ongoing, will now be described.

Developmental screening was first introduced in Britain in the 1950s and 1960s (*Lancet* 1986). However, interest in child development can be traced back more than 200 years. The first known account is that of Tiedmann in Germany, who published a detailed account of the developmental progress of one child in 1787 (Illingworth 1987). Little interest was shown until nearly a century later, with Charles Darwin's account of the development of the eldest of his 10 children in 1877, followed by Shinn publishing one of the most complete accounts of a young child's development in 1893 (Illingworth 1987).

Possible reasons for more interest in children and their development may have been a drop in the infant mortality rate as a result of advances in medical science and changes in the economy, which was previously dependent on child labour. Parents were in less danger of losing their children through early mortality, so could afford to have fewer of them and to become more emotionally involved with them (Kessen 1965). An example of the social and economic climate in 19th-century Britain concerning young children is that as late as the 1840s one in five children died before their first birthday. The Prudential Mutual Insurance, Investment and Loan Association (now the Prudential Corporation) refused to insure the lives of children under the age of 10 for fear of them being murdered so that the insurance could be collected (Dennett 1998).

Pioneering work in developmental testing was carried out mainly by child psychologists, who were interested in designing pass/fail systems to establish 'norms' of intelligence or behaviour. An example is Gesell, who, while studying mentally defective children, began thinking about the early signs of mental deficiency. He set up studies of the normal infant, which led to the establishment of 'norms' (Gesell 1925, 1948, Gesell & Amatruda 1947).

Others who developed developmental testing scales included Stutsman (1931), Buhler & Hetzer (1935) and Cattell (1940) for children under 2 years of age. Binet scales of various types were available for children over 2 years of age (Binet & Simon 1915). Work by Bayley was concentrated on children under the age of 3 years (Bayley 1933, 1940). The Denver Developmental Screening test (DDST), developed in Denver, Colorado (Frankenburg & Dodds 1967), was later revised and abbreviated. The age range covered is 2 weeks to 6.4 years.

A British psychological scale of note produced by Griffiths, a paediatrician, consists of five subscales initially for use with children aged 14 days to 24 months, later extended to 8 years (Griffiths 1954, 1970). These scales were subsequently revised in 1992. In her work, Griffiths changed the emphasis to devising testing procedures to aid in paediatric diagnosis, management of young handicapped children and guidance for parents.

In Britain further work was carried out by Sheridan in development of the psychometric test Stycar developmental sequences (Sheridan 1960). This work drew on the developmental testing scales available in the late 1930s and 1940s (see above; Sheridan 1975). Reasons for this work were that none of the previous scales were British, they did not agree among themselves and there was a lack of graded tests for visual and auditory acuity, necessary for paediatric assessment of young handicapped children. Additionally, the available scales did not cover signs of communication disorders, unstable personality or social maladjustment.

It is from the Sheridan Stycar sequences that the Schedule of Growing Skills (SGS) was developed. Initially it was developed as

Table 9.1 Stycar areas and schedule fields

Stycar areas (Sheridan 1975)	Schedule fields (Bellman & Cash 1987, Bellman et al 1996)
Posture and large movements	Passive postural skills Active postural skills Locomotor skills
Vision and fine movements	Manipulative skills Visual skills
Hearing and speech	Hearing and language skills Speech and language skills
Social behaviour and play	Interactive social skills Self-care social skills

a research instrument, covering children up to 3 years in the National Childhood Encephalopathy study. This was set up in response to alleged neurological reactions to pertussis vaccine (Bellman 1984). It was later developed further up to the age of 5 years, together with the use of the Reynell language scale, as Sheridan was weak in identifying speech and language delay early (Reynell 1969, Bellman & Cash 1987) (Table 9.1).

The tool has been shown through research and validation to be applicable to ethnic minority groups as well as the indigenous population. This is an important issue considering the composition of the child population in the UK today. No child fails, which was a criticism of older tools with a rigid pass/fail system. Nine skill areas are covered, a breakdown of the original Sheridan Stycar areas, creating a much more sensitive tool, yet still quick and easy to administer. The screening results highlight a child's strengths and weaknesses and can be used for health promotion, working in partnership with parents (Bellman & Cash 1987). A copy of the screening results is given to the parent, other copies being available for the GP, the health visitor and for referral if necessary. An example of SGSII paperwork is shown in Figure 9.1.

Prematurity is taken into account at the interpretative stage. Subsequent minor revision of SGS was carried out, together with the

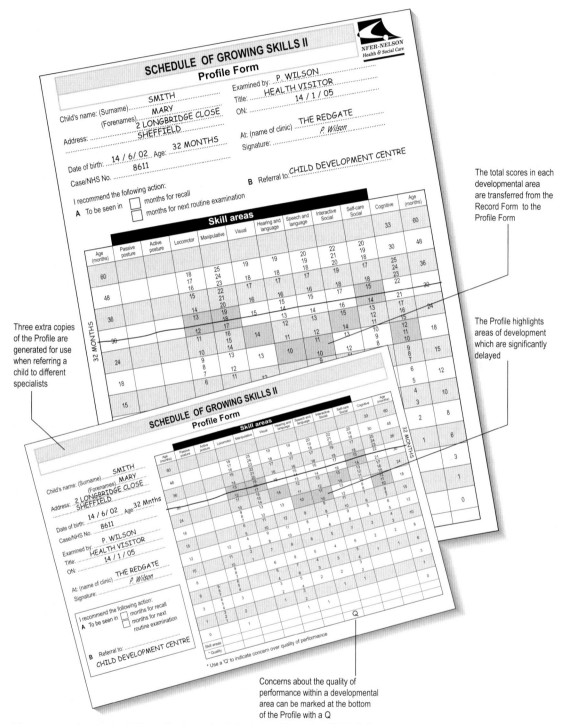

Figure 9.1   A sample child profile from the Schedule of Growing Skills II ©1996 Martin Bellman, Sundara Lungain and Anne Ankett. (Reproduced by permission of the publishers, NFER-Nelson, The Chiswick Centre, 414, Chiswick High Road, London W4 5TF, England. All rights reserved.)

introduction of a cognitive scale (Bellman et al 1996).

THE SCREENING DEBATE

The screening debate has been ongoing over many years, influences upon it including research and moral and ethical considerations, as well as cost and cost-effectiveness. In considering this issue, child health surveillance, child health promotion, screening and developmental screening will be considered.

CHILD HEALTH SURVEILLANCE

This is a broad term including developmental screening and surveillance, immunization, growth monitoring, detection of child abuse and management of chronic and acute illness (*Lancet* 1986). It is a preventive programme aimed at improving all aspect of children's health, which should be carried out in partnership with parents or carers (Birmingham Health Authority 1990).

Hall (1991) broadly agrees with this, also stating that surveillance involves a set of activities initiated by professionals and including oversight of physical, social and emotional health, monitoring of developmental progress, offering and arranging intervention where necessary, and health education. The relationship between primary health care professionals should be one of partnership rather than professional supervision, with parents being enabled to make use of services and expertise in a way most appropriate to their needs.

An example from the health visiting perspective could be where delay in speech and language development has been identified through developmental screening and the professional and parent discuss together possible reasons for this and ways to help the child. It could be that attending a playgroup is the initial agreed course of action: mixing with other children of a similar age could help to stimulate speech and language development. If after further review it is found that satisfactory progress has not been made, parent and professional might then agree that the best course of action

is referral to a speech therapist at a venue convenient for mother and child. A satisfactory outcome for the child is far more likely if parent and professional work in partnership.

CHILD HEALTH PROMOTION

In order to emphasize that preventive health care for children involves more than the detection of defects (implied in the concept of surveillance), Hall (1996) proposed the term 'child health promotion'. 'Child health surveillance' would be retained but would refer specifically to activities designed to achieve early detection (secondary prevention). Hall & Elliman (2003) use the term 'child health promotion', dividing this into primary and secondary prevention.

The following key principles are included in child health promotion: work based on need, partnership between client/carer and professional, primary prevention, a public health approach and teamwork. Hall & Elliman (2003) includes the concept of providing a broad spectrum of services, the child being seen as a member of the family and the family as part of the community.

When applying these two concepts in practice – the core programme for child health surveillance and recommendations on child health promotion (Hall 1996) – the first should be continued and the second used selectively in the light of locally defined need and outcomes (Department of Health Specialist Clinical Services Division 1996).

An example of child health promotion in health visiting practice is anticipatory guidance given to a mother with an 8-month-old child just starting to get around by rolling and squirming. It would be pointed out that soon the child would be crawling, then walking and taking every opportunity to explore the world within his/her reach. Accident prevention in relation to the child's age and stage of development would therefore be a particularly important topic to discuss. Enabling the mother to understand why, for example, a fireguard and safety gate was needed, with assistance given in obtaining these items through a local scheme if the family was on a low income, would be more likely to be effective in promoting child safety in the home than simply telling the mother to purchase them.

DEBATE ON THE VALUE OF SCREENING IN GENERAL

There is ongoing debate about various types of screening relating to child health. Specific examples and conclusions from recent screening research are included here, together with questions raised, in order to explain more clearly why there is debate. The value of continuing research into screening should be recognized, with its potential to add to and improve health care.

We need to question continually what we are doing in relation to screening; not only why we are doing it, or whether we need to do it, but also, if we do, is there a better way?

In many areas these questions are continually being raised, as the following research examples show. As some questions are answered, still others are raised, opening up further debate. It may not simply be a question of whether a particular type of screening is right or wrong but what is best practice in giving value for money. This may conflict with what is considered to be ethically or morally right or wrong.

In developmental screening, as knowledge increases this should be used to inform and change practice. What is important is, not only to use the best tool available, but to acknowledge the importance of continuing research. Older tools need to be subject to ongoing evaluation and changes made as research indicates. The limitations of a screening tool, however good, need to be acknowledged, as the professional's judgement and expertise are of significant importance in interpreting results. A simple example could be where a child is not able to walk alone by the age of 20 months. If the child has been kept strapped in a pushchair for much of each day and not allowed the opportunity to develop gross motor skills, the reason for delay could be environmental rather than medical. This is an important factor that the health visitor may be aware of, and would be an important consideration when making a medical assessment of the child.

Screening for hearing loss (Davis et al 1997), which looked at neonatal screening in detection of congenital hearing loss, shows the complexity of the issues that have to be considered. The research was carried out because of doubt concerning the efficacy of existing programmes – a health visitor distraction test (HVDT) at 7–8 months – in identifying early, permanent hearing impairment. There was growing evidence that new technology available was a more effective option.

Although examples of good practice were found, it was concluded that the health visitor distraction test had poor sensitivity, the median age of identification being 12–20 months. This compared with neonatal screening, which showed high test sensitivity and high specificity, median age of identification being 2 months. However, it was noted that the number of universal neonatal hearing screening programmes being implemented was limited at present.

In terms of cost, universal neonatal screening was approximately half as expensive as the HVDT, with targeted neonatal screening approximately 20% as expensive as universal HVDT. Targeted screening included neonates in whom 'at risk' factors had been identified. Issues here included the high initial cost of equipment for neonatal screening and whether neonatal screening should be universal or targeted, the latter carrying the risk of failing to identify all 'at risk' children, or whether HVDT should be continued, with its comparatively poor rate of early identification of deafness and high cost. Universal neonatal hearing screening is now routinely carried out.

An evaluation of screening for speech and language delay (Law et al 1997) again raises questions as well as providing some answers. It was found that there was insufficient evidence to support formal universal screening for speech and language delay. However, early speech and language delay should be viewed with concern by those undertaking child health surveillance, i.e. health visitors and GPs, because it may indicate both minor and major disabilities. Parents need to be aware of language development in young children and to share any concerns with health visitors and GPs, to allow access to specialist services (Law et al 1997).

Questions that need to be asked here are: how do we ensure that health visitors and GPs have the skills to identify speech and language delays early, and how can parents be educated in language development in young children? Once identified, what happens if there are insufficient resources to cope with identified children in need?

There is a danger in thinking that researchers must always be right: this may not necessarily be the case. Absence of conclusive evidence that a particular type of screening should be stopped when there is some evidence that it is beneficial can be an argument for its continuation, as the following example shows.

Research into pre-school vision screening (Snowdon & Stewart-Brown 1997, 1998) found that little is known about the natural history and treatment of amblyopia and no treatment trials have been identified using a non-treatment control group, which would have been precluded on ethical grounds. Research indicated lack of evidence to support pre-school vision screening in a small-scale trial, but screening by the orthoptist was found to be more effective than screening by a health visitor or GP. In spite of the research findings, Fielder (1997) argued that pre-school vision screening should continue on the grounds that research was small scale. It should have opened up the debate about screening, and the community had in effect been bypassed. Research evidence on the treatment of amblyopia should be obtained and the child with a visual defect should not be ignored.

Issues here, besides dissension about continuing screening while acknowledging the need for early intervention, are effectiveness of a service in ethical terms and cost-effectiveness. Uptake for pre-school vision screening by the orthoptist was poor and more children were seen by the health visitor. Would more children with possible visual defects be identified if health visitors were given specific training in this area, then referred on for specialist assessment and treatment when necessary?

The research detailed in *Population Growth Analysis Using the Child Health Computing System* (Hulse et al 1997, 1998) showed not only how important it is to use the appropriate tools

for a particular type of screening but also the importance of training in their use and accurate recording and interpretation of results. Without these simple safeguards, not only may a particular research project founder and its potential value to child health be lost, but inaccurate measurements may result in inappropriate referrals being made. This may result in unnecessary parent/child anxiety as well as failing to identify children in need of specialist treatment.

The research discovered errors in the way a tool was used, which affected the outcome of the study. It found that there was increasing agreement that children with height below the 0.4th centile or above the 99.6th centile should be evaluated for possible growth disorder. However, there was less agreement about the value of assessing children where height velocity was abnormal, particularly where height was within the normal range. However, at that time there were too many errors on growth data on the child health computing system for it to be of value for screening (Hulse et al 1997). This research was carried out using information from child health records in Kent.

Training for professionals in accurate growth measurement and completion of centile charts, for information to be meaningful, has been long advised by the Child Growth Foundation.

There is a danger in assuming the value of a particular type of screening without its effectiveness having ever been evaluated, as *Screening for Congenital Dislocation of The Hip: A Cost Effective Analysis* (Dezateux et al 1997, 1998) indicates. A national policy for universal neonatal screening for congenital dislocation of the hip (CDH) had been introduced in 1969 but not formally evaluated prior to introduction. Results of the research indicated that the effectiveness in reducing false negatives of universal ultrasound screening, which had been introduced in some European countries, was uncertain. It was the system used in two-thirds of maternity units in the UK but was not the primary screening test. It was used to assess babies with clinically detected hip instability or with high risk factors for CDH. In this case research did not provide a definitive answer but indicated the need for ongoing evaluation of current and alternative primary screening strategies. The best approach was not yet known.

A further example of where research can highlight the need for ongoing research is the national study *Cost Analysis in Child Health Surveillance* (Sanderson 1997). Results indicated that the majority of local policies followed the recommendations of Hall (1996). There was little variation in the number of checks and the ages at which they were undertaken, but two – hearing screening and routine vision checks – were performed in a variety of ways. Ongoing study into the cost of providing child health surveillance and costs to parents, including follow-up visits and referrals, was incomplete.

Neonatal Screening for Inborn Errors of Metabolism (Thomason et al 1997) again indicated that research should be ongoing rather than accepting the effectiveness of a screening method for all time. Findings were that universal screening for phenylketonuria is worthwhile and should be continued. Screening for biotinidase deficiency and congenital adrenal hyperplasia should be introduced, with coordinating evaluation to ensure that the programme is cost-effective and review in 5 years' time. Screening for cystic fibrosis should be encouraged but there was no evidence to support a newborn screening programme for galactosaemia.

From the research examples above, it is evident that screening procedures may be less than perfect and that what was once the most appropriate procedure becomes outdated or is superseded by a more effective method. In practical terms, it is essential to be prepared to change the tool/procedure used in the light of current research. Also, where there is some evidence of its usefulness, a tool should not be dismissed as ineffective without sound research-based evidence to support this.

DEVELOPMENTAL SCREENING

Developmental screening is the process of checking the development of a child whose parents believe it to be normal (Illingworth 1987). It is a rapid application of a test or other tool for the purpose of separating those who

have or are very likely to have developmental delay (Hall 1986, Lynn 1987). Bellman et al (1996) agree with this view, adding that its aim is to check children are developing normally for their age when measured against prescribed criteria, failure to meet these indicating developmental delay or defect.

The prime purpose of a developmental screening tool is to identify children with possible developmental delay early, so that they can quickly be referred to a specialist for the problem to be confirmed or refuted (Frankenburg et al 1973, Bellman & Cash 1987). If it is confirmed, a diagnosis can be made and, where possible, appropriate treatment given to enable the child to achieve his/her potential. In many cases, this can prevent development of special educational needs.

Debate has arisen in recent years as to the value of routine developmental screening of all 0- to 5-year-old children, which was introduced in the late 1950s and early 1960s. The Working Party on Child Health Surveillance (Hall 1989, Hall & Elliman 2003) did not recommend this, nor did it recommend any particular developmental screening tool. It was of the opinion that trained professionals, by using their observational skills, can satisfy themselves in the majority of cases that the child's development is within normal limits. Professional judgement, local policy and needs and wishes of parents should be taken into account when deciding how much time should be spent on developmental screening. Macfarlane (Macfarlane et al 1990, personal communication 1991) endorses this view. The Working Party did not, however, recommend developmental screening (Hall 1991, 1996, Hall & Elliman 2003), although the 1991 report does acknowledge its place in child protection work.

There are a number of people who feel that routine screening of all children is of value in early identification of children with possible developmental delay. These include Frankenburg & Dodds (1967), Bellman & Cash (1987), Illingworth (1987) and Bax et al (1990). Bernice (1986) and Bolton (1986) highlight the importance of hearing and language screening: as delay is often indicative of other disorders, it is also an important part of child health surveillance (Court 1976). Bernice and Bolton's observations are also emphasized by Law et al (1997). Bellman et al (1996) view routine developmental screening as an ethically acceptable part of child health surveillance and promotion provided that appropriate action is taken in terms of prevention and support. While supporting developmental screening for all children, Cash (1991) warns against putting the onus back on parents to report problems, as not all do and the child may suffer as a result. In the Muslim culture, for example, the feeling is that problems are the will of God. In Cash's experience, intervention is allowed if the professional identifies the problem, although there is ambivalence about the result of treatment. Additionally, when working in partnership with parents for the good of their children, it is important to take their views into account. There are indications that they value developmental screening (Sutton et al 1995, Fagan 1997).

Sharples (2004) raises concerns about current recommendations for health visitors to move away from the traditional approach for carrying out routine developmental checks, and about the shortage of health visitors, already alluded to earlier in Chapter 8 and further stretching of their work by new government initiatives. Her argument is that previously health visitors were in a position to identify children with possible autism as well as delay in other areas, but these children may well now be missed. Bearing in mind that Hall & Elliman (2003) likewise advocates early identification of possible problems in pre-school children in order to offer remedial treatment, the question remains as to how this will be achieved as the report advocated no routine screening. Should health visitors consider taking a more managerial role, delegating this task to others, for example nursery nurses, using skill mix within the team, thus continuing to maximize on strengths within the service, while continuing to take on new roles?

The problem of what is normal development and the dangers of assessment by people ignorant of what they are doing and how to do it is discussed by Illingworth (1987). A wrong diagnosis can cause immense trauma to parents and children, yet parents have a right to know as soon as possible if their child is handicapped.

Is routine developmental screening effective? *The Lancet* (1986) argues that studies of children have shown failure to identify physical and developmental problems relating to the pre-school years, but no statistics are given. Aukett (1990) found that the experience of health visitors in a West Midlands area was that about 10% more children with speech and language delay, including Asian children, were identified using SGS than previously with DDST. While studying pre-school children over a 7-year period in Dundee, Drillien & Drummond (1983) found that 9% had moderate to severe developmental delay and 73% were identified through screening. Early intervention reduced the numbers needing special education.

A study in one West Midlands area found that only one child of school age, who had moved into the area, had been missed in the pre-school years, and the two children missed by the doctor were subsequently identified by health visitors through developmental screening (E. Humphries, unpublished PGD thesis 1989).

Although it is felt that more children with developmental delay are being identified early, overall there is a paucity of statistics to prove conclusively the effectiveness of routine developmental screening in the pre-school years (Griffiths 1970, Hall 1989). Yet as Cash (1991) points out, in spite of a lack of research in this area, no research has been carried out to show the difference between two groups of children referred, for example, for speech therapy, where one group was treated and one was not. However, to attempt this would create a moral dilemma. Hall & Elliman (2003) also raises issues over the ethics of identifying a problem and being unable to offer treatment.

Views can change over time, as shown by Hall (1991), in which although routine developmental screening is not supported for all children, support is given to its use in child protection work. Hall (1996), while not advocating the use of any developmental screening tool, noted that SGS and DDST were the most widely used. The report goes on to state that developmental reviews should be aimed at disadvantaged children and those with disabilities. Hall & Elliman (2003) maintain this view, but do not advocate any developmental screening, discussing ethical issues about creating unnecessary anxiety in parents where a problem is falsely identified, and the possibility of litigation. The report does, however, go on to state that further information is required about existing screening programmes and new screening techniques which need to be evaluated not only in terms of effectiveness but also from an ethical viewpoint.

Debate continues as to the value of any psychometric test. Streiner & Norman (1995) have argued that medicine on the one hand and psychology and education on the other have come closer in their understanding of how and why assessment tools are constructed. Traditionally medicine thinks in terms of diagnosis and treatment, the categorical model. A patient either has a disorder or does not. On the other hand, psychology and education think in terms of levels of measurement, the dimensional model. Both sides acknowledge the importance of reliability and validity studies in the construction of screening tools, which in the case of SGS is well documented in both the 1987 studies and in SGS II in 1996.

Arguably health visitors are in a position to understand the stance of both sides as they do not belong to either camp. Through their work their thinking possibly fits more into the dimensional model while at the same time they are in a position to be able to understand the categorical model, having practised as nurses within the acute sector. An example from health visiting practice is when a child is identified as having possible speech and language delay. Although these skills are developing, they are not as far advanced along the developmental continuum as would be expected in terms of their chronological age. In other words it is not a clear-cut case of there is or is not a problem, but a problem on a pathway of development which may be anywhere between severe or mild in nature. What is important is that through early identification appropriate help is given to the child if needed.

Returning to the screening issue with particular groups of children, those who have been subject to abuse can fall into either or both of the groups of those who have been disadvantaged or those with disabilities. The lack of research is again highlighted. It is this issue that research by M. G. Reynolds (unpublished BSc project 1992, unfinished PhD project 2004) has sought to address by implementing small-scale studies in order to open the debate further and stimulate further research.

RATIONALE FOR THE USE OF THE SCHEDULE OF GROWING SKILLS IN CHILD PROTECTION

THE HEALTH VISITOR'S ROLE IN CHILD PROTECTION

Health visitors have a key role in the promotion of children's health and development in child protection (Department of Health/Welsh Office 1995, Department of Health Specialist Clinical Services Division 1996). Health visitors are in a unique position, working with children and families on an ongoing basis. They have knowledge and prior information that may give valuable insight into why crises have occurred. This has implications for ongoing work (Birchall & Hallett 1995).

A fundamental principle of the Children Act 1989 is that the child's welfare is paramount. Accurate, contemporaneous records, including a child's developmental status, that can be clearly understood are likely to be of particular importance in cases of child abuse, which involves working on a multidisciplinary/multi-agency basis. All professionals working in partnership and finding effective ways of working together in practice to serve the child's best interests is a key issue in child protection work (Department of Health/Department of Education and Science/Welsh Office 1991).

DEVELOPMENTAL SCREENING IN THE CONTEXT OF CHILD PROTECTION

Hall (1996, Hall & Elliman 2003) supports developmental reviews for disadvantaged children and those with disabilities. Cash

Refs

(1991) supports developmental screening, considering it to be vital, when assessing children in need, to have a yardstick by which to measure their progress or lack of it. In this context, it is important to use the most appropriate developmental screening tool available. Knowledge of a child's developmental status is viewed as important by social services, hence the inclusion of information relating to child development in the social work assessment guide (Department of Health 1995a). Further support is given in the *Framework for the Assessment of Children in Need and their Families* (Department of Health/Department of Education and Employment 2000), which includes a requirement to assess the developmental status of children in need. This should be considered against the background of the Laming Report (2003) and the plethora of subsequent publications to improve the protection of vulnerable children and young people, including, *What to Do if You're Worried a Child is being Abused* (Department of Health 2003e), *Every Child Matters* (Department of Health 2003a) and *Every Child Matters: Next Steps* (Department for Education and Skills 2004b). A need to understand children's development and positive developmental outcomes is given further weight in Aldgate et al (2004).

We can understand through observation to a certain extent, but more in-depth understanding can only be gained through using a developmental screening tool, for example SGS and SGS11, which has undergone rigorous reliability and validity studies that are well documented, and been shown to be acceptable to both children and their parents (Bellman & Cash 1987, Bellman et al 1996).

Research (M. G. Reynolds, unpublished BSc project 1992) sought to identify the most appropriate developmental screening tool to use with 0- to 5-year-old children in one Midlands area. Tools considered were, first, a very modified form of Griffiths with no recorded research or validation, which was currently being used within the area; and second, the Denver Developmental Screening Test (DDST), with well-recorded research and validation but with a rigid pass/fail system in common with other

older tools and criticized for limitations in its ability to identify speech and language delay early (Lynn 1987). Research by Greer et al (1989) also indicated its failure to identify developmental delay in pre-school children. The third tool was the Schedule of Growing Skills (SGS), a newer tool with well-recorded research and validation, in the development of which health visitors had been involved. Findings indicated that this last was the most appropriate tool for the identified age group in the area. Further research was then carried out to explore its usefulness in the context of child protection (M. G. Reynolds, unfinished PhD project 2004).

A literature search revealed a paucity of information linking child protection with developmental screening in either general or specific terms. Curtis specifies the SGS screening tool for child protection (Curtis 1993, 1995), but no further literature linking the two issues was found. Information from Cainey (M. G. Reynolds, personal communication 1995) indicated that the tool had been used by social workers with 'at risk' children in West Lothian, but no formal evaluation of this work was available.

Current thinking in relation to child protection advocates a change in emphasis. It is being argued that it would be advisable to transfer some of the effort put into investigating child abuse into child and family support. The focus should be on the child's needs, then seeing if there is a protection issue within them. It is by meeting the wider needs – offering the family support services on a multidisciplinary basis following assessment (which includes developmental screening results) – that the risk of abuse to the child can be reduced (Birchall & Hallett 1995).

Parenting skills can profoundly affect the parent–child relationship and the child's social and emotional development (Bowlby 1953). Bowlby is particularly concerned with the importance of the mother–child or mother substitute–child bond in this respect, as well as acknowledging the importance of the father figure and siblings. Ainsworth (1965) points out that subsequent research supports this view. Psychological learning theory, psychoanalytical theory and theories based on the concept of 'sensitive phase' all indicate the potential damage of maternal deprivation to the child's development. Both the child's age at the onset of deprivation and the age at which relief occurs influence future development. The earlier relief occurs the more likely it is that subsequent development will be normal. All areas of development, not only social and emotional, may be affected (Lewis 1988).

Government concerns in relation to parenting skills have initiated a Sure Start programme in which health visitors are heavily involved (Turner 1998).

SGS covers all areas of development, including social and emotional. Results from screening using this tool shared in the multi-agency child protection forum can therefore highlight areas of need at an early stage. Addressing those needs, by professionals working with the family as a whole, as well as specific help for the child, if required, can aid in protecting the child from further abuse.

RESEARCH PROJECT: THE USE OF THE SCHEDULE OF GROWING SKILLS IN CHILD PROTECTION

The project did not seek to establish support for continuing routine developmental screening for all children but to explore its usefulness in child protection work. How reviews of young children are carried out in the light of Hall (1996) is a matter for each area to decide in line with local policy. For the purpose of this study, the original version of SGS was used, as three routine screenings of children in the comparison group were required, at 8, 18 and 30 months, which meant drawing on screening information prior to the introduction of SGS II.

Preliminary work

Prior to the main study, the views of those most likely to be affected by the proposed change were sought. These were all health visitors within the local community trust, 68% of whom responded, and a small sample of convenience of GPs, parents and social workers. The aim was to establish their views on developmental screening of

0- to 5-year-old children and their likelihood of accepting a change of tool to a new, research-based one, results of which could be shared with parents and other professionals if necessary.

Results indicated that a change to SGS would be acceptable to health visitors, and to the small sample groups of parents, GPs and social workers, the majority of the last group perceiving it as beneficial in child protection work. Developmental screening of young children was acknowledged as being of value. It was crucial to establish this before considering possible change or continuing developmental screening at all.

Once all health visitors had been trained in the use of SGS and the tool had been introduced across the trust, a questionnaire was sent to all health visitors 6 weeks and 10 months post introduction to find out their views about its use in practice and whether there were any problems.

Overall findings indicated an increasing acceptance of the SGS tool, familiarity with its use and perception of its value in general use, as well as a reduction in screening time. Children responded well to it, both parents and professionals generally viewing it favourably. From the professional viewpoint comments included its thoroughness, objectivity, being visually graphic and giving a clear picture of a child's developmental status. It was useful for referral and sharing results with parents/other agencies. Additionally, in the second questionnaire comments indicated that it was a good tool to use with children on the Child Protection Register and was useful to teach students about developmental screening.

Main study

Here the overall aim was to explore the usefulness of SGS in child protection work. Evaluation took place over a 6-month period. Routine practice was that screening information was brought to the initial case conference and screening was carried out again prior to the review case conference.

Health visitors whose caseload included a child on the Child Protection Register at the commencement of this stage were identified.

Quantitative data were obtained from SGS scores of subject children and those in the comparison group. Qualitative data were obtained by carrying out semi-structured interviews with participating health visitors at two points: after the initial case conference and after the first review. These two points were chosen because the literature indicated that the greatest volume of work by all agencies was achieved following the child's initial registration. The purpose was to determine:

- health visitors' views about the ability of the tool, in child protection work, to identify need
- how need identified by health visitors fitted in with that identified by other professionals at case conferences
- the success of the child protection plan (anticipated after initial registration and actual after first review)
- whether the system was working in relation to the health visitor contribution
- perceptions as to whether improvements could be made to the health visitor contribution.

Data were collected by interviews with health visitors and from routine anonymous health visiting SGS profiles. There was no access to written health visiting records. Verbal consent was obtained from each health visitor before participation in the study and there was no compulsion to participate.

Children included in the study

In all, six children, boys and girls aged 0–5 years within the trust on the local social services Child Protection Register formed the subject group. The comparison group consisted of 10 children – five boys and five girls – from the caseloads of each of the six health visitors who participated in the study. This was a sample of convenience, matched in terms of age group, social class and ethnicity with each subject child. Additionally, the children in the comparison group were not on the Child Protection Register, were not born prematurely and had no known developmental delay. Three routine screenings were required, at 8, 18 and 30 months, prior to the start of the study. This was so that an estimated SGS score could be calculated that matched the age of each child in the subject group, by a process of statistical regression.

Combination of the qualitative and quantitative approach

Although some continue to argue that qualitative and quantitative research are incompatible, increasingly it is believed that many areas of inquiry can be enriched through the combined approach, using more than one method of data collection in a single investigation (Polit & Hungler 1995). Both numbers and words are needed to understand the world (Miles & Huberman 1994). Miles & Huberman view quantitative and qualitative research as a continuum in the process of inquiry and not as separate entities. In linking quantitative and qualitative data, the four broad reasons described by Rossman & Wilson (1991) were all appropriate to this particular research. These were: to enable confirmation or corroboration of each other via triangulation; to elaborate or develop analysis, providing richer detail; to initiate new lines of thinking through attention to surprises or paradoxes; and to turn ideas around, providing new insight.

With this in mind, the combined approach was used in this study. Qualitative data were obtained by discussing what health visitors felt about the success of the child protection plan after initial and first review case conferences with SGS scores before initial and first review case conferences.

Quantitative data were obtained in two ways. Firstly, scores for each child before initial and first review case conference were discussed to find out whether there were differences and if so in what areas. In SGS, a score for each skill area is obtained. Health visitors' perceptions of the effectiveness or otherwise of the child protection plan were then compared with the screening results. Secondly, screening results of the two groups – children on the Child Protection Register and those who were not – were discussed. This was to find out if there was a difference in the rate of development between the two groups and where such differences were. Lack of research in this area indicated the need for exploration.

Discussion of results

All health visitors involved in the study valued using SGS in child protection work in identifying need and felt the needs they had identified fitted in with those identified by other professionals at the case conference. They felt that ways of meeting those needs were incorporated into the child protection plan.

Perceptions of the effectiveness of the child protection plan indicated that other issues besides content were important. These included the importance of professionals working together, cooperation from the parents and worker planning meetings between case conferences. These could, in effect, provide ongoing monitoring of the plan. The cooperation of parents and professionals was necessary to meet the child's needs, including protection from and prevention of further abuse.

All study participants felt that the SGS tool was of value in child protection and in sharing that information at the case conference. However, the comment was made that although in their view it was the best tool available, as with any tool it had its limitations. The health visitors interpreted the results in the light of their professional judgement, based on experience and expertise; knowledge of the family and child was also very important. This was borne out by their response to the question: Did they feel the child was achieving his/her potential? It was generally felt that the answer was no, apart from the period of time one child was in foster care. This response was given even where children's development appeared to be age appropriate, or even above the chronological age. This was an important finding as, if a child's development appears to be age-appropriate, the case conference may conclude that it is satisfactory. The health visitor needs to put forward her/his view, with reasons as to why this may not be so, in order to look at ways in which the child could be helped further.

One participant experienced difficulties in identifying emotional problems. This linked with a difficulty identified in the pilot study, where a participant felt that an additional tool could be used to identify social and environmental issues. It was acknowledged that the health visitor's knowledge of the family could identify many of these issues but that perhaps more weight should be given to them initially. It is likely that only the health visitor will have this information at the initial case conference stage.

Another participant drew attention to the fact that there was a quality issue in respect of interactive social skills. The level of achievement in this area was not consistent: it was dependent on family circumstances and who was present in the home. The child's behaviour could regress, reflecting the level of emotional instability experienced, which identified a need for planning to provide the stability that such children need. A further comment from participants was concern about parenting skills and the need for improvement in this area.

Comparison of SGS scores of register children and non–register children

These indicated progress relating to the health visitors' perceptions of the effectiveness of the child protection plan. Progress, where it took place, was more rapid than in the general population. Areas where delay was indicated in the subject group included hearing and speech, speech and language, visual comprehension (the child's ability to verbalize and indicate understanding of what they see), interactive social skills and self-care skills. One child had delayed locomotor skills, which proved to be environmental in origin. One child's development was above the chronological age initially. Acknowledgement of the child's needs and subsequent foster placement resulted in further progress being made.

All respondents felt that participating in the study had enabled them to reflect on their work with SGS in child protection and to value it. At the same time, they recognized the limitations of the tool, or any tool. It was the best available that they were aware of, four having used a number of others previously. They were very positive about its use, commenting on its clarity and simplicity when sharing results with other case conference participants. It was useful when working with parents to identify needs and areas of progress. On reflection, one participant felt that she would have valued the actual information generated when giving evidence in court on a previous occasion. Most participants felt that with time a more appropriate tool might be identified through research.

THE FUTURE

Health visiting is a preventive service in which proactive work is of vital importance. A topical example is the government's parenting skills initiative, in which it is anticipated that health visitors will play an important part. The reason why this is important to the health of children is indicated in research by Barlow (1997). Her research indicated that parent training programmes were effective in improving behaviour problems in children aged 3–10 years. This is particularly important as the most important health problems in childhood and adolescence are behaviour and mental health problems. If programmes were set up on a preventive basis, not only where problems have already occurred, this could be an effective way of improving children's health.

Consideration, then, needs to be given not only to teaching those skills but also to giving positive feedback to parents. They need to know how their child is progressing, in what areas they need further help and how to promote further development if their child is to achieve his/her potential. This is another possible area where SGS could be usefully used. In conjunction with this, the parent's level of self-esteem could be assessed as a means of promoting positive parenting. The same approach could be used in a first parenting programme, with assessments taking place at intervals deemed helpful by both parent and professional, as well as with vulnerable families.

Bandura (1977b) felt that people's perceptions of their capabilities affected how they behaved and their level of motivation. In relating this to children and their development, Rotter (1977) pointed out that it was acknowledged that, when a mother felt confident in her ability to help her child, the child picked up those feelings and was likely to do better than a child whose mother had a low self-efficacy level and had difficulty coping.

The partnership approach between client and professional is acknowledged as being particularly important (Billingham 1991). The professional provides expert knowledge, enabling and empowering clients to make informed health choices as individuals and for families as a whole, including young children. This concept can be particularly useful when working to enable parents with poor coping ability and poor parenting skills to change their behaviour and have confidence in themselves. The likely effect would be an improvement in their parenting skills, increasing the potential for their children to grow and develop to realize their potential. Attributes in parents that encourage children's progress include realistic expectations of their child, meeting their need for love and security, provision of an appropriate learning environment and providing opportunities for appropriate socialization (Luker & Orr 1992). Bellman & Cash (1987) and Illingworth (1987) broadly agree with this view.

A suggested scale measuring the mother/carer's level of self-esteem (M. G. Reynolds, unpublished BSc project 1992), based on the Diabetes Self-Efficacy Scale (Padgett 1991), is given in Table 9.2. It is acknowledged that further useful work could be carried out in validating this scale.

The scale is divided into four sub-areas. These are items directly related to: (a) developmental progress; (b) general health (including diet, warmth and appropriate clothing); (c) love and security (including behaviour management and establishment of a routine); (d) provision of an appropriate learning environment (including opportunities for play, socializing and outings to places of interest for the child).

Table 9.2 Scale to measure the self-efficacy of a carer

Scale	Direction	Subarea of scoring	Question
a	+	1.	I find it easy to believe that children have different competencies at different ages
a	+	2.	I know how to choose toys appropriate to my child's age
c	–	3.	I find it difficult to accept when my child does not do what I expect him/her to do
a	+	4.	I know what games to play with my child to help development
c	+	5.	I am able to express my love for my child by cuddling and kissing him/her
b	–	6.	I find it difficult to decide on a proper diet for my child
c	–	7.	I have trouble getting my baby/child into a routine
c	–	8.	I find it difficult to be patient with my child
a	+	9.	I find I have the skills to guide my child to give appropriate activities to encourage development
d	–	10.	I find it difficult to make opportunities for my child to mix and play with other children
b	+	11.	I am confident in my ability to keep my home warm and clean for my child
d	+	12.	I make opportunities to talk to my child and read to him/her
d	–	13.	I find it difficult to find time to take my child out to places of interest to him/her
d	+	14.	I encourage my child to help me when I am doing household chores
b	–	15.	I find it difficult to decide what clothes to dress my child in
c	+	16.	I know when to say 'no' to my child when he/she goes to do something which will harm him/her
b	+	17.	I am confident in my ability to look after my child's health

Key: +, scoring direction strongly agree 5, strongly disagree 1; –, scoring direction strongly agree 1, strongly disagree 5.

Questions in the scale that relate to each of the four sub-areas are: (a) developmental progress – questions 1, 2, 4, 8 and 9; (b) general health – questions 6, 11, 15 and 17; (c) love and security – questions 3, 5, 7, 8 and 16; (d) provision of an appropriate learning environment – questions 10, 12, 13 and 14. A five-point Likert scale was used, ranging from 'strongly agree' to 'strongly disagree', with a similar number of positively and negatively worded questions.

The purpose of the tool is to gain knowledge of the mother/carer's self-efficacy level and insight into their strengths and weaknesses. The raw scores can be converted into a percentage score overall, as well as one for each scale sub-area. The scale could be used as a useful starting point at the commencement of teaching parenting skills and later on to ascertain the level of achievement. If it were used in conjunction with SGS, it could positively reinforce the concept that improved parenting skills can aid a child in achieving his/her potential (Fig. 9.2).

The scale was used with mothers in a small-scale study. It was used initially and then 3 months later following input from the family health visitor in teaching parenting skills. In results shown in Box 9.1, Mother 1 had good parenting skills, a high level of self-esteem and her child appeared to be developing satisfactorily. Mother 2 had low self-esteem, less understanding of parenting skills and her child was exhibiting behaviour problems.

Results after 3 months showed the first mother's improvement in parenting skills and her child's development continued to progress age appropriately. Results for the second mother indicated a marked improvement in parenting skills and improved level of self-esteem, and her child showed improvement in development, particularly in behaviour. Both mothers stated that they appreciated a simple written indication that they had benefited from the programme and the effort they had put in had had beneficial results for both their child and themselves.

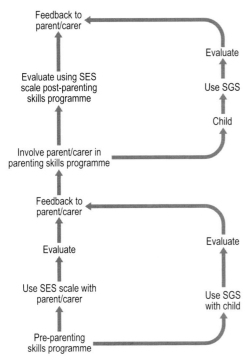

Figure 9.2   How the self-efficacy scale (SES) and SGS could be used in evaluating a parenting skills programme

Box 9.1   Self-efficacy scale results

Maximum score = 85

Total score Mother 1

	First time	Second time
	73 = 85.88%	80 = 94.11%

Total score Mother 2

	First time	Second time
	41 = 48.2%	62 = 72.94%

Score Mother 1

	First time	Second time
a	17 (20) = 85%	20 (20) = 100%
b	17 (20) = 85%	19 (20) = 95%
c	21 (25) = 84%	22 (25) = 88%
d	18 (20) = 90%	19 (20) = 95%
	(86% overall)	(94% overall)

Score Mother 2

	First time	Second time
a	9 (20) = 45%	15 (20) = 75%
b	9 (20) = 45%	14 (20) = 70%
c	16 (25) = 64%	18 (25) = 72%
d	7 (20) = 35%	15 (20) = 75%
	(48% overall)	(73% overall)

SUMMARY

Interest in child development dates back more than 200 years. Work on developing developmental tests and scales was mainly carried out in the 20th century, with DDST and SGS being the most commonly used in the UK today. Debate continues as to whether developmental screening should continue as part of child health promotion/surveillance.

SGS was found to be effective in enabling health visitors within a Midlands Trust to fulfil their role in child protection work, but its limitations were acknowledged. Health visitors' professional judgement and interpretation of results in the light of their knowledge of family circumstances were deemed to be of great importance. Even when a child's development appeared to be normal, this may not mean that the child is achieving his/her potential. This should be acknowledged when considering the child protection plan.

A further possible valuable use of SGS could be in teaching parenting skills. This could be of particular importance in view of the government parenting skills initiative. It could be used in conjunction with a self-efficacy scale, as a positive reinforcement to parents of the benefits to their child following baseline assessment.

As with all screening tests or tools, professionals should use the most appropriate and reliable tool but acknowledge that, with time, existing tools may be improved or be outdated as a result of further research. Prior to using a developmental screening tool thorough familiarization with its use in practice is extremely important if it is to be effective and offer a standardized service in the area in which it is used.

The small-scale study undertaken (M. G. Reynolds, unfinished PhD project 2004), with increasing emphasis being placed on safeguarding children today, could have a valuable role to play in opening the debate further concerning the developmental screening of young children, leading to an increase in the body of knowledge and the development of even more effective tools.

CHILD BEHAVIOUR PROBLEMS

Janice Frost

The most common questions parents ask their health visitor concern the behaviour of their child, whether normal or abnormal. Issues relating to management of sleep problems, toilet training, feeding or tantrums can cause parents much anxiety.

Health visitors' role in teaching parenting skills and behaviour management of children, particularly the under fives, encompasses assessment, recognition, prevention and intervention. Hall & Elliman (2003) state that '20% of children are said to experience psychological problems at any one time', and that 'young people, parents and teachers need to know the services available to support children with emotional and behavioural difficulties and their families'. Health visitors are at the forefront of health care delivery and are often the first professional suitably placed to offer support. Health visitors' knowledge regarding the 'normal development' and expectations of child behaviour enable the assessment of individual children and their families to commence. Recognition and referral of children with abnormal development due to congenital conditions or abuse form part of the health visitor's initial assessment. However, before health visitors contact families it is important to have an awareness of the extrinsic factors that could influence the parents' handling of the child's behaviour.

INFLUENCES ON PARENTING AND BEHAVIOUR

Modern parenthood is too demanding a task to be performed well merely because we have all once been children (Pringle 1975). Memories of our own childhood and the way our parents handled our outbursts influence how we handle our children: the example given by parents and grandparents and how individuals interpret their memories may influence their own parenting style. Health visitors have to be able to challenge familial and cultural parenting practices and offer updated research-based advice. Recent changes within society have had a lasting effect on how parenting must develop in the future: working mothers, child care, the reduction in the role of the extended family and the enlargement of the father's role in child rearing have implications for the management of children. Social trends, including increasing numbers of single parent families through higher divorce rates and lower marriage rates, influence child management; increased stress caused by lone parenting and reduced extended family support add burden to the pressures of modern life. The challenge for the health visitor in relation to child behaviour management is to educate parents in the most effective ways of teaching children desired behaviours.

Much research has been done on the needs and characteristics of children from homeless families and those living in poverty. Poverty influences the growth and development of the child through undernourishment (Pollitt 1994) and also by its effect on parenting. The stress caused to parents by poverty can lead to detrimental parenting practices, which adversely affect the child's well-being and behaviour. High levels of unemployment in turn increase the levels of poverty (Bassuk et al 1997).

Postnatal depression has been identified as a factor in externalizing and internalizing problems in the pre-school and school-age periods (Downey & Coyne 1990). Shaw & Vondra (1995) suggested that early maternal depression interfered with the mother's ability to respond contingently to the infant's cues, thus affecting the infant's attachment. Murrey & Cooper (1997) found an association between early maternal depression and adverse cognitive and emotional infant development.

Evans (2001) highlighted domestic violence as a significant factor of behavioural and emotional disorders in early childhood. The aggressive behaviour of the parents may be copied by the child or the child may be confused and unable to identify behavioural boundaries. Domestic violence or parental disharmony, as often seen when parents separate, may cause a disruption of the boundaries or inconsistency of parental handling of the child's behaviour.

Parental expectations and perceptions of their child will also have an effect upon how a child's behaviour is handled. 'Normal' toddler behaviour may be seen by some as characteristics of a difficult child; parents who identify their child as particularly difficult may respond to the child with less sensitivity, which in turn may intensify the behaviour problems as the child strives to gain parental attention. Perception of behaviour and expectations are also gender linked: what is acceptable boisterous 'boy' behaviour is not deemed correct for a little girl. In educating parents, health visitors can address these gender issues as well as giving accurate expectations of age-related behaviour.

ADDRESSING COMMON BEHAVIOUR PROBLEMS

What is seen as a problem by one parent is not a problem to everyone. It is important that the parents identify what the problem behaviour is and that the health visitor enables them to address the behaviour in a way that is suitable for the individual child and family. The parents' full cooperation is needed to enable a programme of behaviour modification to be developed and completed successfully. There are many books and views available to assist health professionals and parents in the management of child behaviour. Try to select a text that is parent-friendly to reinforce your messages. Before selecting particular management techniques it is important to obtain a full history of the behaviour causing concern and the methods already tried by the parents in order to maximize the effect of a chosen technique.

Behaviour problems such as sleep problems, tantrums and faddy eating often benefit from keeping a diary of the problem behaviour prior to and during the management programme. Keeping a diary enables accurate assessment of the problem, records the progress of failure and

highlights the true nature of the problem for the parents.

BASIC STEPS OF A CHILD BEHAVIOUR MODIFICATION PROGRAMME

- Take a full history, including birth history, medical history, previous medication, help sought relating to the problem and social background. Include specific details pertaining to specific problem behaviour, e.g. sleeping arrangements/room availability for the family for sleep problems, family eating patterns for feeding problems.

- Complete a diary for a minimum of a week prior to dealing with the problem. This will help to identify the problem and highlight the parental difficulties relating to it.

- The parent should identify the 'long-term aim' of the programme.

- Devise a structured 'plan of action' in partnership with the parents that is achievable, not too demanding and takes a step-by-step approach. Basic written instructions for the programme on a week-to-week basis are often needed.

- Review the programme at regular intervals, using diaries to monitor progress, and adjust the plan.

- Remember the child's behaviour has not developed into a problem overnight but has often taken months or years, so do not try to resolve the problem overnight – take time and aim for steady progress.

- Let the parent decide when the problem has resolved to a manageable level for completion of the programme, but offer open access back to the programme if necessary.

SLEEP PROBLEMS IN THE UNDER FIVES

A child who sleeps only for short periods can cause many problems within the family: tired parents and children become irritable, miserable and less able to cope with everyday life and routines. Expectations of how soon a young baby should sleep through the night vary greatly among parents, but a meeting between parents with a wakeful child and parents with a child who has slept through the night since birth is almost guaranteed, thus exacerbating the former's problem. A sleep problem is only a problem when identified as such by the parents, not the professional. Once approached by the parents, follow the basic steps of a child behaviour modification plan.

A sleep diary is a useful tool in the development of a programme (Fig. 9.3).

Behavioural sleep problems can generally be classified into those associated with non-settling, those with a sleep pattern that consists of frequent waking throughout the night, and those

with both settling problems and frequent waking. Health visitors are ideally placed to help the parents of children with disrupted sleep patterns. Many parents have already turned to sedatives to force the child to sleep and have found that, if sedation has been successful, the problem often recurs once it is removed. A planned programme of behaviour modification often helps.

Key strategies include the following:

- 'Cue' the child before bedtime, telling them what is expected – what bedtime is.

- Develop a structured approach to bedtime, e.g. bath, pyjamas, drink, teeth brushed, story and bed.

- Take the child to bed awake – confusion arises in the night if they wake in a different room from the one they went to sleep in.

	Monday	Tuesday	Wednesday	Thursday	Friday	Saturday	Sunday
Time of waking and mood							
Time of daytime naps							
Daytime activities							
Evening bedtime							
Time to sleep in evening							
Time(s) of night waking. What you did. How long to settle							
Parent bedtime							

Figure 9.3   An example of a sleep diary

- Sort out the settling first: this may require a programme in itself, e.g. sit by the bed, move towards the door, leave the room, call, etc. (all the tactics are detailed in many texts); once the settling is sorted the night-time waking often resolves.

- If settling is not the problem but night waking is, find out why, using the diary – what is the parent doing when the child wakes? Giving drinks, getting into the child's bed or taking the child to the parent's bed, putting on the television and taking the child downstairs to play are all rewards for undesirable behaviour.

Helping parents who have a child with a disruptive sleep problem can be time consuming, challenging and very rewarding. Many texts have been written offering guidance on handling sleep problems and must be used as resource material for both professionals and parents.

Children whose sleep problems are medical in origin, e.g. nocturnal epilepsy or sleep apnoea, must be referred on to the medical profession.

EATING PROBLEMS IN THE UNDER FIVES

Many parents get extremely anxious when their child refuses to eat or has a very limited dietary intake. The child who lives on spaghetti hoops only is not uncommon. Often this situation can develop into a battle of wills between parent and child, with the parent finally turning to the health visitor in desperation. It is important that, prior to any intervention with behaviour modification, the health visitor is able to eliminate any failure to thrive or physical reason for the child's behaviour, and must liaise closely with medical staff. In-depth knowledge of the nutritional requirements of children is important (Ministry of Agriculture, Fisheries and Food 1989, Department of Health 1995c). This information, when shared with the parents, offers a basis for adjusting the toddler's diet to incorporate their needs. Again, the use of a diary often helps to identify actual

problems or highlight unreasonably high parental expectations (Fig. 9.4).

Key tactics include the following:

- Make feeding time a fun and sociable activity; eat family meals together if at all possible.

- Let the child eat what the family eats wherever possible – 'What is on your plate must be nicer than what is on mine.'

- Independence is a trait of most toddlers: they like to feed themselves no matter how messy it is – messy eating is not abnormal.

- Many sweet snacks can be nutritious: if the only thing a child will eat are sweets, then put popular cereals in little bags and offer as sweets – most cereals have added vitamins.

- Remember, children do not do the shopping, parents do – if it is not there it cannot be eaten.

- Do not make a big issue of faddy eating: it is usually what it says – a fad that will soon pass if played down.

TANTRUMS AND BEHAVIOUR PROBLEMS IN THE UNDER FIVES

Tantrums and antisocial behaviour in young children often lead to the parent versus child battle of wills. It is health visitors' knowledge of the 'normal developmental stages' of children that enables them to offer advice and reassurance to parents caught in the trap of conflict with a toddler, in order to redress the balance. Biting and kicking, tantrums, head banging and clinging are all behaviours experienced to a greater or lesser extent in normal children. Often, it is the parents' approach in handling these behaviours and high expectations of children to behave as 'little adults' that exacerbate the problem. Use of a diary helps in the recognition of factors associated with the 'bad' behaviour (Fig. 9.5).

It is important to identify what happens immediately before the undesirable behaviour, what exactly the behaviour is and what the parents do about it before any programme of change

	Monday	Tuesday	Wednesday	Thursday	Friday	Saturday	Sunday
Breakfast (a.m.)							
Morning							
Lunch							
Afternoon							
Evening meal							
Supper							
Snacks							

Figure 9.4   An example of a food diary

	Child		Parent	
Day and date	What happened before behaviour?	Behaviour	How did you respond?	Effect of what you did

Figure 9.5   An example of a behaviour diary

can be formulated. Many texts are available as resources to help create specific programmes of behaviour management tailored to the individual child and family, as well as professional help from behavioural psychologists in difficult cases. Techniques such as distraction and positive or negative reinforcement may be used in such behaviour modification programmes.

Key tactics include the following:

- Share information regarding normal child development and behaviour with the parents.

- It is often a change in parental behaviour that brings about change in the child's behaviour.

- Encourage the parents to respond to good behaviour and to look for the positive aspects of their child – even an extremely naughty child has some good points.

- Convince parents of the importance of consistency; they should work as a team, applying the same rules of discipline to the child and not giving out confusing and conflicting information.

GROUPS VERSUS INDIVIDUALS SUPPORT APPROACH

The advantages of a support group approach or an individual approach when dealing with child behaviour problems can be discussed at length; both approaches have benefits and drawbacks.

The group offers release from isolation – often parents feel they are the only ones in the world with a child with a behaviour problem – peer support and the sharing of management skills, which many parents find useful. Parenting groups set up locally by health visitors offer access to a large number of clients in a cost-effective way.

Individual programming in the home is often time consuming for the health visitor but offers continuity to the client. Change in behaviour can be monitored over a long period of time, thus giving the family ongoing support.

An alternative to individual management of behaviour problems in the home is the setting up of clinics aimed at specific behaviour problems, such as sleep clinics. This offers the client access to health visitors who have a special interest in child behaviour and, because of their involvement in the clinics, have developed increased experience and expertise in dealing with the problem.

Health visitors are equipped with the knowledge and communication skills to assess and offer assistance to parents and families experiencing difficult childhood behaviour problems. All behaviour problems can be assessed using a process similar to those discussed above.

CHILD ACCIDENT PREVENTION

Joan Leach

Health visitors are the most appropriate community-based health professionals to promote accident prevention with families. Health visitors' long-term professional association with all families with pre-school children, their community base and detailed knowledge of their clients, the community and local facilities, and their interest and skills in profiling, all place them in an ideal position to be the community's prime workers in the field of child accident prevention. This is supported in the *Health Visitor Practice Development Resource Pack* (Department of Health 2001e).

The principles of health visiting (CETHV 1977) form the conceptual framework for the process of health visiting and have been used to illustrate the role of the health visitor in child accident prevention.

THE SEARCH FOR HEALTH NEEDS

The literature shows convincingly that every area has its own problems in relation to childhood accidents. There are no national statistics that are actually representative of any particular area. Research findings for a socially deprived urban area cannot reflect the same problems as a middle-class rural area.

It is therefore suggested that every area should conduct its own research to enable identification of the needs, trends and problems specific to that area with regard to accidents to children. Collecting local information about accidents is imperative if health visitors are to stand any chance of influencing plans for service provision or initiatives to meet local need.

If a system does not already exist to inform health visitors of accident victims, then communication with other health profession- als and departments needs to be addressed.

A health visitor liaison service with local accident and emergency (A&E) and minor injury hospital departments would inform the health visitor of every hospital attendance for children who have sustained an injury or those who have attended for other reasons. This falls in line with the recommendations of the Laming Report following the death of Victoria Climbié (March 2003). It must be recognized that this information would only provide a partial glimpse of the overall picture because not every child who has an accident is necessarily taken to hospital, particularly if the injury is minor or the family lives outside easy travel- ling distance from a hospital. McKee et al (1990) found that the distance from a patient's home to an A&E department was an important factor in the rate of attendance. Appropriate use of A&E departments is also a factor to con- sider when identifying local need: Ingram et al (1978) found that patients living nearest to an A&E unit tended to use it as a substitute for general practice.

Initiating communication systems within GPs' surgeries (if not already in existence) would also be useful to identify children who are seen or advised within the primary care set- ting following an accident. This would be par- ticularly helpful in rural settings or wherever the nearest A&E unit is not within easy travel- ling distance for the family.

Many minor injuries are dealt with by the family, either because they feel confident and competent to treat minor injuries themselves or because they choose not to seek medical advice or intervention. NHS Direct is becoming a useful resource to some families at times of uncertainty about whether medical treatment is required. Unless accidents are specifically asked about, the health visitor is usually unaware that these children have sustained an injury.

The health visitor must try to find ways to gain more knowledge about the local area and so help to establish a fuller local picture of the 'accident problem'. Caseload profiling should have accidents as an indicator. This would enable the health visitor, exercising statistical expertise, to record data in such a way as to allow meaningful interpretations of hard facts and in time permit monitoring of trends on a caseload, geographical area, Pri- mary Care Trust and Strategic Health Authority area basis.

STIMULATION OF AN AWARENESS OF HEALTH NEED

Having searched out and identified a health need in relation to child accident prevention, it is important that the health visitor has an action plan to address the need. In the past, health visitors have not been seen in a very positive light in this respect. Laidman (1987), the Child Accident Prevention Trust (1989) and Carter et al (1992) all highlight the shortfalls in health visitors' knowledge, training and delivery of safety advice to clients.

Health visitor training was identified as having shortfalls years ago and Laidman (1987) recommended ways of teaching child accident work as a specific topic rather than link- ing it with other course work. Hall & Elliman (2003) supports this by advocating that health care staff need further information and train- ing in injury prevention. He recognizes that suitable materials are available, but their impact has yet to be fully evaluated. Qualified health visitors need to request regular updat- ing and training to improve and update their local knowledge and to improve their skills in delivering this specialized area of work.

Hall (1991) advocated including child acci- dent prevention topics at each child surveil- lance contact that were age and development related. Although better than nothing, it could be argued that surveillance contacts are not the ideal time to be doing specific, detailed acci- dent prevention work. It could be seen as being 'slotted in' and so loses its emphasis and impor- tance, particularly if conducted in clinic or sur- gery settings where the child is not being seen in his/her normal home environment. Home is where potential hazards would be identified more easily and more meaningfully by the health visitor.

It is important that each employing NHS Trust encourages health visitors to work in collaborative groups, as opposed to working in isolation, to address the issues of child accident prevention. When working in groups, ideas can be shared, schemes of work can be piloted and strategies can be formulated more easily. These groups need to be able to monitor their work in a recognized, recordable way so that their outcomes can be readily measured and audited. It is hoped that working collaboratively will not only raise and stimulate awareness of this particular health need but will also result in evidence- and research-based methods of working, and contribute to Hall & Elliman's (2003) recommendations of multi-agency working.

INFLUENCES ON POLICIES AFFECTING HEALTH

The influences on policies that affect health tend to be at the macro level, as most are government generated. *The Health of the Nation* (Department of Health 1992b) aimed at reducing ill health, disability and death caused by accidents. Its main target was to reduce the death rate for accidents among children aged under 15 years by at least 33% by the year 2005. Nurses were encouraged to influence this policy by submitting work they had done that either changed behaviour, changed practice or changed the environment. These initiatives were published in *Targeting Practice: The Contribution of Nurses, Midwives and Health Visitors* (Department of Health 1993b). Although most of this work was done at a micro level, it was hoped to influence the macro problem. An example of these initiatives is given in the following vignette.

The health visitor attached to two general practitioners in the North Staffs area, concerned by the number of children who were sustaining head injuries, set up a research project. The objective was to examine whether providing parents with information on how to prevent accidents that result in an injury to the head, and giving them concrete guidelines as to when to seek medical help or advice should their child sustain a head injury, reduced the number of children presenting at the local accident and emergency department. All children on the GP list for the health visitor's practice were subjects of the study. The method used necessitated establishing the number of children from the district and the study practice who had attended the A&E department following an injury to the head for the period 1991–92. This was achieved through the information supplied by the A&E liaison health visitor. In April 1992 every family on the study caseload was sent a special 'head injuries to children' leaflet. Families joining the practice after that date also had the same leaflet given to them and the contents explained. Every child on the study caseload who presented at the A&E department between May 1992 and April 1993 was followed up with a home visit and a questionnaire was completed.

The results were that the total number of children who attended the A&E department during 1991–92 was roughly the same as previous years, with only a 1% reduction in the total number of children who presented with a head injury. Following the intervention there was a reduction of 17% of children presenting with a head injury for the period of May 1992 to April 1993 on the study caseload when compared with the previous 12 months.

The majority of families interviewed found the head injury leaflet informative and helpful. Some parents said it was instrumental in their decision actually to attend the A&E department with their child. However, overall there was a 17% reduction in attendance with head injuries, allowing more appropriate use of A&E services.

The government Green Paper *Our Healthier Nation* (Department of Health 1998b) also targets accidents. The aim is to reduce the rate of accidents – defined as those that involve a hospital visit or consultation with a family doctor – by at least a fifth (20%) by 2010 from the 1996 baseline.

Saving lives – Our Healthier Nation (Department of Health 1999c) has set tougher but achievable targets in priority areas: by the year 2010 the accident death rate to be reduced by a fifth and serious injury to be reduced by at least a tenth.

Identifying the needs locally and developing strategies to stimulate an awareness of the need should result in local policies being influenced. If local policies are influenced and actioned, this in turn will affect the national situation. Collaborative working must be the key issue if we are to stand any chance of influencing policies that will affect the incidence of accidents to children.

THE FACILITATION OF HEALTH-ENHANCING ACTIVITIES

Most research on childhood accidents states that children from economically deprived backgrounds have a markedly higher death rate from accidents. The Child Accident Prevention Trust (1989) believes that the social-class gradient for deaths due to accident is far steeper than for any other cause of child death; the incidence of non-fatal accidents may also be related to social class. The cause of this relationship is probably a combination of many factors. A fatalistic attitude to accidents among parents in the lower socio-economic groups arising from lack of control over many other aspects of their lives has been suggested as a causal factor.

The Child Accident Prevention Trust illustrates that families in social classes IV and V are likely to be more at risk because of less satisfactory housing in terms of location, overcrowding, space, property maintenance and the lack of money to maintain potentially dangerous equipment and to buy safety equipment such as fireguards. The lack of access to adequate play facilities is frequently associated with poor housing. All contribute to the level of risk.

Our Healthier Nation (Department of Health 1998b) reiterates the health divide: childhood injuries are closely linked to social deprivation. Children from poorer backgrounds are five times more likely to die as a result of an accident than children from better-off families – and the gap is widening. Hall & Elliman (2003)

reiterates the social class and deprivation variables, illustrates parental misconceptions and gives detailed implications of types of injuries. Health needs assessments and caseload profiling will help to identify the vulnerable and will enable health visitors to concentrate their accident prevention work on families and communities known to be vulnerable.

The use of the parent-held record system has enabled the health visitor to work much more effectively with families. Being able to work in partnership with clients helps the health visitor to have a deeper understanding of their health beliefs and knowledge base.

Using a model when working with families would ensure the health visitor has a framework on which to base accident prevention work. Becker's health belief model (1974) would be an appropriate choice, because it identifies the key issues needed in this area of work:

- Individual perceptions: identifies client knowledge base and beliefs
- Modifying factors: identifies what the client believes they must do to make a child's environment safer
- Likelihood of action: clients would have a greater understanding of the possible consequences of their actions or non-actions.

This particular model fits comfortably into the conceptual framework of most care plans. Care plans are a useful tool to use with families where a safety issue has been identified.

Increasing parental knowledge about preventing childhood accidents would seem a sensible route to take when considering facilitation of health-enhancing activities. Health visitors would, at all times, use their professional expertise when delivering this to clients, in a way that has been proved to be most effective with the particular client group. Health visitors are notoriously holistic, and never miss an opportunity to raise preventive health issues when interviewing clients.

As previously stated, it is feared that a lot of accident prevention advice is 'slotted in' with other topics under discussion and families and clients may underestimate the importance of the message. Making accident prevention a specific topic for discussion during appointed home visits to individual families proved to be the most effective way during the Play it Safe campaign (Colver 1983). This study found that even severely disadvantaged families would respond to health education if the education were appropriate. Of families that were given specific advice about hazards present in their homes at the time of a home visit, 60% made at least one change to make their homes safer. This approach to child accident prevention fits comfortably with a recommended core function of *Liberating the Talents* (Department of Health 2002b) – public health/health protection and promoting programmes that improve health and reduce inequalities. Skill mix within a health visiting team could be employed to everyone's advantage when planning strategies to address child accident prevention. It would encourage leadership, planning and identification by the health visitor of families in need and the carrying out of the specific home safety visit by a specially trained nurse member of that team. Discussing and informing during group activities with parents, or holding special health promotional events dealing specifically with child accident prevention, are other examples of facilitating health-enhancing activities to reduce the accident rate among our child population.

INEQUALITIES IN HEALTH

Jean Glynn

When profiling for health needs in Stoke on Trent health visitors are mindful of the fact that Tones & Tilford (1994) found that people in the north of England had poorer diets than those in the south, despite being aware of healthy and unhealthy foods. Individuals are prevented from making healthy choices because there is sometimes a conflict of priorities between paying for food or rent. Low income may therefore prevent women from purchasing a nutritional diet for their family, but this is further compounded by geographical factors. Local shops are more expensive and

sell fewer healthier foods compared to the larger, more distant supermarket where food is cheaper but more difficult to access.

Gender differences have also been noted in health. Women are three times more likely to smoke in the lower classes than in professional households and smoking is increasingly linked to poverty and disadvantage (Roberts 1990, Blackburn 1993). Non-attendance at child health clinics has also been found to be related to maternal smoking (Pitts & Phillips 1991).

In addition to influences of gender, class and geography, health is also determined by an individual's behaviour. The likelihood of an individual performing a behaviour is dependent on privately held attitudes about behaviours and whether positive outcomes can be achieved from performing them (Becker 1974, Broome 1994). Smoking is not always seen by the individual as a negative behaviour because it can give mothers a break from caring, enabling them to cope by resting, and gives positive reinforcement in that psychologically they feel less tense and stressed (Blackburn 1993). Adolescents may seek peer approval and therefore engage in 'risk-taking' behaviour, such as unprotected sex, drug and alcohol abuse (Broome 1994). Individuals may not be interested in future disease prevention if they have other priorities, such as poor housing, unemployment and financial problems (Tones & Tilford 1994). Poor self-esteem, low confidence and lack of self-empowerment are also factors that inhibit individuals from making positive health choices (Ewles & Simnett 2003). The decision to carry out preventive health behaviours may be possible for the individual, but the ability to perform the desired behaviour can therefore be seen to be constrained and limited by social, physical, environmental and emotional factors.

The Department of Health (2001e) outlined key activities for health visitors in their public health role to address some of these problems:

- assessing the health needs of the local population
- planning and implementing programmes that promote and protect health

- identifying inequalities and taking action to address these
- working with others to address the wider threats to health
- using a community development approach to deliver health improvements.

Health visitors are able to target families with greater health and social care needs and offer flexible services, like choice of clinic times, drop-in and evening sessions (North Staffs Combined Healthcare Trust 1996). The flexibility of the health visiting service is an advantage, because health visitors can respond to clients' needs and be accessible because they work in the community in general, in public, the workplace and other settings. Health visiting 'is a unique non-discriminatory professional service', and health visitors are therefore accessible to those who might not otherwise seek health advice (North Staffs Combined Healthcare Trust 1996, p. 3).

IMPACT ON SEXUAL HEALTH

Young girls, once grown out of the childhood infections stage and assuming they have no chronic illness, rarely come into contact with the NHS until they move into the reproductive stage of their lives. It is at this point that many aspects of a female's life are medicalized. The male is seen as the 'norm' in medicine and he is not subjected to the same number of screening programmes, such as cervical smears, breast examination and mammography (Coney 1995). Women have become sought-after 'commodities' in the health service; the reason for this may be that some women are now in a position to pay to improve their health and well-being because they are in paid employment (Coney 1995). Also, many research programmes are now focused on women and their fertility is often determined by medicine (Coney 1995, Roberts 1990). Choice of treatment may also be determined by health economics. The cost of some contraceptives and fertility treatment may limit choices for women. Richardson & Robinson (1993) offer an alternative view: they

consider that woman are prescribed pills so that they remain sexually available to men at all times. Oral contraception can have health risks for some women. Concern has been expressed that injected contraceptives may lead to osteoporosis due to amenorrhoea, and there is an increased risk of arterial disease with the combined pill (Guillebaud 1993). Therefore all women need adequate information, access to appropriate contraceptive services and health promotion clinics in order to feel empowered and in control of their health.

A survey of young people found that the average age they had their first experience of sexual intercourse was 17 and between a third and a half did not use contraception on the first time (Department of Health 2001g). Of particular concern to the government and health professionals was the number of teenage pregnancies resulting from this. The Health of the Nation (Department of Health 1992b) aimed to reduce the number of unwanted pregnancies by reducing the conception rate in under 16-year-olds from 9.5 per 1000 in 1989 to 4.8 by the year 2000 (Department of Health 1993a). However, by 2000 the conception rate in the under 16-year-olds had only fallen to 8.3%, and therefore the national strategy for sexual health and HIV (Department of Health 2001g) has not continued this sexual health target, choosing instead to aim to achieve an established downward trend by 2010. The UK has the highest pregnancy rate among 15- to 19-year-olds in Western Europe and with this is a high percentage of terminations. Half of all conceptions in under 16-year-olds and one-third in 16- to 19-year-olds ended in termination and this had increased to 54% in 2000 (Office of National Statistics 2000). This high termination rate may be due to poor information and low uptake of emergency contraception or, as suggested earlier, be part of the risk-taking behaviour of adolescents (Broome 1989, Fullerton et al 1997). Jones (1996), however, found that teenage pregnancy continued to be a problem despite the availability of reliable contraceptive methods.

Some improvements have been achieved in reducing the number of pregnancies. Programmes that combine sex education with access to contraceptive services have been found to be effective in increasing contraceptive use and have contributed to the lower rate of teenage pregnancies (Fullerton et al 1997). Pregnancy remains higher in socially deprived areas where, for some adolescents, there are positive outcomes despite the risk of adverse health, education, social and economic effects. It is suggested this is because of low expectation of education or job market, lack of knowledge in sexual health and mixed sexual health messages (Department of Health 2001e).

Of recent concern is the rise in sexually transmitted diseases, probably as a result of an increase in diagnosis due to publicity and improved testing (Health Protection Agency 2003). Chlamydia is one of the most common conditions and the rates of infection have almost doubled in recent years, with infection rates up to 12% in women and a significant increase in young people under the age of 20 (Department of Health 2001g). The health visitor has an important role to play in promoting safer sex and explaining the consequences of sexually transmitted diseases, as well as promoting access to screening and supporting the individuals and their families who are affected by infection, infertility and relationship problems. Health visitors need to work in partnership and collaborate with other professionals working in sexual health and youth services to deliver sexual health messages in a variety of settings. The public health role in relation to sexual health is emphasized in the Department of Health Practice Development Toolkit for health visitors (Department of Health 2001e).

To improve the accessibility of services and information for young people it is necessary to take into account local need and circumstances. The compilation of a local profile that includes current service provision and health data provides the basis for a comprehensive needs assessment of the local population. A needs assessment is a complex process involving the determinants of physical, mental, social and environmental factors that may impact on health. It therefore identifies individuals and groups at risk, as well as identifying gaps in the provision of services.

Services need to attract the young and individuals from black and ethnic minorities, give both males and females confidence to attend and ensure confidentiality, while working within the Fraser guidelines and being aware of local and national child protection policies and guidelines (Faculty of Family Planning and Reproductive Health Care 2003). The type of clinic is an important factor and there are many examples of good practice where a variety of approaches and venues have been used by health visitors and other health professionals. Initiatives have included:

- drop-in clinics
- after-school clinics
- one-stop sexual health clinics
- clinic-in-box in schools and youth clubs
- information packs for young people attending their GP
- road shows
- Saturday clinics (Department of Health 1995b, 2001g).

High rates of teenage pregnancy in the Tayside Region in Scotland and the demand from the young for more accessible health care led to the development of drop-in clinics, open days and condom initiatives (Goudie & Redman 1996). An innovation in York targeted young people, advice on sexual health, free condoms, chlamydia screening using a simple urine test and partner notification was carried out in a school (Lewis 2004). Issues of confidentiality and a positive attitude from the staff, as well as better information given on how to access the services, were found to be important for young people in improving attendance at family planning clinics (Jackson & Plant 1996). Similar findings were noted near Glasgow during the development of a teenage club by a health visitor (Little 1997). The service was developed in conjunction with the teenagers, who selected topics about healthy lifestyles, including contraception issues. The teenagers wanted a clinic that was easy to get to, with no appointments, welcoming, somewhere they were able to bring friends, confidential and providing a range of services (Little 1997). Young people's clinics established in general practices found that individuals attended mainly for information on safer sex and contraception. Overall studies have found that attendance is higher and pregnancy rates lower when contraception is provided by clinics specifically for the young, where there is improved access, a relaxed atmosphere achieved through staff attitudes, and where refreshments and music are available (Jackson & Plant 1996, Boston 1997, Little 1997).

Individual support is also needed for young women who find themselves pregnant, so that they are able to make their own decisions, as they usually experience less emotional and practical assistance than older pregnant women (Nolan 1996). Often they are given poor information about their care and are treated as stupid, or it is implied that they should be ashamed of their situation, but teenage mothers should not be stereotyped as they are not all unsupported, single or come from abusive backgrounds (Nolan 1996). Causes of pregnancy in teenagers may include social influences, limited access to appropriate health services, socio-economic factors or individual characteristics. However improvements can be made to reduce pregnancies with good education and access to family planning services developed to meet local need, and the poor socio-economic and health outcomes associated with pregnancy can be reduced with support. The launch of the government's Sure Start Plus initiative in April 2001 located in areas of high teenage pregnancy, such as in Stoke-on-Trent, to which health visitors can refer aims to reduce social exclusion and improve access to services (Teenage Pregnancy Unit 2003).

Health visitors can help to alleviate some of the negative health and social outcomes by devising special antenatal programmes for young expectant mothers, which may include future contraception, sexual health, healthy relationships, women's health in general and parenting. Home visits can support the pregnant teenager and her family, while parenting skills can improve the mother–child interaction (Fullerton et al 1997). Domiciliary services can also help to meet the needs of ethnic minorities and individuals with disabilities (Dwivedi & Varma 1996). Language and cultural barriers, as well as lower expectations and lack of knowledge of services, can compound the problems of accessing services. The current emphasis on improving quality of services may address some of these issues, with the focus on health improvement, fair access, effective delivery of service, client/carer experience and health outcomes (Department of Health 1998a).

CONCLUSION

The use of developmental screening is a dilemma, in that health visitors can see the value of the scientific support in relation to child protection issues. It is unfortunate that the policy in some areas is to minimize the use of screening techniques, considering them overused and expensive, and many health visitors would agree that the child with no problems does not need to be screened on a regular basis. Nevertheless, Reynolds has made a sound argument for the use of developmental screening in child protection. Many parents seek the advice of their health visitor over the issues of behaviour and in enabling them to deal with the issue without seeing it as a problem is an important aspect of good health visiting. Children are very prone to accidents, but the informed carer/parent is empowered to support and prevent accidents to the child. There is much evidence to show the relationship between health inequalities and sexual health problems and this is a public health issue, the reducing of which should be a target of all specialist community public health nurses.

Chapter 10

Violence – debating the issues

Anne Robotham

INTRODUCTION

Definitions of violence can be multiple, ranging from shouting to physical attack, from ostracism to cynical criticism, and victims can be of all ages and from all sections of society.

Most health visitors at one time or another have witnessed acts of violence within the community in which they work. Whereas health visitors up until the 1980s had little education in handling violence and violent situations, the turn of the century has seen a far greater awareness in the need to educate professionals who may meet violence in their work. This chapter will focus primarily on situational causes of violence and will explore issues relating to violence, the knowledge of which will enable the support that health visitors can give to both victims and (occasionally) perpetrators. This is not advocating a specific role for health visitors but helping to recognize that they are in a unique position through their work in homes and schools to detect and if possible prevent violence occurring. To do this the health visitor will use primarily the skills of providing a quiet environment in which to listen to the client, ask direct but non-threatening questions to establish the position, give advice about support and services available and, finally, document carefully with permission. Some discussion of dealing with anger and violence both within work and at work will follow after the main analysis of situational causes of violence.

There are variations around the UK in the types of service available, but the organization Women's Aid covers the whole country, and many inner city areas have hostels for women and children fleeing domestic violence. Housing departments also have a statutory duty to house women who are made homeless by fleeing violent partners. Many cities support a zero tolerance campaign which uses mass media to raise awareness of domestic violence, rape and child sexual abuse. The approach is based on prevention of crimes of violence against women, provision of quality services and appropriate and effective legal protection for women and children experiencing violence. Schools are now involved in the promotion of non-violence and positive relationships, particularly for 14- to 16-year-olds.

VIOLENCE IN CONTEXT

Violence is seen as a breach of the peace rather than a crime against the individual. Since the 13th century the initiative for criminal law has passed to Parliament, and it is Parliament that is responsible for the definition of new crimes. The Department for Education and Employment (1998), the Department of the Environment, Transport and the Regions (1998, 1999), the Department of Social Security (1999), the Health and Safety Executive (1997) and the Home Office (1997, 1998, 1999, 2000) have all produced publications concerning prevention and treatment of violence.

Violence is not a modern phenomenon and the violence of today has parallels in history. The football hooligan differs little from the chariot race hooligan. Violent crime rarely produces a death rate comparable to the death rate in France in the 16th century due to duelling. Violence still can occur within the laws of some countries and is common within judicial processes, e.g. sentencing to lashing or to solitary confinement. The use of 'legal' torture still occurs within 'civilized' countries. In terms of scale, violence in society cannot compete with violence committed by society in the form of warfare.

DIFFERING PERSPECTIVES ON VIOLENCE

History suggests that the root cause for violence can be political, religious, physical or sociological. Modern anthropology suggests that to these must be added psychology and pathology. The following sections will explore the more relevant factors.

HORMONAL INFLUENCES

Considerable biological research has been undertaken on the body's hormone levels and violent behaviour. Most of this research (Rose et al 1971, Doering et al 1974) has been done in relation to the male sex hormones, or androgens. Some work has been done in relation to testosterone but it has not been conclusive. In relation to androgens animal studies (rats) have shown that castrated rats appear to be less aggressive than their unaffected peers. Injections of testosterone to raise levels significantly have shown the development of aggressive behaviour in other animals, while in humans similar studies have been inconclusive – the development of aggressive behaviour in one study was not sustained in others. Studies on premenstrual syndrome in affected women have shown a clear relationship in some women between progesterone levels and aggressive behaviour, to the extent that it has now been accepted in legal judgements that women diagnosed as suffering from premenstrual syndrome are capable of extremely aggressive acts (Owens & Ashcroft 1985).

GENETIC FACTORS

It is possible that certain abnormal chromosome patterns are responsible for aggressive behaviour. Studies on Down's syndrome children have shown that sufferers are particularly characterized by lack of aggressiveness and there may be other anomalies that show the reverse – a characterization of aggressiveness in other chromosomal abnormalities. Owens & Ashcroft (1985) cite several studies that have concentrated on abnormalities in the pairing of the sex chromosomes; in inmates of secure mental hospitals, males with 47 chromosomes (XYY) instead of the normal 46 (XY) occur with something like 30 times the frequency of the incidence in the general population. Further studies on the male inmates of prisons have found that the XYY men are more likely to offend against property than other individuals.

Studies of breeding in animals have shown that in the case of larger mammals – cows, horses, dogs – it is possible to breed for docility or aggression and similar potential may exist in humans.

ANTHROPOLOGICAL STUDIES

Early 19th-century anthropological studies on Tahitians showed them to be very gentle and peaceable people who not only disapproved of violent acts but also considered it shameful to have violent thoughts. However, Western contact changed the culture so that the same people became much more warlike. This was also observed in New Guinea with a change from the hunter-gatherer society to a settled form of food production. At an opposite extreme, some societies have been noted to have extremely warlike and aggressive tendencies. In a study of the Yanomano Indians of northern Brazil it was noted that violent behaviour could be used to express affection. A Yanomano woman, for example, would not believe that a man really loved her unless he left her scarred or bruised.

Attempts have been made to explain the violent behaviour of various groups as adaptive in terms of their individual circumstances but it is important to note that cultural factors do not provide a complete account of violence. Thus within a culture some individuals may act in a way quite different from most of the culture's members. The existence of violent subcultures in larger societies may be a cause for concern if it is accepted that such cultures act as 'breeding grounds' for violent acts. The anthropological evidence provides some support for the notion that action should be taken to avoid the formation of such subcultures, in particular by eliminating contributory factors, e.g. poor housing and overcrowding.

In terms of a more general understanding of violence, the sociological and anthropological work provides strong evidence that a purely biological explanation is inadequate. Reactive aggression has been demonstrated in the laboratory with rats, inducing fighting in otherwise peaceful animals by exposing them to an electric current. Certain drugs appear to affect the probability of fighting in response to aversive stimulation. Seligman (1975) has also pointed out that a person who hits their head on a car door on entering may become furious, yelling at the passengers! The process of reactive aggression provides the beginning of a framework within which to consider the psychological aspects of violence.

THE PSYCHOLOGICAL PERSPECTIVE

Freud attempted to show that energy in some humans was directed towards a drive for death and destruction rather than the pleasures of the 'id' factor of the human personality. However, he found it impossible to validate this theory and few of his contemporaries supported him. Most of the early psychology work was directed more towards attempting to define an aggressive personality. Eysenck (1983) tried to show that a person with an extrovert personality was more likely to indulge in delinquent behaviour but he could make little distinction between crime in general and violent crime. Another researcher (Megargee 1966) came somewhat closer to explaining violence when he postulated personal 'control'. He suggested that there were individuals who were 'under-controlled', who make little or no attempt at self-control when in an aggression-induced situation. In this case these individuals would present with a history of a number of violent episodes and would be characterized by the ease with which violent behaviour could be elicited.

The second type of individual that Megargee (1966) described was the 'over-controlled' individual, who held aggression in check in situations where most individuals would react violently. Certain individuals, it would appear, are normally non-violent but suddenly and unexpectedly may commit an act of extreme violence, often disproportionate to the provocation. Because of their suppressed response to mild aggression, the over-controlled individual would be more likely than the rest of us to be exposed to extended or intense provocation. Eventually, such provocation may reach a point where even the over-controlled person's degree of self-control is inadequate and violence results. An additional factor is introduced by the fact that the over-controlled individual, unlike others, has little 'practice' at being violent. Most people, as a result of some practice, become quite skilled at matching their aggressive responses to the demands of the situation (violent blow to an attacking mugger but only a mild reprimand to a whinging child). Smacking children has long been an acceptable means of controlling undesirable behaviour in all cultures and social classes. Mothers have learnt from their mothers that physical punishment is an appropriate means of correcting one's child. However, there is a fine line between a corrective smack and an escalation into physical abuse. Mention has been made in Chapter 4 of recent work by End Physical Punishment of Children (EPOCH; Cook et al 1991) in raising awareness of smacking escalation, and health visitors are now concerned to help mothers by offering alternative strategies for behaviour modification.

There are a number of problems with accepting the above theory because it is impossible to explain the relationship between situations and human responses in terms of over-control or under-control. Early experimental research showed that experimentally induced frustration could greatly increase aggressive behaviour (Bandura 1973). However, this does not explain how, when aggression occurs, it is not always possible to identify any accompanying frustration factor. Bandura (1973) showed that an alternative consequence to frustration in children was not aggression but regression.

Learned behaviour may play a part in reactive aggression, in that such aggression may be elicited by a stimulus whose aversive properties have been induced by the conditioning process. Much aggressive behaviour appears not to be elicited by any particular prior stimulus but rather to represent an attempt to obtain some subsequent goal, i.e. the behaviour appears to be more under the control of consequences than antecedents. This was seen as an operant conditioning response in Skinner's (1938) work on rats' and pigeons' responses to the need for food. Several behaviourist psychologists in the 1960s were able to show that behaviour could be shaped into more aggressive responses and that children who were victimized at nursery school could be guided into producing more aggressive responses to their attackers, thus changing their behaviour. Similarly, attacking a victim and producing responses of crying, defensiveness and submission may serve as a reinforcing stimulus for maintenance of this type of behaviour in the attacker.

Modelling, as a factor in producing new or altering old behaviours, was demonstrated by Bandura in the 1970s. He showed with the Bobo doll how children would adopt aggressive behaviour in the experimental situation and that this was transferred into real-life situations. Thus it was possible, using this approach, to see that adolescent boys who were non-aggressive had parents who had used no physical punishment in their upbringing, unlike aggressive boys, whose parents had used physical punishment on which the boy then modelled his subsequent behaviour. Thus, imitation as a reason for aggressive behaviour has generated considerable research interest from educationalists and psychologists alike. Detailed research studies into the effect of violent scenes on TV and video on the subsequent behaviour of viewers have shown that in certain individuals it leads to violent behavioural responses (Brody 1977).

Nevertheless, this does not explain why some viewers of violent film scenes do not subsequently act violently. It may have something to do with the argument put forward by TV and video producers that the audience does not see screen violence as part of the 'real' world and thus distinguishes between reality and drama. It is therefore a possibility that individuals in whom it does produce a violent response are those who cannot distinguish between 'reality' and 'drama'. It is also important to consider whether it is a combination of previously learned behaviour and the effect of viewed violence that results in aggression.

Implicit within the discussion above is the concept that it is in the early days of the development of the individual within the family that the seeds of potential violence are sown. In the foreword to the paper *Supporting Families* (Home Office 1999), Jack Straw, the Home Secretary, makes an initial point: 'Family life is the foundation on which our communities, our society and our country are built.'

VULNERABLE AND ABUSING FAMILIES

Many sociologists and psychologists have explored the meaning of family, the differences between families and the way family members interact, and much of the evidence put forward gives the professional an insight into the part that the family might play in relation to domestic violence. Sociologists tend to focus on the group and what makes a family unit, while psychologists explore the interactional and socio-emotional styles within families, and what distinguishes a 'healthy family' from an 'unhealthy family'. Olson et al (1979) used the 'circumplex model' to classify types within two key dimensions of adaptability and cohesion (Fig. 10.1).

Frude (1996) briefly discusses the extremes of these and in the adaptability dimension describes rigid families where each member has an allotted role, the power structure is inflexible and leadership is authoritarian with little compromise. Chaotic families are the reverse, with no clear rules, a power structure that is unstable and support and permission-giving irregular and arbitrary. Children lack guidance and parental discipline is erratic and inconsistent.

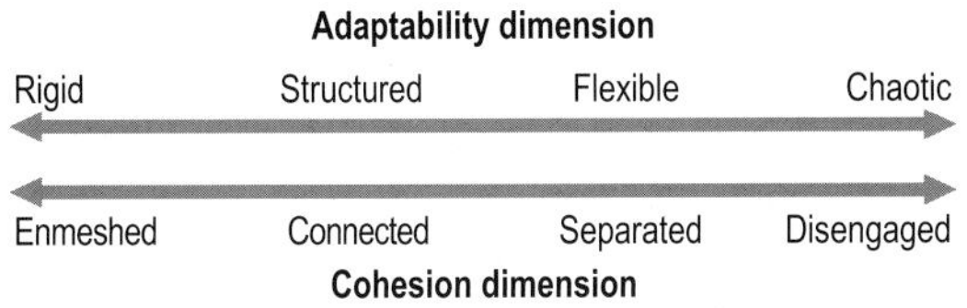

Adaptability dimension

Rigid	Structured	Flexible	Chaotic

Enmeshed	Connected	Separated	Disengaged

Cohesion dimension

Figure 10.1 The circumplex model (reproduced with permission from Olson et al 1979)

The cohesion dimension distinguishes enmeshed families at one end of the spectrum, which are so tightly bonded that the members have little personal identity and are suffocatingly close; while at the other extreme, disengaged families appear to have little unity and no sense of identity.

The use of the term 'dysfunctional families' is premised on the Olson et al (1979) model and these families tend to show extreme positions on one or other of the dimensions or, indeed, extreme positions on both dimensions, e.g. rigid/disengaged or rigid/enmeshed and chaotic/disengaged or chaotic/enmeshed. Families that are dysfunctional tend to develop problems without any outside pressures, so that stress caused by outside pressure quickly becomes intolerable and threatens family health.

FAMILY PATTERNS IN CHILD ABUSE

Crittenden (1988), in discussing family patterns in relation to child abuse, identified four definable patterns of family behaviour that she called 'abusing families', 'neglecting families', 'abusing and neglecting families' and 'marginally maltreating families'. Using her criteria in conjunction with Olson's model, families vulnerable to child abuse would seem to show extremes of dysfunction in either or both of the adaptability and cohesion dimensions, with added criteria relating to one or both parents' personal history of abuse, the parents' socio-economic status and education or the child's health and behaviour.

Child abuse has a number of different categories: for example, there is physical violence, where the child is physically abused and injured. The second category is neglect – not just ignoring a child, which is not usually defined as neglect, but behaviour that may be life-threatening such as not feeding children or keeping them clean. The third category, psychological abuse, which probably includes the greatest number of cases, is the most difficult to identify and may include verbal brutalization and making the child feel inadequate, incompetent and ashamed. Finally, in sexual abuse a child can experience various degrees of interference, from fondling to direct penetration.

Parton (1990), writing for the Violence Against Children Study Group, makes three important observations from the literature. Firstly, the vast majority of sexual abuse of children is committed by men, and girls are abused in greater numbers; secondly, the responsibility for physical abuse is equally distributed between men and women; and thirdly, women predominate in cases of emotional abuse and neglect. Parton highlights the role women play in the abuse of their own children, either directly or indirectly, and suggests that many writers allude to 'the abusing parent' when in reality they mean 'the abusing mother'.

In questioning why some women fail to protect their children feminists argue that the reason lies within women's relative powerlessness within the family and wider society. These women may have had a violent childhood with aggressive fathers, have low self-esteem and experience frequent abuse from their cohabitees. They continue relationships with violent men, even though they may be very frightened of them, at the expense of their children. Ong (1986) argues that coping is seen to be essential for 'successful' motherhood and when a mother neglects or abuses her children this is seen as an individual failing rather than being related to the conditions in which mothering takes place. Yet the pressures upon women to cope with the role of motherhood are powerful, both from society and from within themselves. Ong says that isolation in the home is a major factor in women's violence towards their children and is more likely to be experienced by those women who have least control over where they live and are unable to develop or maintain their links with supportive friends or family through lack of money, a car or baby-sitters. Thus professionals working in child abuse must move away from seeing it as an individual problem and analyse the wider context and confront the issue of violence of the institution of motherhood (Ong 1986).

The incidence and reporting of child sexual abuse is on the increase but it has taken society a long time to recognize the seriousness and scale of the problem and to understand the consequences, both long-term and short-term. Child sexual abuse occurs within the family and, in a sense, the family provides psychological as well as physical resources and also sexual and affectionate needs. The family in Western society has become more isolated – away from the extended family – and thus there is greater pressure on it to cope with its needs with fewer social contacts. Thus the isolation of families may be a factor in child abuse; however, it is frequently the case that the abusing parent was sexually abused. Finkelhor (1986), in the USA, found that, while physical and sexual abuse can be present at all socio-economic levels, the poorer the family the greater the likelihood of child abuse – physical and sexual. He also made the interesting observation that child sexual abuse tended to be found in families with higher incomes, a finding confirmed by Hanks & Stratton (1988) in the UK.

Sexually abused children are put under great pressure to 'keep this as our secret' and it is only recently that as a society, we have been able to believe a child who is able to share this guilty secret. There is evidence that within closed families (see 'enmeshed families' above) all the children may have been sexually abused and each child remains in silent isolation, hoping that they are protecting their siblings and at the same time, possibly, also feeling special (Frude 1996). The physical effects of child abuse may lead to bruising or more serious injuries and some children contract sexually transmitted disease, while older girls who are subjected to intercourse run the risk of pregnancy. However, much child sexual abuse takes the form of masturbation, fondling or indecent exposure and thus there is no physical damage or even forensic evidence. Psychological trauma can be very great, with children requiring long periods of counselling, often many years after the occurrence, but it must be remembered that many children do cope psychologically and appear to be healthy and adjusted. There has been concern among professionals that hunting for hidden psychological trauma may do considerable harm, a criticism levelled against the setting up of Childline by Esther Rantzen, the television personality.

DELINQUENCY

Delinquency by young offenders can be construed as violence towards society and may be defined as involvement in activities that are normally regarded and treated as criminal offences, even if relatively minor ones, e.g. malicious damage to public property, various forms of theft, getting into fights in public and resisting arrest. There are also status offences such as smoking, gambling, under-age drinking, truancy and the increasingly prevalent drug use. These behavioural problems can be analysed in several different ways: for example, it could be argued that they are the result of a constricting society setting standards or restrictions that might be seen as repressive. On the other hand, there is much evidence to show that changes in the fabric of society, in which the family plays a less important role than formerly, mean that the ground rules normally laid down through adequate to good parenting are missing. Thus attitude and personality development is skewed towards the individual and away from care of and within the group.

THE BULLYING PERSONALITY

Randall (1997) has described a number of instances when perpetrators of bullying trace the development of their behaviour back to parental violence towards them as young children. The critical stages in development of aggressive behaviour, beginning with the handling of separation from the prime care-giver (separation anxiety), through the 'terrible twos' and finally the development of skills for entry into pre-schooling or school, are those stages when it is most important that the child is exposed to steady parental handling. Parents who cannot cope with the child's normal developmental stages contribute to deficits in cognitive aspects of behavioural control. Aggression will occur when children do not learn the ability to negotiate within relationships or follow the rules set by adults. Negotiation is very dependent on the development of meaningful language. With the development of language there is a reduction in the physical aspects of aggression such as biting, throwing objects and pulling hair. Language and the ability to play alongside other children without resorting to aggressive behaviour – squabbling over possessions is an example – allows children to begin to show behaviour that relies on empathy and the acceptance of other people's perspectives that differ from their own (Randall 1997).

Parents or primary care-givers play an essential part in helping their children to channel aggressive behaviour into assertive behaviour. Social development in the form of happy social interactions, positive approaches to negative circumstances and calming attitudes and demeanours from the role model are all important factors. Children observe and copy the interactions of their parents and others and learn the ways in which the role model copes with their own emotions (Egeland 1988).

Baumrind's (1967) work on parenting styles has shown how the authoritarian style is not appropriate for children to learn good social interaction skills. Children who are told what to do are often not allowed to try for themselves alternative styles of behaviour or coping strategies and thus don't have the chance to explore the consequences of these.

Children quickly become aware of how parents feel about them and parents' feelings towards their children are often based on whether they perceive them as being 'easy' or 'difficult' to handle from birth. Other researchers have shown that social circumstances of material or financial poverty, poor partner relationships, maternal or paternal depression and low IQ may all create intolerably stressful situations leading to the development of aggression in the home. Conger et al (1992) showed that parents who are cold and rejecting towards their children and are inconsistent in handling them, frequently using physical punishment, are more likely to have aggressive children who, in time, develop the bullying personality.

Gibb & Randall (1989) comment that children who have been handled by assertive parental management need intervention strategies that focus on anger management – particularly where the adult care-giver has portrayed anger. There is also a body of opinion that suggests that not only do these children get faulty signals but their normal development is inhibited and appropriate educational approaches will be required to stimulate age-appropriate development – socially and psychologically.

THE VICTIM PERSONALITY

The development of the victim personality is also centred on parenting of young children and is frequently the result of overprotection, overindulgence and social isolation of the child from the peer group. This results in a child who is totally dependent on others and cannot relate in an independent manner to peers – either in school or later on at work. The alternative cause of victim personality can be as the result of rejection – possibly because of the inability of the parents to see that a child who does not obviously respond to their parenting efforts does, nevertheless, need as much love as the affectionate child who is much easier to love.

Overprotection of children has been seen in several studies as restriction of children's behaviour so that there is less opportunity for social learning outside the home; children are encouraged to stay close to their parents and not allowed to explore novel environments or any type of 'risk-taking' behaviour away from the parent. Studying pre-school children, Hinde et al (1993) suggest that the child seeks the mother's protection frequently and that this dependency is reinforced by the mother's over-solicitous behaviour.

This results in older children in social withdrawal and can be traced back to parenting styles that set down many rules and constraints on children's psychological development, leading to reticent, timid children who cannot cope in settings where there is lack of structure, such as in school playgrounds. This may lead to facial expressions of unhappiness and a capacity to cry easily, making them the likely butt of jokes and thence bullying. Often these children, especially boys, are smaller and weaker than their peers and have a tendency to behave with passivity and submission. They are loners and often seek favour with the teacher in school to get what they want; this will alienate them from their peer group. As these children grow older they attempt to become more assertive but are easily outclassed by their more competent, assertive peers. As the situation continues so these children receive further rebuffs in their attempts to form relationships and in due course begin to think of themselves as worthless, with poor self-perception and low self-esteem. They become more socially withdrawn and depressed and may indeed almost seek out situations where they are bullied simply to get attention from their peer group. It is hardly surprising that this continues into adulthood, when their social ineptitude makes them the victim of bullying in the workplace or neighbourhood (Randall 1997).

It is not particularly easy to identify the symptoms of victim personality and on the whole research studies have resorted to scales for identification of mental disorders to isolate characteristic behaviour of insecurity, timidity, sensitivity, anxiety and cautiousness. Many children display behaviour that is indicative of shy, withdrawn children and yet do not necessarily become victims (Randall 1997). It may be necessary to observe the child over a period of time to see whether certain behaviours develop that appear to be out of character. For example, not wanting to go to school after regular attendance – often accompanied by aches and pains and vomiting; going to school by long routes if going on their own; having relationship problems with the peer group and appearing nervous and jumpy when with peers; or stealing from home in order to pay bullies.

VIOLENCE TOWARDS CHILDREN

That we live in a modern society does little to lessen the amount of violence perpetrated towards children. The rigidity of Victorian society allowed many sadistic and cruel acts towards children in the name of 'correctness', some of which have spilled over into recent times. Classical novelists, such as Charles Dickens, wrote of children being forced up hot chimneys in order to sweep soot. A catalogue of the types of physical, psychological and sociological violence towards children makes sickening reading. Critical analysis of situations surrounding violence towards children allows us to come to some understanding of situational causes. See Chapter 8 for further discussion on causes.

ILL TREATMENT BY MOTIVE AND DEGREE

Following the Laming Report (2003) into the death of Victoria Climbié, Southall et al (2003) proposed that it would be more useful to classify ill treatment of children by motive and degree rather than by the type of injury. They proposed four categories (Box 10.1).

Category A is the premeditated cruel abuse of children for gain; category B is the impulsive active ill treatment of children related to societal and personal pressures; category C is the universal mild hurts inherent in all parenting. Their classification is different from that presently used and based on the mode of ill treatment: physical, sexual and emotional. They defined 'neglect' as the unintentional failure to supply the needs of the child – differentiating it from what they call 'deprivational abuse', where withholding food, care or love is deliberate.

In the same article, Southall et al (2003) discuss certain abuser traits, for example, in category A abuse, child abusers are fully aware of their actions; they know they face retribution if detected. They establish plausible, elaborate explanations for their children's injuries to avoid detection, weaving faint strands of truth into a lattice of lies. In discussing the effect of this type of abuser on the health professional, Southall et al say:

> *Abusers are expert in manipulation. They 'turn on the charm' to entice professionals that show empathy with their fabrications into becoming supporters. When confronted they turn nasty, shout, and use drama to intimidate and isolate the professional who is suspicious. They create doubt and dissent within an overworked team to turn colleague against colleague. Professionals sometimes unwittingly accept lies to make their relationships with such abusers palatable.*
>
> (Southall 2003, p. 102)

In category B abusers, Southall et al (2003) argue that, characteristically, this occurs when parents are themselves under great pressure or depressed, having difficulties with relationships, and lacking family or other support. The actions are impulsive, thoughtless and selfish. The parent lashes out at his/her child when the child is demanding attention, crying or screaming. The act may cause very serious injury, and occasionally death, especially in infants or young children. This type of ill treatment is related to such emotional, social and economic pressures that the parent reaches 'breaking point'. The isolated, inexperienced or poorly educated parent is more likely to reach this stage before the established, supported family. However, most normal parents can behave in this way if sufficient pressures are applied.

In category C violence Southall et al (2003) suggest all loving and caring parents occasionally ill treat their children. Included are: (1) the 'reflex' smack of the badly behaved child; (2) the frustrated aggressive shout that stuns the child; (3) the derogatory remark that demeans hurtfully; and (4) conscious 'disciplinary' acts accepted by some societies as normal or necessary.

Box 10.1 Motivational violence

Four categories of motivational violence

A *Abuse*: premeditated ill treatment undertaken for gain by disturbed, dangerous and manipulative individuals

B *Active ill treatment*: impulsively undertaken because of socio-economic pressures, lack of education, resources, and support, or mental illness

C *Universal mild ill treatment*: behaviour undertaken by all normal caring parents in all societies

D *Neglect*: defined here as an unintentional failure to supply the child's needs

Southall et al (2003, p. 102)

BREAKDOWN IN SAFEGUARDING SYSTEMS

As stated in the foreword to the document *Keeping Children Safe* (2003), the Children Act 1989 is basically sound, but there are serious weaknesses in the way in which it is interpreted, resourced and implemented. Investigative reports carried out in the last decade, culminating in the report *Safeguarding Children* (DH/HO/DFEE 2002), have shown that there are a number of critical reasons why, despite attempts at improving systems for safeguarding children, children are still abused and die. Problems quoted are:

- Organizational
  - staff working to different standards
  - weak Area Child Protection committees
  - systems not focusing on the child's needs
  - managers taking insufficient responsibility for their staff working with children
  - poor assessment by social services staff as to whether a child is 'in need' or 'needs protection'
  - difficulty in recruiting and retaining skilled and qualified staff who are working with children
- Individual practitioner
  - inadequately trained to safeguard children, particularly if staff are not considered to be 'child protection specialists'
  - deficiencies in basic professional practice
  - poor managerial back-up
  - too much local guidance, often out of date
  - staff unsure about the sharing of information – how much and to whom.

Government responses to recent reports and inquiries have been swift and comprehensive, but nevertheless will take time to implement. Improving standards, organization, education and closer working between professionals from the varying backgrounds who deal with children are all seen to be essential and are currently being debated and implemented throughout the UK. The publication of a booklet for all staff, *What to Do if You're Worried a Child is being Abused* (Department of Health 2003e), is helpful in guiding practitioners towards safeguarding children. In particular, the issues of confidentiality and information sharing are raised and discussed.

DOMESTIC VIOLENCE

It is argued that all violence that is perpetrated in the home is domestic violence, be it heterosexual or same-sex, involving children or adolescents, elders, whites, black and minority ethnics or within so-called religious frameworks. However, because the causes are so wide ranging, distinctions will be made between the main types. In the UK violence between adults who are married or in a relatively stable relationship is usually considered by the media and the police to be domestic violence, and this may include same-sex as well as heterosexual clashes. Violence between an adult/adults and a child/children also takes place within the home but is usually called child abuse. Violence between children may occur within the home but also often takes place outside the home and is therefore is not considered to be domestic.

In April 1999 HM Inspector of Constabulary introduced the following definition for the purposes of reported incident:

> The term 'domestic violence' shall be understood to mean any violence between current or former partners in an intimate relationship, wherever and whenever the violence occurs. The violence may include physical, sexual, emotional or finance abuse.
>
> *(Home Office 2000)*

Culture, material circumstances such as bad housing and economic stresses, drug abuse, childhood relational experiences, sexual insecurities and jealousies, deep mistrust and suspicion, misogynist (woman-hating) attitudes and lack of communication are many of the frequent themes that arise from the histories of women involved in domestic violence. Eaton (1994) shows that the abuse of women in the home often takes the form of rape and that violent episodes are often precipitated by the woman becoming pregnant. This suggests that violent behaviour in private spaces is intricately interwoven with male subordination of women.

HOUSING AND DOMESTIC VIOLENCE

It is not suggested that housing problems are the cause of domestic violence, because relationship breakdowns occur before there are any concerns about future accommodation. Nevertheless, evidence is available that if the couple involved had some alternative accommodation to which they could resort, many failed relationships would not lead to violence. Reports abound (Amina Mama 1996) from the women concerned of the partner or cohabitant originally moving into a house where a single mother and her children were the tenants. As it is not housing policy to house single men, if the relationship becomes violent it often has to be the woman and her children who move out because the man refuses to go. Local authorities have a statutory obligation to house people with dependent children, but mothers and their children forced out of Local Authority accommodation have to join the long queues awaiting housing in hostels, reception centres and refuges.

The problems facing women who live secluded lives, as housewives or in more closed communities and who do not have a good command of English, are greater than those who have sought alternative accommodation. These women do not even know about refuges and have little idea from whom they can seek help. Many women from the Asian community do not live in Local Authority housing but with their in-laws or in private rented housing, often as tenants of an Asian landlord. Thus, if they do approach the local housing department they are put at the end of the queue and are possibly referred to a refuge. A 1982 study of women in hostels (Austerberry & Watson 1982) found that relationship breakdown and/or domestic violence was the biggest single cause of women's homelessness. In the case of Asian women without children they were in the desperate position of being unable to return to their families because of the shame brought to the family by their flight from violence – violence that their own families would not acknowledge (Amina Mama 1996).

In 1998 there were media reports (*The Independent*, 13th October) of young male Muslim vigilantes who had set up a business finding Muslim women who had fled from violence, often in arranged marriages, and had gone into hiding because they risked further violence if caught and returned either to their own families or to their husbands and in-laws. Many such women had been subjected to horrendous acts of violence and there were several reports of deaths in what can only be described as suspicious circumstances, reported as accidental, e.g. clothing catching fire or an unexplained fall.

Under the Housing Act 1996, people experiencing domestic violence are defined as homeless. Priority need for accommodation is given to those who are pregnant, have dependent children, are vulnerable or threatened with statutory responses to the abuse of women.

UK law in relation to the protection of women has been criticized by many groups as being slow to modernize; evidence shows that there is substantial room for improvement in the interpretation and enforcement of the law by the police, courts, lawyers and society in general. Historically, both the law and its enforcement have been imbued with patriarchal values that have asserted the necessity and desirability of women's subordination to men (Dobash & Dobash 1980, Edwards 1985).

The Home Office (1998, 1999, 2000) have issued a number of reports relating to domestic violence as a result of the reported incidents of rape, which had trebled during the 1990s decade (Box 10.2).

Box 10.2   Domestic violence in law

Domestic violence falls under several areas of the law

Under *civil law*, relevant legislation includes marital law, assault and trespass law and domestic violence acts; under *criminal law* there are crimes of assault and grievous bodily harm, manslaughter/culpable homicide and murder; *housing law* is relevant to the housing consequences of domestic violence; and, in relation to black women, *immigration law* is also relevant.

The Family Law Act (1996) has introduced two new orders:

- occupation orders, which concern the right to occupy the family home
- non-molestation orders, providing protection against violence and abuse.

The Protection from Harassment Act (1997) provides further protection from abuse through two new criminal offences:

- criminal harassment
- offences involving fear of violence.

It is not the role of health care professionals to offer women legal advice about domestic violence, but it is appropriate to refer them to agencies which can provide such help. The Department of Health (2000a) resource manual *Domestic Violence* gives excellent information on prevalence, health impacts, roles of professionals and multi-agency approaches to domestic violence, as well as details of all agencies and contacts to which victims can be referred.

VIOLENCE AS BULLYING

Modern pluralistic society with its competitiveness and tendency to violence either at the terrorist end of the continuum or the fiction of film Westerns, has raised awareness of different aspects of violence, from verbal abuse and aggression to physical assaults. Harassment at work, indifference to the physical requirements of vulnerable people, rejection within friendships or marriage all lead to the knowledge that these can be interpreted as violence or bullying. The definition of bullying can be seen as a mirror of the definition of aggression. Randall (1997) suggests that a definition of bullying is: 'the aggressive behaviour arising from the deliberate intent to cause physical or psychological distress to others' (p. 4). Randall goes on to consider various types of aggression, and particularly two: affective aggression, which is concerned with strong negative emotions, especially anger; and instrumental aggression, which is behaviour that can be very aggressive but does not have a strong emotional basis. Anger can be the cause of an emotional state that leads

to aggressive behaviour and the end result is the desire to hurt somebody, either physically or psychologically.

Instrumental aggression is also aimed at harming somebody but without necessarily feeling any emotion, anger or otherwise towards the victim. Instrumental aggression can simply be aimed at having power over someone, which is in effect the outcome of a bullying relationship.

Bullying carries with it the connotations of belonging only to childhood and being about teasing or taunting or sly physical attacks such as pinching or punching. However, in many instances there has only been one physical attack by the perpetrator on the victim and yet there is still a bullying relationship present. This is because fear of the bully has been instilled in the victim, which may be termed harassment if carried to extremes. The term 'harassment' is used far more in adult work and certainly has close similarities with the term 'bullying' used in children's work. Yet child bullies, if asked why they use violence against their victims, imply the need for power over their victim – power to make them cry, be subservient or gain material advantage such as pocket money or copying homework.

To establish fear in a victim gives power to the perpetrator and therefore, if a work boss harasses a member of staff and that member of staff fears the consequences if they do not comply, it is very closely akin to bullying and the two situations are coterminous (Randall 1997). This argument suggests that there are two real types of bullying situation that arise in the workplace: premeditated workplace aggression and harassment, which may or may not be sexual in origin. Premeditated workplace aggression often occurs in situations where the organization has small groups of people working on different projects under, for example, the control of a foreman in industry. Further examples could be: a small company of men under a sergeant or NCO in the army; a typing pool/office workers under a senior clerk in business circumstances; workers in service industries under a supervisor, or even nurses in a hospital ward under a senior staff nurse/ward sister. In all these situations and many others there are a variety of reasons why bullying takes place. Perhaps the perpetrator is a highly efficient and effective worker and to increase their effectiveness they have to drive their subordinates to support increased effort, and to do this they resort to bullying behaviour. At the alternative end of the continuum, the perpetrator may use bullying tactics because of their own disaffection about the working situation or have personal problems that result in anger that spills over into the work situation. Recent concerns in the UK have arisen over the stress that teachers experience, particularly in primary schools. As a result of this, there are more cases making the headlines involving senior teachers and junior staff members who are bullied to produce results that are beyond their tolerance or ability. Brady-Wilson (1991) discusses the concept of workplace trauma, in which the victim loses self-esteem and the right to security and contentment in the workplace and which, if persistent over a period of time, can grind down the victim to a state where they exhibit post-traumatic stress disorder.

Workplace aggression can be overt, but this is usually confined to situations where a small group of people are working in a close situation and the perpetrator gets other staff members to collude in his/her activities against the victim, or else the perpetrators are the entire small group of staff, who collectively bully the victim. It is probable that this macho-type of bullying is most prevalent in the armed forces against new recruits or in the prison system against new inmates. Most of the available research cited by Randall (1997) indicates that premeditated aggression is insidiously covert and that the perpetrator often relies on the victim remaining quiet from fear of being disbelieved by others. The circumstances can be many and varied and are usually long-term, e.g. constantly refusing requested changes to a holiday rota or allocating the most boring or dirty jobs to the victim. Preventing opportunities for promotion or constantly demanding increased work output are other examples, as are spreading rumours or gossiping about the victim.

Bullying need not always involve individuals but can be group against group, as in teenage gang warfare, small, highly penetrative groups against large populations, as in terrorism, neighbourhood against small group as with ethnic pockets in a wider population, or one particular family against a neighbourhood. Although these are very different examples they are all reasoned from similar perspectives of power and control.

Power can be pleasurable to the perpetrators and is commonly seen in neighbourhoods where small groups or gangs gain pleasure from harassing a section of the community. This pleasure can stem either from the feeling that the perpetrators have got their own back on the community, with which they are in dispute, or that they have now 'made their mark' on it. Control works on a similar basis but is more about control of resources or territory, e.g. refusing to let a family park outside its own house because the bully next door needs space for two cars (Owens & Ashcroft 1985).

VIOLENCE IN SAME-SEX RELATIONSHIPS

The major factor evident from commentaries on same-sex domestic violence, is that it is obviously premised on power and not gender. In heterosexual relationships it is fundamentally sexism that is at the root of abuse, whereas in homosexual incidents power would appear to be the root cause. Much of the evidence available (Renzetti & Miley 1996) shows that the nature of the abuse is similar: it includes physical, emotional, psychological and sexual abuse (rape).

Physical abuse appears to be the same as in heterosexual violence; it can be verbal as well as involving direct contact and can be serious enough to require medical attention. A number of studies of mysterious deaths show that there is often a sexual attack before the victim is killed, and this is common to both groups: heterosexual and homophobic.

Emotional and psychological abuse are again common to the two groups – threats to the partner's pets or children, constantly demeaning the victim, anger about the victim's friendships, manipulative lies in order to control finances. Renzetti & Miley (1996) suggest that a unique type of psychological abuse in gay or lesbian relationships is the threat of 'outing' to family, landlords, employers and others. As can be imagined, this serves to isolate the couple within the relationship to an even greater extent than women in an abusing heterosexual relationship.

Renzetti & Miley (1996) argue that, in heterosexual abuse, there is a pattern of an abusive incidents followed by a 'honeymoon period' and then another cycle of abuse to gain power or control. Similarly, in same-sex violence there is a recognizable pattern of a violent period followed by a period of calm. What is interesting is a comparable recognizable pattern of behaviour in both heterosexual and same-sex relationships, of victims moving away from one violent relationship only to fall into another. The difference is that in the same-sex repeated violent relationship the victim of one violent relationship may become the perpetrator in the next. This is one of the major reasons why support services are reluctant to support partners in violent lesbian or gay relationships – who is the victim and who the perpetrator? Indeed, if the identified abuser is counselled and supported it is not unknown for the former victim to become their abuser.

There are a number of reasons why same-sex victims stay in violent relationships, such as hope of changing the abuser, fear of reprisal, self-blame or continued love for the batterer. What is very evident is the isolation within which both partners live. To seek help would lead to revelation about the sexual orientation of the victim, very possibly resulting in job loss and exposure to family, friends and social circle.

Most of the work on same-sex violence has taken place in the USA and there has been little work on this topic published in the UK. Elliott (1996) analyses the reasons why it has taken so long to recognize same-sex domestic violence in women and has postulated several ideas. Firstly, she suggests that many battered women's refuge and service providers are themselves lesbians and that these women hide their own sexual orientation and refuse to recognize lesbian battering, although they suspect that it exists. Another reason is that, whatever their sexual orientation, women helpers have accepted the basic philosophy that patriarchy and sexism are responsible for all violence. Having adopted this philosophy it is relatively simple to ignore the issues of power and control that are the particular cause of same-sex violence and concentrate on sexist issues, in so doing, failing to recognize that lesbian violence exists. It is difficult to conceptualize women as batterers and men as victims in same-sex violence. Elliott (1996) also argues that the homosexual community itself perpetrates this illusion that the root cause of violence is sexist in order not to create any further situations that might incite hostility from the heterosexual community.

In the USA work is beginning with lesbian violence through the battered women's movement but there is little evidence of any attempt to follow suit in the UK. As for violence in relationships between gay men, the focus with the gay community appears to be on coping with AIDS and even if gay violence has been recognized there is little evidence of any interest in supporting either the victims or abusers – the attitude is that it is their own problem and they will have to resolve it.

In finding causal explanations for same-sex domestic violence, a study carried out by Farley in 1996 showed that all the men and women who were screened reported having been psychologically abused as children and a high percentage of both groups had also been physically and sexually abused as children. In addition about half of each group had been physically abused as adults and there was evidence of alcohol abuse in the family of origin of just under 50% in both men and women. This particular study also found that gay and lesbian batterers come from all segments of society and represent all ethnic and racial groups in all economic situations and from all educational and occupational backgrounds. Further work is necessary to confirm that the childhood abuse seen as the background of all the participants in the study, is reflected in other studies and also that a high incidence of substance abuse in the partners, cited as a cause in another study, is also significant.

Some work has been done to explore lesbianism in women of all racial and ethnic origins. These women are incredibly isolated by virtue of the sexism, racism and homophobia present both in society and the helping agencies. It has been suggested in the literature that abusive black women use the threats of breaking of trust and what society will think to force the victim to remain silent. However, racism and homophobia are the prevailing concerns of black lesbian couples and this is used as a weapon by the primary aggressor in a domestic violence situation, leading to the victim maintaining a protective attitude towards them (Kivel 1996).

To accept the evidence that violence in lesbian relationships is a possibility means that health visitors may be in a position to help women trapped in such a situation. Clearly, the help available ought to be the same as for women trapped in violent heterosexual relationships, but drawing on the evidence from the USA, there are attitude problems to be overcome by the helpers involved. There are probably two main ways in which health visitors can help black lesbians in violent relationships. The first is by allowing the victim to talk about the circumstances, encouraging them to see what is happening and helping them to recognize the root cause for the violence: power. It calls for the health visitor to be aware of their own feelings about same-sex violence and for honest personal reflection to identify any racism, sexism or homophobia within themselves. Secondly, the health visitor can become an advocate for the victim with the support services available for battered women in heterosexual relations. It calls for health visitors who are working with victims to encourage the community to talk about problems and recognize the meaning of healthy relationships – especially same-sex relationships – and generally to recognize that the tip of the iceberg is hardly to be seen at this time.

If it is difficult to identify and support lesbian victims of domestic violence it is even more difficult to work with gay victims of domestic violence. The main focus of concern among gay men has been the incidence of HIV and support has involved identifying and treating infection. However, evidence from the USA indicates that HIV concerns have been used as a weapon of control between gay partners – it is the control preventing a man from leaving his violent partner. Again, research in the USA (Renzetti & Miley 1996) suggests that a sizeable minority of gay and bisexual men have to contend with both HIV and partner abuse as part of their daily lives. It is important to realize that HIV itself is not a cause of physical abuse within the relationship but may well be the cause of psychological abuse, being used either to control the victim or to prevent him from leaving his violent partner.

Merrill's (1996) work shows that the 'control' identified above works in several ways; for example, both HIV-positive and HIV-negative men report that their HIV-infected partners will feign illness in order to convince them not to leave or to entice them back once they have left. Both often have low self-esteem and tend to blame themselves for their partner's violence. In addition, the attitudes of society in general towards gay men and people with AIDS, contributes towards their low self-esteem and reduces their psychological ability to escape from violent partners.

Letellier (1996) reports that there is a growing body of evidence about serious psychological problems experienced by HIV-negative men. They are prone to chronic anxiety, depression, sleep disorders, impaired concentration, feelings of shame, fear, helplessness and hopelessness – a list of problems not dissimilar to those experienced by victims of domestic violence. In addition, they suffer feelings of guilt for not having contracted the condition themselves or, alternatively, for having contracted the condition and survived when those they loved have died. As the feelings outlined above can be experienced by victims as well as the guilt of either not having contracted the disease or, alternatively, having left an abuser who is affected; it is not difficult to see the overwhelming emotional and psychological stresses that leave the victim in isolation.

For HIV-positive men there is a similar set of psychological problems, compounded by the knowledge that they have little hope of any new same-sex relationship because of their HIV status. Unless their anger at being HIV positive is such that they wish to take it out on the gay community and have no compunction about singles dating, many HIV-positive men have strong feelings of responsibility towards their community. They are thus prepared to stay in an abusive relationship rather than lose the security of being in a relationship, albeit one that sometimes is violent.

Letellier (1996) discusses the level of care that battered heterosexual women can expect from health care providers and suggests that these women need to be able to question health care workers about domestic abuse. In turn, they expect health care workers to respond to their questions in a caring and non-judgemental manner. Battered gay and bisexual men deserve the same level of care and Letellier suggests that the communication can go something like: 'Some of the men I work with are hurt by their male partners. Are you in a relationship with a man? Does he hurt you? Are you afraid of him?' or 'Many gay men are hurt by their partners. Did your boyfriend/lover hurt you?'

What is very important in this type of communication exchange is that the professional/ care worker concerned, is fully aware of their own values and attitudes to this type of situation and that they can cope with the responses that may come back from the abused person. Equally and on a similar level of importance is the knowledge that the professional worker can transmit to the abused person that they really care and understand.

As well as the type of communication between care worker and victim outlined above, there is also a need for exploration of feelings concerning HIV and AIDS within the victim themselves, and this includes separating out the two factors in the situation between abuser and victim, that of violence and the epidemic itself. Helping a victim to work through guilt about the situation requires considerable self-awareness on the part of the professional, and appropriate courses on HIV and AIDS are very useful for professionals intending to work with domestic violence in gay and lesbian communities.

HEALTH AND ABUSE IN THE CARE OF OLDER PEOPLE

Elder abuse and neglect as a phenomenon was first described in the UK in the mid 1970s but little acknowledgement and research work was apparent until 1989, when the Department of Health recognized elder abuse and neglect as a new field of social concern. Since then the learning curve for the professionals involved has been steep but this has not been reflected in the formal education systems, which still allocate insufficient curriculum time to do more than pay lip service to family violence or elder abuse. The bulk of curriculum time is still spent on child abuse/protection matters. Yet clearly there is a growing body of evidence illustrating the size of the problem, to the extent that it should now be recognized as a major public health issue (Eastman 1984, Bennett 1990, Biggs et al 1995).

Institutional abuse of older people has been described in history and was particularly seen in relation to practices within workhouses, none of which was ever challenged. Still today, a number of scandals reach the media, and only as recently as 1994 the Professional Misconduct Committee of the UKCC saw a rise in referrals, mostly cases of ill treatment of older people in private nursing homes. It is probably accurate to say that the number of cases of elder abuse within the family that reach the media are the merest fraction of those that occur. In the majority of cases the old person will never complain, from fear of losing their home and/or care. What is very interesting is the basis from which professionals view abuse: Bennett et al (1997) analyse the current approaches, showing that child abuse and elder abuse are seen as a medical problem whereas family violence is considered to be a social problem.

The organization Action on Elder Abuse (2000) analysed 1421 calls received during 2 years (1997–1999) by their confidential telephone help line, and the following factors emerged:

- Two-thirds of calls came from older people or their relatives.
- Most calls were about abuse in people's own homes but a quarter of calls referred

to abuse in hospitals, nursing and residential homes.

- Two-thirds of the calls reported psychological abuse, one-fifth each physical and financial abuse. One call in ten was about neglect and nearly 2 calls in 10 calls were about sexual abuse. Calls frequently reported more than one type of abuse going on at once.
- Three times as many calls reported women as being abused as men.
- Abuse appears to increase with age.
- Over a quarter of calls identified workers as the abuser.
- Very few family members who were the main carers were reported as abusing.
- In people's own homes they were most likely to be subjected to psychological and financial abuse by other family members, most commonly the children. Where spouses abused it was likely to be psychological or physical.
- Almost equal numbers of male and female family members were reported as abusing older people.
- In a care setting, abuse was most likely to be physical or neglect and to be perpetrated by a worker.
- The greatest number of calls reported care workers as the abuser. Nurses were the second largest group. In either case about half the perpetrators were men.

There are five main types of abuse:

1. Physical, e.g. hitting, slapping, burning, pushing, restraining or giving too much medication or the wrong medication.
2. Psychological, e.g. shouting, swearing, frightening, blaming, ignoring or humiliating a person.
3. Financial, e.g. illegal or unauthorized use of a person's property, money, pension book or other valuables.
4. Sexual, e.g. forcing a person to take part in any sexual activity without his or her consent; this can occur within any relationship.
5. Neglect, e.g. where a person is deprived of food, heat, clothing, comfort or essential medication
                    (Action on Elder Abuse, 1998).

ELDER ABUSE AS PART OF FAMILY VIOLENCE

Frude (1996) states that the family is the setting for a substantial proportion of the violence that occurs within society and suggests that family aggression is relatively common, because a good deal of anger is generated in family situations and there are relatively few inhibitions to prevent this anger from being expressed as physical aggression. He makes an interesting distinction between hostile and instrumental violence. Hostile violence is driven by anger and the principal motive is to hurt the victim. Instrumental violence is driven principally by a desire for 'gain' and is used merely as a means to an end. Thus instrumental violence may be used to maintain a dominant role or to teach a family member (usually a woman) a lesson.

Family life is governed by rules, which are often related to allocation of space, duties, responsibilities, household chores, money and other resources, and anger is often preceded by the judgement that someone has broken a rule. Anger over rule-breaking is not the only reason for family violence, because the fact that people have relatively few inhibitions in the home situation also plays a large part. Family members know each other's vulnerabilities and are therefore in a prime position to inflict maximum hurt, which can lead to self-blame and stigma, a lowering of self-esteem and a reduction in general coping skills. Other affects may be sleep disturbance, depression, a sense of isolation and despair and an increase in feelings of dependence. It is this latter aspect that may be a major factor in abuse of elders within the family and in many ways this reflects the situation regarding child abuse (Blakemore & Boneham 1994, Slater 1995).

Detection of elder abuse within families is difficult because elderly people do not live public lives and there is far less likelihood of contact with external agencies. In addition, there are few developmental parameters against which one can measure adult progress and thus there are problems in discerning the difference between frailty caused by age and/or illness and the effects of abuse.

Elder abuse is unlikely to arise suddenly as a new phenomenon within a family but is more likely to be a gradual deterioration of what has been a difficult relationship for many years, although it is possible that 'overload' due to other problems may suddenly change a relationship from difficult to abusive. Detection rates of elder abuse tend to be most effective in circumstances where there are other social factors such as poverty, unemployment and difficult social situations, and where they come to the attention of the authorities. Despite the previous comments, violence is not confined to families in lower social classes although rates of family violence appear to be highest in poorer urban families with high rates of unemployment (Bennett et al 1997).

OLDER PEOPLE IN RESIDENTIAL/NURSING CARE

Only 5% of the population aged 75–84 years enter residential care, although the figure rises to 21% for those aged 85 years and over (Department of Health 1996b). Yet despite these figures the view that institutional care is desirable for older people has been created and is perpetuated in society at large. This, however, is not the view of older people currently, whose view of institutional care is coloured by images of the workhouse – although none of them is old enough to have experienced the workhouse at first hand.

Discussion still revolves around the social and financial circumstances in which older people can gain access to private residential care or care in nursing homes. As a result of community care reforms and accompanying investigative reports (Wagner Report 1988, Griffiths Report 1988) it has become apparent that both institutionalized care and the provision of care for people living in their own homes are expensive and complex resource issues. There are also issues concerning regulation of homes. The Department of Health

(1996c) produced a White Paper about changing the requirement for residential and nursing homes to register with either the Health Authority (for nursing homes) or the Local Authority social services department (for residential homes) to registration with the Health Authority only. Some homes can remain registered with both bodies and arrangements are made to ensure that dual registration can be undergone with cooperation between both inspection bodies. Following the publication of *The National Service Framework for Older People* (Department of Health 2001b), under the Care Standards Act 2000, the government issued a set of national minimum standards for *Care Homes for Older People* (2001, 2002, 2003). These cover:

- age discrimination in relation to criteria for access to health and social care
- better administrative policies in relation to health and social care
- better services in relation to preventive measures in strokes and falls; better protocols relating to mental health care; and general improvements in prevention of illness and promotion of health and well-being.

In all of these standards there have been dates set for performance and outcome measures, mostly to be completed by 2005. While there is always criticism of measurement and the potential for manipulation of achievements, nevertheless many of the protocols identified have raised awareness of the need for standards amongst carers and users alike.

As with any type of institutional care, there is always the danger of neglect or abuse of inmates, but it would appear that, far from such occurrences becoming rarer, there is a steady recording of a wide range of episodes. Many of the instances of abuse take place within the context of a relationship in the institutional setting and such relationships may be between a staff member and an inmate, a volunteer and an inmate, two inmates or possibly an inmate and friends or relatives who are visiting. Such abuse can be physical, psychopathological, deliberate neglect, neglect through omission due to poor organization, lack of basic standards, erosion of individuality of care, physical restraint, drug-induced restraint, fraud or theft, or the taking of life. This catalogue of violence may be directed towards one inmate within the institution or all the inmates and may result from lack of staff training, serious staff shortages or poor management. This does not apply only to private homes but also to long-stay NHS hospitals, which are often regarded as the Cinderella of the hospital service, suffering from overcrowding, substandard furnishings, poor-quality limited-choice meals and little or no stimulation.

In the USA a number of research studies have assessed the predictors of physical abuse of older people in institutional care and found that staff burnout, patient aggression and conflict between staff and patients are the most significant predictors. Work done in the UK is further behind and limited, but there is evidence from the UKCC Professional Conduct Committee of a rise in the numbers of nurses appearing before the committee who work in the nursing home sector, and that these appearances are greater than any other area of practice (UKCC 1994b).

Ways to reduce abuse and neglect are rarely discussed openly and in fact there is evidence of the minimization of what is an endemic problem. Clearly, much can be done in terms of education and training both of qualified and unqualified staff and better supervisory processes will also help, as will support and training for stress handling and relief. There is a need to raise staff self-esteem and morale and this may be done as a result of better and more imaginative management, particularly when taking into consideration budgets and resource costs. It is also important to recognize the need for good quality control in both the NHS and the private sector, the latter requiring better inspection and registration, the former using clinical governance and well-implemented clinical supervision.

MEDICAL ISSUES IN OLDER PEOPLE

The percentage of the population now living to old age is rising and is a world problem. In Europe the highest proportions of older people are found in Scandinavia and the UK; on average in these countries 26% of the population are over the age of 65. In terms of the availability of medical care, older people in the UK feel marginalized and in the current market economy in health care are seen as expensive to treat. The emphasis on health care is still that we should enable frail older people to remain living in the community by successful management of their care needs in such settings. In reality, packages of care, which should be appropriate for each individual and planned before hospital discharge, tend to be care-manager determined from a financial perspective rather than a true needs-assessed package. Patient and carer have to carry on as best they can. If the situation deteriorates into an abusive one, the same realities prevent intervention and help.

Work undertaken in the USA by Jones (1990) suggested that there are a number of situations when an older person is seen in an A&E department and questions could be asked about possible abuse/neglect, for example:

- differing histories given by the patient and carer, either in explanation of injury or about its timing
- delays between injury/illness and seeking medical attention
- vague explanations for (for instance) a fracture
- frequent A&E department visits, often due to lack of medicines or their administration, despite a care plan and available resources
- a functionally impaired patient who arrives without the main carer present
- sub-therapeutic drug levels on laboratory findings despite carer-reported compliance.

Two major concerns that the literature identifies (Bennett et al 1997) are: lack of knowledge on the part of both the medical and nursing professions in how to recognize abuse; and ageist attitudes in such professionals, who assume that older people naturally have health deficits due to their age. Some fairly recent studies in the UK (Smith et al 1992) found that 5% of people attending A&E departments in Leicester who were 59 years and older, were victims of domestic abuse. The aspects of the identification of abuse suggest that protocols should be produced, using questions such as: 'The injuries you have are like bruises and lacerations people get when someone hits them. Did someone hit you? Are you afraid?' or 'Sometimes patients tell me they have been hurt by someone close to them. Could this be happening to you?' (Jezierski 1992, Snyder 1994). It is suggested that history-taking should be done independently with both patient and carer where there is any suspicion of an abusive situation and that particular attention should be paid to the possibility of both overt and covert physical and psychological signs of abuse.

PROTECTION OF ABUSED OLDER PEOPLE

One of the main issues in offering support to potentially abused older people is that they have every right to refuse protection and this can be frustrating for professionals concerned who feel rejected, particularly if they have worked for a long period with a person. Older people often have a fierce sense of self-determination and may well feel that the possibility of abuse or danger is less important than their independence. Professionals have to accept the decision even if they do not agree with it, provided there are no grounds for suspecting mental incompetence and thus an approach under the terms of the Mental Health Act 1983. However, this does not mean that older people should be left with no provision if they wish to change their minds, and professionals need to make very clear the ways in which the person can gain support and further assistance. Bennett et al (1997) make the important point that older people need to understand that abusive situations rarely consist of single acts and that as time goes on the abuse generally becomes more severe and more frequent. It is also important for the person to recognize that they are one of many older people who have experienced abusive situations and that many have managed to alter their circumstances and been able to live free from abuse and neglect.

Perceptions and attitudes in professionals who work with older people are a major factor in determining how best to intervene in potentially difficult situations. The education of professionals concerned needs to be wide ranging, covering reflection, self-awareness and self-knowledge as well as knowledge of systems and policies. Professionals working in these areas of practice should have developed the skills of reflection and should practise these regularly. It is also important to understand how we develop attitudes towards older people and what creates bias within cultures. Knowledge of abuse within families, particularly of a long-standing nature, is important, as is the need to recognize what might be construed as positive intervention as opposed to interference. The difference between positive intervention and interference is one of perception on both sides – professional and family/client – and it is important for professionals to understand how families or victims may feel and to recognize what might be construed as overprotective or paternalistic. Phillipson (1992) argues coherently for the professional to work with the client through a process of advocacy, enablement and empowerment, particularly when the client is marginalized.

The Department of Health and Social Services Inspectorate (1993) issued guidelines for the assessment of older people who are suspected of being victims of an abusive situation, and they strongly advocated a multidisciplinary approach individually adapted and carried out by experienced practitioners. It is necessary to take time and care in assessment, given that many older people are reluctant to discuss abuse or abusive situations.

Assessment needs to include:

- an in-depth history both of family dynamics and relationships and of the current situation
- an idea of the everyday functioning of the family or of the carer and abused
- the dependency of the abused and the stressors to the situation
- the views, beliefs and attitudes of the key players
- the ways in which the abused person has so far coped with the situation.

The Department of Health stresses the importance of assessing the needs of the individuals concerned rather than needs for service provision. It may be necessary to use a needs-led assessment, but ensure that it is abuse focused.

An aspect of protection that often causes health visitors great concern is that it can be seen as paternalistic and disempowering, but it has to be remembered that older people belong to a different generation from their carers and are often more receptive to the notion of compliance and acceptance. These attitudes themselves often create vulnerability in older people and thus protective services are necessary. In some instances, older people are not totally dependent and with appropriate support may become empowered enough to be able to avoid risk situations and, recognizing the precedent factors, may be able to take avoiding action.

A holistic approach to potentially abusing situations means that a range of intervention strategies matching the differing causes of abuse is necessary. These will extend from education and counselling to speedy access to emergency services, from safe havens for the abused older person to alternative accommodation for the abuser who cannot get out of the situation. The provision of a practical service such as a lifting aid may be as helpful, as may provision of carer relief through a sitting service. Bennett et al (1997) cite the work of Gelles (1983) in considering the value of a social exchange as a trade-off from an alteration in the abusive situation. It may mean, in a sense, that it would be more profitable for an abuser to accept a 'reward' than to continue in the abuser role. Likewise, it may be more profitable for the abused elder to adopt a less vulnerable subservient attitude and thus 'gain' from the acceptance of an alteration in the situation.

Practical support as an effective intervention can be material, for example the provision of finance or equipment such as a continence service or a laundry facility, respite care in an alternative situation for both the older person and their carer, or a sitting service; finally, therapeutic interventions such as stress reduction techniques or anger management programmes.

Therapeutic interventions require an education approach and the opportunity to see an endpoint, otherwise they may well be considered of little value. They may include the understanding of the difference between protection and personal liberty and how to introduce these. Other education approaches include advice and information on a wide range of issues, which may include medical information about health maintenance, illness, housing or financial benefit advice, or ways in which the employment of the carer can be maintained. Another major benefit can be gained from multi-agency support and this in itself is fraught with difficulty where there is no key worker who can act as coordinator to ensure a smooth service.

Violence towards older people from people outside the home is still relatively rare. However, there are regular reports in the press of older people being subjected to violence during a burglary. Much of this violence would appear to be spontaneous and greater force is often used, sometimes resulting in death, either directly or as a result of the accompanying shock leading to a stroke or heart attack. Health visitors can assist in prevention of such incidents by raising awareness of the importance of not displaying signs of affluence, encouraging neighbourhood support, mounting anti-crime campaigns, or attempting to reduce the social isolation of older people.

The preceding sections have covered the theories of violence. The next section turns to practical aspects of working with potentially violent clients.

PROFESSIONAL SKILLS FOR WORKING WITH VICTIMS OR POTENTIALLY VIOLENT CLIENTS

Always ensure that you record and report all aspects of potential or violent situations.

WORKING WITH VICTIMS

As the professional making contact with identified victims of (domestic) violence it is likely that the health visitor may be visiting the client in a refuge or hostel. In these situations the skills required will particularly focus on empathetic listening. Victims of domestic violence who have been brought outside the situation are often confused as to why they have allowed the situation to occur, and angry with themselves for being seen in their current situation and possibly for having lost their home. Their self-esteem is lowered and they may be clinically depressed. Continued listening by the health visitor and encouragement to plan for the next step forward can be of immense support to women. There are also children to be concerned about, immediate care, future housing and future schooling/nursery care.

The broad approach to working with a victim of violence is not dissimilar to general health visiting communication strategies in most situations (Box 10.3).

The health visitor who might be going into the home where suspected violence has occurred must be particularly mindful of their own safety. It is of paramount importance that someone at the work base knows when a health visitor is going into a doubtful domestic situation. The time of a visit should be known; when the visit is completed the contact at base office must be informed of the completion of the visit, and the departure from the clients home address must

be notified. Where there is particular concern about a potentially violent situation, the health visitor working with the client must take a colleague with them. It is probably wise for the colleague to remain outside in the car and the length of the visit to be agreed between health visitor and colleague. There is research evidence to show that if two health visitors go into a potentially violent situation the weight of numbers may exacerbate aggressive responses from the partner of the victim, should they be present. The alternative is for the health visitor to arrange the visit and indicate from the outset that he or

---

Box 10.3   Communication strategy

1. Allow the person space and time:
   'Tell me how it happened'
2. Show concern and understanding:
   'I can see that you are very upset'
3. Communicate clearly:
   'I want to make sure that I've understood this properly'
4. Convey your desire to reduce stress:
   'I'm sure that something can be sorted out'
5. Avoid escalating by confrontation:
   'I think your partner is right and you are wrong'
6. Avoid provocative phrases:
   'I can tell you, I have known other people to have worse problems'
7. Be ruthless with the issue, gracious with people:
   'Although this cannot be changed at the moment you are coping well'

Davies & Frude (1995)

Box 10.4   Possible options in potentially dangerous situations

Play for time ... *don't insist on maintaining your authority, don't be afraid to lose face. Promise anything – 'I'll make sure that by the end of the week you will have the house you want.' The moral obligation does not exist in a violent situation.*

Keep talking ... *try to ask relevant questions which put you back in control: 'Has she gone missing before?'*

Try diversionary tactics:

- Humour ... *'And I thought this was going to be a boring day'*
- Distracting activity ... *'Why don't we have a break? Let's have a cup of coffee'*
- Feign distraction ... *Put your hand up, be still, looking puzzled – 'I'm sorry, I thought I heard someone shouting'*
- Keep your distance ... *It is suggested that aggressive people often have body buffer zones that are bigger than those of other people*
- Stay controlled and concerned ... *'I wish you would stop pacing around like that, it's really worrying me.'*

Locate and move towards the escape exit (covertly)

Tell the person to put any weapon down – repeatedly if necessary ... *'Put the ashtray down ... put it down over there ... '* etc.

Davies & Frude (1995)

she will be bringing a colleague along as well. Do ensure that you park your car in a position where you can make an immediate get-away, e.g. not facing the wrong way in a cul-de-sac.

There are times, although rare, when someone's behaviour really gets out of hand. Attempts at calming the situation will not have worked and it is necessary to escape or raise the alarm or seek help. If it is possible, just leave if you can, telling the person it would be better to resume another time. However, good manners are secondary to safety.

If your exit is blocked then the situation has become more dangerous but there are still a number of options that you can use (Box 10.4). The scenario suggestions in Box 10.4 are taken from a course on dealing with anger and aggression at work and do not represent the whole course. However, all professionals who are visiting people at home should be aware that they are in a possibly dangerous situation if they are working with clients who are linked with violence. The prepared professional is the one who has thought through possibly dangerous situations and who has developed strategies for ensuring minimum risk. The more prepared we are, the less likely we need to use the above strategies.

Again, at the risk of endlessly repeating it: immediate and contemporaneous recording of situations that could escalate into violence is essential, as is ensuring that line managers are fully aware of the situation.

CONCLUSION

Health visitors are increasingly becoming aware of the need to increase their knowledge of many aspects of violence. James-Hanman of the Greater London Domestic Violence Project, in a conference paper in 1998, accused the NHS of being very slow to respond to violence, in particular domestic violence. She particularly commented that the NHS was accident-focused rather than injury-focused, deals with consequences rather than causes, and that staff do not know of practical solutions to situations. Other factors that James-Hanman highlighted are lack of education and training, embarrassment about asking direct questions and concerns about upsetting relationships.

This chapter has tried to cover the range of violent issues that health visitors may be exposed to, often as a consequence of a home or clinic intervention or other reasons, e.g. a child health surveillance visit. Asking direct questions should not necessarily be seen as leading to intervention, but the opportunity for a victim to talk to an outsider may be more helpful than any formal response. If health visitors feel secure that they have sufficient knowledge about violence to be able to listen to victims without experiencing an overwhelming sense of powerlessness, then their response to victims is often more measured and empathetic, giving the victim a feeling of support. Health visitors should also recognize that they can be very effective in maintaining family dynamics and helping families to understand themselves, especially along the lines of the circumplex model of Olson et al (1979), providing families with insight into their own evolution.

The skills of intervention that may be appropriate have also been touched on, although it is worthwhile considering attending a course on aggression if you are particularly concerned about your own handling skills.

Chapter **11**

Reflective practice

Anne Robotham and Doreen Sheldrake

INTRODUCTION

Health visitor education has for many years taught its new practitioners to evaluate their work during debriefing sessions. At different stages of the educational process, students are encouraged by the practice teacher to describe what they have done with the client and relate it to their current knowledge. The debriefing sessions allow the community practice teacher to explore with the student the content of their intervention work with the client, the relationship between the work done and their present state of knowledge, and finally their own feelings about the experience. These feelings include an assessment of the purpose and outcomes of the intervention, all aspects of communication with the client and an analysis of the student's values and behaviour in relation to the client contact. These debriefing sessions between community practice teacher and student begin as regular, frequent meetings on an ongoing basis, initially between visits/contacts in clinic, but as time goes on, their structure changes from description to critical analysis and evaluation.

This chapter is designed to follow the process of education of a student health visitor, including theory of practice, reflective practice, knowledge, critical analysis, conceptual frameworks and mapping, and finally creative thinking.

To begin any process of evaluation or reflection one must initially consider what health visiting is, its principles and what its practice consists of.

THE PRINCIPLES OF HEALTH VISITING

Health visitor skills are founded on four principles of practice that have stood the test of time since their definition by the CETHV in 1974. They were adopted by the UKCC for post-registration education and were quoted in *Making it Happen* (SNMAC 1995) in relation to child health promotion, good parenting and family health visiting. The SNMAC believes that the skills that health visitors apply to their practice equips them to assess the health needs of communities. NMC (2003a) have further underlined the importance of the principles of health visiting by using them as the basis for the framework for registration for the third part of the Register as a specialist community public health nurse.

The principles of health visiting, which were re-examined in 1977 and 1992, have remained unchanged and are:

- the search for health needs
- stimulation of an awareness of health needs
- influencing policies affecting health
- facilitation of health-enhancing activities.

These principles will each be examined in detail.

THE SEARCH FOR HEALTH NEEDS

In a re-examination of the principles of health visiting (Twinn & Cowley 1992) there is a discussion of the interpretation of the words 'search' and 'needs'. At that time it was felt that the words should be left unchanged but many health visitors have expressed concern that 'search' implies that this is not the basis for their work in health needs. Search can be based only on what is overt; however, health visitors use all their senses to assist them to identify and explore what is actually worrying the client. Thus, where the needs are not obvious to either client or health visitor, the process of discussion and enabling the client to draw out their beliefs and values creates a partnership in which client and professional both search for covert health needs. If covert health needs are uncovered the client may be enabled to understand their significance on both an individual and a family basis.

Health visitors use advanced skills of listening and empathy to practise in partnership with individual clients and community groups during this searching process. A model may be the tool outlined by Carnwell in Chapter 3, identifying stressors using Neuman's (1989) systems model.

It is important in the planning of health visiting practice to consider whether health visiting focuses on targeted intervention or maintains a generalist approach. If the organization of health visiting is based on targeted intervention where there are known areas of vulnerability, then the importance of this principle is lost. In other words, generalist health visiting practice allows for every opportunity to search for health needs, whereas targeted practice is based on overt health needs.

Health visitors use both qualitative and quantitative research methods to collect epidemiological data to establish community health needs, as discussed in Chapter 2, but the uniqueness of the work that health visitors undertake with individuals realizes the richness of the methodology in establishing health needs.

Continued health visiting practice in relation to the principle of searching for health needs means that health visitors should take every opportunity to keep Primary Care Trusts informed of health needs that are uncovered.

STIMULATION OF AN AWARENESS OF HEALTH NEEDS

Past NHS planning did not allow for those health needs associated with demographic changes, specific life-situations (such as poverty, homelessness and unemployment) and ethnicity to be readily identified and included in the business plans and subsequent service provision. This emphasizes the importance of alerting people to health needs and any potential help that may be available. The stimulation of awareness of health needs by health visitors encompasses three different levels of action: clients (individuals and communities), health service managers (commissioning authorities and provider units) and politicians and policy-makers at a national level (Twinn & Cowley 1992).

From a superficial point of view there would seem to be little difference between searching for health needs and stimulating awareness of health needs and yet health visiting has always differentiated between these two terms. Stimulation of awareness of health needs is at the heart of why, in many ways, the medical model/approach to health care is only semi-successful. This is because it fails to do more than acknowledge health needs resulting from social inequalities, need and deprivation. The only way in which the medical model approach will ever be entirely successful is if social needs are not only acknowledged but also acted upon. The Labour Government, in its two documents *A New NHS* (Department of Health 1997a) and *Our Healthier Nation* (Department of Health 1998b), has grasped the nettle in accepting that for health care to succeed there are social factors that must be dealt with. This is where health visiting has always striven to play a part – in raising awareness of inequality; badgering agencies on behalf of the disadvantaged; encouraging and empowering individuals and communities to demand equal opportunities for health care. It is to be hoped that the new Primary Care Trusts will be more focused on redressing social inequality issues, and, with their fundamental skills, health visitors will continue to stimulate the awareness of primary care groups of such inequalities.

INFLUENCING POLICIES AFFECTING HEALTH

In *Making it Happen* the SNMAC committee (1995) made the following statement: 'SNMAC believes that the skills that health visitors apply to their practice equips them to assess the health needs of communities, and that this should be built upon for locality-based health need assessment and primary care purchasing' (p. 16). Since the adoption of the 'New NHS' this has become an even more important statement in relation to influencing policies affecting health. As discussed in Chapter 2, health needs assessment is an integral part of public health delivery and the current movement towards Primary Care Trusts as the hub of public health means that health visitors, through their membership of them, are in an even stronger position to influence policies affecting health.

Health visitors have consistently and persistently used their professional bodies to lobby Members of Parliament, local government officials and, indirectly, from time to time, the public through press releases and other statements. An example of a press release has been criticism by health visitors of prominent advertising of artificial infant formula milks, to the detriment of breast-feeding. A further example is the strong support voiced by health visitors of stop-smacking campaigns – *End Physical Punishment of Children* (EPOCH, Cook et al 1991).

Health visitors are natural cross-boundary workers with experience in networking across health care and other statutory and voluntary sectors, thus enabling them to influence other agencies and professional groups in relation to health care needs and provisions. Health visiting provides a voice for women and their concerns and, as a predominantly woman-based profession, is instrumental in highlighting the real concerns of women.

Health visitors practise in managed primary health care teams and are responsible for developing teamwork and responding to the policies of the Health Authority/Primary Care Trust. They are thus in a position to promote innovative practice development in response to general practice and primary health care needs. The marketing process (de la Cuesta 1994) can be used to develop a relationship with the purchaser/GP in order to agree a service package. This should be based on outcome measures specific to the requirements of the Children Act 1989, *Caring for People* (Department of Health 1989c), *The Patient's Charter* (Department of Health 1991) and *Our Healthier Nation* (Department of Health 1998b).

THE FACILITATION OF HEALTH-ENHANCING ACTIVITIES

More than ever before, this health visiting principle is central to the concept of public health. Personal confidence and self-esteem are crucial to individual client development and in many instances are developed through group settings.

Health visitor stimulation of lay and community groups can improve health facilities in an area and also lead to safety and environmental campaigns.

The promotion of health is central and pivotal to all the principles of health visiting practice, particularly when it is associated with primary prevention and with creating structural or community change.

The specialist health promotion roles of health visitors in general practice may involve health-enhancing activities for individuals or in response to a specific need, such as stress or anxiety management. It might mean targeting wider groups across GP practice boundaries, e.g. a mobile clinic site for travellers or a monthly health market stall (Twinn & Cowley 1992). It could also mean campaigning for resources to help people to live more healthily – safer roads, better housing, more realistic levels of income support.

Our Healthier Nation (Department of Health 1998b) makes the point that previous health strategy – *The Health of the Nation* (Department of Health 1992b) – was limited because of its reluctance to acknowledge the social, economic and environmental causes of ill health. The redefined targets in relation to heart disease and stroke, accidents, cancer and mental health each have an attached national contract. Within these there is very clear scope for health visitors to introduce health-enhancing activities and empower the public to take these up or introduce new ones themselves.

HEALTH VISITING PRACTICE

The purpose of health visiting (DH 2001e) is to improve health and social well-being through identifying health needs, raising awareness of health and social well-being, influencing the broader context which affects health and social well-being, and enabling people to improve their own health. This is achieved through the health visiting contribution to public health which takes account of the different dynamics and needs of individuals, families and groups, and the community as a whole.

Robinson (1982), in a masterly work on the evaluation of health visiting, struggled with the idea that health visiting contains a body of knowledge upon which practice is built, and over the past 18 years there have been many attempts to evaluate health visiting practice (Luker 1982, Robinson 1982, Dobby 1986, Twinn 1989, Cowley 1991, Chalmers 1992). Despite these and other careful analyses, there has been no clear articulation of the body of knowledge unique to health visiting. Robinson (1982) and Twinn (1991) consider that health visiting practice is both a science and an art. Goodwin (1988) suggests that health visiting, as a science alone without the art, becomes mechanistic, routine and even mindless, with the measurable product being a numerical list of contacts. It could be argued that skills and knowledge are fundamentally entwined in the philosophy of health visiting and that to disentangle these within the individuality of practice will reveal both the science and artistry that Robinson (1982) and Twinn (1989) discuss.

The opening statement in this chapter recognizes the practice teacher as pivotal in teaching health visiting practice. In the very title 'practice teacher' lies an assumption that there is a definable type of work in professional life that is called practice and means just that – practice of an art or science. Jarvis (1992) suggests a theory of practice, and that to understand professional practice it is necessary to understand health visiting action with which to underpin the theory. He draws on the work of Schutz (1972) to posit an idea of meaningful social action that he argues is an adequate description of professional practice. However, many professional practitioners would challenge the notion that practice is all action, and Jarvis accepts this point and suggests that within professional practice there is also non-action.

On the basis of this it might now be appropriate to identify categories of action as part of practice (Table 11.1).

ACTION IN PRACTICE

In identifying categories of *non-action* it is important to recognize their value in eliciting what

Table 11.1   A theoretical analysis of conscious action (Jarvis 1992)

Category of action	Level of consciousness		
	Planning	Monitoring	Retrospecting
Non–action			
Anomic	None	None	High
Prohibited	Low–high	None	None–high
Non–response	None–high	None	None–high
Action			
Experimental	High	High	High
Repetitive	High–none	High–low	High–none
Presumptive	None–low	None–low	None
Ritualistic	None	None–low	None–high
Alienating	None	None–low	None–high

has occurred (or not) in practice – i.e. what was considered by the practitioner but rejected because intuitively it was felt that alternative actions would be more appropriate in the circumstances. It is recognized that all activities ought to be client-led. However, there are many situations where the health visitor suggests a variety of options, one of which the client selects. Within these options are categories of action and, if considered, they reach the level of conscious planning by both client and health visitor. It still means that there may be unexpressed options that fall into the *anomic* (no name) category with its attendant consciousness level.

For example, in a moment of desperation the client may fleetingly consider suicide. It is neither expressed to the health visitor nor, indeed, seriously planned by the client. It thus becomes an *anomic* action because the health visitor, reflecting on the situation, has the sensitivity and perception to recognize that it could have been an option. In other words, at the time, the health visitor and client did not plan or monitor the option but retrospection suggested the possibility. Each health visiting situation is unique, with attendant unique categories of non-action.

It is necessary to consider levels of consciousness because it is only on the basis of their recognition that reflection can take place. Thus reflection must encompass the ability to articulate consciousness levels – was something planned, was it monitored by the practitioner (or client), was retrospective thought given to the process within the situation?

The premise that there is an art and a science to health visiting was mentioned earlier. Using analysis of categories of action enables the reflective practitioner to recognize that one can only measure action, not *non-action*. Thus *non-action*, which is an essential part of health visiting practice through its consideration and rejection by practitioner and client, becomes part of the art of health visiting because the nature of science is that it is measurable. Continuing with this theme, the measurement of the scientific aspect is, in effect, the measurement of tasks undertaken because the categories of action are all based on visible planning with clearly identified outcomes.

The two other categories of non-action identified in Table 11.1 can be treated similarly. For example, a health visitor who is a community practice teacher is running late for a planned appointment with a client. She drives over the speed limit and arrives at the venue reasonably promptly. A later debriefing session with her student focuses on time management. The health visitor uses as an analogy the difficulty of keeping to planned visits and realizes that in reaching her earlier appointment on time she has used a *prohibited* category of action. To help the student to understand the process they consider together whether consciousness levels are part of this category of action. Together they consider whether driving within the law is part of health visiting practice. They also consider whether breaking the law was conscious or unconscious – simply being so focused on the management of her work that an unconscious action occurred. In the normal course of events the community practice teacher would not have given this another thought, but in searching for an example to illustrate levels of consciousness to the student she has selected this example and thus there was a retrospective level of consciousness.

Non-response is, for example, when people involved in situations do know how to respond but choose not to at that time. A health visitor is passing through the GP surgery waiting-room when she sees a client at reception whom she knows is coming to her with a difficult problem. She decides not to approach the client in anticipation and to wait until the receptionist rings through to say that the client is waiting to see her. She selects this non-action in the knowledge (high-planning level) that she can check her records in order to prepare herself for the intervention.

Turning to categories of action, it is useful to be able to discuss them all, finding examples in practice to enable the student to recognize that level of consciousness is essential to the reflective process.

Experimental action is seen as being creative, new actions being worked out in the process of health visiting practice. This typifies health visiting because each intervention is practised within a new contextual situation and, for practice to be relevant, previously tried methods will have to be modified (experimented with) to satisfy the new situation. For this process to be effective a high level of consciousness is required at all stages. This could be interpreted as the artistry within experimental action.

Repetitive action can be either highly conscious, as in Table 11.1, or involve limited levels of consciousness. Highly conscious repetitive actions in health visiting include the constant repetition of feeding or weaning advice, e.g. in the well baby clinic, articulated to suit each individual client. Poor practice would be to repeat the same advice irrespective of client individuality; good practice means that the entire

communication is consciously underpinned by being tailored to the client taking into account cultural issues and anti-discriminatory practice.

Presumptive action has little place in sensitive and perceptive health visiting. There are few, if any, instances when a health visitor would programme an action with the client without a detailed communication process to ascertain its appropriateness to their needs. All communicative action is therefore assumed to have a higher level of consciousness than that identified with presumptive action.

Ritualistic action has been seen as the bedrock of past traditional health visiting practice – 'we do it this way because we have always done it this way'. The importance of research-based practice carried out in a challenging and questioning atmosphere is to eradicate all ritualistic practice. Again, the low levels of consciousness required are inappropriate except in retrospection, which is the hub of reflection. Reflection, therefore, is the safeguard against ritualistic practice.

Finally, *alienating action* mitigates against any meaningful further work with the client. As discussed in Chapter 4, effective initial entry work by health visitors will ensure the continuation of planned programmes of activity.

It is also useful here to discuss the dangers to practice of:

- experiment without safeguards or experience
- repetition without consciousness
- presumption without communication and checking-out
- ritual without conscious thought – habitual practice may be dangerous practice
- alienating, which will prevent client participation and empowerment.

Discussion of action moves the process of reflection through learning from action.

LEARNING FROM ACTION

Retrospection (Table 11.1) can be seen as the precursor to reflection, which is most likely to occur when retrospection indicates that the action has not produced the expected outcome, e.g. when the probability factor has been greater than was anticipated. Learning occurs during the process of translating retrospection to reflection. Dictionary definitions (*Penguin English Dictionary*) identify the process:

- *retrospect*: to look back
- *retrospection*: act of looking back on past experience
- *reflection*: act of reflecting, thoughtful consideration, meditation.

Thus, moving from retrospection to reflection must include learning from the experience, and to learn from experience there must be an analysis of that experience from which to learn. Learning from practice is experience and therefore becomes experiential learning.

Argyris & Schön (1974) conducted a number of studies across a variety of professional groups to develop a theory of competent interpersonal practice and explain how individuals learn in practice situations. They concluded that there are theories of action, including values, strategies and underlying assumptions, that form individuals' patterns of personal behaviour in professional practice. Argyris & Schön identified two levels of theories in action: espoused theory and theory-in-use.

They suggested that espoused theory is what an individual, when questioned, says he or she would do, and theory-in-use is what the individual, when observed in practice, actually does. Argyris (1982) later challenged this by showing the incongruity between espoused theory and theory-in-use and suggested that espoused theories may be seen as a representation of the accepted norms of a profession and theories-in-use the practitioner's intuitive response to the particulars of a given situation, which are difficult to describe but can be observed in the practitioner's behaviour.

Twinn (1991) used Schön's (1983) work to argue that intuition and artistry are complex aspects of professional practice but are nevertheless fundamental to the process of professional judgement, which is essential to effective action in professional practice and can only be learned from experience.

An example of Schön's (1983) reflection in action could be as follows: a student plans to do a new birth visit with a list of objectives in line with Trust policy. When she arrives, however, the mother is in tears and so she reflects in action and actively listens to the mother's worries. She later reflects with her practice teacher, who confirms that user-centred care is in line with current government directives (*Liberating the Talents*, Department of Health 2002b), and in addition the student action will have helped to build a trusting relationship.

Jarvis's earlier work (Jarvis 1987) demonstrated how reflective skills and reflective knowledge stem from disjuncture, i.e. questioning why the outcome has occurred, particularly if something has gone wrong. From this premise he formed a typology of learning (Table 11.2).

Each of the reflective forms of learning can have two possible outcomes: conformity or change. Scrutiny of Table 11.2 in relation to health visiting suggests that there is a similar process in non-learning to the non-action in Table 11.1 and that therefore the same analysis is appropriate.

Non-reflective learning belongs to the early days of student health visiting practice where the knowledge level is insufficient to work without pre-conscious skills of briefing, prior to an intervention, as the result of the preparation between community practice teacher and student. This is part of the early shadowing process essential to building experiential knowledge. Thus, during debriefing sessions in these early days, the community practice teacher and student identify the action/non-action processes

Table 11.2 A typology of learning (Jarvis 1992)

Category of learning	Type of learning
Non-learning	Presumption
	Non-consideration
	Rejection
Non-reflective learning	Preconscious skills
	Memorization
Reflective learning	Contemplation
	Reflective skills
	Experimental knowledge

is the learning/non-learning processes flow. Moving through the *non-reflective* learning aspect of Table 11.2 enables student *reflective learning* and making sense of situations as they evolve.

Boyd & Fales (1983), considering the link between knowledge and learning, examined learning from experience and argued that research on learning from experience tended to focus on the outcomes of such learning, rather than the process. They contended that experiential learning must be conceptualized as a process and that most of this type of learning goes on without the benefit of a structured learning environment, much of it is unintentional and some of it is even unconscious. The main advantage of the teacher/practitioner–student relationship is that the environment is structured to a greater or lesser extent, and for this reason the student may learn more quickly from experiential learning – particularly when there is active reflection through the debriefing process. This process requires the use of a reflective journal (see p. 278).

TEACHING LEARNING BY INTERPRETING REFLECTION

To facilitate the preceding discussion, it is recommended that the student uses the model illustrated in Figure 11.1 during shadowing, for reflecting with the community practice teacher. With the client's permission the student records the visit in the journal, including as many aspects of the cycle as possible. The journal entry for this visit is discussed using Socratic dialogue. The community practice teacher adds further comment, using his or her professional knowledge and judgement, to explore all aspects of the visit from the perspective of all the participants concerned, using the Gibbs categories outlined in the cycle. This process is time consuming but the community practice teacher who makes time in the early days will find that this is compensated for by the speed with which the student absorbs experiential learning. Empirical evidence (Sheldrake et al 1998) shows that students move far more quickly through the stages of

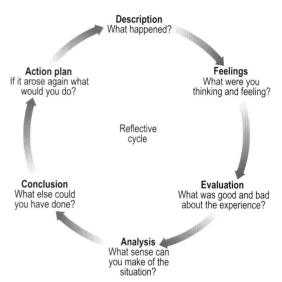

Figure 11.1 The reflective cycle (redrawn from Gibbs 1988)

novice to advanced beginner and hence to competence, as suggested by Benner (1984), by using this method.

Reflective learning is the *process* of learning and makes the difference between whether a person repeats the same experience several times, becoming highly proficient at one behaviour, or learns from experience in such a way that he or she is cognitively or affectively changed. To explore the process of learning how to reflect, Boyd & Fales (1983) used qualified counsellors who were accepted by their peers as 'reflective persons'. In repeated interviews with nine counsellors, Boyd & Fales showed a progression of focus-shifts within the activity of reflecting on the process of reflection and these are represented in Figure 11.2.

To examine this figure briefly:

- *Stage 1.* Defining reflection means initially exploring its parameters. The greatest difficulty is pinning down what we mean by reflection: What is it? What is it not?

- *Stage 2.* proceeds in the light of Stage 1: one is now more conscious of reflecting even if not sure what it is. A suggestion is that it is self-revealing, i.e. that really it is all about ourselves and our response to a situation.

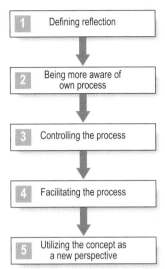

1   Defining reflection

2   Being more aware of
     own process

3   Controlling the process

4   Facilitating the process

5   Utilizing the concept as
     a new perspective

Figure 11.2   Towards a progression of reflection
(redrawn with kind permission from Boyd & Fales 1983)

- *Stage 3.* Boyd & Fales's group found that with this emphasis on reflection they were actively able to control decision-making – the reflective process enabled them to speed up active thinking. They did, however, feel the need to control the process and, if they were stuck, to stop going round in circles. Interestingly, the counsellors felt that at times the focus on reflection was unwelcome and they had to learn how to turn it off – to distract themselves.

- *Stage 4.* created some excitement in the counsellors as they allowed clients/students to become more aware of what they do and let them come to their own conclusions.

- *Stage 5.* The study group found they had used reflecting as a concept to enhance existing knowledge and understanding.

As a result of this initial study with their group, Boyd & Fales were able to construct a set of components of the process of reflection based on an analysis of 'self' (Table 11.3). Clearly, this is based on a counselling process, and the teaching of health visiting practice is similar because the demands of counselling mirror the demands of the unique health visiting context. In teaching the practice of health

visiting it is impossible to divorce the influence of self (i.e. the practitioner) from the structured enablement of client power.

To extend the above discussion, Saylor (1990) described research analysis of student nurses' ability to evaluate 'self' in terms of a job well done. Students from early seniority levels were most likely to base their evaluations on positive reactions from the client, contrasting with experienced seniors, who were most likely to base their evaluations on 'objective' data. For example, they often described thinking back on the day and reviewing vital signs, pain and level of anxiety, understanding the rationale for procedures and medication as a measure of competency. On the basis of this work, Saylor suggested that reflective self-evaluation, using appropriate indicators, is essential for professional education. In addition to being a means of appropriate self-evaluation, reflection is also necessary for experiential learning.

THOUGHT PROCESSES IN LEARNING

In developing a theory of reflection and teacher education, Goodman (1984) was concerned that the meaning of the term 'reflection' should be clarified and his argument focused on the need to recognize that reflection is not just quiet rumination. If reflection is to be a worthwhile goal within teacher education (and thus health visitor education), our notion of it must be comprehensive.

Firstly, reflection suggests a need to focus on substantive rather than utilitarian concerns, i.e. the categories of action/non-action. Secondly, a theory of reflection must be legitimate and integrate both intuitive and rational thinking, i.e. the categories of conscious thinking. Finally, certain underlying attitudes are necessary in order to be truly reflective, i.e. the process descriptors of Boyd & Fales' (1983) stages of reflection.

Dewey (1933) referred to routine thought, which is a process of thinking and may lead to problem-solving but is in direct opposition to that of reflection. Routine thought is about how we confront, manage and deal with immediate situations, but it does not allow time to reflect because it lacks the patience necessary to work

Table 11.3 The process of reflection based on the analysis of self (Boyd & Fales 1983)

	Stage of reflection	Process descriptors
1.	A sense of inner discomfort	Awareness that something doesn't 'fit'. A feeling as though we have 'forgotten' something
2.	Identification or clarification of the concern	A key characteristic appears to be that, unlike thinking or problem solving, the reflective process is conceptualized in relation to self
3.	Openness to new information from internal and external sources, with ability to observe and take in from a variety of perspectives	Openness taking the form of reviewing past experience, foregoing the need for immediate closure on the issue (i.e. forming a conclusion), intentionally structured lateral thinking, intentionally setting aside the problem. For the community practice teacher/counsellor this is a useful intervention stage by enabling the collecting of this information but without forcing it into a pattern
4.	Resolution, expressed as 'integration', 'coming together', 'acceptance of self-reality' and 'creative synthesis'	This is the 'eureka' stage of reflection, when insight is gained and at which point people experience themselves as changed, having learned or having come to a satisfactory point of closure in relation to the issue (i.e. reached a satisfactory endpoint or conclusion)
5.	Establishing continuity of self with past, present and future	There is a recognition in terms of similar solutions from past experience, reviewing past values in relation to the changed perspective, evaluating the change as better for self, applying the new perspective to a variety of additional issues in the present self-structure, planning for future behaviour consistent with the changed perspective, or examining the implications of the change for future behaviour
6.	Deciding whether to act on the outcome of the reflective process	The change or resolution is evaluated in terms of the individual's own subjective criteria, the intensity of the subjective sense of the rightness of the resolution, its consistency with the individual's existing or aspired value structure, and with other desired goals of the self. The need to test one's self-changes against the mirror of others is an essential component of all growth

through one's doubts and perplexity. Goodman (1984) identifies rational thought, which is clearly distinguishable from routine thought and which some observers equate to reflection. However, Goodman argues that rational thought does not encompass intuitive thought, which is associated with the spark of creative ideas, insight and empathy. He thus posits reflective thinking as occurring with the integration of rational and intuitive thought processes. It is possible that this is the art and science of thinking in health visiting practice.

Up to this point the emphasis has been on the student, but it is important that the ability of the community practice teacher is not forgotten: drawing again on Dewey (1933), Goodman identifies three attitudes as prerequisites for reflective teaching:

- *open-mindedness*: an active desire to listen to more than one side
- *responsibility*: there must be a desire to synthesize ideas, to make sense out of nonsense and to apply information in an

Table 11.4   Comparative examination of levels of thought and reflection

Level	Levels of thought (Dewey 1933/Goodman 1984)	Levels of reflection (Goodman 1984)
1.	*Thinking encompasses formulations of ideas (routine thought)*: Criteria for thinking include situational observation, previous and current knowledge	*Reflection to reach given objectives*: Criteria for reflection are limited to technocratic issues of efficiency, effectiveness and accountability
2.	*Thinking is about processing the information (rational thought)*: Criteria for thinking include the absorption and assimilation of all evidence (including policies) to formulate a recognizable structure for strategic action	*Reflection on the relationship between principles and practice*: There is an assessment of the implications and consequences of actions and beliefs as well as the underlying rationale for practice
3.	*Thinking is about creating and using information for new ideas (intuitive thought)*: Criteria for thinking include assimilated evidence within research-based knowledge: it relies on the ability to rise above policy and organizational constraints to allow far-sighted flexible practice	*Reflection which, besides the above, incorporates ethical and political concerns*: Issues of justice and emancipation enter deliberations over the value of professional goals and practice and the practitioner makes links between the setting of everyday practice and broader social structures and forces

aspired direction. This attitude fosters consideration of the consequences and implications beyond questions of immediate utility

- *whole-heartedness*: the internal strength necessary for genuine reflection and the ability to work through fears and insecurities.

It is suggested that both teacher and student work within these parameters and that enthusiasm for learning with the provision of a quality learning environment is possibly an interpretation of 'whole-heartedness'. Goodman identified three levels of reflection. In the light of the analysis of thought processes, these could be assigned similar levels (Table 11.4).

At the third level, if practitioners relied on reflective criteria only, then there might be a constraint in the development of practice. Heath (1998) uses Porter & Ryan (1996) to postulate that reflection is not necessarily the dominant factor in higher-level practice and that it is the combination with a comparable level of rational thought that spearheads expert practice. If reflection only is used, then practitioners may conclude that practice cannot be developed because of the constraints of organization or policy and go no further. Thus creative

thinking (level 3 thought) must be seen to precede level 3 reflection in order that practice can move forward, albeit on the basis of reflection. This suggests that levels of thought might be one step ahead of levels of reflection. However, creative thought requires high levels of reflection. To explore this further, other models of reflectivity should be examined.

LEVELS OF REFLECTIVITY

In writing on a critical theory of adult education and learning Mezirow (1981) proposed levels of reflectivity within the learning process (Box 11.1). Mezirow (1981) proposes that the first four levels are of a lower order, likening these to consciousness. The remaining three are thus at a higher level, likened to critical consciousness. The link between Mezirow's proposition and reflection via consciousness is illuminated by the statement made in the first section of the chapter, here repeated: 'It is necessary to consider [the] levels of consciousness because it is only on the basis of their recognition that reflection can take place. Thus reflection must encompass the ability to articulate consciousness levels – was something planned, was it monitored by the practitioner (or client), was retrospective thought given to the process within the situation?'

Box 11.1 Levels of reflectivity (Mezirow 1981)

- **Reflectivity** – awareness of specific perception, meaning or behaviour of our own or of habits we have of seeing, thinking or acting
- **Affective reflectivity** – becoming aware of how we feel about the way we are perceiving, thinking or acting or about our habits of doing so
- **Discriminant reflectivity** – we assess the efficacy of our perceptions, thoughts, actions and habits of doing things; identify immediate causes; recognize reality contexts in which we are functioning (play, dream, religious, musical or drug experience) and identify our relationships in the situation
- **Judgmental reflectivity** – involves making and becoming aware of our value judgements about our perceptions, thoughts, actions and habits in terms of their being liked or disliked, beautiful or ugly, positive or negative
- **Conceptual reflectivity** – becoming aware of our awareness and critiquing it, i.e. critical awareness or critical consciousness
- **Psychic reflectivity** – this leads one to recognize in oneself the habit of making precipitate judgements about people on the basis of limited information about them
- **Theoretical reflectivity** – differs from the previous two in that it encompasses them both in a process central to perspective transformation. Theoretical reflectivity represents a uniquely adult capacity and, as such, becomes realized through perspective transformation

It is assumed, therefore, that using the technique above to compare Goodman's three levels of reflectivity with the levels of thought process, it should be possible to identify seven levels of thought process. However, the exercise is not conducive to the momentum of the chapter and it will therefore be left to the reader to attempt this task.

A more recent hierarchy of levels of reflection has been identified in Table 11.5, which is a model proposed by Kitchener & King (1990) to facilitate learners to become critically reflective. The reflective judgement model describes changes in assumptions about sources and certainty of knowledge and how decisions are justified in the light of these assumptions. That is, the model focuses on describing the development of epistemological (theory and nature of knowledge) assumptions and how these act as 'meaning perspectives' that radically affect the way individuals understand and subsequently solve problems. The model has seven stages, and each stage includes assumptions about what can be known and how certain one can be about knowing it; it also includes assumptions about the role of evidence, authority and interpretation in the formation of solutions to problems. This model goes beyond the first tentative stages for student learning, but can certainly be used by the time they are halfway through their practicum.

Clearly, Table 11.5 has led us into an extension of the reflecting and thinking processes into an analysis of knowledge; whether there is a body of knowledge called health visiting and whether it is possible to reflect on knowledge identified as belonging to one professional discipline alone.

KNOWLEDGE

Knowledge has been discussed in Chapter 1 in relation to professionalism; that is, identifiable professions will have recognizable knowledge which is used specifically for professional practice. Schön (1983) proposes that the professions are bound by a form of professional knowledge that fails to take into account the indeterminacy of practice. Schön argues that the dominant epistemology (a branch of philosophy that deals with the nature and validity of knowledge) of practice is technical rationality, which relies on the assumption that empirical science – based on positive facts and observable phenomena – is the only source of objective knowledge about the world. Schön suggests that there is an area in professional practice where practitioners can make use of research-based theory and

Table 11.5 The reflective judgement model (Kitchener & King 1990)

Stage of reflective judgement	Characteristics (modified to suit health visiting)
Stage 1	Knowing is characterized by a concrete, single-belief system: what the person knows to be true is true. Knowledge is both absolute and concrete: beliefs do not need to be justified. This is unlikely to be seen in student health visitors as it probably only belongs to young children
Stage 2	Knowing takes on more complexity since individuals assume that, while truth is ultimately accessible, it may not be directly and immediately known to everyone – some people hold 'right' beliefs while others hold 'wrong' ones. There is an assumption that the source of a knowledgeable answer will be an authority, e.g. teacher, doctor. This might be apparent in initial nurse training. It can concern the student health visitor because they may have to revisit this level having come into training as an experienced practitioner. The client might expect knowledgeable answers from them in this new professional approach
Stage 3	There is a belief that authorities/professionals hold the truth although it may be at times inaccessible. However, they believe that absolute truth will be manifest in concrete data some time in the future and argue that, since evidence is currently incomplete, no one can claim any authority beyond his or her own impressions or feelings. Individuals at this stage do not understand or acknowledge any basis for evaluation beyond these feelings. This may well be seen during the first semester in average and above students and for weaker students may last considerably longer
Stage 4	The uncertainty of knowing is initially acknowledged at this stage and usually attributed to the limitations of the knower. Without certainty, individuals argue that knowledge cannot be validated externally; thus, they argue, it is idiosyncratic. The fact that uncertainty is clearly accepted at this stage as an intrinsic characteristic of knowing is, however, an important development. It allows individuals to distinguish between well- and ill-structured problems (Churchman 1971, Kitchener 1983, Wood 1983). Well-structured problems, e.g. an arithmetic problem, can be described completely and solved with certainty. Ill-structured, real-world problems, e.g. how to reduce pollution, are such because all the parameters are seldom clear or available and it is difficult to determine when and whether an adequate solution has been identified. When students in stages 1, 2 and 3 cannot acknowledge that some problems do not have an absolutely correct solution, they cannot acknowledge the existence of real, ill-structured problems. This stage may be seen in the student health visitor prior to health visiting practice
Stage 5	Individuals believe that knowledge must be placed within a context, an assumption deriving from the understanding that interpretation plays a role in what a person perceives. This is beyond the idiosyncratic justifications of stage 4: it is only at stage 5 that they are able to compare and evaluate the relative merits of two alternative interpretations of the same issue. This should be typical of all students about to complete the health visitor course
Stage 6	Knowing is uncertain and knowledge must be understood in relation to the context from which it was derived. Knowing involves evaluation and some perspectives, arguments or points of view may be evaluated as better than others. These evaluations involve comparing evidence and opinion across

(Continued)

Table 11.5 (Continued)	
Stage of reflective judgement	Characteristics (modified to suit health visiting)
	contexts, which allows an initial basis for forming judgements about ill-structured problems
Stage 7	Individuals still believe that knowing is uncertain and subject to interpretation, but they can argue that epistemically justifiable claims can be made about the better or best solution to the problem under consideration. As with Dewey's (1933) description of reflective thinking, individuals claim that knowledge can be constructed via critical inquiry and through the synthesis of existing evidence and opinion into claims that can be evaluated as having greater 'truth value' or being more 'warranted' than others

technique, but equally there are other areas where there are uncertainties and value conflicts that are incapable of technical solution. Benner (1984) also makes the point that not all knowledge embedded in expertise can be captured in theoretical propositions or in analytical strategies that depend on identifying all the elements that go into a clinical decision.

Eraut (1985) argues that there are different kinds of professional knowledge. He suggests that there is knowledge of the kind that does not normally get included in syllabi. This knowledge may be as significant as the quality of 'getting on with people', which may simply be assumed as part of the job, although it could be theorised as 'interpersonal skills' or 'psychology' and is the basis of Chapter 1. Another form of knowledge, Eraut claims, is professional codified knowledge derived from an analysis of such activities as problem-solving, decision-making and communication, and is clearly different in kind from the experience-derived know-how that professionals intuitively use. Eraut quotes Oakeshott (1962), following Aristotle, as making a clear distinction between 'technical knowledge' and 'practical knowledge'. Technical knowledge is capable of written codification but practical knowledge is expressed only in practice and is learned only through experience with practice. If Eraut is right in his analysis, therefore, the relationship between these two is difficult to assess and is called the theory–practice gap. Similarly, and much later, Heath (1998) uses Moch (1990) to compare the knowledge that evolves within research-based

practice and the theory that might stem from practice, or is derived separately from it. She suggests that during the reflective process the professional may recognize that the knowledge he or she is identifying has evolved from within that very practice.

Meerabeau (1992) draws on the work of Polanyi (1958, 1967) to describe 'tacit knowledge': experts do not use the same pattern of skills as learners but they view situations holistically and much of their knowledge is embedded in practice. It would seem that the embedded knowledge that Meerabeau describes is the intuitive knowledge suggested by other writers. Eraut (1985) draws on the work of Broudy et al (1964), who suggest that this intuitive mode of knowledge (called semi-conscious) often involves metaphors or images that do not derive only from practical experience but also serve as carriers for theoretical ideas. As metaphor can only be articulated in language the argument is carried into the necessary recognition that language use is of considerable importance in espousing knowledge.

Deshler (1990a) suggested that metaphor is the means whereby critical reflection and transformative learning can be recognized and identified. Metaphors can assist us to reflect on personal, popular-cultural and organizational socialization. Through 'unpacking' the meaning associated with these domains, metaphors uncover frames of reference or structures of assumptions that have influenced the way we perceive, think, decide, feel and act upon our experience. Deshler states that metaphors are concrete images that require us to find threads of continuity and congruence between the metaphor and the primary object.

Mezirow (1981) argues that perspectives are constitutive of experience. They determine how we see, think, feel and behave. Human experience is brought into being through language. Restrictive language codes can arbitrarily distort experience so that it gets shoehorned into categories of meanings or typifications. Meaning perspectives can incorporate fragmented, incomplete experience involving areas of meaninglessness, and typification is the process of categorizing our perceptions.

MODELS AND TOOLS TO AID EFFECTIVE REFLECTION

The chapter has so far worked through some major concepts related to learning, reflection, judgement and knowledge, and the next step in the process of using reflection in practice is to look at ways in which these concepts might be structured in the thinking process. There are some useful flow diagrams of processes of reflection and three in particular are shown in order to aid understanding. The Gibbs (1988) reflective cycle is set out in Figure 11.1 and is the most useful for the early days of learning reflection and reflective processes. Boyd & Fales' (1983) progression process seen in Figure 11.2 and Table 11.3 has already been described and is useful to aid recognition of the possible depths of the process.

Structured reflection is of great value in the early days of learning reflective practice and in Boxes 11.2 and 11.3 two models of structured reflection are shown. They are both self-explanatory by the very nature of their structured process, and their great value is in providing cues to link an experience with an analysis of its outcomes. However, in order to ensure best use of a model students should use a reflective journal (Box 11.4).

The community practice teacher plays an important part in unpacking the reflective journal jointly with the student. Language and metaphor use in the journal requires exploration and checking back with student

---

Box 11.2   A model of structured reflection (Carper 1978, Johns 1992)

Description of the experience
1. Phenomenon – describe the here and now experience
2. Causal – what essential factors contributed to the experience?
3. Context – what/who are the significant background actors in the experience?
4. Clarifying – what are the key processes (for reflection) in this experience?

Reflection
1. What was I trying to achieve?
2. Why did I intervene as I did?
3. What are the consequences of my action for:
   – myself?
   – the client/family?
   – the people I work with?
4. How did I feel about this experience when it was happening?
5. How did the client feel about it?
6. How do I know how the client felt about it?

Influencing factors
1. What internal factors influenced my decision-making?
2. What external factors influenced my decision-making?
3. What sources of knowledge did/should have influence(d) my decision-making?

Could I have dealt better with the situation?
1. What other choices did I have?
2. What would be the consequences of those choices?

Learning
1. How do I now feel about this experience?
2. How have I made sense of this experience in the light of past experience and future practices?
3. How has this experience changed my ways of knowing:
   – empirics?
   – aesthetics?
   – ethics?
   – personal?

Box 11.3 The stage model of reflection (Dudley 1994)

This model was devised for students undertaking a course in theatre studies and, although apparently a different perspective from health visiting, nevertheless it has a basic structure that lends itself to health visiting practice.

Stage 1. Description
What was the situation, where and when? Who was there? Why?

Stage 2. Analysis
What did I contribute? What did I think – feel? Is this surprising, i.e. what would I have expected or what would others have expected of me?

Stage 3. Skill analysis
What skills/behaviours did I bring to the situation?
What skills/behaviours did I notice in others?
What skills/behaviours were needed in the situation?
What skills/behaviours would I have liked to have been able to demonstrate?

Stage 4. Evaluation
What judgements do I wish to make about my contribution to this event?
How will I measure my performance against my expectations and against standards/criteria set by others?
What views and perspectives will I adopt to evaluate the norms and expectations of other behavioural frameworks?

Stage 5. Research
What resources are available to help me integrate the changes I want to make?
Make lists of people, readings, recordings, courses, other experiences.

Stage 6. Action plan
What steps will I take to avail myself of these resources and use them? Make an action schedule indicating (a) what resources, (b) how and when I plan to access each one.

Box 11.4 Guidelines for keeping a reflective journal (Johns 1994)

1. Use an A4 notebook
2. Split each page vertically
3. Write up diary events on the left side
4. Use right-hand side for further reflection
5. Write up experience the same day if possible
6. Use actual dialogue wherever possible to capture the situation
7. Make a habit of writing up at least one experience per day
8. Balance problematic experiences with a satisfying experience
9. Challenge yourself at least once a day about something that you normally do without thought/take for granted – ask yourself: 'Why did I do that?' (i.e. make the normal problematic)
10. Always endeavour to be open and honest with yourself – find the 'authentic you' to do the writing

conceptualization of the experience articulated. Initially, of course, this process is a shared process during the period of shadowing of the community practice teacher by the student. However, later, when the student is practising alone and articulating the content of the practice intervention, it is essential to explore the meaning of language and metaphor used. This entire process should be normalized to the extent that it becomes totally integrated into the student's subsequent qualified practice. Good health visiting practice should always be managed in such a way that the practitioner deliberately allows time for reflection and this may need to be written rather than just mused upon.

Currently, the effectiveness of health visiting practice is based on a quantification of task analysis in those areas of practice visible to the Primary Care Trust. As yet unexplored is the entirely new concept of the purchase of reflective practice. If, as is well articulated in the literature, good professional practice is research-based reflective practice, this should be the practice that purchasers use for client/patient care. It is really only in the practicum that reflective journals are regularly used. To carry this argument a stage further therefore, it would appear that to show quality reflective practice a journal-type approach should be the basis of all recording, and yet this is clearly impracticable for everyday documentation. In addition, the quality of reflection of the learning student is probably clearer than that of the practising professional, whose work will be far more contextually and experientially premised.

It is thus more practical to suggest that where there is extensive intervention work with a client (or clients) then the additional supplementary records should contain a considerably greater amount of reflection, this of course, being shared with the client. This whole discussion is now leading towards the handling of reflection and thinking in everyday practice.

THE DEVELOPMENT OF CRITICAL THINKING IN HEALTH VISITING PRACTICE

Critical thinking has been the domain of philosophers and analysts since humans began to question. Daly (1998) suggests that critical thinking is purposeful, towards an end rather than the routine thought identified by Dewey (1933). Glen (1995) used Gallie's (1955) work to suggest that critical thinking is a contested concept. Critical thinking, therefore, can be seen as the art or science of productive thought, and if it is considered as such then it must be identifiable and tangible. Productive thought can be defined as thinking that has an end-product, which could be a decision made, an idea created and processes for action identified, a brainstorm leading to management of a situation. Non-productive thought is definable and can best be described as rumination or ruminative thought, when our mental processes churn over problems without coming to any end (productive) result. Referring back to Table 11.3 (p. 272), the third level of reflection identified by Boyd & Fales (1983) could be compared to ruminative thought processes.

Critical thinking is seen, in the developing academic processes of the modern nursing world, as necessary for research-based practice and informed care. Many commentators (Watson & Glaser 1964, Glen 1995, Daly 1998) argue coherently that critical thinking must be a taught or guided process; others, including Mezirow (1981), suggest that it should be left to the individual in competency-based programmes, particularly in technical or instrumental learning, such as learning to use a computer.

Taking into consideration the discussion above, as health visiting is such an abstract process with problem-solving requirements, it clearly requires guided techniques of reflection and conceptual mapping in order to facilitate the process in the individual learner. Both processes are now discussed, using critical incident analysis, through critical reflection and concept analysis.

CRITICAL INCIDENT ANALYSIS

The critical incident technique is described by Dunn & Hamilton (1986) as a sophisticated method for collecting behavioural data about the ingredients of competent behaviour in a profession. They cite Ingalsbe & Spears (1979) as proposing that the strategy of critical incident analysis, when compared with other methods of performance evaluation, is a more objective and efficient method of determining performance effectiveness. Critical incident technique was devised by Flanagan in 1947 as a method of training air pilots – by collecting information based on first-hand observation. Flanagan constructed a short questionnaire to distribute to the instructors:

> *Think of the last time you saw a trainee pilot do something that was effective/ineffective.*
> *What led up to this situation?*
> *Exactly what did the man do?*
> *Why was it effective/ineffective?*

These questions required answers based neither on intuition nor on opinion but on observed fact. As a result of this work Flanagan

(1954, 1963) made a clear statement of definition of a critical incident:

> By an incident is meant any observable activity that is sufficiently complete in itself to permit inferences and predictions to be made about the person performing the act. To be critical, an incident must occur in a situation where the purpose of the act seems fairly clear to the observer and where its consequences are sufficiently definite to leave little doubt concerning its effects. The main concern is always with the incident, never with the individuals concerned except as a means whereby they might learn from the incident.

Dunn & Hamilton (1986) suggest that the main value of critical incident technique lies in the three areas of competency-based education, priority areas in education and problem-solving material. Brookfield (1990) suggests that the process of critical reflection can be viewed as comprising three interrelated phases:

- identifying the assumptions that underlie our thoughts and actions
- scrutinizing the accuracy and validity of these in terms of how they connect to, or are discrepant with, our experience of reality
- reconstituting these assumptions to make them more inclusive and integrative.

Critical incident analysis is a technique that seeks to highlight particular, concrete and contextually specific aspects of people's experiences. It is often threatening to the learner to ask for their assumptions in response to a direct question on a general issue. For educators to help develop critical thinking in others they must be able to do this for themselves and this often works well with a small group of educators and learners. In practical terms it is often useful to describe an incident or set of circumstances in relation to your work with a client, and then analyse and examine the assumptions underlying the intimate relationship with the client. Once this is done it can then be thrown to the group to take up particular points and learn to challenge assumptions made. It is interesting to look for commonalities and differences in the assumptions that each person identifies. If there are commonly held assumptions, do they represent what passes for conventional wisdom in your field of practice? If there are major differences, to what extent might these signify divergent views in the field at large? Or might the differences be the result of contextual variations? As this is done within a climate of trust which has been engendered by the initial self-exposure of the educator, student response is often relaxed and perceptive.

Benner (1984) uses critical incident technique to identify the difference in the behaviour of nurses with different levels of experience within the acute field and it translates easily to community health care, where many assumptions are made and the working time with clients is generally irregular and often sporadic.

Dunn & Hamilton (1986) used critical incident technique to ascertain and identify the competencies of the pharmaceutical profession, and much depended on the ability of the interviewer to gain the trust of the professional so that the interview itself became more of an anecdotal dialogue, but one containing concrete examples of carefully described detailed incidents. The interviewee was then asked for any incidents they had observed or participated in when the pharmacist could have done a little better. In this way, the interviewers were able to identify important competencies of the profession and in compiling something like 700 incidents were able to say that these were the competencies of the profession.

It can be seen, therefore, that critical incident analysis is a basis for two strategies: an 'objective' and efficient method of determining performance effectiveness, and contributing towards determination of the competencies of a profession. However, critical incident analysis can also be valuable to explore the assumptions of the student in relation to their knowledge (see Table 11.5).

Watson & Glaser (1964) developed a list of abilities that comprise critical thinking:

- the ability to define a problem
- the ability to select pertinent information for the solution of the problem

- the ability to recognize stated and unstated assumptions
- the ability to formulate and select relevant hypotheses
- the ability to draw valid conclusions and to judge the validity of inferences.

This vignette is used to explore the five aspects of critical thinking.

> The student health visitor is approached by the GP, who has been visited by a mother with a 15-month-old child with apparent sleep problems. The community practice teacher has previously tried to help the family with this problem. The student health visitor suggests to the GP that she spend some time with the mother, who is still in the waiting room. Private and gentle discussion with the mother gradually took her back to pre-conception life, pregnancy and the early postnatal period following a Caesarean section. The mother said that the child's sleeping problem was creating big difficulties in her family life.

THE ABILITY TO DEFINE THE PROBLEM

Later, using Watson and Glaser's abilities list and guiding the student through this critical incident analysis, the initial process was to determine and define the problem. The student was encouraged to consider the behaviour of the mother as a result of actually questioning her problem. In many situations a client comes with a problem and is not well known to the health visitor whom s/he is consulting, who initially can only work with the client on the expressed problem. The student needs to be aware that although the expressed need is identified as the problem there may well be underlying issues such as relationship problems, lack of social networks, noisy neighbours, overcrowding, and so forth.

THE ABILITY TO SELECT PERTINENT INFORMATION

The student has encouraged the client to consider what would be an acceptable solution. Within her own knowledge framework the

student is encouraged to consider whether what the mother wants is achievable. The student would be encouraged to explore a more in-depth history of the problem. S/he would ask about support, beliefs, attitudes, significant other family members, family routines and so forth.

THE ABILITY TO RECOGNIZE STATED AND UNSTATED ASSUMPTIONS

Using this incident the student would be encouraged to question the presenting problem and consider whether beginning some work on it is the best way forward at this stage. Is it better to go along a management path, aware that in time more relevant information may be revealed and the basic problem exposed, or not to initiate anything immediately, except the maintenance of a sleep diary, which would precipitate further exploration?

THE ABILITY TO SELECT RELEVANT AND PROMISING HYPOTHESES

The use of a sleep diary could lead to: non-completion of the diary; completion revealing a very disturbed sleep pattern; completion revealing infrequent waking patterns; completion showing extended daytime sleep; completion showing unsettled family rhythms; and others. On the basis of these suggestions the student is then guided into selecting several hypotheses. Non-completion could suggest that the child's sleep problem is not the main difficulty. Very disturbed sleeping patterns may mean that it is the prime problem and needs sleep management techniques; extended daytime sleep may reveal little or no parent–child interaction; unsettled family rhythms may suggest discussion of parenting skills and their relationship to settled child rearing, etc.

THE ABILITY TO DRAW VALID CONCLUSIONS

The student will recognize that s/he will be unable to draw valid conclusions unless her/his knowledge level is appropriate to the incident. The application of reflection processes and techniques will facilitate this conclusion. The student will also recognize where his/her own thoughts about the origin of the problem are in relation to those presented by the client, and any mismatch between cause and effect. Using a reflection process on evaluating his/her own potential communication processes, the student is guided to recognize the validity of the inferences s/he has drawn in relation to the original incident experienced by the community practice teacher and used as a teaching tool to guide the whole analytical reflecting process.

Using a phenomenological approach there is the assumption that specific responses to critical incidents often have the generic embedded within them. In other words, critical incident analysis does not necessarily mean that general conclusions can be made from one analysis. Critical incident responses alone as primary data sources give insights into learners' assumptive worlds in expressions that are indisputably the learners' own and have not been taken from other sources.

CRITICAL REFLECTION

Mezirow et al (1990) suggest that critical incident analysis challenges the reflecting practitioner to question the presumptions that are brought to the process. Are the assumptions the analyst is starting from appropriate to the critical incident situation? They may have been acquired in a different context and therefore do not 'fit' the present situation. This suggests that the reflecting practitioner then has to go back to stage 5 of the reflective judgement model (Table 11.5) and realize that knowledge (and thus assumptions) must be placed in context. The context must be ascertained in critical incident analysis before reflection can really take place. Critical incident analysis is therefore an important prerequisite for valid and accurate critical reflection processes.

The process of critical reflection can be viewed as comprising three interrelated phases (Brookfield 1990):

- identifying the assumptions that underlie our thoughts and actions
- scrutinizing the accuracy and validity of these in terms of how they connect to, or

are discrepant with, our experience of reality (frequently through comparing our experience with others in similar contexts)
- reconstituting these assumptions to make them more inclusive and integrative.

Central to the process of critical reflection is the recognition and analysis of assumptions. An assumption is one of those taken-for-granted ideas, common-sense beliefs and self-evident rules of thumb that inform our thoughts and actions.

Before asking others to be critically reflective of their assumptions and meaning perspectives, practitioners must be able to do this for themselves. To do this, model the kinds of critical reflection that students might be asked to explore by taking something you have written or said and analysing it publicly for its distortions, inaccuracies, oversimplifications, contradictions and ambiguities. The focal point behind this exercise is to teach recognition of the ways in which assumptions become distorted within the contexts of situations. This is not particularly easy to do, but the very process will enable students to move forward in their critical reflection methods.

CONCEPT ANALYSIS AND CONCEPTUAL MAPPING

Conceptual analysis and conceptual mapping are tools used not only to develop and consolidate critical reflection, but also to develop creative thought. The use of conceptual analysis and conceptual mapping in relation to reflection will be considered first. Conceptual analysis has been defined from a number of perspectives, two of which will be considered here. Norris (1982) used a definition: 'Concepts are abstractions of concrete events. They represent ways of perceiving phenomena. Concepts are generalisations about particulars, such as cause and effect, duration, dimension, attributes, and continua of phenomena or objects'; and Meleis's (1985) definition adds the following:

Concepts are a mental image of reality tinted with the theorist's perception, experience and philosophical bent. They function as a reservoir and an organisational entity and bring order to observation and perceptions. They help to flag related ideas and perceptions without going into detailed descriptions.

There is a close relationship between this and the use of metaphor in reflective learning as suggested by Deshler (1990a) in the earlier discussion on knowledge. Both metaphor and concepts help to classify and distinguish between ideas and primary and secondary subjects, by a process of highlighting the primary subject and suppressing the secondary and less important features, recognizing the congruence between them. Thus in critical reflection the community practice teacher guides the student to identify and tease out the apparent merger of several different threads of thought. The difference between using metaphor and concept analysis is that concepts classify and organize and metaphor articulates this.

The use of the concept analysis has enabled health visitors to articulate and disentangle information that comes from several different sources during one single incident (observation, sensory, knowledge, assumptions and intuition). The community practice teacher assists the student to interpret metaphors used to illustrate meaning. These will include the assumptions, values and beliefs of the student. For example, in discussing mothers' uses of the descriptors 'diarrhoea' and 'constipation' the community practice teacher helps the student to see that these are metaphors (concepts) for apparent bowel dysfunction. Once unpicked, the student can then work to enable the mother to understand that for her child not to have a daily bowel movement does not necessarily signify constipation, or that breast-fed babies tend to have either frequent or infrequent bowel movements. These are perfectly normal for breast fed babies and rarely linked to the mother's diet.

Carrying and guiding the student into these advanced areas of critical, analytic reflection, is aided by the use of *conceptual mapping.* Conceptual mapping is a practical technique that can be used to reflect critically upon our concepts, their relationship to each other and

our underlying assumptions and values about the matters under consideration. This technique can be applied to a broad range of subject matter to assist in making explicit to ourselves the taken-for-granted frameworks, propositions and structures of assumption that influence the way we perceive, feel, and act upon our experience.

Our critical reflections on these maps reveal new pathways we may take to connect meanings among concepts in propositions. (Definition of proposition: statement, suggestion, statement of a theorem or problem.) Also revealed to us may be omissions and missing links, inconsistencies, false assumptions and previously unrecognised relationships.

A concept map is a schematic device for representing sets of concept meanings, embedded in the framework of propositions (Novak & Gowan 1984). Flow charts or other organizational charts are not really concept maps because their key words are usually not concepts with meanings. Concept maps are holistic, spatial, hierarchically constructed representations of the relationships among essential concepts.

Concept maps can be read as compound sentences that visually depict subordinate concepts and operations. Thus, complex multiple relationships can be displayed. Written or spoken concepts usually come to us in the form of linear propositions. Conceptual thinking, on the other hand, is more hierarchical or holographic (Novak & Gowan 1984). Concept maps assist us in transforming linear material into more holistic visual imagery and therefore help us to evaluate, synthesize and perceive in new ways.

The process of creating concept maps, critically reflecting upon them and reconstructing and validating them can contribute to transformative learning and emancipatory education. Using the same sleep example, a simple analogy here is the concept of an infant's sleep. The patterns of infant sleep vary and although they may be dependent on management, for this example we are interested only in the concept of sleep. A mother comes to the health visitor concerned that her infant has a sleep problem. On inquiry the mother states the infant wakes several times during the night. The mother wakes with her infant and worries that the infant is not sleeping; therefore he must have a sleeping problem and she is concerned. The health visitor suggests that the mother keeps a sleep diary for several nights and they then discuss the situation again. When they analyse the diary together the infant appears to wake twice during the night but is not distressed or crying. The health visitor then analyses the concept of sleep with the mother and she realizes that sleep does not necessarily mean unconsciousness but may include restful waking. In addition, waking actually only occurs twice a night and the infant appears even-tempered and happy most of the time. He does not appear fractious from lack of sleep. The mother then realizes that her interpretation of events arose from her lack of understanding of what sleep meant. In using this type of concept map the health visitor and mother work together to appreciate the understanding of sleep behaviour as a pattern and not a problem (Figs 11.3 and 11.4).

The use of the above as an example is to help change concepts or assumptions within them.

Some mothers may understand the process of concept mapping but it is more likely that the community practice teacher will use this tool with the student to enable the student to recognize the conceptual changes that need to be made in order to cope with events that challenge assumptions.

CREATING INITIAL CONCEPT MAPS

The purpose of an initial concept map is to confront ourselves with the current structure of our knowledge about the subject under discussion. It is not, at this point, an attempt to be critical about what we know but to describe our ideas and assumptions as they are.

To introduce conceptual mapping, we should begin with content of concern to students:

- concerns with which students are personally struggling
- concerns about what other people think about them, which may have an unrecognized influence on their behaviour

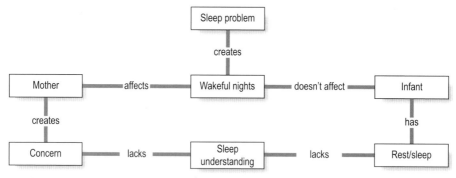

Figure 11.3   A concept map of a sleep problem (based on an original idea in Deshler 1990b)

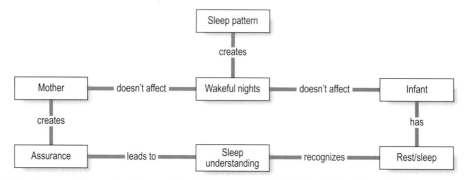

Figure 11.4   A concept map of a sleep pattern (based on an original idea in Deshler 1990b)

- concerns about theory/practice
- concerns about professional decision-making.

We can introduce current dilemmas that will provoke the need to reflect critically through the creation of concept maps. Transformative learning (Deshler 1990b) is most likely to occur through concept mapping when the focus is on concerns that we as learners recognize as:

- *important*, so that learning which is central to our future situations, environmental conditions, lifestyle or ethical behaviour can occur
- *puzzling* or cognitively dissonant, so that learning can result in a new synthesis of knowledge, ideas or feelings
- *constraining*, so that learning can result in the expansion and emancipation of choice.

Deshler (1990b) suggests that, after the focus of concern has been identified, the procedures for creating initial concept maps include the following steps:

- write or talk about the subject of concern
- understand the difference between concepts, names and linking words

- make lists of the key concepts
- select the one concept that is most general
- arrange the other concepts underneath the general concept
- draw linking lines between concepts and write linking words
- consider the maps as temporary, pliable, in-process and never finished.

The concept map of a sleep problem/pattern shows evidence of transformatory learning resulting from critical reflection on the initial map, which led to a more specific step for critical reflection.

Here is another example of a concept map in relation to student health visitor education. In this example the student in possession of a good honours first degree elected to undertake health visitor education at postgraduate diploma level. The community practice teacher was concerned that, although the student was functioning well in the practicum, it was apparent that a minimum of effort was being put into academic work – merely sufficient to scrape a pass. The community practice teacher brought this up in discussion and suggested a concept

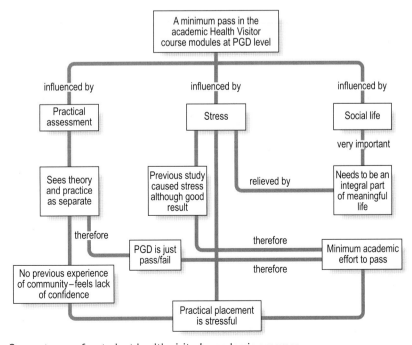

Figure 11.5   Concept map of a student health visitor's academic progress

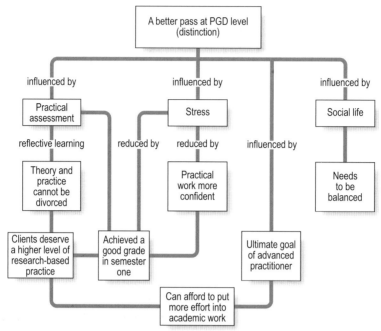

Figure 11.6 Reconstructed progress map of the concept of academic work effort

map approach, and the student complied by producing Figures 11.5 and 11.6.

What the student had not been aware of was that the academic level achievement could be raised to distinction and not just pass/fail. The student had also failed to see that practice could only be enhanced by academic comparability, and therefore had not realized that a bare pass in academic level could be reflected by a bare pass in practice. As it happened, the student did well in the first part of practice, but having recognized that it was possible to achieve this without becoming too stressed, it was also possible to work harder at academic work without becoming too stressed. The student's confidence level received a boost at the first practice assessment and thus a PGD distinction was within the bounds of possibility.

CONCLUSION

Health visiting has always used reflection, but originally in a cruder form. A criticism made

of health visitors practising in the 1960s–1970s was that they were always contemplating their navels – the premise being that health visitors were very good at evaluating themselves but much less able to evaluate their work. Formalization of this process by using reflection to both teach and learn health visiting has meant that there has been a forward movement into linking the evaluation of professional self to the evaluation of effective practice. The processes of understanding reflective practice in health visiting as critically discussed throughout this chapter must now be carried into a formal logging of the process so that discerning purchasers can recognize the value of purchasing specialist community public health nursing – health visiting. The principles of health visiting must always be seen to be underlying all aspects of reflective practice.

Chapter 12

Ethical issues in prevention of ill health and health promotion

Jan Rose

CHAPTER CONTENTS

INTRODUCTION

It is the intention of this chapter to raise awareness of ethical issues surrounding the practice of promoting health in its widest sense. Do not expect to be supplied with answers, since ethical dilemmas are intensely personal and there are no right solutions. What is hoped is that this chapter will increase moral reasoning, thus improving the quality of decision-making. Some of the ethical issues germane to the practice of health visiting that carry a potential for harm are health education and health screening, including immunization.

Ethics is a much used word and as such is open to individual interpretation. Ethical choice is influenced by personal values and personal values are usually learned through the process of socialization. This means that what may be ethical to one individual could be considered immoral by another. As health visitors you are warned about not imposing middle class values on your clients (at least, I was when I trained back in the 1970s), so can one rely on just one's own personal values and beliefs when faced with a dilemma that impacts on the client? Many health care practitioners may take comfort from the thought that they need only comply with the *Code of Professional Conduct* (2002) to practise ethically, but the code of conduct is provided for guidance only. The diversity of the various disciplines within nursing means that specific rules cannot be applied. The code of conduct therefore, of necessity, is couched in very general terms and when faced with a particular dilemma it is up to the individual to make the final decision as to the best way to act, or not act, as the case may be. Codes of conduct are therefore of limited value in helping to resolve ethical dilemmas. Consider the guidance set down within the code:

You are personally accountable for your practice. This means that you are answerable for your actions and omissions, regardless of advice or directions from another professional.

This is quite a heavy responsibility and, as Bergman (1981) points out, to be accountable one needs to have the ability to decide and act on a specific issue; ability requires knowledge, skills and values. The knowledge should be research based and up to date. The responsibility for keeping up to date is the individual's; when workloads are excessive and it is a struggle to get through the day's work, how feasible is it also to keep up with reading relevant literature? As Sieghart (1982) pointed out:

professional codes, if they are to be worth anything, cannot merely confine themselves to asserting that there is a problem and leave it at that – let alone leaving it to individual members of the profession to solve the dilemma as best they can, after consulting their unguided conscience and perhaps a few respected colleagues. At least such a code must say something about how to approach this kind of problem.

The Nursing and Midwifery Council, which came into being in 2001, published the new *Code of Professional Conduct* (NMC 2002a), replacing the previous *Code of Professional Conduct* (UKCC 1992), the *Scope of Professional Practice* (UKCC 1992) and the *Guidelines for Professional Practice* (UKCC 1996). In its new *Standards of Proficiency for Specialist Community Public Health Nurses* (NMC 2004a), the NMC point out in the introduction:

The NMC is required by the Nursing and Midwifery Order 2001 (the Order) to establish and maintain a register of qualified nurses and midwives [Article 5(1)], and from time to time establish standards of proficiency to be met by applicants to different parts of the register, being the standards it considers necessary for safe and effective practice [Article 5(2)(a)].

Elsewhere NMC (2004b) point out that the new third part of the register has been established to cover a form of practice that has distinct characteristics that require public protection, working with both individuals and a population. This is tighter than previous standards statements, but it does not provide definitive answers to the ethical dimension of working with individuals and populations. Although the NMC has set out standards it does not state the meaning of the term proficiency, or how it is achieved and maintained.

The health visitor enjoys more autonomy than other community disciplines. This is a double-edged sword since more autonomy means more accountability and more responsibility. As an example of some of the difficulties that may be encountered let us consider a prime concern for all health visitors: child protection. The concept of childhood is relatively new. Up until the latter half of the 19th century children were regarded as chattels or the property of their parents. When tracing genealogy it is quite common to find the same forename occurring several times within the same family. When a child died the next child born of the same sex was given the first child's name. Thus one supposes that the child was not valued as an individual but merely as an heir or for providing future support for the parents. As Aristotle put it: 'there can be no injustice in the unqualified sense towards things that are one's own, but a man's chattel, and his child until it reaches a certain age and sets up for itself, is as it were a part of himself.'

Children are perceived in the light of cultural values and mores. It is the culture of a particular society that defines the meaning and essential nature of childhood and the length that childhood should last. Children have been subject to abuse for centuries and before children were given recognition through legislation such as the Children Act 1989 the extent of abuse was not documented. Historically, awareness of child abuse came through the writings of social reformers such as Charles Dickens.

With child abuse the abiding decision is when (and how) to intervene. Health visitors may often find that they are 'damned if they do and damned if they don't'. There are horrific examples of the results of failing to intervene, as in the many recent cases where a young child has been killed. Alternatively, the effects on both parents and children of leaping to conclusions with too rigorous an approach, as in the Cleveland case, are still coming to light. In many cases, permanent damage to the family unit may result.

One problem with dealing with child abuse is that once the referral has been made to social services the prevailing attitude appears to be that the parent(s) or abusing adult(s) is guilty until proven innocent. Where there is clear evidence of physical harm to a child, no one would argue that it is imperative to act quickly and either remove the child or the alleged abuser as soon as possible. The issue is not quite so clear when there is suspected sexual abuse without physical violence or actual penetration. As with any form of suspected abuse, if there is evidence of actual harm then immediate action must be taken, but when does a cuddle become covertly sexual in nature? Who can decide this? How much evidence is required before action can be taken? Is there a cut-off age when fathers should stop bathing their daughters or should fathers not be allowed to bathe their female children at all? How practical would it be to impose rules like this when it may be that traditional family roles have been reversed and the mother is the breadwinner? What of male children? Should the same restrictions apply? When do photographs taken by proud parents become pornographic? Incest is taboo in our society but is it necessarily so in other cultures? The ancient Egyptians considered that incest was the only way to keep the royal blood-line uncontaminated.

While not condoning incest, one could argue that it is learned attitudes within the UK towards this practice that colour the health care professional's judgement when dealing with a suspected case. It is vital that action should be taken when there is a suspicion that an incestuous relationship with a minor may exist, but potential harm may be done to the innocent victim by a 'shock! horror!' reaction and insensitive probing. The child may perceive what has happened as an expression of love (provided that rape or coercion is not involved); indeed, it may be the only show of love or affection that the child receives. How much damage can be done by rushing in to remove either the child or the alleged abuser because our society abhors the concept of incestuous relationships! As John Harris (1985) puts it: 'There is nothing wrong with sex of any kind … There is lots wrong with violation, exploitation, the infliction of harm, pain, suffering and so on' (p. 191). Harris goes on to suggest that the sexual preferences of health professionals should not influence their treatment of those whose preferences differ. So it is important not to let distaste colour judgement.

When should the health visitor refer in order to protect the child? Because of an intuitive feeling? Can one take comfort from relinquishing responsibility to the social worker and thus taking no responsibility for subsequent adverse results should the suspicion be unfounded and false? But what if one fails to pass on concerns regarding a child? Failure to act (an omission) could result in considerable harm being done. Obviously, one should take action if there is anything in the child's demeanour that strongly suggests that a violation has taken place, but if this is not the case then the risk is that reporting your suspicions may adversely affect future relationships within that family unit. This situation is typical of an ethical dilemma where two equally unacceptable outcomes are likely whether an act or omission is undertaken by the health care professional. What help is needed in decision-making where ethical dilemmas exist? Is intuition enough? How can we judge when an action is right or good and how do we decide what we ought to do? How helpful is the *Code of Professional Conduct* (NMC 2002a) and the subsequent *Standards of Proficiency for Specialist Community Public Health Nurses* (NMC 2004a).

Allmark (1992) suggests that the two main approaches to the application of ethics in nursing are to examine the normative philo-sophical theories or, more commonly, to ignore any insights philosophy may offer and follow a systematic approach based on a form of the nursing process: assess, judge, plan, implement, evaluate. While Allmark admits that the second approach is tempting for nurses, being prag-matic and practical, he warns that nurses who ignore philosophical ideas on ethics are doomed to repeat the mistakes of the past. So before going any further it is pertinent to consider the philosophical basis of what is understood by ethics.

Ethics has been defined as a generic term for several ways of examining the moral life. Originally, 'morals' and 'ethics' were Greek and Roman terms meaning a code of acceptable con-duct within the constraints of society. Latterly, morals have taken on more of a religious con-notation. When we deliberate about whether a judgement is morally right, we are considering which judgement is morally justified, i.e. which has the strongest moral reasons behind it. Ethics is not one body of thought but a range of dif-ferent theories from which many other moral philosophies have been derived. There are many books written on ethical theory and it is not the intention to discuss ethical theories in any depth other than to distinguish between two main philosophies and explore ethical principles. (Those interested in studying ethical theory in greater depth are recommended to read Gillon 1986, Seedhouse 1988 and Beauchamp & Childress 1989.)

Deontology is derived from the Greek word *deon*, meaning 'duty', and is sometimes referred to as rights- or duty-based ethics – that what matters most is that a person acts accord-ing to a perceived duty and intends that some good should come about. Central to the philoso-phy of deontology is the idea that to be moral a person must perform his or her ordained duty. In its purest or most extreme form a deontolo-gist would always do what was perceived as the 'right' action, regardless of the conse-quences. Tell the absolute and unvarnished truth and be damned to the consequences is one example of this duty-based philosophy, which can cause considerable harm.

The best-known proponent of deontology was Immanuel Kant, an 18th-century German philosopher (a devout Christian), who identi-fied what he referred to as the 'categorical imperative' or moral law – categorical because it admits no exceptions and is absolutely bind-ing, and imperative because there are instruc-tions on how one should act. 'To duty every other motive must give place because duty is a condition of will good in itself whose worth transcends everything' (Kant 1964). Kant con-sidered that an action only had moral worth if a person who had a 'good will' carried it out and that a person only has a good will if a moral duty based on a valid rule is the only motive of action. The concept of a valid moral rule was presumably based upon the biblical Ten Commandments; deontology thus has its roots in Judo-Christianity. One should always take the right option regardless of the good or harm it might do.

Deontology aims to establish universal stand-ards of justice and embodies ultimate prin-ciples such as truth-telling and promise-keeping. One could not argue that such principles are less than admirable, and deontology has many strengths. Most importantly, this philosophy embraces respect for persons: it is always wrong to treat people as if they were mere objects to be used to further one's own ends. Deontology therefore rejects the concept that the end justifies the means and will not allow minorities to be disadvantaged for the sake of the majority. Deontology also addresses the question of what ought to be done. It is very comforting to be able to apply a universal moral rule, but even the right to life is not absolute and who decides, when two Christian countries are at war, which side is right? No doubt priests for both sides send the respective armies off with prayers that good will triumph over evil and God will protect the right side! Which raises the question of which rights are moral rights? How can one trace the route from abstract first principles to determine policies, practices and ways of life? With regard to health care practice, how can such rigid principles be adhered to? The process of social-ization and the needs of the society in which we live affect moral codes and ideologies. Is it possible to adhere to a philosophy based on Judo-Christian moral rules in today's multi-racial, multicultural society?

The other major philosophy is teleology, derived from the Greek word *telos* meaning 'ends', in other words, 'the ends justify the means'. This philosophy is also referred to as consequentialism and ethical dilemmas are resolved by consideration of the consequences of an action rather than its inherent goodness; actions are right or wrong according to the outcome. Consequentialism is based on the concept that value, pleasure, friendship, knowledge or health are the goals of any society. The most prominent consequentialist theory is utilitarianism. Utilitarians maintain that the moral rightness of actions is that they should create the greatest benefit for society as a whole. Utilitarianism does not always assume that there are morally 'right' actions. A person ought always to act in such a way that will produce the greatest balance of good over evil – 'the greatest good for the greatest number' or what is most useful is right, hence use of the term 'utility'. A major strength of this philosophy is that all options can be evaluated and the best outcomes identified. Decisions are focused on the results of actions so that the philosophy is forward looking; whatever dilemma presents (and with increasing technological advances there will always be new ethical dilemmas) the results of actions can be set down and the best possible option decided before action is taken. One problem with this philosophy is that it can allow for cost–benefit evaluations and one can see the potential for harm in health care, which may become routinized, especially when considering allocation of scarce resources. The rule of utility may create an excess of good over evil for the population as a whole but consideration of maximizing good for the majority could result in a proportion of the population being disadvantaged, so the potential for discrimination exists.

In order to avoid the pitfalls of advocating either deontology or utilitarianism as providing the answer to all ethical dilemmas, David Seedhouse (1988) has devised a tool which he calls the Ethical Grid (Fig. 12.1). This grid uses concepts from both philosophies but also incorporates four well-known ethical principles: autonomy, beneficence, non-maleficence and justice, first espoused by Beauchamp & Childress (1989) and used thereafter by many philosophers and medical ethicists. The principles have been taken from medical ethical codes, notably the Hippocratic Oath; the explanations are therefore couched in terms of doctor–patient relationships but the concepts can be widely applied to all health professional–client interactions. Before consideration of the Ethical Grid these four principles will be outlined.

THE PRINCIPLE OF AUTONOMY

Autonomy is derived from two Greek words: *autos* ('self') and *nomos* ('rule, governance or law'; Beauchamp & Childress 1989). So the literal meaning is 'self-rule'. Autonomy is also defined as self-determination. Gillon (1991) defines autonomy as 'the capacity to think, decide and act on the basis of such thought and decision freely and independently and without let or hindrance' (p. 60). Creating and respecting autonomy, Seedhouse (1988) considers, is at the very heart of health care. To respect a person's autonomy means respecting the decisions they make about themselves even though you may disagree with them. There can be no autonomy where pressure or coercion is used to gain consent to a procedure (immunization, for example). It has been suggested that 'it must be the right of every grown human being to be foolish if that is what he or she chooses to be' (Matthews 1986). Matthews maintains that however foolish a physician considers the decisions of any person to be with regard to their health care, the doctor has no right to override those decisions. Matthews uses the analogy of a garage mechanic who may inform him that his car brakes are in a dangerous condition but has no right to take the car away in order to repair it against his expressed wishes. For a person to exercise his autonomy he must be treated with respect. If you feel that you have the right to make decisions for yourself, e.g. what to wear, what to eat, where to send your child to school, where to live, then you should respect others' decisions about their life and how they live it. One problem that health professionals have is that, because they have a certain amount of expertise due to their education and training, they sometimes assume that they know what is best for their patient/client. Provided that there are no defects in autonomy, if full information is given then the decision must rest with the individual, galling though that may be if we disagree.

One problem for the health practitioner is in deciding when autonomy is impaired, or not desired. It is possible to respect autonomy by not disclosing all to the patient/client who has expressed a desire not to be informed. In this case, if the patient has autonomously decided to let the doctor make any decision and has expressly stated that he or she does not want to be given distressing news, then health professionals clearly would not be respecting the patient's autonomy if they insisted on telling them all the facts. Harris (1985) disagrees with this opinion and argues that it is doubtful whether the patient possesses a 'right' not to be told; he maintains that there are all sorts of unpleasant things in life that we do not want to be informed about but this does not mean that we have a right not to be informed about them. He does concede that it is a difficult area to discuss, but maintains that it is very clear that people do have a right to be told if they expressly wish it. Harris also considers that consent should not be 'once and for all' and that we have an obligation to keep seeking consent whenever the circumstances change.

Competence, or rather lack of it, is the reason given for overriding patient/client autonomy. But what do we understand by competence? When is a person judged not to be competent? Harris (1985) sets down what he terms defects in autonomy. These, he maintains, occur when an individual's autonomy is undermined and diminished by four different kinds of defect. Firstly, there are defects in the individual's ability to control desires or actions, as in mental illness or when under the influence of drugs or medication. A second way in which there may be defects in reasoning is uncritical acceptance of traditional views ('My mother and grandmother told me that the best way to keep the baby from crying was to put a dab of honey on a dummy – and it works'), prejudice or 'gut' reaction, and beliefs that have no foundation in fact ('My grandfather smoked 60 cigarettes a day and died at 95, so why should I stop?'). The third defect is in the information received: it may be false or incomplete, even deliberate deception, or there may be lack of adequate understanding or comprehension. The fourth defect Harris calls defects in stability. He points out that our likes, dislikes and values alter over time and that decisions made when we are young may be regretted later in life. This excuse is often used to overrule autonomy – 'You are wrong and I know what is best and you will thank me later when you realize this' – sound familiar? The only true justification for ever overriding autonomy is where there is the risk or likelihood of substantial harm to third persons. Unfortunately, health professionals are often guilty of acting paternalistically. Paternalism, sometimes referred to as parentalism, means, as the word implies, behaving like a father or parent. Paternalism, Tschudin & Marks-Maran (1993) maintain, is not only the province of doctors; maternalism is alive and well within the nursing profession, therefore parentalism is perhaps a more accurate word to use. Parentalism means treating patients or clients like children (for their own good) and so overruling autonomy by invoking the next ethical principle, that of beneficence.

THE PRINCIPLE OF BENEFICENCE

The principle of doing your best for others is embodied in the Hippocratic Oath: 'I will prescribe regimen for the good of my patients according to my ability and judgement … in every house where I come I will enter only for the good of my patients'. It is easy to see how the desire to do what is best for the patient/client can result in paternalistic decisions. As with the principle of autonomy the principle of beneficence is not absolute. The price of doing good must not be too high and taking the autonomy of the client into consideration is paramount. Doing what is best then depends upon consideration of the principle of autonomy and the next principle, sometimes referred to by the Latin tag *primum non nocere* – 'above all, do no harm'. Perhaps this principle should be given a higher priority, since much harm can be done by the enthusiastic practitioner intending only beneficence.

THE PRINCIPLE OF NON-MALEFICENCE

Like the principle of beneficence, this principle may well have its origins in the Hippocratic Oath, which requires doctors to 'abstain from whatever is deleterious or mischievous'. The first conflict that occurs when considering this principle is that many interventions do harm in that they may cause pain, but the intention is that a greater good will result. An obvious example is public health medicine, where the greater good of society is considered above the needs of the individual (a typical utilitarian standpoint). Take, for instance, vaccination and immunization, where the procedure is painful and the risk of an adverse reaction is considered to be justified in order to convey 'herd' immunity and protect the population at large. With this principle there is a moral obligation to weigh the expected bad effects of any intervention against the intended good effects. There is also a need to consider autonomy as a component of non-maleficence since the concept of what is harmful is intensely personal.

THE PRINCIPLE OF JUSTICE

There is some controversy as to whether this principle can be applied in ethical debate. Justice implies that there should be fairness or equity; the dictionary states that to be just is to be fair or impartial in action or judgement or awarding what is due. With the current management of NHS provision it is difficult to see how justice can be applied to the population as a whole. There is considerable disparity in allocation of resources and the quality of the service differs according to where you live and sometimes according to the whim of the medical consultant, who decides on the type of treatment on offer (as in breast cancer, for example). The concept of 'to each according to his need' was the principle upon which the NHS was set up in 1948. Since then the cost of health care continues to rise, demand is infinite and yet resources are finite, so rationing is a reality. How can there be justice where rationing exists? Be that as it may, it is still incumbent upon all health professionals to treat clients with equity.

DAVID SEEDHOUSE'S ETHICAL GRID

The theories and principles outlined above are by no means exhaustive. There are a plethora of opinions; many of them conflict with one another. It was in an attempt to improve on moral reasoning and aid ethical decision-making that Seedhouse devised his Ethical Grid (Seedhouse 1988).

According to Seedhouse, we are constantly faced with a range of choices that shape our destiny – we may have our paths limited by what we have done already, by our talents, our education and the historical era in which we exist. But we always have a choice about what to do, what to believe, how to act towards others and what to say. It therefore becomes vital, Seedhouse states, that health workers not only speak of 'positive health' and 'empowering' but also act according to richer ideas rather than according to the tenets of the old, medically dominated paradigm. A person's actions, he says, are the acid test of his beliefs. It is not enough to believe that individual autonomy should be a major priority for health work – even to the extent that it should be placed above the duty to prolong life – and yet conform in practice to the latter principle.

Seedhouse has developed an instrument, which, he suggests, helps health care professionals to develop a powerful health work skill,

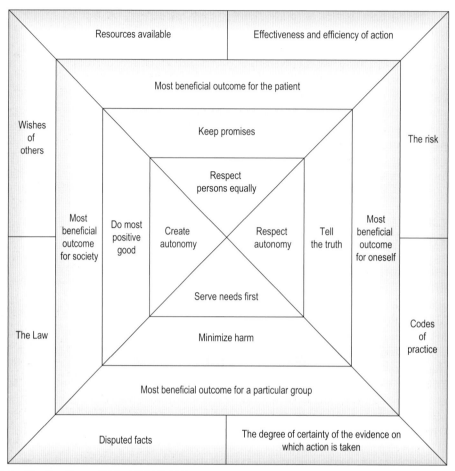

Figure 12.1   The Seedhouse Ethical Grid (1988)

which is the ability to reason morally. This tool he calls the Ethical Grid, suggesting that it is not a tool in the same way as a conveyor belt, for example, but rather as a spade that a gardener uses to cultivate his land. As the good gardener knows the best way to use a spade, so, Seedhouse suggests, the health care professional will understand the best way to use the grid in order to get the best out of the situation. One needs to understand that the end results are never entirely predictable and that even the most conscientious use of the grid may not produce the most practical results.

There are four different layers to the grid, which Seedhouse has identified by the use of different colours – blue, red, green and black – to aid differentiation. Each of the boxes is independent and detachable. Although each box can stand independently all the boxes have strong relationships with one another.

The grid is an artificial device and is not an exact representation of the mental processes that make up moral reasoning. In order to provide a practical and accessible route into the complexity of moral reasoning, Seedhouse has separated out the layers of the grid and distinguished each layer by the use of colour.

Four distinct layers of the grid are shown in order to show that at least four different sets of elements make up comprehensive ethical deliberation. As Seedhouse maintains, a deliberation that examines only the consequences of actions, or only the law, or only duties, might happen to produce good results on occasion but it will not be a deliberation carried through with integrity. Deliberations made in the context of health work should always acknowledge at least one box from the blue layer, since, according to Seedhouse, the need to create and respect autonomy is at the very heart of health care.

Seedhouse maintains that the Ethical Grid can improve moral reasoning, but it cannot take its place. The responsibility, he says, lies with the user and not with the grid. In ethical reflection much depends upon personal values, preferences and mode of thought of each individual and these cannot be represented graphically. Seedhouse states that each box cannot be considered in isolation; inevitably all the other factors listed in the grid will have to be taken into account. To take a box on its own, without considering the boxes in other layers, Seedhouse maintains is both hollow and impractical.

THE BLUE LAYER

Within this layer appear four boxes. Each box clearly represents the principle of autonomy by the provisos that one should create autonomy, respect autonomy, respect persons equally and serve needs first. These, according to Seedhouse, represent the basic principles behind health work. The blue layer is set at the centre of the grid since it provides the core rationale, the notions that make up the richest idea of health. To create and respect autonomy is essential for the creation of full personhood. To serve needs before wants and respect persons equally is essential for basic personhood. Associated ideas of enablement, personhood and enhancing potential are more likely to produce benefits that can be shared by all than any other option.

THE RED LAYER

This layer focuses on duties and motives. It adheres strongly to deontological principles. The layer includes the consideration of duties during moral deliberation. The four boxes are: minimize harm, do the most positive good, tell the truth and keep promises. In addition to a requirement to adhere to moral duties the red layer also invokes the principle of non-maleficence (minimize harm) and beneficence (do the most positive good).

THE GREEN LAYER

This part of the grid states that one should consider what action will have the most beneficial outcome for the patient, most beneficial outcome for society, most beneficial outcome for a particular group and finally the most beneficial outcome for oneself. This last adjunct allows for consideration of one's personal values. This layer, as can be seen, considers the general nature of the outcome and focuses on various aspects of consequentialism, i.e. the necessity to consider the consequences of any proposed intervention. It encourages reflection about whether the 'good' (specified in advance) is increased for humanity or society as a whole, for a particular group, for an individual or for the agent him/herself. While focusing on outcomes, this layer is not strongly utilitarian in that there is consideration of the most beneficial outcome for oneself and the individual. It adheres almost entirely to the principle of beneficence. It is in this layer that conflicts of interest can arise. Increase of social good will rightly take priority over individual good in cases of danger to others, e.g. the individual with homicidal tendencies or the HIV-positive individual determined to spread the virus far and wide.

An example of conflict when using this layer occurs in cases of child abuse. The boxes 'increase of benefit for self' and 'best outcome for society' may not be considered, or alternatively they may. For example, removing the child to a place of safety may result in family disintegration or the family may benefit by the intervention. Would the best outcome be to remove the abuser? The decision will be affected by many factors, including the family dynamics, and the health visitor is often involved in the case conference to decide which is the best outcome.

THE BLACK LAYER

This is the layer of practicality and contains the pertinent practical features. As such, it is plainly the layer which is the most utilitarian. This layer contains external constraints, which include legal rights. It could be said that in the real world this layer contains the most important factors of all and may effectively take the decision about what to do out of the hands of the health care professional. The layer requires consideration of: resources available, effectiveness and efficiency of action, the risk, codes of practice, the degree of certainty of the evidence on which action is taken, disputed facts, the law, and wishes of others. One could argue that, through consideration of disputed facts, effectiveness and efficiency of action, together with the law and wishes of others, this layer also supports the principle of justice.

The Ethical Grid is simply a tool; used competently it can help make certain tasks easier but it cannot direct the tasks, nor can it help decide which tasks are the most important. The grid cannot replace moral reasoning; the responsibilities, Seedhouse (1988) states, lie with the user and not with the grid.

HEALTH SCREENING

Health screening forms a large part of the health visitor's role. Ethical dilemmas regarding health screening have been, and still are, the subject of fierce debate. The rationale for health screening is that it will be of ultimate benefit to the recipient. It is generally perceived to be 'a good thing to do'. Prevention of ill health by detecting disease at the early, pre-symptomatic stage, before the disease process has caused irredeemable damage, is an admirable philosophy and one with which most health care practitioners would agree. Advocates of health screening claim that through early diagnosis the condition is cheaper to treat and the outcome more likely to be successful. Another popular belief is that there are only two possible outcomes of screening: benefit or no effect.

This has not always been the case: the earliest recorded health screening was in a brothel in Avignon in France in 1347. This was clearly for the benefit of the clients only – if one considers the lack of effective treatment for venereal disease at that time, this screening certainly could not have benefited the recipients. Early preventive medicine was synonymous with medical policing and screening for disease was initially used as a sieve to separate the healthy and useful from the weak and useless. This latter use, it could be argued, is still a reason for carrying out pre-employment screening, at least as far as the employer is concerned.

In 1973, Sackett looked at motives for carrying out health screening and came up with three: to influence the gamble of life insurance, to protect third parties – as in public health screening – and to do the patient some good. It can be seen from the order in which these are set down that doing good appears to be low on the priority list.

As far back as 1968 Wilson & Jungner laid down a set of principles for pre-symptomatic screening that are still applicable today: the condition should be serious with a recognizable early stage; early treatment should be available and of more benefit than later; there should be a suitable test that is acceptable to the population; the chance of physical or psychological harm should be less than the chance of benefit; and finally the cost of the programme should be balanced against the benefit it provides. The current literature available would suggest that these criteria are not always adhered to.

Downie & Calman (1989) identify four main areas of concern with health screening: the false-negative test, which could lead to a false sense of security and may lead the practitioner into unjustified reassurance, which will doubly disadvantage the person when the true facts emerge; the false-positive test, which creates unnecessary anxiety that is not always resolved; ineffective treatment for the condition (hence the reluctance among the medical profession to test routinely for HIV positivity, despite pressure from interested bodies such as insurance companies); and the high-risk groups who usually fail to attend for screening. The last group are already disadvantaged as they invariably have low socio-economic status.

Shickle & Chadwick (1994) point out that, as well as the problems inherent in false-positive and false-negative results, there are also costs with true-positive and true-negative results. A true-positive result is beneficial in that earlier treatment is more likely to be effective and improve the prognosis, usually less invasive and cheaper. There are also advantages of the sick role, for example, being excused social responsibilities. However, the costs could be stigmatization, anxiety (the worried ill) and the possibility of living longer with the diagnosis. True-negative results, Shickle & Chadwick maintain, may legitimize an 'unhealthy' lifestyle. If a negative result is given without explanation or advice then there is a risk of reinforcing an unhealthy lifestyle, bolstering a pre-existing sense of invulnerability and making participants less likely to return for subsequent testing. Duncan (1990) suggests that it is very difficult to measure the benefits of screening since there is no clear causal link between risk factors and ill health and no guarantee that screening will lead to health improvement.

What are the unwanted ill-health effects of screening? Should clients be informed that they are at high risk of developing a particular illness or disease? The principle of beneficence might lead one to consider that it should be of benefit, either by more effective treatment through early intervention or by changing to a healthier, less risky lifestyle. Alternatively it could be argued that the increased awareness of mortality and anxieties raised by positive results (false or otherwise) is diametrically opposed to the principle of non-maleficence. What evidence is there to support this supposition? Stoate (1989) cites an earlier example from Haynes et al (1978) that illustrates 'that the labelling of previously undiagnosed hypertensives, detected by screening in the work place, results in increased absenteeism from work' and argues that detecting abnormalities may have significant costs to the patient. Stoate also maintains that systematic screening may result in making people more aware of their mortality and increase hypochondria, which could lead to greater psychological distress. This viewpoint is also supported by Marteau (1989), who reports that high levels of anxiety are experienced by people participating in many screening programmes. Marteau (1990) states that anxiety is not only an undesirable effect in itself but also has a 'knock-on' effect on physical health, increasing consultation rates while at the same time reducing the patient's ability to recall or act on any advice given. It may also be argued

that costs are increased, as many doctors prescribe expensive medication for anxiety, which may not have occurred had the screening not been available. Marteau also discusses a study concerning a group of pregnant women with false alpha-fetoprotein results, who were found to be significantly more anxious 3 weeks later, when subsequent testing had shown the foetuses to be unaffected, than women who had originally received a negative result.

Peter Skrabanek (1990) uses several examples to voice his concern: the tragedy of a trial for clofibrate, a drug that lowers blood cholesterol, in which more healthy men treated with clofibrate died than the controls. It is unlikely that the men were fully informed of the danger from this drug before participating in the trial. Skrabanek also cites the case against screening for hypertension and states: 'The effects of such labelling are serious: they include the erosion of the sense of well-being, lowered sense of self-esteem, marital problems, reduction in earning power, and the adoption of a "sick role" in a previously healthy person' (Skrabanek 1990).

Women are a particularly vulnerable group (Skrabanek 1990): pressure is put on them to undergo regular gynaecological examinations. Cervical cytology is one screening procedure that is considered worthwhile and has been well documented but even so there is disparity in the service offered depending on where you live. Some areas of the country have such poor funding that it can be as long as 3 months before the results are known, with all the attendant worry and anxiety that are incurred until the all-clear is received. Breast screening is another doubtful area: risks include unnecessary surgery and needle biopsy. One claim is that for each woman who benefits from screening, 18 women have to live longer with the knowledge of their incurable disease because of earlier diagnosis (Marteau 1989). There is pressure on women to attend for breast screening and the implication is that if you attend the outcome will be good (Roberts 1989) – this is by no means necessarily so. There is no empirical evidence that treatment is successful; different surgeons will carry out different procedures and the current strongly implied statement that everything will be all right if women present themselves for screening is therefore unacceptable. Skrabanek (1990) also considers that breast self-examination is unlikely to reduce mortality from breast cancer, because by the time the tumour is palpable it will have been growing for a long time, and that it could be argued that self-examination is actually harmful, particularly for younger women, because it leads to unnecessary anxiety, with surgical and medical intervention.

Developmental screening, one could maintain, is the *raison d'être* of health visitors. Although the health visitor role has been extended and expanded, historically, it was concern about the neonatal and infant mortality and poor child health of those in lower socio-economic classes that led to the original inception of the health visitor. The intention of developmental screening, as with all screening procedures, is adhering to the principle of beneficence with early identification of health problems. Hearing tests are of proven value: early identification of hearing problems can prevent communication difficulties, especially with the development of speech. So with this particular test Wilson & Jungner's (1968) principle that effective treatment is available is met. What of other tests? In some areas they are still being carried out routinely despite the Hall recommendations. Where a mother knows that a screening test is being carried out there is bound to be a certain amount of anxiety and tension that the child will pass.

If there is some slight concern on the part of the health visitor that there may be a problem, what is he or she to do? The Ethical Grid advocates truth-telling, and sharing and openness is vital to ensure trust between health visitor and client. The principle of beneficence and non-maleficence could be in conflict here. Will more harm result by sharing your concerns and creating anxiety or should you decide not to mention your worries and risk being accused of secrecy (or even negligence) at a later date? Where routine tests are not carried out but the health visitor remains vigilant and merely observes the young child's developmental progress, when should delays in achieving milestones be shared with the parent? If the parent is not aware that the child's progress is being monitored, does that alter one's responsibilities? Even the most sensitive handling of the situation will be likely to create anxieties. Once the decision has been made that a referral is necessary, then telling the parent is much easier: a problem has been identified and a solution proposed. It is not so easy when the evidence is not clear and the feeling that all is not well is intuitive only. The dilemma is at what stage concern should be verbalized. It has been demonstrated in the literature (Marteau 1989, Skrabanek 1990) that significant psychological harm can occur through false-positive tests. Labelling a child as having slow cognitive development, for example, could impact on that child's future, particularly when starting school. The teaching staff may have low expectations of the child's ability. The health visitor may well keep the information confidential, but the client may be so worried that other family members or friends may be told. The parent may even tell other professionals what the health visitor has told them.

The Human Genome Project, currently being undertaken in several countries, including the UK, is providing data on genetic susceptibility to disease. When genetic monitoring is available, will pressure be put on 'at-risk' groups? Where a history exists of Huntington's chorea, will family members be coerced into taking the test? Will health visitors be encouraged to promote genetic screening in much the same way that they are encouraged to gain consent to immunizations? Which is worse, living with the possibility that you might get the disease, or living with the certain knowledge that you will? Knowledge of carrying the defective gene could lead to eradicating certain conditions within a couple of generations; however, the evidence is that the majority would prefer to live with the uncertainty. In a survey carried out in 1990 (Hatchwell 1992), most people (86%) would not take the test and 15% of those studied said that if the test was positive they would consider suicide. If mandatory genetic screening is introduced, there are considerable resource implications for provision of counselling and support. Health visitors already carry considerable caseloads; what will be the impact on health visiting practice of introducing genetic screening?

Where health screening is offered on a voluntary basis, or even implicitly suggested as beneficial, the uptake will be by self-selection. These individuals are therefore not a representative cross-section of the population and are likely to be of a higher socio-economic status, better educated and more health-conscious than non-participants. This raises the question of whether health screening is 'just' or 'fair'. Clearly, imposed screening procedures are unjust in that they take away an individual's autonomy.

Health screening contains many ethical dilemmas. The principle of justice is not adhered to, particularly when there is a bias towards self-selection, which excludes many within the population who are at risk. Beneficence is often outweighed by the harmful effects of false-positive results, which cause anxiety and fear. Certainly it can be argued that, where research has demonstrated that there is no suitable and successful treatment available, screening for disease is positively detrimental and gives longer 'sickness years'. There is also conflict in respecting the autonomy of the individual. It has been suggested that screening militates against respect and freedom of choice, thus reducing autonomy.

IMMUNIZATION AND VACCINATION

One of the most powerful weapons in preventing ill health and promoting health is vaccination against infectious diseases. Immunization meets utilitarian principles of creating the greatest good for the greatest number. The more children that are vaccinated, the greater the 'herd' immunity. That smallpox has been eradicated from the UK has been attributed to successful campaigns for vaccination in infancy. Therefore immunization is ethically beneficial – or is it?

Even smallpox efficacy is not totally supported by the facts. The Vaccination Act 1871 made smallpox vaccination compulsory, with over 90% vaccination rates achieved. Because of the strength of the anti-vaccination lobby the compulsory nature of the system was modified in 1898, when subsequent legislation allowed for a principle of conscientious objection, although parents had to appear before two justices or stipendiary magistrates and convince them of their belief that vaccination would be bad for their children's health. A further Act in 1907 relaxed the compulsory nature even further by making the parents' declaration before one magistrate or justice of the peace sufficient (Ottewill & Wall 1990). From 1905 to 1918 the rates of smallpox vaccination fell. One might expect that the incidence of smallpox cases would correspondingly rise, but this was not the case. The trend of reported cases was downwards; severe cases were few and the outbreaks that did occur were mainly due to imported cases that had managed to evade port sanitary authorities (Frazer 1950, cited in Ottewill & Wall 1990). It may well be that the fall in smallpox incidence had more to do with improved standards of hygiene and nutrition than smallpox vaccination. However, smallpox vaccination has historically been credited with eradication of the disease from Britain.

Thus vaccination was perceived as a beneficent intervention and opened the door for subsequent vaccines to be developed. Since smallpox vaccination was initiated, vaccination against other diseases followed. Diphtheria vaccination grew in importance during the 1940s and in 1946 the National Health Service Act repealed all previous legislation concerning vaccination and immunization. Compulsion was removed in respect of smallpox vaccination and vaccination against diphtheria was specifically included. Section 26 of the 1946 Act allowed local health authorities to make similar provisions against any other disease. Thus in 1955 tetanus and poliomyelitis were classified as immunizable diseases and in 1957 were joined by pertussis. Despite BCG being available in the 1940s and, considering the limited treatment options for tuberculosis at that time, it is surprising that it was not until 1956 that this vaccine was given to school children routinely.

All these diseases were life threatening and also had severe complications, leaving those affected with a range of disabilities (provided they survived). So one could argue that vaccination has been one of the most successful methods of preventing ill health since the Second World War. But since the 1950s vaccines have been developed for diseases in which, while unpleasant, the severe complications of death and disability are comparatively rare. If these vaccines were free from side effects then there would be little controversy, but unfortunately there are concerns that the vaccines themselves are not without risk. This raises the dilemma for many as to which carries the most benefit and which has the potential for most harm – a direct conflict between the principles of beneficence and non-maleficence. Should one consider the most beneficial outcome for society or the most beneficial outcome for the individual?

The measles vaccine was developed during the 1960s; rubella for 11- to 14-year-old girls followed from 1970. Since then the triple vaccine measles, mumps and rubella (MMR) has been developed and is routinely offered to children in their second year.

During the 1970s pertussis vaccine was suspected of causing brain damage in susceptible children. The media attention created a scare that resulted in a dramatic fall in vaccination rates for pertussis, with a corresponding rise in the incidence of whooping cough. Most of the evidence supporting the argument for brain damage was based on anecdotal case studies, according to Nicoll et al (1998). Nicoll et al cite a national study carried out by Miller et al (1993), which found that there was a temporal association with encephalopathy but that the risk of lasting damage was so rare as to be unquantifiable. It is interesting to note, however, that encephalopathy is still listed as a side effect of the pertussis vaccine in a table produced for the National Vaccine Injury Compensation Program (Health Resources and Service Administration 1997), which presumably means that vaccine-induced encephalopathy resulting in lasting brain damage is recognized in the USA if not in Britain.

Currently, there are concerns regarding the MMR vaccine; most recently the onset of autism has been attributed to this vaccine. Wakefield et al (1998) carried out a study of 12 children who had been vaccinated with MMR, of whom nine had been diagnosed as autistic. All 12 children had developed normally prior to having the MMR vaccine and subsequently all developed intestinal disorders. In eight of the cases the parents or the child's GP said that the changes in behaviour and health followed the MMR vaccination. Wakefield concedes that his research has failed to prove empirically that there is a link; however, he considers that there is sufficient evidence to justify an independent government review. Due to his concern that multi-component vaccines may overload the immune system of some infants, Wakefield also recommended that the vaccines should be given separately at yearly intervals. The media attention that followed the publication of this article in *The Lancet* resulted in such an increase in parents requesting the separate vaccines that supplies ran out.

Publication of this article released a storm of protest from the medical profession. Letters to the *British Medical Journal* in response to Wakefield's article in *The Lancet* pointed out the value of the vaccine. Young (1998) challenged the methodology of Wakefield et al's research: a cohort of only 12 subjects certainly raises questions about bias and validity. Caldwell (1998) considers that the MMR vaccine has prevented thousands of sick children, thus reducing GPs' workloads, reducing sleepless nights (the GPs', presumably!) and eliminating stress for parents. In a subsequent editorial in the *British Medical Journal*, Nicoll et al (1998) argue that over 600 000 British children receive MMR in their second year, and that since this is the age at which autism typically manifests itself it is likely that some cases will appear shortly after vaccination, and that this is a mere chance association and not a causal link. Kiln (1998) asks why the expert committee convened by the Medical Research Council to investigate Wakefield's findings failed to include GPs, health visitors and practice nurses, who have day-to-day experience of the MMR vaccines. Kiln states that what is required is straightforward figures to help parents understand why their child should have the vaccine. It has subsequently been found that contributors to the research study undertaken by Wakefield were the company producing single vaccination doses.

How can parents get accurate information? The medical profession takes a utilitarian stance and encourages immunization on the grounds of achieving herd immunity. What of other health professionals? In a study carried out in Leeds (Hatton 1990), an audit of the knowledge of health professionals (which included health visitors) of contraindications to the MMR vaccine was carried out. The results were somewhat alarming. Some health professionals, it appeared, would happily give the vaccine to children when it was contraindicated. Other health professionals were applying the contraindications of the pertussis vaccine to MMR and some would not give the vaccine even when there were no valid contraindications to its use. How can parents decide when there appears to be confusion and, it would appear, a lack of knowledge among those who should be well informed?

The debate continues despite the fact that the Government have gone to great lengths to publish detailed information about the efficacy of MMR (www.mmrthefacts.nhs.uk/).

Dyson (1995) argues that infectious diseases such as whooping cough have declined in the context of particular historical and social conditions and persist in the context of particular types of social inequality, and that the respective risks of the vaccine and the disease are still unresolved owing to methodological limitations of studies on both sides of the argument. Dyson also questions the questionable ethics of one-sided health campaigns. This is supported by a letter from a parent to the magazine *Health Matters*, who considers that the decision whether or not to vaccinate a child can only be made when all the information is made available, not just that supplied by the Health Education Authority (Easy 1995).

Sadly, information is difficult to come by: on searching the Internet it is clear that most anti-vaccination information comes from non-medical sources and as such is denigrated by

doctors and epidemiologists. Information from the medical profession highlights the rarity of suspected side effects and points out the benefits of the vaccine, putting the emphasis on the likelihood of increased death rates and other serious complications should parents stop having their children vaccinated. Begg et al (1998) provide a graph demonstrating how deaths from measles have decreased in the UK (as a result, of course, of increased vaccination rates), as opposed to Italy and France. Total death rates in other European countries may be affected by other socio-economic factors. The graph demonstrates that the death rate from measles fell from 4 during the period 1986–88 and 4 during 1989–91 to 2 for the period 1992–94 but no mention is made of adverse reactions to the vaccine. The Centers for Disease Control (January 1999) list the complications of measles: ear infection, pneumonia, seizures, brain damage and death, with no information as to the incidence of these. Similarly, for mumps the complications of ear infection, meningitis and painful swollen testicles are listed without incidence data. As one might expect from a service devoted to disease control, the benefits of the vaccine are emphasized. On discussing the risks of the vaccines, prevalence figures are provided for all the milder side effects, e.g. a fever of 103°F or higher in 5–15 per 100 doses, but for seizures, severe allergic reactions or coma only the comment that they are rare is made. Surely an official source should provide the actual incidence rates for the more serious side effects in order that parents may make a fully informed choice.

It appears that vaccination will create the most beneficial outcome for society as a whole but is it the most beneficial outcome for the individual? There is strong opposition from the medical fraternity to the idea that vaccines are dangerous, but it needs to be borne in mind that much of the outcry comes from public health physicians and epidemiologists, who are concerned with controlling epidemics of infectious disease. Calman on ITN News (1998) advocated that it is vital that parents continue to give their consent to vaccinate their children. Calman was the government's Chief Medical

Officer and had a wider brief: that of protecting society. No surprise then that he took the utilitarian standpoint of the greatest good for the greatest number and was prepared to risk what is considered to be a small minority of children. GPs receive remuneration for every child vaccinated at their practice; a considerable fall in vaccination uptake will essentially result in reduced income. This must be a consideration, however many altruistic reasons are given for encouraging parents into giving consent for vaccination. Pilgrim & Rogers (1995) argue that the financial inducements given to GPs to meet immunization targets have reinforced suppression of the right to parental dissent and that some families are being removed from GP lists in order to maintain target levels. In terms of financial gain, the pharmaceutical companies that produce these vaccines also have a vested interest in continuing their manufacture. If they could be proved to be safe, there would be no ethical dilemma about advocating their use, but there seems to be a coyness about revealing the actual incidence of brain damage resulting from vaccines.

If the various parts of Seedhouse's Ethical Grid (1988) are applied to the dilemma of vaccination, several conflicts appear. In the blue layer, health professionals cannot create or respect autonomy if they themselves lack sufficient information, and in any case the recipients are young children who are not able to make an informed choice for themselves. The medical profession would argue that they are serving needs first, but whose needs? The red or duty-based layer states, 'tell the truth', but what is the truth in respect of vaccines? Can the health visitor truthfully state that there are no risks from the MMR vaccination? Doctors would maintain that vaccination does the most positive good and that they are minimizing harm by reducing the incidence of these three diseases, but would the parent of a damaged child feel the same way? The consequentialist green layer would appear to support vaccination, but then it is the utilitarian layer of the grid. The only conflict could arise when there was an adverse reaction to MMR: then clearly the most beneficial outcome for the patient

could not be claimed. Consideration of the boxes in the black layer of practicality highlights the conflicts in using the grid. Disputed facts, the degree of certainty of the evidence on which action is taken, the effectiveness and efficacy of action and the risk all need to be taken into account.

Much of the information about brain damage is accused of being anecdotal, is reported by parents or other non-professionals, and therefore lacks scientific validity. If this is the case, then why does encephalopathy manifesting between 5 and 15 days following administration of the vaccine appear as a side effect not only of pertussis vaccine but also of MMR (Health Resources and Service Administration 1997)? Compensation is paid to parents in the USA if this is proved. It is difficult to believe that compensation would be paid out without sound empirical evidence. Is there any validity in Wakefield's (1998) claim that multi-component vaccines overload the immature immune system? Multi-component vaccines are popular with health officials because they require fewer clinic visits (Day 1998), thus saving costs. But if multi-component vaccines increase the risk of side effects, then, in the long term, separate vaccinations may be more cost effective by reducing side effects and encouraging increased immunization rates. What none of the debates in the literature seems to address is that measles vaccine was given on its own for many years before the MMR vaccine was developed. There was no public outcry about adverse reaction to immunization against measles before the triple vaccine was introduced. The other suspect vaccine, pertussis, is also given as part of a multi-component vaccine. Might Wakefield et al (1998) be right?

Pilgrim & Rogers (1995) consider that immunization policies are driven by propaganda that reviews advantages and disadvantages of vaccination or non-vaccination, and that this is deceitful and simplistic. Natural acquired immunity is better than artificially acquired immunity. How effective are these vaccines? How long will the protection last? If a child gets the disease as a young adult will the effects be worse? Will a vaccine-resistant strain develop? These are all questions that need to be addressed before full information can be given to parents. Seedhouse (1988) considers that creating and respecting autonomy is the core rationale behind health work and conveys the richest notion of health. A component of autonomy is the need for full information. How can autonomy be created or respected and a fully autonomous decision be made if some information is withheld? As Easy (1995) pointed out, since parents are asked to give consent to vaccination, they must also take full responsibility for the subsequent effects of that vaccination. One should not expect to take on responsibility without adequate knowledge. The current market-led health service places pressures on health professionals to pursue population targets (Pilgrim & Rogers 1995). This pressure on health professionals leads them into the dangerous moral minefield of failing to respect individual autonomy.

HEALTH PROMOTION VERSUS HEALTH EDUCATION

Health education and health promotion have often been taken to mean the same thing. Both are concerned with improving health status. However, health education is a term that has fallen out of favour, since it has gained the reputation of didactic instruction rather than the sharing of knowledge, thus empowering the individual to make more informed choices about their lifestyle. Although the words have changed, has this resulted in a change in the way the health professional approaches clients?

The recent emphasis on health promotion and teaching constantly raises questions about justifiable paternalism (Benjamin & Curtis 1992). Thomas & Wainwright (1996) suggest that the approach of many nurses to health promotion has tended to be either somewhat naïve or authoritarian and didactic, and that there has been little discussion in the nursing literature of ethical aspects of health promotion. Thomas & Wainwright also suggest that community nurses fall into two distinct groups in terms of their health promotion

interventions: health visitors take a deontological stance whereas district nurses tend to be utilitarian in their approach. This does not mean that health visitors are more parentalistic than district nurses, for both the main ethical theories have fostered this approach. Deontologists would maintain that it is your duty to behave in a certain manner – 'you ought to do this' (Tschudin & Marks-Maran 1993) – whereas teleologists would consider that you should consider the consequences of your actions. How many health visitors can honestly state that they have never used the phrases 'you ought to' or 'you should not'? How far should one go in trying to alter a client's way of living in the name of better health? What form should it take? Are exaggerated threats acceptable if nothing else proves effective? When information and advice are given, it is easy to imply that dire consequences will result if that advice is not followed. Because of the experience and knowledge held by the health professional, it is extremely difficult not to behave in a paternalist manner.

Benjamin & Curtis (1992) maintain that, in order to respect the client's personhood, health professionals must allow the client to express their views. They refer to this process as rational persuasion, i.e. appealing to another person's rational capacities in order to influence them into changing their behaviour, providing reasons and information for or against certain courses of action with a view to changing the person's beliefs without indulging in scare tactics. It is important that the person attempting to persuade recognizes that the person they are debating with is their equal as a person. It is extremely frustrating to observe clients indulging in risk-taking behaviour after advising them of the potential ill-health effects, but it is better by far to respect their autonomy than explicitly or implicitly to show disapproval of their behaviour, however subtly this is done.

Traditionally, health promotion aims at changing individual behaviour by increasing knowledge: this implies that people have a free choice and does not take into account socioeconomic factors. The previous government produced the document *The Health of the Nation*

(Department of Health 1992b) to prove their commitment to preventive medicine and promoting good health. In it they identified several areas of concern and recommended reduction of the incidence of these conditions by a certain period of time. They emphasized that health was the responsibility of the individual. This is classical victim blaming, taking the assumption that people are always responsible for their actions. Clarke (1999) warns that health professionals need to be critical of their approach to health promotion, especially with relation to the emphasis on individual responsibility. The *Health of the Nation* placed the onus on health professionals to meet these targets laid down by the government. How feasible was this?

Smoking is a good example of typical victim blaming and a perpetual bone of contention. Smokers are denigrated by society generally. Fears of the effects of passive smoking on non-smokers has increased intolerance of smokers. Although there are conflicts as to whether passive smoke is carcinogenic or not, cigarette smoke is unpleasant and irritant to others. Employers are liable under the Health and Safety at Work Act 1974 (HSC 1974) to provide a safe environment. This includes eliminating atmospheric pollutants, which includes cigarette smoke. Many employers are imposing non-smoking policies and places of entertainment are increasing the areas where smoking is not allowed. For non-smokers this is excellent and is a good example of when overruling the autonomy of individuals (the smokers) is justified under the principle of beneficence and utilitarian principles of the greatest good for the greatest number. What it does result in, however, is an increase in victim blaming. Smokers are perceived as weak willed, self-indulgent and feckless; after all, the effects of smoking have been well documented since the 1950s, haven't they? There have been instances of smokers being refused cardiovascular surgery. Whereas this can be justified on clinical and utilitarian grounds, the smoker feels victimized. There is a feeling that blame is being attributed to the individual. Health promotion activity is targeted at the smoker. Smoking is a pleasurable experience for those who smoke.

Of course it is – nicotine is an addictive substance. Smokers do not want to know about the ill-health effects. Smoking is associated with social activity, naughty but nice and, in the case of under-age smokers, there is the illicit thrill of indulging in a forbidden activity. Even those smokers who want to give up experience the greatest difficulty because they are addicted to the nicotine content. There is an acceptance that alcoholics are not to blame for their addiction, that drug addicts have been led astray by unscrupulous drug pushers, but it is not accepted that smokers are equally helpless in the throes of their particular addiction.

Health education campaigns have failed to affect the numbers of obese people in our society. There are ethical dilemmas in giving dietary advice, as in any aspect of health-promoting activity – that of coercion and manipulation by a paternalistic approach. A stock answer that is given time after time is that the health visitor should empower the client by providing knowledge and information. Sounds wonderful, does it not? But beware that the word 'empower' does not become a weasel word, overuse of which renders it meaningless.

The health visitor is ideally placed to encourage mothers to feed their children healthy choices, since they are available for advice on infant feeding very shortly after the mother comes home. If the advice given is successful and the baby thrives, then why are unhealthy choices given once the child is weaned? Why is the advice of the health visitor, so sought after when the child was an infant, ignored once solid foods are introduced? The lure of sweet, fatty convenience foods is too great, it would appear. Perhaps health visitors would be better advised to start a campaign to ban food advertising on television. Advice to individuals may be seen as interfering with individual autonomy, but reducing the number of advertisements could have a considerable impact on consumption of fattening goodies. Campaigning against food advertising would be the most beneficial outcome for society even if it were not the most beneficial outcome for a particular group (the food manufacturer). It would minimize harm by cutting down on obesity and do the most positive good by removing the temptation to snack between meals.

Much advice given regarding exercise is well founded and research based, but how ethical is it? Walking at least 15 minutes a day is commonly advocated as a way to keep healthy, lose weight and stay fit. In inner city areas, how ethical is it to encourage the daily walk, let alone jogging? The exercise may be beneficial but exercise increases the heart rate, which increases respiration and results in more air intake. Within cities and towns the air is contaminated by many pollutants. Fresh air has always been perceived as beneficial: grandmothers may talk their daughters into believing that the baby should spend part of every day in the open air. That's fine if you live in the comparative peace of a rural area or a nice suburb with large gardens and very little traffic pollution. If, on the other hand you happen to live within 500 metres of Spaghetti Junction in Birmingham, putting the baby outside is more likely to result in lead poisoning. Basic advice, such as the daily walk, is only ethically sound advice if you live in a pollution-free area.

CONCLUSION

There is a basic assumption made by health professionals that individuals have a choice about choosing a healthy or an unhealthy lifestyle. This assumption does not consider the political and social context in which we live and, without this consideration, health promotion goals may be unrealistic and thus unethical. Social scientists highlight social inequalities in health (Townsend & Davidson 1982) as having a major effect on the efficacy of health-promoting activities. However, little has been achieved in terms of redressing the balance. Achieving change is never easy, and the current government have recognized that their support is necessary if change is to be achieved. This has resulted in a plethora of publications and letters of guidance, many of which have been helpful in their approaches, and others simply add to the weight of paper needing to be read and absorbed. This has also led to criticism that the government is set to create a 'nanny state'. In other words, they're damned if they will and they're damned if they won't!

Currently, achieving improved health goals is left to health professionals. There are ethical dilemmas in attempting to promote health by improving activities without changing the socio-political climate. People do not always have a choice about where they live or where they work. Access to education is restricted for certain groups within our society. Empowering clients through health promotion should consider the ability of the client to benefit from that knowledge.

Chapter **13**

Nurse prescribing

Ann Clarridge

INTRODUCTION

One of the most important developments within community nursing practice has been the implementation of prescribing by health care professionals other than doctors or dentists. According to the Chief Nursing Officer, nurse prescribing is 'an essential skill of the future nurse and is an important component in the nurse's toolkit, vital to providing comprehensive care' (Mullally, Department of Health 2003d). After a cautious beginning the rate of progress has gathered momentum with a number of government policies that have encouraged and supported the implementation of nurse prescribing. *The NHS Plan* (Department of Health 2000c) and *Liberating the Talents* (Department of Health 2002b) are concerned with the development of nurses' roles and the use of their skills to improve the health of the population, with nurse prescribing as one of the 10 key roles within *The NHS Plan*.

This chapter looks at the role of the nurse prescriber and gives an outline of the historical background to its development. There is a discussion of the general principles of good practice in prescribing together with some of the challenges that the nurse prescriber will encounter. Some guidelines and suggestions are offered for consideration as to how such challenges may be met. There is a discussion of the accountability of nurses and the legal implications that need to be taken into account when prescribing. Finally, issues are raised relating to the further education and training and the professional development of nurses of the future who are likely to have access to a wider formulary for prescribing. Two case studies are used to illustrate some of the points in the discussions.

THE HISTORICAL CONTEXT

It is important to understand the development and history of nurse prescribing in order to gain an insight into the present situation (Baird 2003). A long and tortuous campaign was initiated by Julia Cumberlege in 1986, supported by many health care professionals, which resulted in legislation that permitted nurse prescribing finally reaching the statute book in early 1992. This statement does not, however, convey the extent of the contributions made by officials and activists at the Royal College of Nursing (RCN) nor the continuous publicity and lobbying by supporters within Parliament to bring about the success of placing nurse prescribing on the statute book (Sims 1999).

In 1986 it was suggested by Julia Cumberlege in the *Neighbourhood Nursing Review* (DHSS, 1986) that experienced district nurses working in the community were wasting their valuable time waiting outside GPs' doorways for prescriptions for clients whom they had already assessed and diagnosed without the involvement of the medical practitioner. The Cumberlege Report recommended that qualified community nurses should be able to prescribe from a limited formulary of medicines, appliances and dressings. Government response was to set up an advisory group under the leadership of Dr June Crown to review the necessary arrangements for nurses to be able to prescribe from a limited formulary. As Jones (1999) points out, it is interesting that the advisory group at that time did not limit their undertaking to a specific group, for example district nurses or health visitors, when considering whether community nurses should be able to prescribe. The recommendations from the Review (DHSS 1986) were further extended in the first *Crown Report* (Department of Health 1989b), which proposed that a limited list of items could be prescribed by nurses with a district nurse (DN) or health visitor (HV)

qualification. District nurses and health visitors were so designated since they were the only community nurses at that time with a recognized post-initial qualification. Furthermore, it was a way of limiting a proposed formulary to the specific needs of this group of nurses. However, Crown (Department of Health 1989b) did recognize that, in the future, it might be possible to extend the formulary and prescribing rights to other groups of nurses.

The intention was to implement the recommendations of the report as soon as the necessary legislation was in place but there was a delay arising from governmental concerns regarding the cost of prescribing by doctors (Baird 2003). It was recognized that district nurses and health visitors were wasting time waiting for GPs to endorse their prescribing decisions but it was difficult to quantify the costs involved. The money saved was not 'real money'; it was already within the National Health Service (NHS) budget. The cost–benefit analysis undertaken by Touche Ross (1991) was inconclusive in terms of estimating the true cost of prescribing but it did point out the savings in time for the clients and the practitioners. Despite government support and willingness for nurse prescribing there was an overriding concern at the steadily increasing NHS drugs bill which prevented the release of more money in an 'open-ended budget' to permit nurses to prescribe (Jones 1999, p. 12).

The United Kingdom Central Council and the National Boards developed a limited formulary of medicines, appliances and dressings and made recommendations to the government. It was this formulary that was used in the 1994 pilot sites selected to implement nurse prescribing by district nurses and health visitors. The eight sites were representative of the whole of England: four fund-holding general practices in the north and four in the south. The nurses in the pilot sites had either a district nurse or health visitor qualification and had completed the approved prescribing education and training prior to prescribing from the Nurse Prescribers' Formulary (NPF). The NPF comprised those items highlighted as being most useful for district nurses and health visitors and included such items as are used in the management of wounds, constipation, scabies and threadworms, head louse infections, urinary incontinence and mild to moderate pain.

In 1992 the English National Board for Nursing, Midwifery and Health Visiting (ENB) developed a short-course curriculum for the education and training of district nurses and health visitors. Successful completion of the course would qualify them as nurse prescribers. Students undertaking the course received an open learning pack 2 months before the commencement of the taught programme, with the expectation that they would engage in a self-assessment questionnaire. The focus of the open learning pack was to encourage students to identify their learning needs in relation to issues around prescribing, accountability and prescribing safely and effectively. The 2-day taught component of the programme developed these issues further and also included elements of basic pharmacology. However, as Banning (1999) suggests, undertaking this programme proved to be problematic for students: they were in full-time employment with little support and limited access to library facilities. In addition, many had not undertaken any formal studying for some years and found the course challenging. It is now the practice to incorporate the learning outcomes for the District Nurse and Health Visitor Prescribing Programme into the Specialist Practitioner Programme that has changed the nature of the qualification. District nurses and health visitors now only qualify as a Specialist Practitioner with successful completion of the prescribing component of the programme.

The evaluation of nurse prescribing undertaken in the eight pilot sites found that 'prescribing by nurses was considered to be an undoubted success' (Luker et al 1997b, p. 37), with benefits to clients, nurses and other health care professionals. In particular it was found that nurses, after appropriate education and training in nurse prescribing, were able to make prescribing decisions within their area of expertise. However, the evaluation raised the issue of the limited range of the NPF and the continuing dependence of district nurses and health visitors on their GPs for authorization of products not contained in the NPF (Luker et al 1997). On the strength of the very positive evaluation from the pilot sites it was subsequently agreed to 'roll out' the prescribing programme for all qualified district nurses and health visitors. On successful completion of the programme all district nurses and health visitors are now able to prescribe from the NPF. It had taken 12 years for Julia Cumberlege's recommendation to come into effect, for nurses to be able to prescribe in order to improve the care of clients in their own homes.

PRINCIPLES OF GOOD PRESCRIBING – THE SEVEN STEPS

Writing a prescription starts a process that will have an impact upon the client, the carer, the prescriber and the NHS in a number of different and important ways. The success of the process is entirely dependent on the decision made by the prescriber and the factors that have informed that decision.

Exercise: Consider a decision you have made recently, perhaps going on holiday. What are the questions that you have asked yourself? What steps have you taken to arrive at your decision?

Where shall I go, what shall I do, what do I need to think about, what factors do I need to take into account? These and many others might lead you to make a final decision regarding your holiday.

This is how we all make most of our everyday decisions but without necessarily being aware of the process we are using. However, the decisions made as a prescribing nurse must be taken with a full awareness of all the numerous and complex factors involved in safe, effective and appropriate prescribing.

The National Prescribing Centre (1999) (www.npc.co.uk) produced a series of *Prescribing Nurse Bulletins* as teaching and learning guides to aid the implementation of nurse prescribing for district nurses and health visitors. The first of these bulletins provides guidelines to assist with decision making and is entitled 'Signposts for prescribing nurses – general principles of good prescribing'. It outlines seven principles of good prescribing in a step-by-step approach (National Prescribing Centre 1999) that will be explored in more detail below. The seven principles or steps provide a framework to structure the decisions that need to be made when prescribing. They are:

- consider the client
- which strategy
- consider the choice of product
- negotiate a 'contract'
- review
- record keeping
- reflect.

ILLUSTRATIVE CASE STUDIES

Case study one: You are doing a home visit to Lucy and her son Raj who is 3 years of age and attends the local nursery. Lucy is upset as she has received a letter from the nursery class leader to say that several of the children have head lice and that all parents are requested to check their children's hair weekly. She is worried because Raj has been scratching his head for the last few days.

Case study two: Jane, who is a single parent, brings her baby Tom, aged 6 months, to the child health clinic. You observe that Tom has very dry, flaky skin on his abdomen and face. When asked, Jane reports that she has been applying baby oil to his skin for the last 2 weeks as advised by her mother but there has been no improvement. She wonders whether you can suggest any other treatment.

Step 1 – Considering the client

Children or their parents are individuals with specific needs, and in order to make a diagnosis and subsequent decision regarding their care the prescribing nurse needs information, some of it in depth. Much is dependent on good communication skills and the ability of the nurse to elicit information during the consultation process, including listening to the client's viewpoint. There are a number of consultation

models in use. The most successful are drawn from general practice where the interaction and decision-making between client and health care professional is reduced to a limited period of time (Baird 2004). Three different models are outlined here for consideration:

- Gask and Usherwood (2002) identified a 'three-function' model that includes building the relationship with the client, collecting data and finally agreeing a management plan. Within these three functions is the recognition that clients are active participants in the interaction as well as potentially passive recipients of professional care.

- Byrne and Long (1976) identified six phases to the consultation: establishing a relationship with the client, discovering the reason for the client's visit, conducting a verbal or physical examination or both, consideration of the condition, the need for further treatment or further investigations, ending the consultation with a final stage: the 'parting shot' when the client reveals the real reason for the consultation.

- Neighbour (1987) describes the consultation between client and the professional as a journey with 'checkpoints' along the way, connecting, summarizing, handing over, safety netting and housekeeping (Baird 2004).

In addition, a helpful mnemonic used by pharmacists for decision-making regarding 'over the counter' (OTC) therapeutics is 'WWHAM': who is the client; what are the symptoms; how long have the symptoms been present; action taken so far and by whom; medication – any other prescribed medicine and OTC (NPC 1999).

It is a matter of personal preference as to which model is followed. What is important is that the approach should be systematic, thus ensuring that all relevant information is gathered to help the professional in the diagnosis and decision-making process. The prescribing nurse must keep in mind at all times that prescribing should be safe, effective and appropriate. It is also important to gather information regarding the clients' ability to access relevant services and their social networks.

Mention is made here of some of the areas of information that should be recorded.

- The client's current and anticipated health status including diet, fluid intake, psychological and social well-being, and their ability to access social networks.
- The client's financial status.

The relevance of this information relates to the professional's decision whether to issue a prescription or whether to obtain OTC medicines that might prove more cost effective.

- The client's medication history.

It is essential that it should include whether the client is taking OTCs or alternative therapies such as herbal remedies or homoeopathic remedies such as the use of tea tree oil for the removal of head lice and which might involve contraindications. Any identified medicine allergy must also be included in the client's medical records.

There are several issues here that need to be considered further as they are vital to ensure that prescribing is safe, effective and appropriate. Most failures occur in the therapeutic process because not enough attention has been given to what else is happening when the prescription is written. Good prescribing practice should take into account any other medication the client may be taking. This may be prescribed medication, OTC medicines and herbal or complementary medicines. For example, Lucy may have considered using 'tea tree oil' as a treatment for removal of head lice. Alternatively, consider the prescribing of paracetamol for a child. Many OTC medicines containing paracetamol can be purchased from a corner shop or supermarket. Parents are not likely to be aware that if taken with prescribed paracetamol there is the risk of overdose occurring.

Herbal medicines are not subject to the same rigorous legislation that applies to licensed medicines. It is easy to forget that many herbal medicines often interact with drugs. For example, St John's wort binds to microsomal liver enzymes involved in the metabolic process. The effect of its presence could cause a host of commonly prescribed drugs at standard doses to reach toxic levels or alternatively to be ineffective. Even foods can cause problems for the unwary. Grapefruit or cranberry juice can also interfere with drug metabolism in certain cases.

Step 2 – Selecting a strategy

Selecting an appropriate strategy is not straightforward and depends on a variety of factors. In the past it was considered that making a diagnosis of a client's condition and selecting an appropriate strategy was solely the domain of the doctor. However, in a small study undertaken by Baird (2001) it was found that the nurses were involved in diagnosis on a day-to-day basis but would not diagnose out of their area of expertise. Also they were clearly aware of their accountability (Baird 2001).

The first concern of the nurse prescriber must be whether the assessment of the client on the basis of information gained from the consultation is sufficient to make a diagnosis. At this stage it might be appropriate to refer the client to another professional because the required medication is not available to a nurse prescriber to prescribe, or because the situation does not fall within the nurse's area of expertise.

Another concern for the nurse prescriber is to be aware of the client's non-verbal communication as well as the verbal comments when considering which strategy to adopt. Clients may find it difficult to express themselves and their true concerns; what clients say may not be confirmed by how they are behaving. Lack of awareness could lead to inappropriate or unsafe prescribing. Research undertaken by Stewart looking at the relationship between consultation and outcomes of care found that effective communication between the professional, in this case the doctor, and the client leads to improved outcomes for many common diseases (Stewart 1995).

In addition, the nurse prescriber needs to appreciate that perceptions of what it means to be healthy are not the same as they were. Changes in society and health care have meant that people have different ideas about health and may have very different expectations of the health care professional. The emphasis of health care has shifted to encourage individuals to take preventive action and avoid risks to health rather than adopt a reactive approach when problems arise (Gask & Usherwood 2002). It might be that the client requires health advice, dietary or lifestyle advice and does not require a prescription.

The nurse prescriber must be very clear about who the prescription is intended for. There might be expectations by the client that other members of the family can be prescribed for in their absence. However, a nurse must not prescribe without undertaking a full assessment of the client: to prescribe for other family members without seeing them is not within the scope of professional practice.

> Reference case study one: While Raj will be prescribed a suitable product if a live head louse is found, Lucy might expect to receive a prescription for children in the family other than Raj.

The nurse prescriber must also be aware that a client may wish to receive a prescription for some reason other than to gain treatment for the stated complaint. Alternatively, the client may be seeking help for another issue but uses the request for a prescription as a means of gaining attention: the 'parting shot'.

Step 3 – Choosing a product

The primary consideration when choosing a product is its clinical effectiveness. One of the key government directives enshrined in the documents *A First Class Service* (Department of Health 1998a) and the *NHS Plan* (Department of Health 2000c) is the need for quality and clinical effectiveness in the NHS. Clinical effectiveness is about 'doing the right thing, in the right way, and at the right time, for the right client' (RCN 1996). In the context of prescribing a medication for a client it means the extent to which a specified clinical intervention does what it is intended to do: maintain and improve health and secure the greatest possible health gain from the available resources. When considering a product or item to prescribe, another helpful

mnemonic is EASE (NPC 1999): is the product effective, appropriate, safe and cost effective?

The dilemma for practitioners is how to ensure that practice is both clinically appropriate and effective. They must be prepared to be self-critical and consider a number of questions that can help to clarify the issues involved in ensuring clinical effectiveness within practice generally and prescribing in particular. It is important for the practitioner to focus on particular aspects of day-to-day care and to question whether practice is maintaining traditional methods and ideas or is based upon sound evidence. The practitioner should be prepared to question the current status of practice: Is it up to date? Is it regularly evaluated and audited? Perhaps more difficult for the practitioner to evaluate is the evidence gained from research regarding the effectiveness and benefit to clients. Was the research thorough and was it subjected to a systematic review?

There are a number of reference sources that practitioners can go to when seeking the information they need to help them make informed choices. The government has promoted clinical effectiveness through the development of NHS frameworks, the formation of the National Institute of Clinical Excellence and the Commission for Health Improvement. There are guidelines and protocols for particular diseases that have been developed on the basis of evidence of effectiveness as assessed following randomized controlled trials, meta-analyses and systematic reviews (Starey 2003). Professional journals that have been reviewed by practising peers also offer a more readily available source of information that can be of practical use. Nevertheless, it must be stressed that all data should be approached with a critical mind.

When considering the appropriateness of treatment it is important to be aware of any contraindications that might exist. There might be other conditions present that could include pregnancy, renal or hepatic impairment or the potential for drug interaction. Special consideration needs to be given when prescribing to some particular groups of clients, such as the very young or older people. In these cases factors relating to drug absorption and metabolism come into play.

Reference case study one: How to treat
Raj provides an instance of the effect of
contraindications on choosing a product. It
illustrates the kind of information that the
practitioner needs to have available to be
able to prescribe appropriately. The prescriber
needs to know that there are a number of
contraindications regarding the use of
insecticides for head lice. For example,
phenothrin is not recommended in severe
eczema or asthma. There is limited good-quality
published evidence on the treatment of head
lice and the policy of rotating insecticides on
a regular basis is no longer recommended.
The current approach taken to manage the
treatment of head lice is to use a 'mosaic' of
treatments (Boardman 1999). This involves the
use of a particular insecticide initially, followed
by a second application. If at the follow-up
assessment live lice are still visible, then a
different insecticide should be prescribed
(Courtney & Butler 1999).

Reference case study two: Water-based
emollients may not be preferable where the
skin is broken. Additionally, some people are
sensitive to emollients that contain excipients
such as lanolin. (For further information
regarding contraindications refer to the BNF.)

Safety of prescribing is a critical issue since all
drugs have the potential for undesired side
effects or adverse drug reactions (ADRs). Prescribers must know where in the British National
Formulary they can find all relevant information.
There are also a number of guiding general principles with regard to avoiding ADRs. These are:

- Use as few concurrent drugs as possible.
- Use the lowest effective doses.
- Check if the client is pregnant or breast-
  feeding.
- Is the client at either extreme of age?
- Do you know of all the drugs used by the
  client?
- Check for OTC drugs.
- Check for previous adverse drug reactions
  (NPC 1999).

It should also be noted that all ADRs must
be reported using the Yellow Card system.

There are two other important factors for the
prescriber to take into account when considering safety and effectiveness: the pathophysiology of the condition to be treated and the mode
of action of the drug. Pathophysiology is the
characteristic of a disorder and how it relates
to our physiology; what causes it and what
changes take place in the body; how it manifests and why. Finally, of course, what is the
prognosis and why? This is vital information
since it helps the prescriber to make an informed
choice and allows information to be confidently
conveyed to the client, thus improving concordance. As regards the mode of action of a drug,
it should be inconceivable that the prescriber
when considering the use of a particular treatment would not have some idea as to how it
works. Knowledge of how drugs work enables
the prescribers to build a skill base from which
they can spot a potential problem with an interaction or detect the worsening of an unrelated
concomitant illness.

An example would be the prescribing of
aspirin as an analgesic. Would it be prudent to
prescribe if the client reports an episode of bron-
chospasm after self-medicating with ibuprofen?
The point here is that the prescriber should be
aware that both drugs work essentially in the
same way and adverse events may well be
common to both.

The cost-effectiveness of treatment also has
to be taken into account. Many items can be
purchased over the counter by clients and may
cost less than a prescription charge, which could
be relevant bearing in mind the financial status
of some clients. In the interests of economy for
the NHS, practitioners are encouraged when
prescribing a drug to use its generic name in
order to minimize the cost. This does not apply
to the prescribing of dressings and appliances.
The need for Primary Care Trusts to manage
their own prescribing has led to the considerable
development of local prescribing formularies.
The aim is that these formularies should become
standardized for different health care settings
and thus ensure that prescribing is rational,
cost effective and evidence based (NPC 2001).
Therefore it is important that all prescribers
should know the formulary that is indicated

for use within their employing Primary Care Trust.

Step 4 – Negotiating a contract

The importance of client-centred care within a partnership approach to care is at the heart of government policy and is emphasized in *The NHS Plan* (Department of Health 2000c). According to statistics, around 70% of the UK population are on a prescribed or OTC medication at any one time (Office of National Statistics 1997) but as many as 30–45% of the people on long-term prescribed treatment do not get their repeat prescriptions dispensed (Schering 1987, in Tsoneva 2004), which gives cause for concern. Research undertaken by Roter et al (1998) found that clients' concordance with treatment would be improved if the management plan had been negotiated jointly (Gask & Usherwood 2002).

Concordance refers to the outcome of the consultation process between the client and the health care professional. It is the agreement 'reached after negotiation that takes account of the wishes and beliefs of the client in determining whether, when and how their medicine is taken' (Bond 2003, p. 496). The key characteristics of concordance are: the sharing of power in the professional–client interaction, the valuing of clients' perspectives, the acknowledgement of clients' expertise in their experience of illness and response to treatment, and the inclusion of both clients' and professionals' views in the decision-making process (Weiss & Britten 2003). When concordance is achieved the degree of clients' satisfaction with care is enhanced together with a greater knowledge and understanding of their own condition and treatment. Furthermore, they suggest that where there is such concordance there will be fewer medication-related problems, fewer drug administration errors and less drug wastage.

A qualitative study of children's perceptions and attitudes to health, disease and drug use found that when seeking to initiate concordance with a child it is important to include that child in the decision-making (Sanz 2003). The best approach to illness is more than finding the best 'technical solution, but also how to live with it, in terms of the mind, the heart, the soul, and the psyche' (Sanz 2003, p. 860). Health visitors might find this philosophy a valuable addition to their approach since a significant area of their practice is with families with young children.

Successful concordance is about stating the risks and benefits of treatment, knowledge of what is being prescribed, why and how it will work, giving accurate, relevant and accessible information and above all listening to what the client has to say (Murphy & Tallis 2003). Therefore, to achieve a successful outcome for both client and practitioner it is critical that any prescribing decision is made in partnership with the client and that any potential problems are fully explored. According to Boardman (1998) it is essential that the client is involved in choosing the product. For instance, in the case of prescribing an emollient for Tom, while the choice should be for the least expensive one it should also be the one most acceptable to the client, or carer in the case of a young child, that will be used willingly on a regular basis (Boardman 1998, p. 46). In this way it is more likely that concordance will be achieved. Clients or carers will feel more involved and have a greater understanding of the information being given to them.

An important aspect of the prescribing process that should be taken into account is the attitude of clients towards illness, their individual beliefs and behaviours regarding medication. A client's acceptance of the prescribed medication is vital to the final outcome. Emollients provide a prime example of the way a client might be affected regarding the efficacy of a product. There is a vast range of emollients available and they vary considerably in their properties. Some will be greasier and may mark clothing and others will be absorbed rapidly into the skin. However, there are many more factors that will affect how the emollient is received by the client and this will affect concordance. In the final analysis, what one person finds pleasing and acceptable another will discard as useless, so it is important to encourage the client to try several different preparations to find which one suits them. Of course, there are one or two rules of play that help in the decision-making process: dry and thickened skin often responds better to greasy barrier preparations rather than to a water-based emollient. The point here is that the client should have a full explanation in order to make an informed choice.

> Reference case studies: For both Raj and Tom there would need to be a thorough discussion with both mothers so that informed choices could be made regarding treatment. Additionally, in the case of Tom, his mother is aware of the aspects of safety when bathing Tom, and use of an emollient in the bath may cause slipping.

An essential part of the prescribing process is that the client should have understood the information being given. Within the *Code of Professional Conduct* (NMC 2002a) nurses are held accountable for their actions and this includes ensuring that any information given to a client is clearly understood. The client's use and understanding of spoken English or the written form might be a factor to be taken into account. The client must be clear about a number of points: the dose of the drug to take and how to take it, over how long a period, what the prescriptions are for it and if there are likely to be any side effects (NPC 1999). For example, the instructions for a course of treatment for head lice for Raj are very specific and would need to be followed precisely in order to ensure treatment effectiveness. With regard to the use of an emollient for Tom, it would be important that a correct diagnosis had been made so that the appropriate treatment could be prescribed. In any skin condition, if there is a possibility of an additional infection it would need to be correctly diagnosed, particularly if there were an open wound. An adverse effect might occur as a result of the increase of absorption of the drug applied (Courtney & Butler 1999). Generally however, emollients are safe to use unless the client is sensitive to the constituents in the preparation, for example, lanolin (Courtney & Butler 1999). The issue of accountability will be discussed in more detail later in the chapter.

As part of negotiating the contract it is important that the client, or carer in the case of a young child, should know the procedure for contacting the health care professional in the case of a reaction or problem regarding the medication.

Step 5 – Reviewing the situation

The review has its place in the process of prescribing by providing an opportunity to establish whether prescribed treatment is effective, safe and acceptable (NPC 1999). The importance of the review is that it offers a way to ensure continuity of care, to repeat a prescription for ongoing care if appropriate, to consider an alternative treatment or to refer the client to another professional. It is also the time when problems emerge if the treatment is not having the desired effect. This could well be despite all the information that will have been discussed and established by client and nurse at the initial assessment regarding what to do and who to contact in the event of an adverse reaction. The reviewing process carried out on a regular basis by health professionals presents a valuable opportunity to further develop the client/professional relationship. Luker et al (1998) found that a number of clients raised the issues of continuity of care and a stable relationship as being important and advantageous when the nurse prescriber was involved. The long-term relationship that develops between the health visitor and the family was seen as a 'good thing' because the clients felt able to confide more in the health visitor regarding the children and their problems.

Step 6 – Keeping a record

The keeping of records is an integral part of nursing and midwifery practice and should not be regarded as 'an optional extra' to be completed as and when it is convenient to do so (NMC 2002b). Good record keeping is essential to protect the welfare of the client. It promotes high standards of care through accurate accounts of treatment and its effectiveness. It also ensures continuity of care by making available all necessary information to each professional involved (NMC 2002b). Furthermore, there are legal implications for keeping good records, particularly in relation to prescribing. Records that refer to a client's care may be required as evidence in a court of law in a case of negligence or by the Professional Conduct Committee (NMC 2002b) in the case of a complaint, therefore, it is critical that records should contain a full account of all relevant information.

There are some key principles that underpin what constitutes a good record and its contents: a record should be factual, should be accurate, clearly written without abbreviations, and should be dated and signed. It should include a full account of the initial assessment, all pertinent information obtained from the client, the measures taken, which should include any prescription of medication together, with specific instructions to the client regarding its administration and, finally, the review of the client. It is essential that all treatment prescribed by nurse prescribers should be included in the client's records. Where there are different practices and procedures in place to meet the local needs of practitioners it is the prescriber's responsibility to know what these are and to adhere to them.

The introduction of IT into general practice has resulted in the use of computer-held records and computer-generated prescriptions. For those nurse prescribers who are beginning to make use of them it is important to remember that the same principles of good record keeping apply and that it is their responsibility to follow local policies and procedures. For further information see NMC Guidelines for Records and Record Keeping (April 2002b).

The Crown Report (Department of Health 1989b), Sections 14 and 19, emphasizes the importance of shared information and its communication between involved professionals by means of clients' records.

> Good communication between health professionals and clients, and between different professionals, is essential for high quality care. All health professionals empowered to prescribe for a client should have access to the relevant client records.
>
> Clients' personal record cards showing the timing and dosage of all medication, and other relevant information, should be completed by each professional who prescribes for the clients and updated to show any changes. They should be available to doctors and nurses treating the client, and to pharmacists issuing medicines. Client-held records should be used wherever possible. (Department of Health 1989b)

The Nursing and Midwifery Council Guidelines for Records and Record Keeping (NMC 2002b) emphasizes the need for a professional standard of record keeping. It clearly states that it is part of the health practitioner's responsibility to maintain up-to-date, accurate records of all client–professional interactions. Maintaining records at an acceptable professional standard together with competent safe practice should 'place the health professional in the position of being able to refute any criticism effectively' Preece (2002, p. 42).

Step 7 – Time for reflection

Reflection is an important component of professional practice in order to maintain knowledge and competence in practice. It will also improve practice through identification of areas for further development. In particular, reflection can highlight lack of knowledge and be used as a strategy for maintaining prescribing competence, which is every nurse's responsibility under the Code of Professional Conduct (NMC 2002a). There are many models of reflection and it will be for nurse prescribers to identify and use the one that is most appropriate for their needs.

All health care professionals have a responsibility to work within a framework of clinical governance (Department of Health 1998a). At the same time it is essential that every organization should have a 'coherent education and development strategy' within the clinical governance agenda that is visible and understood by all members of the workforce (Basford 2003, pp. 40–45). As part of the NHS workforce it is right that nurse prescribers should be supported in their new role by the organization. However, it is also the prescriber's responsibility to ensure that they access those structures, such as clinical supervision, that are put in place for their professional support by the organization. A small-scale study was carried out to explore the 'lived experience' of nurse prescribers in maintaining competency for practice. It was found that workplace mentoring and support were important factors in the maintenance of nurse prescribing competence (Basford 2003). Winstanley (2000) identified specific goals for successful clinical supervision: to expand the practitioner's knowledge base, to assist in developing clinical proficiency and to develop autonomy and self-esteem. Nevertheless, clinical supervision represents only part of the framework for maintaining competency.

There is a need for support mechanisms that are specifically aimed at helping practitioners through the transition to their new and demanding role as prescribers. The provision of a forum where prescribing practitioners could come together to address problems and concerns relating to their prescribing role would be of great value. An aim of the forum might be to include opportunities to discuss critical incidents, to identify further training needs, to share and debate local and specific concerns, to consider national prescribing issues, and to devise and implement local guidelines and policies relevant to their area of practice (Collins & George 2003). Such a forum would not only provide support for prescribers but would also enable them to be proactive in identifying relevant additions to the limited formularies at present available to health visitors and district nurses.

In a consideration of the demands associated with achieving and maintaining competency Basford (2003) suggested that there are three strands: professional competency, occupational competency and behavioural competency. Professional competence is achieved by undertaking an educational programme that is governed by statutory legislation and regulations through the relevant professional body. Occupational competence is predetermined by criteria or benchmarks against which performance can be assessed in a detailed manner (Basford 2003). Behavioural competency is attained when the practitioner works within a 'framework of moral obligation' demonstrating evidence-based knowledge and a range of skills, motives and personal traits (NPC 2001). To assist nurse prescribers the NPC have issued an outline framework of competencies that relate to prescribing practice and this provides a reference when determining their own levels of competency (NPC 2001). In the research undertaken to evaluate the eight nurse-prescribing pilot sites reference was made in particular to the nurses' prescribing behaviour. It was found that nurses would only prescribe products of which they had knowledge, and that they were able to distinguish and discriminate against those that were outside their area of expertise and competence (Luker 1997). Basford (2003) concluded that while some nurses were aware of the need to maintain competence, others were not. These were generally nurses who perceived prescribing as a 'chore' rather than as a task they would choose to undertake.

Crucial to prescribing, however, is the need to receive adequate and appropriate education to achieve safe, competent practice. At the same time it is of paramount importance that practitioners maintain their competence throughout their professional careers to ensure the principles of clinical governance. The delivery of high-quality health care based on the best available evidence is a key aspect of the government's modernization agenda (Department of Health 2002b) as well as being part of professional accountability.

ACCOUNTABILITY

Accountability in prescribing, as in other nursing practice, means that the nurse prescriber is answerable to the client and also to the employing organizations, colleagues, the NMC and the law. Nurse prescribing is a new skill and as it is incorporated into health visiting and nursing practice so the scope and range of the professional responsibility and accountability for their actions and practice is extended (Groves 2002). A qualified nurse prescriber will be eligible to make a prescribing decision and will therefore be both legally and professionally accountable for all aspects of the decision-making process. This process encompasses the initial consultation, the advice given to the client or carer and the review of the client to ensure treatment is effective. The nurse prescriber is accountable for the information given to the client or carer regarding the administration of the medication. The Code of Professional Conduct (NMC 2002a) sets the standard of criteria for good nursing practice against which any allegations of misconduct would be measured. It clearly states that 'as a registered nurse, midwife or health visitor you are personally accountable for your practice'. Thus, accountability must be seen in terms of respect for the client as an individual, informed consent, confidentiality, cooperation with other professionals, the maintenance of professional knowledge and competence, and finally the identification and minimizing of risk to clients and their carers (NMC 2002a). Fundamental to nurse prescribing is the decision-making process, and nurse prescribers are individually accountable for their decisions and for their practice. By adhering to the Code of Professional Conduct (NMC 2002a) in their practice nurse prescribers will ensure that their decisions will uphold the ethical principles of autonomy, respect for autonomy, beneficence (to do good), non-maleficence (to do no harm) and justice.

THE NURSE PRESCRIBER AND THE LAW

The legal aspects of nurse prescribing are different from any other areas of clinical practice because of the detailed legislation relating to medicines. The Medicine Act 1968 is the primary legislation that sets out the exact details regarding the 'manufacture, testing, research, distribution, sale, supply and administration of drugs' (Caulfield 2004, p. 20). Deviation or misinterpretation of any part of the rules enshrined within the Act will result potentially in committing a criminal offence. Since nurses were not allowed to prescribe under the Medicine Act there was a need for new legislation. The Medicines Products: Prescribing by Nurses etc. Act (Department of Health 1992a) permitted nurses to prescribe from the Nurse Prescribers' Formulary (NPF).

This Act was limited to district nurses and health visitors only but further legislative changes under the Health and Social Care Act 2001 have since provided a legislative framework for a new structure for statutory prescribing. It allows nurses to prescribe from an Extended Nurse Prescribers' Formulary, within certain clinical conditions, as 'Independent prescribers'. It also allows access to the whole of the BNF by nurses as 'Supplementary Prescribers' but within very clear guidelines and criteria (Department of Health 2003d). These guidelines set out in precise terms what the legislation means for nurses acting appropriately as part of their professional duties.

Preece (2002) is of the opinion that nurses have a legal accountability to the courts in both criminal and in civil law and that they also have 'contractual accountability to their employer' (Preece 2002, p. 36). It is imperative that nurse prescribers are aware of the other legal issues relating to practice generally and prescribing specifically: consent, record keeping, vicarious liability and product liability. Nurse prescribers must ensure that they practice within the scope designated for health visitors and district nurses. For those nurses who have undertaken further education and training in prescribing, their scope of practice is either the Extended Nurse Prescribers' Formulary or the BNF depending on their qualification as Extended Nurse Prescriber and/or Supplementary Prescriber. Failure to practise within their scope will result in an infringement of the Medicines Act and will be seen as a criminal offence (Preece 2002). The more likely event, however, is that a nurse might be facing a case of negligence and would be held accountable to the civil courts. The principles of civil law to which nurse prescribers must adhere are that professionals will practise to a reasonable standard and must not act outside their competence. Thus the standard applying to a nurse prescriber would be the same as that applicable to a doctor prescribing medication (Preece 2002).

In a case of negligence the client would be seeking compensation for the injury they have received. The law will decide who was responsible for causing the harm by asking certain questions of the nurse prescriber related to a duty of care (Caulfield 2004a).

Consent is a complex issue and is based upon the understanding that a client is not obliged to receive treatment if they do not wish to or agree to (Preece 2002). There are a number of types of consent and each one is valid in law: implied consent, oral and written consent. Clearly, to have written consent is the most advantageous option. The important issue for nurse prescribers is to ensure that the client and the carer, where appropriate, really do understand the information and instructions being given to them. 'Safety-netting' is an important stage in the consultation process and refers to checking that clients know and understand what the treatment is for, how it will work and any risks or possible adverse reactions. The client also needs to be clear about what to do in the case of any of those occurring (Neighbour 1987).

Children are judged to be competent to consent to treatment if 'they are mature and capable of understanding the situation' and this principle is emphasized within the Children Act 1989. The phrase a 'Gillick-competent child' previously used in any case should be replaced by the phrase 'a child competent according to Lord Fraser Guidelines' (Dimond 2005, p. 328).

Vicarious liability gives clinical staff indemnity 'in respect of their NHS duties by their employing authority' (Preece 2002, p. 43). However, nurse prescribers must accept responsibility for acting within their employment contract and job description and in accordance with their employers' policies and procedures. It is advisable that all nurses ensure that they have professional indemnity cover in place. According to Caulfield (2004b) the main professional organizations, such as the Royal College of Nursing, the Community and District Nurse Association and the Community Practitioner and Health Visitor Association, provide indemnity as part of the membership fee. Additionally the Medical Defence Union provides indemnity with respect to professional practice and especially for those involved in the practice of prescribing.

Contractual law will be concerned with the detail of individual contracts of employment.

Thus it is the responsibility of nurse prescribers to ensure that the relevant qualification is within their employment contract and job description. It must be stressed that with regard to contractual law it is critical that practitioners adhere to all policies and procedures.

EDUCATION AND TRAINING

The present education and training for district nurses and health visitors is through the specialist practitioner programme, which incorporates the nurse-prescribing curriculum approved by the NMC. The structure, content and standard of the curricula are validated and regularly monitored for quality by the NMC. All specialist practitioner programmes have specific outcomes and competencies for their respective disciplines and include competencies for prescribing. In this way, specialist practitioners on successful completion of the course with either the district nurse or health visiting qualification can be deemed both professionally and occupationally competent in prescribing from the NPF.

CHANGING AGENDA IN PRESCRIBING PRACTICE

Since the implementation of the Medicines Products: Prescribing by Nurses etc., Act 1992 allowing nurses to prescribe, the development of prescribing professionals other than doctors and dentists has been significant. There are now a further two categories of prescriber to add to the independent prescribing of district nurses and health visitors: Extended Nurse Prescribers (ENP) and Supplementary Prescribers (SP). Additionally, Section 63 of the Health and Social Care Act 2001 provides for a new group of professionals including pharmacists.

Extended nurse prescribing is an extension of independent prescribing and enables nurses to prescribe from a wider range of prescription only medicines as well as pharmacy and general sales list treatments, within a specified range of therapeutic areas. The full list of conditions and drugs available to the ENP is in the British National Formulary.

Supplementary prescribing is defined as 'a voluntary partnership between an independent prescriber (doctor or dentist) and a supplementary prescriber to implement a client-specific clinical management plan (CMP) and with the clients' agreement' (Department of Health 2003d). There are no legal restrictions on the clinical conditions that may be treated under supplementary prescribing. Supplementary prescribing is most appropriate for the ongoing care of clients with chronic diseases such as diabetes, asthma or Parkinson's disease.

Both extended nurse prescribing and supplementary prescribing require additional education and training, and practitioners must have their qualification recorded by their appropriate professional body: the Nursing and Midwifery Council for nurses and the Royal Pharmaceutical Society of Great Britain for pharmacists.

Supplementary prescribing is to be extended to allied health professionals and it is also likely that other health professionals will access independent prescribing at some future date. The possible result of the different forms and categories of prescribing is likely to be confusing for both clients and health care professionals. It is also likely that dispensing pharmacists may be unclear about the type of prescribing authority held by the prescriber, thus potentially undermining the client's confidence in the prescriber (Baird 2003).

CONCLUSION

Clearly prescribing is an essential skill of the future nurse, but prescribing is not without risks, and nurses and pharmacists and other allied health professionals who undertake this new role must 'remain alert' to the limits of their scope of professional practice and ensure that they remain within their competency. However, the benefits for clients are recognized, which is a key government aim within the *NHS Plan*, and perhaps most specifically in the extent of the client/professional relationship and the effect of this on client concordance and, ultimately, the cost of medicines in the NHS.

FURTHER READING

Jones M (ed) 1999 Nurse prescribing: politics to practice. Baillière Tindall, London, Chs 1, 4, 5

Chapter **14**

Complementary therapies and health visiting

Pat Alexander

There is one thing stronger than all the armies of the world, and that is an idea whose time has come.

Victor Hugo

INTRODUCTION

It is my privilege in the following pages to explore the birth and growth of complementary medicine within the realms of health visiting and its integration into the NHS. We are standing on the brink of an exciting new approach to specialist community public health–health visiting: one which will enable us to deepen further our philosophy of preventive care, of partnership with clients and of empowerment.

At the same time it is essential to acknowledge our role in the primary health care team, where we may act as a catalyst for change, a coordinator and a key worker for client care.

One of our vital roles embraced under the umbrella of 'coordinator' will be that of a link person with GPs so that complementary medicine is seen as complementary rather than alternative. Unfortunately, as a result of lack of consultation, discussion and mutual respect, complementary medicine continues to be regarded as 'witchcraft' with little scientific backup to support its work. There is a long way to go and there are many obstacles to be tackled but all is possible with the right approach and positive attitudes.

Health visitors are seen as advocates for the clients they visit. They will now become advocates for complementary medicines using the basic tools learned from their training and field-work experience, of listening, respect, teaching and planning, both short and long term, based on research. In this way they will not only assist in deepening the understanding of complementary medicine by health care professionals but will also work towards creating a harmonious marriage between orthodox and complementary health care and an integrated health care service.

INTEGRATED HEALTH CARE – DO WE NEED IT?

Over the last 50 years there have been tremendous improvements in the treatment of illness but unfortunately this has led to increasing demands on limited resources, resulting in waiting lists and long delays for treatment. There is also growing concern regarding the potential side effects of drugs used to combat ill health. These two major drawbacks in health care have spearheaded the work of the Foundation for Integrated Medicine, which believes that the integration of orthodox and complementary medicine can help to provide a solution. The House of Lords Select Committee on Science and Technology has recognized this move towards integration in its report on Complementary and Alternative Medicine (2000).

HOW TO ACHIEVE INTEGRATION?

The Foundation for Integrated Medicine, a charity initiated at the suggestion of HRH the Prince of Wales in 1994, holds the vision that integration will be achieved only by 'the close working together of orthodox and complementary medical practitioners, with mutual respect and understanding'. It is hoped that this vision will be realized by the attainment of the following objectives:

- to promote awareness of the clinical and economic benefits of effective integrated health and medical practices
- to promote scientific research into complementary medicine
- to collaborate with other medical and complementary organizations
- to collect, codify and disseminate knowledge of complementary medical practices
- to promote educational programmes in integrated medicine.

The goals of the Foundation offer a holistic approach to the care of the client:

- to promote health and well-being in addition to treating illness
- to deal with people as whole individuals, obtaining their confidence and trust, building inner strength for the treatment of their illness
- to restore to people their feeling of self-worth and esteem through active participation in their own treatment, which is often essential for recovery.

THE ROLE OF SCIENTIFIC RESEARCH

The Foundation for Integrated Medicine acknowledges research as one of its important objectives. It pays special attention to cost–benefit analysis and the efficacy of treatments.

It supports the following approaches to research:

- to undertake pilot research studies into new areas of integrated medicine

- to support research into the efficacy of complementary medicine for common debilitating ailments such as childhood asthma, irritable bowel syndrome, hypertension, menopausal syndromes and back pain

- to review previous research work to establish the complementary treatments that have reasonably good evidence for efficacy and to note gaps where new research might be beneficial.

The above objectives are of crucial importance as at present there is virtually no information, treatment trials or research on good integrated medical practice.

THE ROLE OF EDUCATION

If integration is to take place it is necessary to facilitate this through easily available study days and pertinent literature to help doctors and health professionals to become familiar with complementary therapies. As a result of an initiative stemming from the British Medical Association's 1993 publication *Complementary Medicine: New Approaches to Good Practice*, the Research Council for Complementary Medicine is assessing the best methods of educating conventional practitioners about complementary medicine and increasing the awareness and understanding of GPs.

In a comparative study carried out by Perkin et al in 1994, which involved a random sample of 100 GPs and 100 hospital doctors in the South West Thames Regional Health Authority and 237 pre-clinical medical students at St George's Hospital Medical School, it was found that the majority of the respondents felt that complementary medicine should be available on the NHS and that medical students should receive some tuition about it. Some 70% of hospital doctors and 93% of GPs had on at least one occasion suggested a referral for complementary treatment, and 12% of hospital doctors and 20% of GPs were practising complementary medicine.

It is one of the recommendations of the House of Lords (2000) that familiarization with Complementary and Alternative Medicine (CAM) be made available in schools of medicine and nursing in addition to its inclusion within Continuing Professional Development.

RESEARCH METHODS

On a practical level it is necessary that complementary therapists are suitably trained in research methods in order that data can be processed and analysed. The Research Council for Complementary Medicine has acknowledged that research is a complicated and technical procedure and to this end has been involved in a number of educational initiatives to teach research skills to practitioners of complementary medicine. First-time researchers gain experience in simple research designs before seeking funds for larger scale projects.

Some examples of research funded by the Research Council are:

- 'An evaluation in atopic eczema of topical treatments containing Chinese medicinal herbs'
- 'The fragrance component of aromatherapy in anxiety'
- 'Anti-nausea effect of acupuncture'
- 'Controlled trial of yoga for stress related ailments'
- 'Assessment of osteopathic manipulation for acute back pain'.

The Universities of Exeter and Plymouth, under the auspices of the Peninsula Medical School, provide documentation on clinically relevant research between 1993 and 2003 in their report *Complementary Medicine: The Evidence So Far*.

THE RELATIONSHIP BETWEEN HEALTH VISITORS, ALLOPATHIC MEDICINE AND COMPLEMENTARY MEDICINE

The greatest unifying factor of this multidisciplinary approach is the well-being of the client. In theory, this should override any differing opinions as long as the treatment is supported by the appropriate research and all practice is evidence based.

The needs of an individual are many and complex and any imbalance in the fulfilment of these needs can cause ill health. This is symbolized in Figure 14.1.

Holistic medicine would take an overall view of the whole flower, as would a health visitor, whereas in orthodox medicine, frequently as a result of time restrictions, only one petal of the flower would be scrutinized. Both approaches are of vital importance to the client and, if combined, form a powerful force towards eliminating the causes of ill health.

Holistic care involves:

- responding to the person as a whole (body, mind and spirit) within the context of their environment (family, culture and ecology)
- a willingness to use a wide range of interventions, from drugs and surgery to meditation and diet
- an emphasis on a more participatory relationship between doctor and patient
- an awareness of the impact of the 'health' of the practitioner on the patient.

WORKING TOGETHER

In the NHS Executive document *Primary Care: The Future* (Department of Health 1996a) it is recognized that the best services are provided when there is a spirit of collaboration and cooperation not only among professionals but also with the client and the carers if applicable. It cites the importance of understanding and appreciating the roles and skills of each member of the primary health care team in order to cultivate an atmosphere that is both positive and therapeutic for those involved in treatment. The document

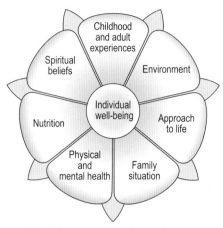

Figure 14.1 The holistic medicine flower

explores the option of direct self-referral plus the use of a health care worker to advise people on the range and types of help available.

It is a well-known fact that complementary therapies present a confusing and somewhat frightening picture to the lay person, not to mention the trial of finding a reputable and trustworthy specialist. The specialist health visitor for complementary medicine would be sufficiently trained to fulfil this role, acting as a link between orthodox and complementary treatments and as an advisor to the client (Fig. 14.2).

This would ensure an integrated health service, providing local people with access to qualified professionals in the type of complementary medicine best suited to treat their condition. The House of Lords Select Committee (2000) acknowledges the importance of a central resource person within the NHS to provide guidance to the public on complementary and alternative medicine (CAM).

CLIENT–HELD RECORDS

At the moment the only documentation retained by clients in the community are:

- child health records
- maternity records
- pilot projects in which the client records reactions to treatment.

If relationships are to be addressed seriously by professionals and clients, it is imperative that the

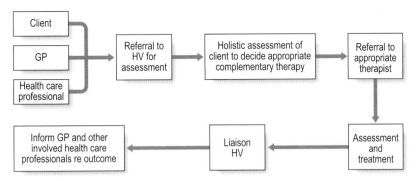

Figure 14.2   Health visitor/key worker referral/discharge procedure

client retains a permanent record of his general health plus details of ongoing treatment. As health visitors, key words such as 'empowerment', 'partnership', 'self-esteem' and 'shared responsibility' slip easily off our tongues and it is through the establishment of a comprehensive health record that these ideals may be achieved. A sample of such a client-held record could be as shown in Figure 14.3 (see also Ch. 15).

This would form a basis for partnership in care, a copy being kept by the client and another by the key health worker, who may be the health visitor or another appointed person. These details might be in the form of a small booklet, similar to the child health records, and would ideally also contain details on:

- recommended weights, according to height
- nutritional advice on healthy diets related to weight control, heart disease, diabetes, bowel disorders and allergic conditions
- alcohol consumption, with recommended daily intakes
- the importance of exercise and types of relaxation
- management of stress
- coping with minor illnesses (e.g. colds, flu)
- health checks for men and women
- family planning
- advice on smoking cessation.

The booklet would thus serve as a useful reference for the client regarding the maintenance of a healthy lifestyle in addition to promoting a sense of personal responsibility and involvement in the treatment of ill health. It would also

---

Client Health Record

Name:

Address:

Telephone no:

Date of birth:

Next of kin:

GP:

Health visitor:

Key worker:

Other health care professionals, for example:
1. District nurse, practice nurse
2. Obstetrician, midwife
3. Mental health team
4. Complementary therapist

Date	Health concerns	Treatment	Outcome	Health care plan

Figure 14.3   An example of a client-held record

---

contain a list of useful contact numbers where further advice and support might be accessed.

By fulfilment of the key worker role in complementary medicine the health visitor will be exploiting the four principles of practice defined by the CETHV (1977) and now part of the *Standards of Proficiency* (NMC 2004a) – the search for health needs, the stimulation of the awareness of health, the influence of policies affecting health and the facilitation of health-enhancing activities.

It is important to remember that the most powerful way a health visitor is able to influence policies affecting health, especially in relation to the successful treatment of certain ailments through the use of complementary medicine, is through the collection of evidence-based practice. An integrated health care service will only develop through the collection of reliable and proven research-based documentation.

HEALTH MAINTENANCE BEHAVIOURS AND THE USE OF COMPLEMENTARY THERAPY

What is 'health maintenance behaviour'? Simply put, it is creating a healthy lifestyle and approach to life through the elimination of disease and negative attitudes.

It is the role of the GP to treat ill health, but the issues of maintaining good health for the local population exist in a vacuum. Health visitors adopt the role of preventive health care but, as mentioned in the *Code of Professional Conduct* (NMC 2002a), there are many instances where their skills and experience are not used to their full potential. At present, in the majority of cases, health visitors concentrate on work with families of children under 5, which, although vitally important, results in other community needs being neglected. In *Liberating the Talents* (Department of Health 2002b), it is clearly recommended that practice should be broadened with suitable education and training.

In response to this innovative and encouraging statement it is clearly evident that health visiting may break free from its stereotyped 'under-fives' role to adopt a wider perspective in its approach to work within the community. A health visitor specialist in complementary medicine is just one example of how community needs may be met by assisting the client to make more informed choices and thereby create a better relationship with all those involved in optimal health. This also works towards raising the client's self-esteem and sense of responsibility to enable them to become an active member of the multidisciplinary health team.

It is important that the advice put forward to the client by the health visitor is research based

to maintain credibility both within the medical profession and among the community. To this end the Foundation for Integrated Medicine is at present funding six research projects:

- 'Reflexology for childhood asthma'
- 'Homeopathy for childhood asthma'
- 'Osteopathy for asthma'
- 'The Alexander technique for Parkinson's disease'
- 'Marma therapy for stroke victims'
- 'A diagnostic test for lower back pain'.

Through its Research Committee the Foundation assists potential researchers in the production of sound protocols, and it is the duty of the health visitor to ensure that the practitioners to whom he or she refers adhere to such protocols in addition to carrying out research projects.

It is important that the role of the specialist health visitor is far reaching in order to create maximum awareness of the complementary therapy treatments available in both professionals and lay people alike (Fig. 14.4).

There needs also to be the backdrop of ongoing research in order to guarantee evidence-based practice, which may be coordinated with the research project supported by the Research Committee of the Foundation for Integrated Medicine. The health visitor should also ensure that clear policies exist within the practice area

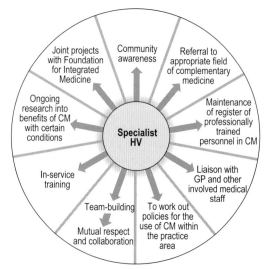

Figure 14.4 The role of the specialist health visitor in complementary medicine

to safeguard both the client and practitioner and to give credibility to the field of complementary therapy.

INTEGRATING COMPLEMENTARY THERAPIES WITHIN THE PRIMARY CARE TRUST

The philosophy behind the setting up of Primary Care Trusts mirrors that of complementary therapies:

- to work in partnership with others
- to promote health
- to share skills.

Some of the qualities brought to the groups by health visitor specialists include:

- good communication skills
- holistic assessments
- integrated care
- resource management
- sensitivity to ethnic issues
- evidence-based practice.

The hope is that professionals will maintain mutual respect for each other's roles according to the overall plan of the White Paper (Department of Health 1997a), which is:

- to improve the health of the nation as a whole
- to improve the health of the less privileged, thus decreasing the health divide.

It is well known that at present complementary therapies remain the luxury of the privileged few, with the occasional exception where they are accessed through the NHS. The integration of orthodox medicine with complementary therapies would be instrumental in removing this divide.

In order to bring the aims of the White Paper down to grass roots level it is necessary to look at the common denominator for most people in Britain as regards health issues – the GP. It is the GP who decides, following an initial assessment, whether the client might be best suited for orthodox or complementary medicine. This ensures that any health problems requiring immediate medical or surgical intervention receive attention with the minimum delay. However, some clients may still wish to combine orthodox and complementary medicine for the treatment of life-threatening conditions if the choice is available. For example, after cardiac surgery where the patient might also attend yoga classes to encourage relaxation and decrease stress or, alternatively, receive aromatherapy treatment to lower blood pressure and encourage a sense of well-being. Integrated medicine within primary care groups is thus able to address the health priorities listed in the national targets – heart disease, stroke, accidents, mental health and cancer.

THE USE OF COMPLEMENTARY THERAPIES WITHIN THE PRIMARY CARE TRUST

The type of therapy used is dependent initially upon those who have been accepted by the health authority concerned. For example, South Birmingham Mental Health Trust approved the following therapies in a draft policy dated January 1996: acupuncture, the Alexander technique, aromatherapy, art therapy, auricular acupuncture, counselling, drama therapy, herbalism, homeopathy, massage, movement therapy, music therapy, reflexology, sports therapy and yoga. In order to have a brief overview we will look at five therapies and their application in practice in greater detail: aromatherapy, reiki, yoga, touch – baby massage and nutritional medicine.

It is to be remembered that the principles behind all good primary care are those quoted by the NHS Executive in their information booklet *Primary Care: The Future* (Department of Health 1996a). These are as follows:

- Quality
  - Professionals should be knowledgeable about the conditions that present in primary care and skilled in their treatment.
  - Professionals should be knowledgeable about the people to whom they are offering services.
  - Services should be coordinated with professionals aware of each other's

contributions (including inter-professional working) and no service gaps.
- Premises and facilities should be of a good standard and fit for their purpose, and equipment should be up to date, well maintained and safe to use.

- Fairness
  - Services should not vary widely in range or quality in different parts of the country.
  - Primary care should receive an appropriate share of overall NHS resources.

- Accessibility
  - Services should be reasonably accessible when clinically needed.
  - Necessary services should be accessible to people regardless of age, sex, ethnicity or health status.

- Responsiveness
  - Services should reflect the needs and preferences of the individuals using them.
  - Services should reflect the demographic and social needs of the area they serve.

- Efficiency
  - Primary care services should be based on scientific evidence.
  - Primary care resources should be used efficiently.

AROMATHERAPY

Aromatherapy is one of the most popular forms of complementary therapy in the UK and USA and is frequently being employed by nurses and other health care professionals in hospital, hospice and community settings.

Aromatherapy uses potent substances and therefore comprehensive training is essential. The therapist should be a member of a reputable professional body, e.g. the International Federation of Professional Aromatherapists (IFPA), and have full insurance cover.

HOW ESSENTIAL OILS WORK

Essential oils enter the body by inhalation plus transference to the bloodstream via the nose, lungs and skin by means of vaporizers, massage and baths. Essential oils, when inhaled, affect the brain directly by means of neurochemical messages that are picked up by the olfactory nerve endings in the nose and passed to the limbic area, which forms part of our complex brain. From there they rapidly affect our moods and emotions, giving rise to complex chemical changes in the body. The release of encephalins and endorphins, which act as the body's natural painkillers, produce sensations of well-being and calm. During respiration the molecules of oil pass into the lungs and thence by diffusion into the bloodstream with oxygen. This is facilitated by the small molecular size of essential oils and the single-cell thickness of the alveoli and blood capillaries of the lungs.

During massage oils pass by diffusion into the skin, crossing the stratum corneum, the outer layer of the skin, entering the epidermis and the dermis and thence into the capillary circulation. Essential oils can act very quickly as well as over a period of time, being released into the bloodstream and distributed around the body. They are then excreted in respiration, sweat, urine or faeces.

APPLICATION

Aromatherapy is definitely a complementary therapy in that it can be used alongside allopathic medicine and most other therapies. One exception may be homeopathy, as there is a risk of the essential oils nullifying the effect of the homeopathic remedy. Research is currently being carried out in this area.

In Appendix 2 the properties of lavender oil have been examined in detail in order to demonstrate the in-depth knowledge that is required, not only for the practice of aromatherapy but indeed for the practice of all forms of complementary therapy.

SAFETY

In cases where adults/children have an allergy to some or all fragrances, it is wise to carry out patch testing before administering an oil. It is important to note that, where essential oils are used knowledgeably and with due caution, there is no threat to health. An in-depth guide to essential oil safety is provided by Tisserand et al (1995) and Price et al (1995), referred to at the end of this chapter.

REIKI

The practice of reiki is an original method of healing, developed by Mikao Usui in Japan in the early 20th century, which is activated by intention. Reiki's natural healing energy is said to work on every level, not just the physical, promoting the body's regenerative self-healing ability. The Japanese word *reiki* means 'universal energy'. Eastern medicine has always recognized and worked with this energy, believed to flow through all living things and being a vital part of well-being. It is known as *ki* in Japan, *chi* in China and *prana* in India. There is no belief system to reiki; the only prerequisite is the desire to be healed.

BENEFITS

The energy of reiki is used to help accelerate the healing of physical problems, balance the emotions and address any restrictive mental attitudes. It is a non-invasive therapy and may be used alongside orthodox medicine. At present it is being used in various settings including private practice, complementary centres, GP surgeries, hospitals, cancer support groups, care of the elderly and drug rehabilitation units.

TREATMENT

A session is usually carried out with the client lying down or sitting, in a comfortable and peaceful environment; there is no need to remove clothing. The practitioner places their hands gently, in a series of positions, on or over the body. Reiki may be felt as a flow of energy, mild tingling or other sensations or perhaps nothing at all.

SAFETY

Conscious of the emerging need to regulate the practice of reiki following the House of Lords *Report on Complementary and Alternative Medicine* (2000), the UK Reiki Federation has been involved in the development of the Complementary and Alternative Medicine templates for National Occupational Standards in conjunction with Skills for Health, the standard-setting body relating to qualifications in health care.

YOGA

Many people who consult an aromatherapist or a reiki practitioner do so because they are under stress or because they are suffering from physical symptoms that are the result of stress and anxiety. While the aromatherapist can help to reduce stress and bring about a state of calm and relaxation in the short term, it is important to look to a long-term solution for this problem. Yoga fulfils this need by teaching the stressed person active methods to help himself.

Yoga, as aromatherapy, works on many levels. It may be viewed simply as a system of physical exercise or as a profound philosophy, and yoga teachers vary in the amount of emphasis they place on the different aspects.

Classical yoga dates back to 2000 BC when an Indian scholar called Patanjali recorded in minute detail the means of attaining 'enlightenment' or a oneness with oneself and the world. His teachings are holistic and embrace physical and mental health, aiming to create a humble, positive and sincere approach to life. Simplistically his works may be summarized in the 'eightfold path of yoga': yama = restraints, e.g. non-violence; niyama = observances, e.g. self-study; asana = good health through physical education; pranayama = regulation of bioenergy (respiratory) practices; pratyahara = the process of abstraction; dharana = concentration; dhyana = meditation; samadhi = self-realization (Fig. 14.5).

PHYSICAL BENEFITS

Research has revealed that meditation is the most effective technique for decreasing anxiety levels, reducing alcohol, cigarette and drug intake and improving psychological health (Thomas 1997).

INTEGRATION

From the above results it is clear that it would be of benefit to clients in the community setting to be taught the art of meditation as part of a health promotion programme either by a health visitor specialist or by a suitably trained professional. At present this is being carried out on a one-to-one basis by a health visitor trained to teach yoga in:

- postnatal and general depression affecting the client's self-esteem, confidence and ability to socialize
- stress causing anxiety attacks and insomnia.

However, meditation would also be ideal for small-group teaching, as illustrated in Figure 14.6.

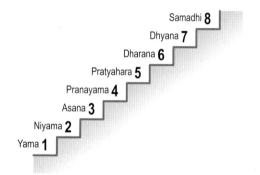

Figure 14.5 The eightfold path of yoga

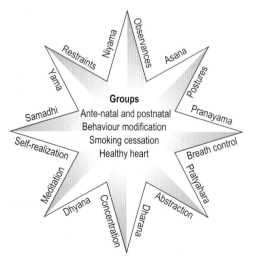

Figure 14.6 Meditation in small-group teaching

It should be noted that in the teachings of classical yoga no step is taken in isolation. Clients therefore study the full eightfold path in order to reach the seventh step, meditation (dhyana). This would ensure a holistic approach to each individual covering the well-being of the person physically, mentally, psychologically and spiritually. The client would be reassured that yoga is not a religion, as some imagine, and in no way clashes with any religious beliefs. It is a way of life that creates a positive approach to life and a sense of inner calm.

TOUCH – BABY MASSAGE

Anna Freud writes that being stroked, cuddled and soothed by touch helps to build up a healthy baby image and body ego, cementing the intimate relationship between child and parents. It is this relationship that the health visitor works towards establishing through encouragement and support in the early months of parenthood. Teaching the parents the art of massaging their baby may further enhance this.

The health visiting principles of raising clients' awareness of health needs and facilitating health-enhancing activities (Twinn et al 1992) are embodied in the teaching of infant massage skills to new parents (Fig. 14.7).

Sue Moloney, health visitor and certified infant massage instructor who works with Harlow Primary Care Trust, shares her

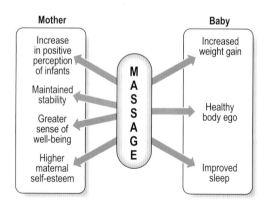

Figure 14.7 The benefits of massage for mother and baby

knowledge and experience in the following writings on baby massage.

DEFINITION

Baby or infant massage is the building of parent–baby communication through the baby's most highly developed sense, the sense of touch. It is an interactive process between a parent/carer and their baby, where the baby receives respectful nurturing touch through learned strokes from the care-giver.

BENEFITS

The simple loving touch between a baby and its parents has physical and psychological benefits, which are reflected in many areas:

- interactive communication strengthening the emotional attachment needed for feelings of security and optimum development

- stimulation of all the body systems: circulatory, lymphatic, digestive, eliminatory, muscular and immune

- relaxation for parent and baby: when baby massage is carried out with love, value and respect, this can result in not only a feeling of security for the baby but also relaxation of body and mind for both the person giving the massage and the recipient

- relief from minor ailments such as colic and constipation.

TRAINING

There are many courses available to become an infant massage instructor; however, it is important to select a parent-based education programme in contrast to a therapy-based one as this includes the underlying principle of supporting and encouraging parents to trust their abilities and intuition. The parents are recognized as the experts with their babies. The International Association of Infant Massage (www.iaim.org.uk) meets such requirements.

GROUP FACILITATION

When baby massage is taught in a group situation there are the additional benefits of the provision of social support, increasing parental confidence in their own abilities, relaxation techniques and opportunities for discussion on health or family-related topics which all take place within a warm, safe environment created by the instructor. Groups normally consist of 5–10 parents who meet on a weekly basis for one and a half hours over 4–5 weeks.

SAFETY

This is ensured by a sound understanding, recognition and awareness of infant cues. Massage should only take place when the baby is in a quiet, alert state and not if the baby is showing signs of disengagement with the parent.

Oil is used to massage the baby, in order to facilitate smooth flow of the strokes. However, caution is given regarding the use of oils with a nut origin (such as almond oil) in case of an allergic response.

RESEARCH

'Improving mother–baby interaction for mothers with post-natal depression', a small randomized control trial conducted at Queen Charlotte's and Chelsea Hospital, London, involved two groups of mothers suffering from postnatal depression. Each group was allocated randomly to either (a) attend infant massage classes and a support group or (b) only attend the directed support group (as a control group). Each group attended five weekly sessions. Measures of the Edinburgh Postnatal Depression Scale (Cox et al 1987) and Mother–Infant Interaction (video recording) were made at the beginning and the end of the sessions. Results revealed an improvement in depression for both groups but, most significantly, in the baby massage group, a marked improvement was noted in mother–infant interaction which was not apparent in the control group. A longer-term study is now in progress which will look at the mother–infant interaction scores at 1 year as well as after the five massage sessions (Adams et al 2003).

'Infant massage: developing an evidence-base for health visiting practice': this study explores the efficacy of health visitor-run baby massage classes in relation to social interaction in parenting. It specifically demonstrates that these classes act as a vehicle for developing parent–child relationships in addition to delivering health promotion activities (Clarke et al 2003).

NUTRITIONAL MEDICINE

The basis of holistic health care is that the whole person requires attention, so it would be negligent if the aspect of dietary intake is ignored. Every practitioner therefore, whatever the therapy, should have a sound understanding of dietary therapy and its practical application in both general and specific conditions.

In cases of stress the body requires an increase in vitamins, minerals and trace elements to enable the organism to cope with the additional demands. This is because prolonged stress causes both biochemical and neurochemical imbalances within the bodily systems. Deficiency progressively leads to disease, which is the principal reason why the health practitioner needs to become aware of dietary needs.

'Contemporary foods are nutritionally deficient because of the consumption of de-nutritionalised, processed foods, imbalanced by an excess of animal fats and an under-consumption of fibres and fresh vegetables. They are unnatural because of the excessive use of additives at all levels of the food chain and all categories of food' (Bennett 1992). It is a fact well known to the health visitor that colourings and additives in the diet of some children can lead to the following problems:

- behavioural problems
- night terrors
- infantile colic
- hyperactivity.

In adults dietary deficiencies manifest themselves in numerous conditions. In the postnatal period examples are anaemia, depression, irritability and insomnia, and dietary deficiency is a contributory factor in postnatal depression. It is therefore an important role of the health visitor to create an awareness of the curative aspects of a healthy diet in order to assist clients to take responsibility for their own health. This may be done at all minimal surveillance checks arranged for the child, where the contact provides an ideal opportunity to learn about the family's health and probable manifestations of vitamin or mineral deficiency, allergy or food intolerance. This is often seen in the following conditions:

- skin disorders
- gastrointestinal disturbances
- respiratory problems
- behavioural difficulties.

The health visitor needs therefore to possess an in-depth knowledge of nutritional needs, which differs remarkably from the more basic knowledge conveyed in health promotion sessions.

INTEGRATING COMPLEMENTARY MEDICINE INTO THE MEDICAL FIELD

Complementary therapies that may be considered for integration into the roles of various health professionals are illustrated in Figures 14.8 and 14.9.

An example of a complementary therapy being successfully integrated into the medical field is at the Neuropsychiatry and Seizure Clinic based at the Queen Elizabeth Psychiatric Hospital in Birmingham by Dr Tim Betts (1995), a consultant neuropsychiatrist. Dr Betts uses aromatherapy and hypnosis in the treatment of epilepsy. In one case study he writes:

Using a diary for 2 or 3 months Glynis was able to recognise that her tonic–clonic seizures were occurring in association with anxiety triggered off by problems in her relationship. She was able to recognise when she was becoming anxious (massages with camomile taught her for the first time what it was like to be relaxed and were invaluable in teaching her to discriminate between tension and relaxation). By using the smell of camomile as a countermeasure whenever she felt herself become tense she was able to completely stop her seizures and has been seizure-free for over 3 years and has regained her driving licence.

It should be noted that the types of therapy suggested in Figures 14.8 and 14.9 are only suggestions. There are many other excellent complementary therapies, which are too numerous to mention. More details on complementary

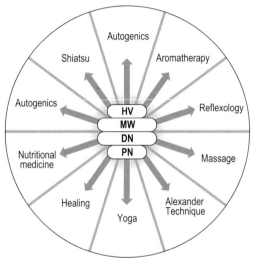

Figure 14.8 Types of complementary therapy appropriate for primary care teams (DN, district nurse; HV, health visitor; MW, midwife; PN, practice nurse)

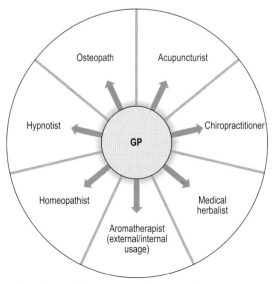

Figure 14.9 Types of complementary therapy contingent with the GP role

therapies may be obtained from the Research Council for Complementary Medicine, 60 Great Ormond Street, London WC1N 3JF.

For the reader's convenience a short summary of the complementary therapies mentioned in this chapter is included in Appendix 1.

HEALTH VISITING CASE STUDIES IN THE COMMUNITY SETTING

The following are case studies recently carried out, with the permission of the GP, on clients in the Hertfordshire and Essex Health Authority.

CASE STUDY 1

History

Child A was admitted to hospital in August 1997 at the age of 15 months with initially acute onset of complete flaccid paralysis of both upper limbs and respiratory embarrassment. He was transferred to the paediatric intensive care unit with the diagnosis of acute transverse myelitis; in addition he had some bladder weakness. He was discharged home 6 weeks later with the support of the GP, physiotherapist, occupational therapist, speech and language therapist, community paediatric nurses, social worker and health visitor.

Parental concerns

Mr & Mrs A highlighted the following problems since their child's discharge from hospital: muscle stiffness (there was a possibility that he would not be able to walk again); lowered resistance to infection; disturbed sleep; increased mucoid secretions with respiratory difficulties; bladder instability.

Treatment

Essential oils were selected to embrace the concerns mentioned above as follows:

- to strengthen the immune system
  - *Lavandula angustifolia* (lavender)
  - *Melaleuca alternifolia* (tea tree)

- to relax the muscle stiffness
  - *Origanum marjoram* (sweet marjoram)
  - *Lavandula angustifolia* (lavender)
- to help regulate bladder activity
  - *Cedrus atlanticus* (cedarwood)
  - *Santalum album* (sandalwood)
- to decrease mucoid secretions and assist respiration
  - *Eucalyptus smithii* (eucalyptus)
  - *Santalum album* (sandalwood)
  - *Melaleuca alternifolia* (tea tree)
  - *Cedrus atlanticus* (cedarwood).

These were mixed together in grapeseed oil to form a synergistic blend. The effect of synergy is that when two or more oils are combined a greater effect is achieved. For example, the bactericidal effect of several oils combined is greater than the effect of any of the individual oils.

A second mixture was also made to assist child A's sleep. This comprised the following oils: *Santalum album* (sandalwood) and *Cananga odorata* (ylang ylang). Instructions were given to the parents regarding application and massage techniques for the mixtures, which were applied once daily.

Outcome

This case study is an excellent example of complementary medicine: the treatment of Child A was carried out alongside allopathic medicine. As a result of this partnership, in August 1998 Child A was beginning to take steps on his own, his breathing had greatly improved and he no longer attended the GP surgery weekly because of infections. The parents are delighted with his progress, which is attributed to a holistic health approach to the child's care whereby professionals have worked alongside each other with mutual respect. Figure 14.10 shows a very proud little boy taking his first few steps since his illness.

CASE STUDY 2

History

Child B was admitted to hospital at the age of 2½ years with a viral infection but following

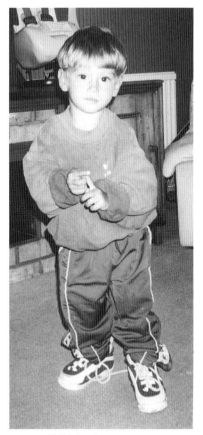

Figure 14.10 Child A after treatment

discharge hair loss occurred, leaving the child with very fine downy hair resembling that of patients who had undergone chemotherapy. She was seen in hospital regarding the hair loss and no cause could be diagnosed. Child B's mother was reassured that her child had no serious illness and that the hair would either grow back or fall out completely. She was advised there were good wigs available.

Parental concerns

The main concern was regarding the reaction of other children when Child B started school and the psychological damage it would cause to her personality and general self-esteem.

Treatment

With the permission of the GP a holistic assessment was carried out on Child B, looking at her

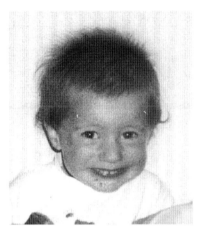

Figure 14.11   Child B before treatment (reproduced by kind permission of the child's parents)

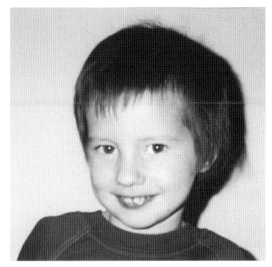

Figure 14.12   Child B after treatment

lifestyle, diet, personality and general health. In partnership with the parents the following were agreed:

- to massage the scalp each evening with the lotion given, rinsing this off the following morning and brushing the hair well; the lotion contained the following essential oils to help stimulate hair growth and improve the circulation:
  - *Cananga odorata* (ylang ylang)
  - *Rosmarinus officinalis* (rosemary)
  - *Cedrus atlanticus* (cedarwood)
- to ensure the diet contained foods rich in iron, zinc, vitamins B and C, and protein.

Outcome

After only 2 weeks of the above treatment the hair had started to thicken and Child B's scalp could no longer be seen through her hair. A side effect was also that she was beginning to sleep more soundly! Figures 14.11 and 14.12 show Child B before and after treatment.

Other conditions treated by aromatherapy in the community are insomnia in children, head lice, postnatal depression and stress in adults.

CASE STUDY 3

The following includes extracts from a thesis prepared by Jean Gonella, health visitor in Harrow Community Health Trust, which looks at the effectiveness of treating stress using aromatherapy massage.

Massage was used on a group of women where stress had become distress, who volunteered to try aromatherapy in place of or to reduce medications such as tranquillisers and analgesics.

This pilot study was targeted at women's health and continued for a period of 6 months. It was supported by senior management and all treatment was expected to be carried out within working hours. In total, 16 clients took part in the study, attending for 4–10 sessions each, for a duration of 1–1½ hours per session.

We would like to stress that, although a minimum of 1 hour is needed for a full body massage, it is not at all unusual for health visitors to spend an hour per visit with families with problems needing counselling and support. We see it as offering another approach to stress management, giving our clients a new dimension on their outlook and attitude towards their health.

The criteria for selection for treatment by massage are given in Figure 14.13.

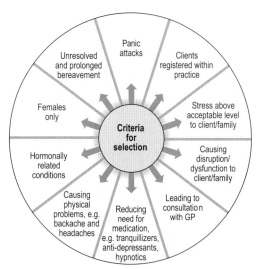

Figure 14.13 Criteria for selection for treatment by massage

Objectives

- To alleviate stress through the use of aromatic oils with massage in order to create a sense of well-being on physical, psychological and emotional levels
- To increase self-awareness in relation to the effects of stress on the body
- To reduce GP consultation time
- To offer a more economic alternative to drug usage.

In summary, all clients reported that they felt more in control when placed in stressful situations; the quality of sleep had improved and generally they felt more confident in themselves. All except one client had great improvement in all areas.

GP PRACTICE

The project was fully supported by the GPs. Consultations on the whole were considerably reduced – one patient had not seen her GP since commencing aromatherapy treatment; two patients took the option of massage rather than medication; one patient began to reduce her medication with her GP's permission.

RECOMMENDATIONS

- It might be more cost effective if treatments were carried out on a sessional basis.
- It would save both time and money if treatments were given on the clinic premises rather than in the client's home.
- Oils would need to be purchased, consisting of at least 12 basic essential oils and a large bottle of grapeseed or base oil.

CONCLUSION

The practical project proved 99% successful and involved 16 women over a period of 6 months. However, a much larger cohort study, using at least 100 clients and a control group, would be necessary to prove that aromatherapy could replace drug therapy.

Such replacement would naturally be decided by the GP according to the severity of the problem at hand. It is to be remembered that, if the client's health needs are going to be fully addressed, complementary therapy can only exist in partnership with orthodox medicine.

SUMMARY

The above case studies merely reflect the possibilities of integrated care in the community. The choice of aromatherapy as a complementary therapy is due to the author's experience in this field and is in no way intended to create a preference for a particular therapy.

In order to help demonstrate the in-depth knowledge required to practise any branch of complementary medicine a snapshot of aromatherapy is presented in Appendix 2.

THE NHS AND COMPLEMENTARY THERAPIES

At the moment there is no provision within primary legislation for patients to seek treatment from a complementary therapist under the auspices of the NHS. The only exception to this is through referral by a GP or hospital doctor to one of the five NHS homeopathic hospitals in the UK, where doctors are all conventionally trained with orthodox qualifications.

However, with changing public opinion it is likely that new legislation will be introduced. In 1991 the Consumers Association reported that one in four of their readers visited an alternative or complementary practitioner, which is double the number found in a survey in 1986. In 1990 a Medical Research Council study (Meade et al 1990) recommended that chiropractic should be available on the NHS, which has resulted in a Bill being put before Parliament for a statutory council to regulate the profession because of the demand for and use of chiropractors and osteopaths.

There have been many studies carried out by prominent medical journals such as the *British Medical Journal* over the last 10 years looking at the use of complementary therapies and doctors' attitudes to them. Attitudes have consistently been both positive and supportive. A list of these studies is included in Appendix 3.

CURRENT OPINION

In September 1992 Dr Gwen Cameron-Blackie, a senior registrar in public health medicine, and Yvonne Mouncer, a health service consultant, carried out a national survey of district health authorities (DHAs), family health service authorities (FHSAs) and GP fundholders to examine purchasers' attitudes towards the availability of complementary therapies on the NHS and to establish current and future approaches to purchasing and funding such therapies. Questionnaires were sent to all DHAs and FHSAs and a sample of GP fundholders. Response rates were: 57% (110/192), 75% (74/99) and 43% respectively; a sample of the results is illustrated in Figures 14.14–14.20.

From studying these results it is apparent that homeopathy, acupuncture, osteopathy and chiropractic are viewed more favourably than aromatherapy or reflexology. However, the researchers believe this may be caused by the fact that:

- homeopathy has always been available on the NHS
- acupuncture is frequently used within the NHS

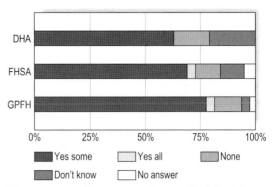

Figure 14.14 Response to the question 'Should complementary therapies be available on the NHS?' (DHA, district health authorities; FHSA, family health service authorities; GPFH, GP fundholders) (reproduced with kind permission from Cameron-Blackie & Mouncer 1992)

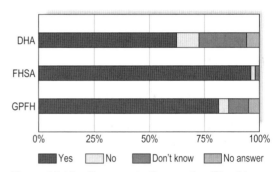

Figure 14.15 Response to the question 'Should acupuncture be available on the NHS?' (DHA, district health authorities; FHSA, family health service authorities; GPFH, GP fundholders) (reproduced with kind permission from Cameron-Blackie & Mouncer 1992)

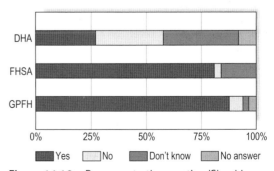

Figure 14.16 Response to the question 'Should osteopathy be available on the NHS?' (DHA, district health authorities; FHSA, family health service authorities; GPFH, GP fundholders) (reproduced with kind permission from Cameron-Blackie & Mouncer 1992)

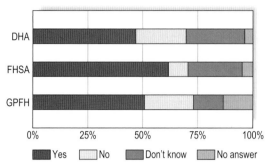

Figure 14.17 Response to the question 'Should chiropractic be available on the NHS?' (DHA, district health authorities; FHSA, family health service authorities; GPFH, GP fundholders) (reproduced with kind permission from Cameron-Blackie & Mouncer 1992)

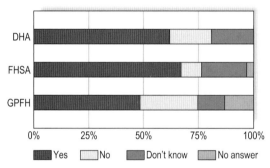

Figure 14.18 Response to the question 'Should homeopathy be available on the NHS?' (DHA, district health authorities; FHSA, family health service authorities; GPFH, GP fundholders) (reproduced with kind permission from Cameron-Blackie & Mouncer 1992)

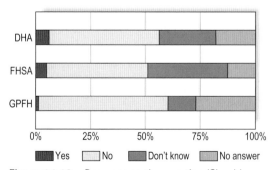

Figure 14.19 Response to the question 'Should reflexology be available on the NHS?' (DHA, district health authorities; FHSA, family health service authorities; GPFH, GP fundholders) (reproduced with kind permission from Cameron-Blackie & Mouncer 1992)

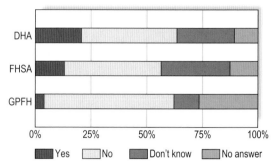

Figure 14.20 Response to the question 'Should aromatherapy be available on the NHS?' (DHA, district health authorities; FHSA, family health service authorities; GPFH, GP fundholders) (reproduced with kind permission from Cameron-Blackie & Mouncer 1992)

- patients are often referred by GPs privately to osteopaths and chiropractors
- reflexology and aromatherapy may be seen as relatively 'new age' therapies.

From the graphs there is also a noticeable percentage of authorities who remain unsure as to whether the therapies should or should not be available on the NHS. This is reflected by the number of 'don't knows' and 'no answers' in the results.

GP FUNDHOLDERS: AVAILABILITY AND APPROPRIATE USE OF COMPLEMENTARY THERAPIES

The study revealed that complementary therapies were available in 34% of the GP fundholder practices responding to the questionnaire. Therapies being used were hypnosis, osteopathy, spinal manipulation, homeopathy, aromatherapy and counselling. The majority of these therapies were provided by a member of the primary health care team, which proves that integrated health care is already being practised, albeit in a small way, and should offer encouragement to any health visitor wishing to specialize in a complementary therapy.

Table 14.1 shows the types of therapy that GP fundholders consider could appropriately be used in the management of 10 conditions

Table 14.1 The therapies GP fundholders consider could appropriately be used in the management of conditions commonly encountered in general practice (from Cameron-Blackie & Mouncer 1992)

Therapy	Acupuncture	Osteopathy	Chiropractic	Homeopathy	Reflexology	Aromatherapy	None	Don't know	No answer
Chronic back pain	59	74	41	9	3	1	8	1	2
Osteoarthritis	59	36	17	15	1	1	14	4	6
Rheumatoid arthritis	47	21	10	30	1	5	24	5	7
Hay fever	14	0	0	40	1	1	32	5	13
Anxiety	23	0	0	32	10	14	22	7	11
Insomnia	20	0	0	32	7	10	24	7	10
Obesity	18	0	0	1	0	1	41	7	20
Smoking	54	0	0	9	0	1	28	7	6
Peptic ulceration	5	0	0	12	0	0	51	9	20
Maturity-onset diabetes	2	0	1	6	1	1	61	8	18

Table 14.2 The factors stated by purchasers to be important to decision-making on complementary therapies (from Cameron-Blackie & Mouncer 1992)

Factor	%
District health authorities	
Lack of information on effectiveness	66
Lack of resources	24
Lack of demand	20
Lack of information/knowledge	14
Other priorities	14
Demand by GPs/public	10
High cost	8
Professional scepticism	8
GP fundholders	
Lack of information on effectiveness	48
Lack of information/knowledge	36
Lack of resources	31
Patient demand	16
Low priority	7
Lack of district health authority provision	7
Family health service authorities	
Lack of information on effectiveness	59
Lack of information/knowledge	25
Lack of resources	25
Public/GP opinion	20
Lack of information re quality/training	17
Lack of demand from GPs/public	13
Lack of support from GPs	13
Low priority	11

commonly encountered in general practice. Table 14.2 shows the factors said by each purchaser to be important to their decision-making on complementary therapies.

All three groups of purchasers were concerned about the lack of evidence on effectiveness, which is caused by various factors:

- There have been few randomized control trials.
- The majority of the literature is on holistic studies or anecdotal evidence.
- The majority of reports appear in complementary therapy journals, which are not readily available in local, medical, hospital or university libraries.

The above comments reflect the need for research as an ongoing duty for any health professional becoming involved in complementary medicine. It also highlights the importance of supplying accurate information on therapies to purchasers so that they are able to make informed decisions. The information requested covered:

- a basic understanding of what the therapy involves
- the principles/theoretical basis underlying the therapy
- the appropriate qualifications/training of therapist
- the medico-legal implications.

FUNDING

GP fundholders commented that funding complementary therapies would be dependent upon demonstrable cost-effectiveness and savings in other budgets, e.g. drug budgets or reductions in referrals.

RECOMMENDATIONS

- Additional research into the effectiveness of complementary medicines
- Evaluation of complementary therapy services currently available within the NHS
- Research into the cost/benefits of complementary therapies
- Development of standards for training and qualification
- All research findings and general information to be disseminated widely.

GOVERNMENTAL REGULATION, SAFETY AND ACCOUNTABILITY

Complementary medicine is moving towards being fully recognised by law in order to ensure that:

- all practitioners have passed basic levels of competence and remain up to date with current developments
- clients can turn to a statutory system of safeguards in the event of dissatisfaction
- clients have a full understanding of the treatment they wish to undertake.

Osteopathy and chiropractic are already registered under the General Osteopathy and Chiropractic Councils. The Department of Health is now examining proposals to regulate acupuncturists and herbalists. One strong suggestion is that they be brought under the umbrella of a new organization, the Complementary and Alternative Medicine Council, which would be set up with powers similar to those of the General Medical Council regarding the establishment of minimum training standards

and striking off anyone guilty of malpractice. The government will use these ideas as a basis for consultation on new laws in the coming months.

The Foundation for Integrated Health is soon to publish guidelines on 'How to choose a practitioner' in an effort to assist the public with their search for well-trained and reputable complementary therapists.

CONCLUSION

It is vital that complementary medicine is seen and understood as complementary: it is not alternative nor competitive but wishes to work alongside orthodox medicine. The only way forward is through mutual respect for the role each health professional plays in the prevention of disease, the maintenance of good health and the treatment of ill health. Without this professional integrity the client will become a victim in the battleground for medical supremacy. However, there is no ideal therapy; we are all individuals reacting to the stresses and strains of the world in different ways. We need to celebrate this diversity and, at the same time, celebrate the fact that, for each unique person, there is a unique therapy that will meet their needs perfectly. 'What is required is a humble realisation that we are but partners in a healing relationship. There is no doctor alive who has ever cured anyone of anything. Only the body heals. Our part is to support the body in its cleansing and regenerative processes. We should strive to be part of the solution and not part of the problem' (Bennett 1992).

It is clear that there are many amazing possibilities ahead in the health field and it is hoped that this chapter may serve as a springboard for action for those health professionals who wish to pursue a specialism in complementary medicine. It is also clear that, while there are thousands of studies showing the efficacy of various complementary therapies, many of them are uncontrolled, involve small experimental groups or lack objective measurement criteria. The need for well-researched evidence-based practice is paramount.

Health visitors are in a privileged and exciting position in the field of preventive care and, through choosing to extend their role by specializing in an area of complementary medicine or becoming a liaison specialist, may serve as pathfinders for the profession.

Live your beliefs and you can turn the World around.

Henry Thoreau

Appendix 1: AN OVERVIEW OF COMPLEMENTARY THERAPIES

- **Acupuncture** literally means 'needle insertion'. There are two main forms of acupuncture, the first using traditional methods of needle insertion and selection of acupuncture points following traditional Chinese principles of diagnosis and disease classification based on the need to restore the balance of chi energy, which is considered essential to good health. The second form uses a modified form of acupuncture in which selection of points is based on dermatomal distributions of pain.

- The **Alexander technique** is a type of therapy that aims to prevent and treat a range of disorders using a system of postural changes. The principle is that habit influences the use of the body and that use in turn affects the way in which the body functions.

- **Aromatherapy** is most often used to describe a particular type of treatment in which essential oils or aromatic essences are massaged into the skin, inhaled or occasionally ingested.

- **Autogenics** consists of a series of easy mental exercises designed to switch off the stress 'flight or fight' responses of the body and switch on the rest, relaxation and recreation system.

- **Chiropractic**. Chiropractors specialize in the diagnosis and treatment of mechanical disorders of the joints, especially those of the spine, and their effects on the nervous system. Chiropractic is mainly used in the treatment of common musculoskeletal complaints.

- **Healing**. Most healers call themselves simply 'healers' although some add the qualification 'spiritual'. All healers believe in the existence of a healing force that can be channelled through them to patients. Some believe it to be channelled through God, while others believe the force to be more natural but not yet recognized by science.

- **Homeopathy** is a system of medicine based on the principle of 'like curing like'. Homeopathic remedies are believed to assist the body's tendency to heal itself. Symptoms are believed to be the result of the body's defence mechanisms resisting attack; therefore homeopaths prescribe substances which, if used in a healthy person, would produce symptoms and signs similar to those presented by the patient. Remedies are prepared from repeatedly diluted extracts from, for example, minerals and plants. However, the effectiveness of a remedy is not directly related to its 'strength' as measured conventionally, and may in fact increase in potency with increasing dilution.

- **Hypnotherapy**. There are two main types of hypnotherapy. In the first the patient is put into a trance and the therapist suggests that their symptoms will disappear. In the second type they are put into a trance to facilitate the psychological treatment being used, e.g. to enable the therapist to explore what is going on in their subconscious mind.

- **Medical herbalism**. There are two main strands of herbal medicine: Western and Chinese. Both work from the basic principle that the symptoms of illness are a sign of underlying disharmony and are the physical manifestations of the body's attempts to heal itself. The herbs prescribed by the practitioner help this self-healing process.

- **Nutritional medicine**. Therapists believe that an unhealthy body is partly due to an inadequate diet. They aim to restore health by altering the body's biochemistry through dietary changes. The changes are determined by pinpointing whether an individual is suffering from vitamin or mineral deficiencies

Table 14.3 The uses of lavender oil

Body system	Properties	Conditions treated	Method of use
Circulation	Hypotensive sedative and decongestant; alleviates fluid retention	Hypertension; stress	Baths, massage, application
Digestion	Cleansing and calming	Indigestion, colic, nausea, flatulence, mouth ulcers	Compresses, massage, application
Emotional/nervous system	Sedative; nerve tonic	Nervous tension, stress, insomnia, headaches, migraine, depression	Inhalations, vaporizers, baths, massage, application
Genitourinary and endocrine systems	Antispasmodic; bactericidal; antiviral	Dysmenorrhoea, labour pains, genital injections	Compresses, inhalations, vaporizers, baths, applications, douche
Immune system	Antispasmodic; antiviral	Colds, flu, infections	Compresses, inhalations, vaporizers, baths, applications
The mind	Affects memory and emotions (two olfactory nerve tracts run into the limbic system)	Dementia, epilepsy	Inhalations, vaporizers, applications
Muscles and joints	Analgesic; anti-inflammatory	Muscular sprains, aches and pains, rheumatism	Compresses, baths, application, massage
Respiratory system	Analgesic; anti-inflammatory	Colds, flu, sinusitis, throat infections	Inhalation, vaporizers, application
The skin	Analgesic; anti-inflammatory; fungicidal; regenerative	Cuts, insect bites, eczema, infected wounds, athletes foot, head lice, herpes simplex, burns	Application, massage, compresses

and whether certain foods are acting on the body as a mild poison.

- **Osteopathy** is based on the principle that 'structure governs function'. The osteopath is concerned with identifying and treating 'osteopathic lesions', primarily by manipulating joints in order to restore them to their normal positions and mobility. Such manipulation is intended to relieve tension in muscle and ligaments and thereby alleviate dysfunction.

- **Reflexology** involves a method of treatment using massage to reflex areas found in the feet and hands – most commonly the feet are treated. It is based on the proposition that energy/life forces run through channels and that each channel relates to a zone of the body. It is believed that each organ or part of the body is mirrored on the foot and that organs that lie in the same zone are represented in the same segment of the foot. By feeling people's feet reflexologists can detect which energy channels are blocked and by massaging appropriate areas the channels can be unblocked.

- **Reiki** (pronounced Ray-key) is a Japanese word meaning 'universal life energy', an energy that is all around us. It is a system of natural healing which works on every level, not just the physical, and promotes the body's regenerative self-healing ability.

- **Shiatsu** means 'finger pressure'. The therapy incorporates aspects of acupressure and, like acupuncture, is based on promoting health by stimulating chi energy using pressure on the skin at various points along meridians associated with the function of vital organs.

- **Yoga** implies perfect harmony of body, mind and spirit. On a physical level it implies glowing health attained through exercise with controlled breathing and relaxation techniques. On a mental level, it implies the harmonious integration of the personality and the corresponding elimination of psychological 'complexes'. On the soul level, yoga implies union of the little self with the greater self, of the ego with the vastness of cosmic awareness.

Appendix 2: THE USE OF LAVENDER OIL IN AROMATHERAPY – A SNAPSHOT

In order to highlight the complexity of essential oils, lavender has been chosen as an example because it is one of the most versatile and well known of all essential oils. It is hoped that this will demonstrate the in-depth knowledge that is required not only for the practice of aromatherapy but indeed for the practice of all forms of complementary therapy.

LAVENDER, TRUE (LAVANDULA ANGUSTIFOLIA)

Plant family: Lamiaceae (Labiatae).
Method of extraction: Essential oil by steam distillation from the fresh flowering tops.
Volatility (speed of evaporation): Middle note.
Safety data: Non-toxic, non-irritant, non-sensitizing.
Principal constituents: Over 100 constituents including linalyl acetate (up to 40%), linalol, lavandulol, lavandulyl acetate, terpineol, cineol, limonene, ocimene and caryophyllene, among others. Constituents vary

according to source – high altitudes generally produce more esters.

The high percentage of terpenes and alcohols makes lavender a safe oil to use.

The terpenes (hydrocarbons) give a mild therapeutic effect, as do the alcohols, which are also calming, soothing and antibacterial. The additions of the esters encourages cell regeneration, which is why lavender is often used in healing wounds and burns (Table 14.3).

Appendix 3: RESEARCH ON COMPLEMENTARY THERAPIES AND FURTHER READING

Research on complementary therapies and doctors' attitudes to them

Aldridge D, Pietroni P 1987 Clinical assessment of acupuncture in asthma therapy: discussion paper. Journal of the Royal Society of Medicine 80:222–224

Anderson E, Anderson P 1987 GPs and alternative medicine. Journal of the Royal College of General Practitioners 37:52–55

Fulder S J, Munro R E 1985 Complementary medicine in the United Kingdom: patients, practitioners, and consultations. Lancet ii:542–545

Peninsula Medical School 2003 Complementary medicine: the evidence so far (a documentation on clinically relevant research 1993–2003). University of Exeter

Pietroni P M 1987 Holistic medicine: new lessons to be learned. Practitioner 231:1386–1390

Reilly D T 1983 Young doctors' views on alternative medicine. British Medical Journal 287: 337–339

Steehan M P et al 1992 Efficacy of traditional Chinese herbal therapy in adult atopic dermatitis. Lancet 340:13–17

Swayne J 1989 Survey of the use of homeopathic medicine in the UK health system. Journal of the Royal College of General Practitioners 39: 503–506

Symposium 1990 Practitioner 234:111–125

Thomas K J, Carr J, Westlake L, Williams B T 1991 Use of non-orthodox and conventional healthcare in Great Britain. Br Med J 302: 207–210

Wharton R, Lewith G 1986 Complementary medicine and the general practitioner. British Medical Journal 292:1498–1500

FURTHER READING

Davis P 1996 Aromatherapy: an A–Z. C W Daniel, London

Davies S, Stewart A 1987 Nutritional medicine. Pan Books, London

Featherstone C, Forsyth L 1997 Medical marriage. Findhorn Press, Forres

Foundation for Integrated Medicine 1997 Integrated healthcare: the way forward for the next 5 years. Foundation for Integrated Medicine, London

House of Lords Select Committee on Science and Technology 2000 Complementary and alternative medicine 6th report Session 1999–2000 (HL Paper 123). London

Lawless J 1992 Encyclopaedia of essential oils. Element Books, Shaftesbury

Montagu A 1978 Touching. Harper & Row, London

Price S 1991 Aromatherapy for common ailments. Gaia Books, London

Price S, Price L 1995 Aromatherapy for health professionals. Livingstone, Edinburgh

Sturgess S 1997 The yoga book. Element Books, Shaftesbury

Tisserand R, Balacs T 1995 Essential oil safety. Churchill Livingstone, Edinburgh

Wilson E, Lewith G 1997 Natural born healers. Collins & Brown, London

Yoga Sadhak Group 1975 Patanjali's yoga sutras. AH Pawaskar, Bombay

Chapter 15

The use of health informatics in practice

Ruth Wain and Randa Charles

DEDICATION

I would like to dedicate this chapter to my friend and colleague, Judith Shuttleworth, who was the co-author of this chapter in the first edition of this book. Sadly she died just after the publication of the book in 2000.

Ruth Wain

INTRODUCTION

In this chapter, the current and potential use of health informatics in health visiting will be reviewed. First, it is important to define the concept of health informatics and to consider the background to the development of health informatics in the NHS as a whole and in the community setting in particular. The reasons why development in this area has been slower than elsewhere are discussed, and then the potential uses of information and the vision for health visiting are outlined and put into the wider context of the NHS as a whole. Finally, the National Programme for IT (NPfIT) is outlined and the potential for health visiting to harness the potential provided by IT to bring it into the 21st century is discussed.

The main theme of this chapter is to determine how information can best be used to improve patient care, both at the individual and population level. The White Paper, *The New NHS: Modern, Dependable* (Department of Health 1997a) states that 'better care for patients, and improved health for everyone depends on the availability of good information, accessible, when and where it is needed'.

Central to this development has been the new NHS strategy, Information for Health (NHS Executive 1998a), which outlines the development path for information for the period 1998–2005. Frank Dobson, in the foreword to this document, describes the strategy as 'a radical programme to provide NHS staff with the most modern tools to improve the treatment and care of patients and to be able to narrow inequalities in health by identifying individuals, groups and neighbourhoods whose health care needs particular attention'. These business objectives are not only relevant to the NHS as a whole, but to health visitors in particular as they are in the unique position of carrying out all of these functions at a local level. However, the strategy was the vision and the realization of that vision is dependent on successful implementation. This is a crucial time in the realization of the strategy and it is crucially important that health visitors play their role in determining future development and implementation of systems, so that both their needs are met and they are able to meet the information requirements of others.

DEFINITIONS

What is health informatics? It can be described as 'the defining, storage, processing, analysing and retrieval of information, either in the form of data or knowledge' and encompasses the different aspects of people, skills, processes, systems and technology required to carry out these functions. Wyatt (1996) defines it as 'the term used to describe the science of information management in health care and its applications to support clinical research, decision-making and practice', and the *Enabling People Programme* (1997) as 'making effective use of information and technology for communication, decision-making and learning in health delivery and management'.

The kinds of activity encompassed by this view of health informatics include:

- audit
- management of resources

- self-management and professional development
- research
- communication among health care professionals/organizations
- using information for managing services
- using information for patient management
- decision support
- evidence-based clinical practice
- activity analysis
- monitoring quality of care
- epidemiology
- tracking patients
- development of clinical services.

The term 'health informatics' is synonymous with 'information management and technology' (IM&T) and the more recently used term 'information communication technology' (ICT). However, because of the way that IM&T has developed, in that it has concentrated on the development of information systems and technology and has failed to address the issue of information management, it has not been seen as part of the domain of those primarily involved in the delivery and management of health care. As a result of this, health informatics tends to be a term with which clinicians can more readily identify, as it may be seen to be approaching the subject from the information management perspective, although in reality the content is the same.

However, IM&T should not be seen as an entity in itself but as an integral part of the delivery of health care services. According to the study of the Massachusetts Institute of Technology, *Management in the 90s*, in rapidly changing organizations it is essential that there is effective planning and integration of the strategies for business activity, human resources, and for information management, systems and supporting technology (Adams et al 1992). This concept is illustrated in Figure 15.1, and maintains that if any of the circles representing the three strategies shift in relation to the others there will be a consequent effect on the ability of the organization to streamline, innovate or respond to change.

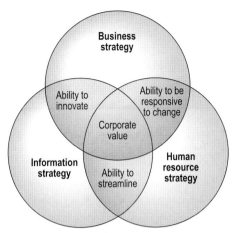

Figure 15.1   The strategic alignment model (Adams et al 1992)

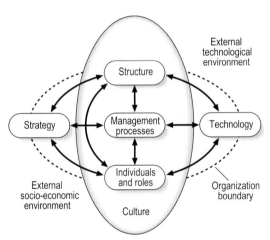

Figure 15.2   The management in the 90s framework (Adams et al 1992)

The process of strategic alignment is related to a conceptual framework. On one side of the framework is the organization's business domain and on the other side are the information systems, their management framework, IM&T specialist staff and supporting technology. In the middle of the framework sits the human resources domain reflecting the culture of the organization (Fig. 15.2). It is within this framework that the role of IM&T in health care, with particular reference to health visiting, will be considered.

BACKGROUND

The computing revolution which engulfed the health service during the early 1990s has had little impact on community services in general and health visiting in particular. The majority of the investment in IM&T has been in the acute sector – this may be partly due to the fact that community services are still seen as the 'Cinderella services', and therefore have not been able to accrue the enormous financial investment in IT that has happened in the acute sector, but also to the fact that it is much easier to implement IT systems in a single-site hospital than in community services. These are not only multi-site but also consist of large numbers of domiciliary workers such as health visitors and district nurses. An additional factor is undoubtedly the dearth of information systems available to support community services. However, this is a cyclical argument, as with no commitment to investment in IM&T in this area there is little incentive for systems suppliers to develop these systems, nor is there any clear national picture as to the sorts of system that are required. The fact that patient care in the community can be greatly improved by better information is well recognized: the Audit Commission (1997) estimated that improving information could save Community Trusts in England and Wales up to £30 m annually through reduction in administrative support. A further £180 m of clinical time could be released to invest in patient care. This represented an average avoidable cost of £200 000, plus £1.2 m in clinical time that could be released in each Trust annually. Apart from the financial gains there are also, and more importantly, the gains which could be made in terms of client/patient care at both the individual and population level. At the population level this is not quantifiable and even at the individual level the benefits cannot be measured, but when things go wrong, such as in the tragic death of Victoria Climbié, the suffering of this little girl cannot be imagined. Several recommendations of the Laming Report (2003) suggest that the collection and sharing of information both within and across organizations were part of the whole system failure.

The key principles that information should be person based, shared, derived from operational systems and secure, together with the philosophy of the new strategy *Information for Health* (NHS Executive 1998a) of providing access to clinical information to support patient care and the development of the electronic patient record (EPR), are fundamental to all parts of the NHS. They have real potential benefits for health visiting should they be embraced by the profession. In addition, the infrastructure that was developed and implemented as part of the first national IM&T strategy (Adams et al 1992) – the new NHS number, the use of national definitions such as read-coded clinical terms, and electronic communications via the NHS Net – provide the central building blocks on which to base any future developments.

However, the reluctance of community health professionals to accept this new technology is to some extent understandable, as it is obvious that their previous experience of computer technology has not enthused them. They have become fatigued by what is commonly termed 'feeding the beast', the process by which they have been required to complete diary sheets for input to the legacy systems mainly for staff activity monitoring purposes, and from which they have been unable to extract any useful information about their clients. This has made them feel that it has been a futile exercise and one that has used valuable time better spent on patient care. There are two issues identified here: first, it is only by 'closing the loop', i.e. feeding back information to those who provide it, that the quality of the information improves; and second, the information itself needs to be of use to the health professional in supporting the delivery of clinical care. Such clinical information is currently mainly kept on the parent-held record rather than by the health visitors themselves. A further problem is the nature of the health visitor's record, which is fundamentally different from other health records that focus much more on illness and disease. The type of information kept about children under 5 is more about objectives for child stimulation and development, along with psychosocial and physical dimensions. Records also contain information about immunization status,

level of growth and development attainments and other factors relating to parenting skills. We will now discuss the principles of paper-based record keeping before going on to discuss issues around electronic record keeping and the challenges that brings.

RECORD KEEPING BY HEALTH VISITORS

With an increasing demand for health-related data, practitioners must examine the issues to get the balance of the need for information right. There are many different types of record used by practitioners in different Trusts and health care settings. It would be unrealistic to assume that a standard universal record might emerge to suit the information needs of all. However, basic principles of good record keeping should underpin the development of records used by practitioners, focusing on an accurate account of the interaction with the client. The focus when considering documentation is the recording of relevant information upon which professional decisions are made and not solely the need for information or data collection.

The public health agenda and developments of Primary Care Trusts put the focus on assessing the health needs of the population. Innovative practice, progress in information technology and team working, such as Sure Start, are yet more drivers for change. Practitioners must, therefore, be aware of the potential of professional records to collect other relevant information and look critically at existing records to decide if current documentation does assist practitioners to assemble data from which health needs may be identified.

THE PURPOSE OF RECORDS

The purpose of a record developed for and written by nurses and health visitors is to document the professional interaction between client and professional. The NMC (2002b) maintains that this record must provide 'accurate, current, comprehensive and consistent information' about the assessment of the client. This interaction leads the practitioner to identify the health needs of the client/family and to record the action taken in response to those needs. The record should be written in such a way that the 'chronology of events' is clear to anyone looking at the record. It is good practice for records to be written contemporaneously and for the practitioner making the entry to date, time and sign it.

Record keeping should be supported by locally agreed standards developed by health visitors and their managers about the types of record issued and how they are used in practice. This standard-setting process considers quality issues and audit to ensure that local standards are being met while responding to developments in practice. Audit and the review of the processes for using records allow practitioners the opportunity to share good practice and to identify problems in using the documentation. The use of parent-held records, for example, identified a need to review other health visiting documentation to meet changing practice and need for information (Charles 1996).

Working in partnership with clients indicates a fundamental shift in practice towards records being written with clients. This ensures that both parties are clear about their role within the partnership and what the issues or concerns may be. This type of working creates the environment in which inaccuracies can be corrected – this may be factual information contained within the record but equally it may be inaccurate views the client may hold about the service offered. This raises training issues about using appropriate language, documenting interaction, sharing information, recording difficult issues/concerns and child protection.

Practitioners not only assemble information but also must be skilled in managing the data they gather. This management of information is a function critical to both practitioners and their managers in the current climate of NHS reforms. The collection and presentation of this data assist practitioners and managers within the organization/practice with three main functions (Torrington et al 1989, p. 338):

- planning
- control
- decision-making.

PLANNING

For practitioners, this can mean recording the assessment of a client using a structured approach from which a health visiting care pathway emerges. An example could be the need for additional support for a mother with postnatal depression, reflect the agreed intervention with the client, the time committed to offer counselling and a measure of outcome – a repeat Edinburgh Postnatal Depression Scale Scoring. For managers, the data about health visiting activity forms a part of the information for strategic planning of the nursing service for the organization. This can be achieved by looking at activity data of community practitioners and setting these against local and national policy, but used alone is not the best tool for planning purposes. The current focus on inequalities, parenting issues, nutrition, accident prevention and mental health gives tremendous opportunities for health visitors and managers to link practice to research evidence reflecting positive health outcomes. Records developed to assist data collection on an individual and population basis can provide managers and health visitors with powerful information on which to support investment and service development. An example of this could be health visitors developing a means of recording the identification, intervention and outcome measures of supporting women with postnatal depression and measuring this against referral patterns to secondary services. Practitioners must therefore be aware of the planning process and use opportunities proactively to present 'good' information to managers on positive health outcomes for clients arising from health visiting intervention.

CONTROL

Torrington et al (1989) also suggest that controlling (or evaluating) information influences operational issues and how the overall strategy is carried out. Managers must ensure that information collected reflects the need of the organization to demonstrate to commissioners of the service that the contracts are being met.

Ensuring quality is a major factor here and audit may identify poor performance – possibly due to covering vacant caseloads or unequal distribution of workload among staff. From a practitioner's perspective, evaluation must reflect how identified client health needs are being met; for example, have the child surveillances due been identified, completed, actioned and documented. Practitioners can use this statistical data to identify unmet health needs, excess demands within a workload or innovation in response to demand and articulate this case to managers and colleagues.

DECISION-MAKING

This is concerned with 'the day-to-day execution of activities' – the action of delivering a service (Torrington 1989). Practitioners must keep an accurate account of their interactions with clients as an 'aide memoire' so that these can be reviewed at the next contact and progress can be measured. This professional record would be part of any investigation of a problem or complaint about professional practice.

Good practice in record keeping is essential and critical in terms of accountability and 'is not an optional extra' (NMC 2002b).

The NMC Code of Professional Conduct (NMC 2002a) state that 'as a registered nurse you are personally accountable for your practice, your actions and omissions'. It is therefore essential that local records, policies and standards reflect this professional accountability by focusing on documenting clinical decisions related to patient care and raising the awareness of responsibilities in terms of record keeping.

TYPES OF RECORD

Professionally held records may take the form of manually or electronically held records. The type of record is determined by local agreements within organizations. When developing any type of documentation communication must take place between managers and practitioners to identify issues and ensure that both the organization's and practitioners' needs for

information are taken into account as well as reflecting professional accountability requirements and developments in practice.

The NMC makes it clear that the prime importance of nursing and health visiting records is to communicate factual data to team members and others – what has been observed or done. In the absence of contemporaneous records, a court must assume that no action was taken – 'if it is not recorded, it has not been done' (NMC 2002b, Fletcher & Buka 1999). Completing professional records with clients is considered good practice, allowing them an opportunity to correct inaccuracies (Baldry et al 1985, Naish 1991). Information is power and working in partnership implies equality and this must include health information. The Human Rights Act 1998 is relevant to all practitioners because it gives clients legal rights, such as being adequately informed, involved in decision-making and giving valid consent for health care (Jacks 2004). Clients must therefore have access to information on which to make informed choices about their health.

There are several formats used when documenting in records (Fischbach 1991, Iyer & Camp 1991). The narrative and problem-oriented approaches are possibly the two most common methods used in health visiting.

The narrative technique is the most traditional method of recording information in health records. The information is recorded in chronological order but the style will differ depending on who is recording the information. Fischbach (1991) suggests that the advantages are in chronology and sequence of patient events and allowing practitioners to determine how the information is recorded. The disadvantage in this type of recording is in quality of information, which may be disjointed, with 'buried information', and time consuming. In addition there are difficulties in information retrieval, such as in determining and tracking the health status of the client. As can be seen from the vignette below, hidden information may surround areas of concern about the child: poor parenting, lack of routine, safety issues. The tendency with the narrative format is to record less factual information and to record opinions instead, which are less likely to be shared by clients.

> Claire and Ben are a very young couple with their first baby. Claire does have some contact with her mother but Ben resents her 'interfering'. Baby Rebecca is 8 weeks old and the health visitor has concerns about her: her feeding pattern is erratic, she is not gaining much weight and she has nappy rash. Claire had not brought Rebecca for her check-up because she said the surgery was fully booked. The surgery had sent an appointment but the baby did not attend.

The problem-orientated system – the most familiar to many practitioners – is the SOAP/SOAPIER method of recording data relating to client interaction. SOAP is a process of recording that focuses on:

S subjective information, and
O objective information, forming the basis of the
A assessment; a problem list is developed from which a
P plan is developed for the client. The extended SOAPIER documents the planned/agreed intervention, and
I implementation recording the actions taken by practitioners to carry out the plan. This approach also makes the practitioner focus on planning
E evaluation of the interaction and future
R reviews.

A simple adaptation of this format applied to the vignette appears in Table 15.1.

A benefit of this format is the focus on the patient's health need/concerns and details of the interaction to address the need. The agreed actions of both client and health visitor are explicit, and realistic outcome measures have been put in place. This type of recording helps to define the professional role and explain to others how the job is done at a micro level – something

Table 15.1   A problem-oriented system

Actual/potential need (subjective/objective data)	Agreed action (action planning/implementation)	Date of review of plan	Evaluation/outcome of agreed plan
For Rebecca to have regular feeds	1. Claire and Ben know how to sterilize bottles and make feeds		
	2. To offer feeds to Rebecca every *n* number of hours		
	3. Parents to keep a feeding diary		3. Diary sheet discussed with parents
	4. HV to visit and talk about progress on (enter time and date)	Enter date of action 4	4. Plan amended if necessary
	5. Weigh baby at (time and date)	Enter date of action 5	5. Baby has gained weight
	6. Claire and Ben have HV contact number		6. Claire contacted HV for advice re night feeds
For Rebecca to have her check-up and receive treatment for nappy rash	1. Parents contact surgery to make appointment	Enter date of action 1	1. Rebecca attends appointment
	2. Claire's mother willing to drive them to surgery		
	3. HV to remind Claire about appointment	Enter date of action 3	
	4. Go over previous advice about cleaning skin and nappy changing		4. Nappy rash treated and improving

that is often difficult or perceived as too complex to attempt.

Fischbach (1991) acknowledges that focusing on problems can 'foster a negative approach to treatment', but this must not overshadow the benefits in recording in such a way (Table 15.2). This method of documenting care does require a change in the way we think about practice and recording care. It requires a corporate approach to risk management in record keeping. Practitioners should seek out and read PCT standards and policies on records management.

The family-centred public health agenda, health needs assessment and developments such as Sure Start in the community, setting have an impact on community practitioner documentation. Profile information about the health of the individual/caseload/population, together with a system for recording an effective outcome of interaction, helps practitioners to link the health needs of clients and communities within their specialist area and the effectiveness of their clinical intervention. These outcomes should demonstrate activity to help meet PCT objectives in local delivery plans. The changing need for different data should encourage professionals to review existing documentation and develop or test modifications to existing systems. Any review in terms of data collection must be underpinned by two factors. First, the information must be realistic, meaningful and inform individual practice, and second, it must be realistic in quantity. We must consider the extent to which the information we collect can

contribute to public health and commissioning responsibilities within primary care organizations. The information assembled by practitioners in this way is much more meaningful than 'the focus on achieving a maximum number of contacts' (Health Education Authority 1997).

HEALTH VISITOR INDEX CARD

The health visitor index card (Fig. 15.3) was developed by practitioners and built on work within the Trust by health visitor colleagues developing a tool for profiling (Watts 1992) and performance outcomes (Plant 1992).

The catalyst for change was a successful pilot of child health parent-held records with a planned implementation across the district. This represented a change in practice towards an overt partnership with clients and included the use other documentation. These changes ran alongside the development of a customized electronic information system to help health visitors manage their data. Practitioners identified a need for a record that would assemble meaningful data on an ongoing basis in a format ready for input, allow updating and represent a reduction in clerical activity. The record also had to meet practitioners' needs concerning accountability. What a challenge!

The project began with consultation at a local level with managers, health visitors, child protection advisors and the school health service. This was to ensure that the need for information through the potential pathways was taken into account. It was anticipated that change in health visitor documentation would have an impact on other nursing records used within the Trust.

PROFILE AND OUTCOME DATA

Health visitor profile and outcome data is assembled on the front of the card in a coded format for easy computer input. This information is confidential and used for providing baseline information, care planning, access to health/other services and measuring impact on health gain.

Table 15.2   The value of problem-oriented system records

Professional requirement in record keeping	Does the problem–oriented system fit?
Identifies problem/need	Yes
Records action/plan	Yes
Measures outcome/progress	Yes
Information easily retrievable	Yes
Factual, concise, consistent information	Yes
Involve/share with client	Yes

HEALTH VISITING INDEX CARD   CONFIDENTIAL   North Staffordshire Primary Care Trusts **NHS**

LABEL

Address
1 ....
2 ....
3 ....
4 ....

G.P.
1 ....
2 ....
3 ....
4 ....

Reference Address
1 ....
2 ....

Health Visitor
Clinic
1 ....
2 ....
3 ....
4 ....

Child - Known allergy or Hypersensitivity

PROFILE

A/N	Breast Fed	Vit K	Breast 6 wks	Breast 4 mths	Breast 6 mths	Age weaned	S/C	CPR	LAC	Disability L/P	Unsupp	Cult/ Lang Diff	Accom T/U	Eth

Risk Markers
( ) Environmental   ( ) Animal
( ) Property Hazard   ( ) Do Not Visit Alone
( ) Contact Notifier

CHILD HEALTH SURVEILLANCE: SPTORN

	Initial HV Assessment	6 wks	8 mths	18 mths	3 yrs	Orth	Pelvic Floor Advice
Newborn Hearing Screening							

Pelvic Floor Advice
Advice Given
Problem
Referred

SMOKING

	Main Carer Smokes	Other Smoker in Household	Brief Intervention
Initial Assessment			
6 Weeks			
8 Months			
18/24 Months			
3 Years			

S - satisfactory P - problem T - treatment O - observation R - referred N - not examined

ACCIDENT PREVENTION

	Advice Given	Attended A&E
Initial Assessment		
6 Weeks		
8 Months		
18/24 Mths		
3 Years		

Accident Prevention Pack
Date Issued:

Immunisation 0 full consent   date
0 part consent   date

Date Issued:
Bookstart:
1.
2.

Dental Pack
1.

LABEL

Registered for Sure Start
Y or N
Date:

MENTAL HEALTH

	EPDS	DATE DONE
5 - 8 Weeks		
Repeat		
3 - 6 Months		
Repeat		

Figure 15.3   Health visitor index card developed by North Staffordshire Primary Care Trusts

Research suggests that there are major health gains from breast-feeding for both mother and child, which could represent a cost saving to the NHS. A health visitor performance outcome related to breast-feeding was developed by Plant (1992) and can be applied to the use of the record and data collection in the index card. Baseline data is collected at the first health visitor contact on the method of feeding. Health visitors offer an intervention to breast-feeding women in the form of advice, support and expertise, access to support networks and specialist services needed. Health visitors then measure the prevalence of breast-feeding at 6 weeks, 4 and 6 months as an indication of the efficacy of their interactions. Data can be compared on an annual basis to individual, team, PCT and district statistics. This represents a potentially powerful tool enabling practitioners to demonstrate health gains linked to health visitor intervention, contribute to PCT targets, and identify and potentially influence other variables related to this public health issue within the community.

Information on contact data and forward planning is recorded on the back cover of the record card. The record is reviewed and updated annually in response to consultation and practice developments. The index card is supported by guidelines for practitioners for its use, updating training sessions and PCT health visiting standards on record keeping.

Evaluation of the index card showed that it was successful in recording contacts with clients, assisted in collection of profile and outcome data and was useful as a forward planner for intervention (Charles 1996). Clients accepted the use of the index card in practice.

FAMILY HEALTH PLANS

The family-centred public health role for health visitors presents new challenges in the development of documentation with integration of the population-based public health approach and the work health visitors undertake with individuals and families.

A family health plan is a core tool for health visitors to work with parents to explore their health and parenting needs (Department of Health 2001e). The plan identifies need, as the family perceives it, and an action plan for the family, the interaction and support given to achieve this and an evaluation mechanism to measure progress. The family health plan helps explore some of the wider determinants of health: family issues such as work, relationships, income, disability, bringing up children with a focus on behaviour, parenthood, nutrition, safety, managing illness and community issues, for example, housing, education, transport, crime and isolation.

Garside (2000) suggests that the use of family health plans has the potential to involve parents in local developments, promote a non-directive approach to practice, deliver the public health role and make services more relevant to the needs of families. She suggests families welcome the opportunity to explore their own health and their community's health and appears to enable them to plan change. Garside suggests that family health plans cannot be introduced as an extra to the health visitor's current role. It represents new ways of working based on the needs and views of parents and the development of multi-agency working. Garside states that a facilitated approach is needed for the successful introduction of the family health plans with release from the traditional ways of working.

HEALTH NEEDS ASSESSMENT TOOL

Another model for the assessment of health need has been developed based on the *Framework for the Assessment of Children in Need and their Families* (Department of Health 2000b). This model provides a 'systematic way of understanding and recording what is happening to children within their families and the wider context of the communities in which they live'. The framework presents three interrelated domains: the child's developmental needs, family and environmental factors and parenting capacity. The framework document further explores dimensions within these three main domains.

The electronic health needs assessment tool used in one area identified that it enabled the development of a family health plan, empowered both parents and professionals and encouraged early intervention (Shariatmadari and Miller 2003). The use of the tool was also considered to strengthen the public health role and demonstrate effectiveness.

PERSONAL CHILD HEALTH RECORDS (PCHR)

The British Paediatric Association, with the support of other professional nursing and medical associations, launched PCHRs in 1990. The ethos supporting the introduction of the parent-held record was to encourage partnership with parents, improve communication, enhance continuity of care and increase parents' understanding of their child's health and development (Hall & Elliman 2003). The record is intended as the main record of the child's health, initially developed for the period between birth and 5 years of age. School-age modules have been developed.

The PCHR serves two main functions: first as a resource containing information and advice given by professionals, outcomes of health checks and details of immunizations, weights and measurements. Information for parents, observations and checklists are also included. This sharing of information facilitates working in partnership as a two-way process. Secondly, the record can be used as a teaching tool using the basic health education material contained within it. This information may be tailored to identify local health needs and may be a means of universally targeting health messages to all parents.

Parents need information on which to make choices about the health of their children. This process cannot be achieved by issuing a record alone but must embrace the concept of working in partnership with parents in an open and participatory way (CPHVA 1999). The change means that parents are more involved in decision-making related to the health and well-being of their children. Professionals with experience of parent-held records are in favour of parents holding the main child health record and suggest that they are less likely to lose them

than health professionals (Macfarlene & Saffin 1990, Pearson & Waterson 1992, Charles 1994)! From the professionals' perspective, use of the record enhances communication, is a comprehensive record of immunization and surveillance and may improve uptake of screening and immunization by opportunistic review and offer of such services (Charles 1994).

The PCHR can be a means to promote mutual trust and respect between parents and professionals. For this to happen, professionals must actively encourage parents to bring the PCHR and consider making it a part of booking-in procedures at clinics and surgeries. Professionals should ask to read relevant parents' entries and observations and record the advice given in the PCHR. Parents have highlighted the benefits, e.g. helping them to remember advice and 'important things' and feeling more actively involved in their child's health care; parents value the record and have no difficulty in remembering to bring it to child health clinics (Charles 1994). Health visitors and school nurses can affect the use and value of the record by including the use of the PCHR in standards and protocols related to children. Advice given to parents should be recorded using appropriate language so that carers have the opportunity to review advice given; this advice is also available to other professionals who may be involved in the child's care.

When issuing the PCHR to parents and carers, the time spent by health visitors promoting the importance of the record and their responsibilities in keeping it safe is a valuable investment and directly affects the importance the parents place on it and its subsequent use (Charles 1996).

ADDITIONAL DOCUMENTATION

The type of information and record will differ from organization to organization depending on interpretation of guidelines and local and national policies. Occasions may arise when more detailed documentation is needed for some clients. Health visitors and managers should work together to develop guidance criteria for the introduction of additional records, in order that practitioners can feel safe in practice and to reduce the risk of informal and unofficial records being kept. Some issues to consider may involve children with multiple or chronic health needs, and complex needs due to socio-economic factors or child protection concerns (Charles 1996). This additional documentation helps to clarify for the client and other professionals the nature of the intervention and measure of outcome within a complex multi-agency intervention. This documentation should also be completed with parents.

The NMC (2002b) suggests that supplementary records kept without access by the client or family members should be the exception rather than the norm. A way forward may be to use a carbon-duplicated care plan with a copy each for professional and parent. An agreed action between client and practitioner is written and any dissent is recorded. The document is signed and dated and a copy kept in the professional's record. The client also has a copy of this detailed plan to keep. The difficulty for some practitioners lies in setting out and writing care plans that act as a working document and training may be required (Charles 1996).

LEGAL ISSUES

Professional records are legal documents and can be required before a court of law. It is essential that practitioners recognize their responsibility for accurately recording not only care given but also 'identify problems that have arisen and action taken to rectify them' and 'the care delivered and the information shared' (NMC 2002b). Practitioners must be aware of local policies relating to the retention of records.

The Data Protection Act 1998 give patients/clients the right to request access to information about themselves whether it is in a manual or a computer record – this includes health records (CPHVA 1999). Applications for access to health records must be made in writing and health organizations have to respond within a certain time-frame. The suggested good practice of health visitors writing and sharing their professional records and reports with clients

should reduce the incidence of clients needing to proceed along this legal avenue.

Parent-held records (parent child health records) are the property of the issuing Trust although held by the parents. Confidentiality about the information held within the record therefore rests with the parent as they choose with whom the record is shared. The CPHVA (1999) suggests that it should be made clear to carers of the child that access to the record may be 'sought for purposes of audit, profiling, data collection or legal matters'. Access to the record can be requested and enforced by law if necessary. Health professionals are not liable if the record is lost by parents, but are responsible for her/his own entries in the record and recording in the professionally held baseline data in the event of a loss of the parent held records.

This has attempted to raise some of the issues around records and record keeping in practice. Records are not static but must be the subject of review and development in response to innovation and developments in practice. Health visitors and community practitioners must critically analyse their documentation in the light of changes in working practices, team working and working across traditional boundaries. Does it reflect the patient's outcome? Can it contribute to research evidence of practice? Is it acceptable to both clients and practitioners? Has it considered professional accountability? Does it measure quality in a meaningful way? Is the information collected used? Do records meet the clinical governance requirements? These questions form an ongoing debate as to what information should be collected. In the next section, the background to the development of electronic patient records is discussed.

THE NEW NATIONAL IM&T STRATEGY

As part of its modernization plans, the government set out its information strategy for the modern NHS in the document *Information for Health: An Information Strategy for the Modern NHS 1998–2005* (NHS Executive 1998). The purpose of the new strategy is to ensure that information is used to help patients receive the best possible care by enabling NHS professionals to have the information they need both to provide that care and to play their part in improving the public's health.

In order to do this, the strategy commits to:

- lifelong electronic health records for every person in the country
- round-the-clock on-line access to patient records and information about best clinical practice for all NHS clinicians
- genuine seamless care for patients through GPs, hospitals and community services sharing information across the NHS information highway
- the effective use of NHS resources by providing health care planners and managers with the information they need.

The key issues which the strategy supports are:

- tackling inequalities in health as outlined in the Green Paper *Our Healthier Nation* (Department of Health 1998b)
- a primary care-led NHS
- collaboration between the NHS, local authorities and others in order to improve health
- preparation and evaluation of health improvement programmes
- development of primary care groups/trusts
- improving the quality of care and supporting clinical governance arrangements.

The information principles on which the strategy is based are as follows:

- information will be person based
- systems will be integrated
- management information will be derived from operational systems
- information will be shared across the NHS
- information will be secure and confidential.

These support the concept of 'integrated care' and are based on the fundamental premise that good clinical practice and service performance management will only flow if the strategy is focused on delivering the information required to support day-to-day clinical practice.

The strategy states that health care professionals need:

- fast, reliable and accurate information about the individual patients in their care
- fast, easy access to local and national knowledge bases that support the direct care of patients and clinical management decision-making
- access to information to support them in the evaluation of the care they give, underpinning clinical governance, planning and research, and helping with their continuing professional development

and that policy-makers and managers need to have good-quality information to help them better target and use the resources deployed in the NHS and to improve the quality of life of patients and local communities.

ELECTRONIC RECORDS

Central to the strategy is a move towards electronic records, as they are likely to be more legible, accurate, safe, secure, to be available when required, and can be more readily and rapidly retrieved and communicated. Also, they can be integrated with other records and made available for audit, research and quality assurance purposes. The strategy clearly defines the terms *electronic patient record* (EPR) and *electronic health record* (EHR) – phrases often used to define similar concepts. The EPR describes the record of the periodic care provided mainly by one institution, whereas the EHR is used to describe the concept of a longitudinal record of a patient's health and health care – from cradle to grave. It is defined as a combination of information about patient contacts with primary health care and subsets of information associated with the outcomes of periodic care held in the EPRs, as illustrated in Figure 15.4.

This model can be seen to be flawed, however, as it represents the primary care record as an EHR when in fact it is an EPR in its

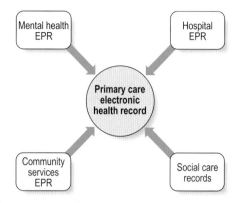

Figure 15.4 *Information for Health:* electronic health record (From NHS Executive 1998a)

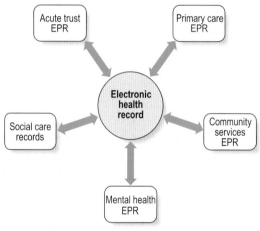

Figure 15.5 Electronic health record: an alternative view

own right. An alternative model is shown in Figure 15.5, in which the EHR is seen to be made up of all of the constituent parts and data can flow in both directions so that all NHS providers can both provide data for and view the EHR.

Whether the EHR is 'real' (i.e. is held centrally in a data warehouse) or virtual, in that the various components are kept by the supplying organizations but can be viewed by means of an interface, is still under debate. Regardless of how the data are to be held, it is essential that health professionals agree the nature and content of the component data sets so that a consistent model of EHRs can be constructed. The unique NHS number will play a crucial role in facilitating linkage and in improving confidentiality in data transfers and the use of data for audit and research purposes.

The main use of the electronic health record is for providing routine patient care, and one of its main benefits is seen as improving the integration of care across organizational boundaries. In addition, aggregated anonymized subsets of the EHRs can be used for other purposes, as shown in Figure 15.6.

For EHRs to benefit patient care it is essential to create and maintain accurate, complete, relevant, up-to-date and accessible data sets. However, currently there is no agreement on either the content, structure or potential use of individual patient summary records.

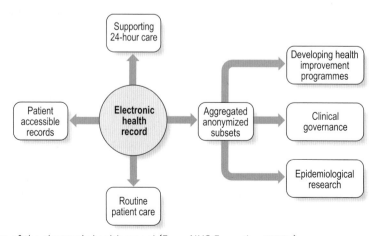

Figure 15.6 Use of the electronic health record (From NHS Executive 1998a)

From its inception the NHS has pursued the goal of seamless care. In most aspects it has been hampered by the sheer volume of communications about patients, coupled with the number of organizations and professional boundaries involved. Where co-ordination and communication between different parts falls down, the consequence is inevitably poorer care. Considerable time and costs are involved in chasing up information and resolving problems caused by incomplete information. Developing EHRs was seen as the mechanism by which to facilitate the shift from profession-specific and institutional records to integrated lifelong person-based records. As a minimum, coordination of care was expected to improve across the following organizational boundaries:

- within the full primary care team
- between hospitals and general practice
- between health and social care.

The failure of the NHS to make progress with the electronic health record, combined with the recommendations of the Wanless Report (April 2002), resulted in the revised national strategy *Delivering 21st Century IT Support for the NHS*, which set out the scope and first steps for the nationally directed National Programme for IT (NPfIT) (DH 2002a). Wanless recommended doubling and protecting IT spend in the NHS, stringent centrally managed national standards for data and IT and the better management of IT implementation in the NHS including a national programme. It stated: 'Without a major advance in the effective use of information and communications technology, the health services will find it increasingly difficult to deliver the efficient, high quality service which the public will demand. This is a major priority, which will have a crucial impact on the health service over future years'.

The shift has begun from systems running along institutional lines, dealing with only a portion of patient interactions, to whole systems that track and record a user, or a patient's progress across care services. It involves creating a national care records service (CRS) to provide a live, interactive patient record service accessible 24 hours a day, 7 days a week, covering hospital, primary care and community services.

The main criticism of existing systems is that they do not support care professionals in the delivery of care. The processes involved in the delivery of care can be grouped into six high-level areas:

- Delivering proactive services. Covering the care involved in health promotion, prevention, and screening and surveillance services
- Delivering responsive services covering a wide range of simple and complex situations, where advice is provided, assessments undertaken, care planned and provided in response to an inquiry, presentation or referral initiated by the patient or service user, a carer or other care professional
- Managing care professional, covering team management activities such as reallocating caseloads due to staff absence
- Managing information to support care processes, covering the maintenance of information that underpins the care processes listed above, such as maintaining the service register
- Managing providers, covering the monitoring of provider performance and calculating payments to providers
- Auditing and monitoring services, covering the extraction and provision of information to support the monitoring of targets, production of statutory returns and clinical audit.

Source: National Specification for Integrated Care Records Service (Department of Health 2004a).

The National Specification for Integrated Care Records Service also states that the purpose of and Integrated Care Record Service (ICRS) is to support the provision of high-quality care across the whole of the health community, linked to national services and conformant to national standards. ICRS should therefore be looking to support a seamless continuum of care for an individual patient or service user across all care settings within a care community and across care communities (Box 15.1).

Box 15.1   What we want from an Integrated Care Records Service

For patients, a modern IT-enabled NHS will directly and visibly impact on how they interact with the care system and on their experience as consumers of care services to:

1. Feel confident that information about them and their history of care is accurate and easily accessible to any other professional involved with their care and with a need to know, except where the patient has expressed a view to the contrary
2. Be reassured that their professionals have access to information about the latest care knowledge and practice
3. Be reassured that the information that they provide at any health care encounter is kept secure
4. Be able to look at their records and have the ability to amend or add information (taking into account the legal implications)
5. Be able to understand their care process through use of 'patient-friendly care pathway views'
6. Be offered the opportunity to exercise choice over date, time and place of future encounters with care services
7. Be offered choice over where to pick up prescriptions
8. Be able to use a range of technologies – PCs, phones, digital TV – to interact with care services and at times that are convenient to them
9. Have access to evidence of the quality of care provided to them or by local providers
10. Be able to understand their records and to derive beneficial advice and support from them
11. Provide links to patient communities and support groups

For professionals involved with direct patient and service user care, to have safe, fast, modern IT systems to support them routinely in their work and to:

1. Have ready access to information about their patients when they want it, from wherever they want it (including peripatetic staff), and structured in a format they want
2. Have ready access to the knowledge, clinical tools and related services they need to support their clinical decision-making process
3. Be able to use high-quality information in support of the implementation of audit, peer review, clinical effectiveness and other aspects of Clinical Governance
4. Be able to rely on the fact that they will be notified about responses to service requests – which could be referrals or test requests – or lack of response within an appropriate time period
5. Be assured that their records and communications with patients and colleagues are secure and conformant with agreed information-sharing protocols
6. Be able to participate in lifelong learning through access to education, training and development services

For managers, researchers and other professionals not involved in direct patient care – for example, epidemiologists – to:

1. Have ready access to aggregated and anonymized information to support research, planning and management of care services
2. Be able to use high-quality information in support of the implementation of clinical governance and improvement of public health
3. Be able to participate in lifelong learning through access to education, training and development services

ACCESSING PRIMARY CARE DATA

Developing these new sources of data will take some time and an urgent issue for PCTs is the relative lack of access they normally have to information about primary and community care. At present much of the Korner data is of little value – knowing how many patients actually received a particular service is not the same as knowing that patients who need the service actually received it.

A real concern of community-based clinicians is the substantial amount of time taken up by recording data for central statistical returns that does not flow naturally from the care process and is of little or no value to their treatment of individuals or for retrospective evaluation. There is little evidence that the collection of Korner data in community services offers managers anything useful for gauging either value for money or effectiveness in community services.

The successful development of the EPR and EHR requires a common-coded clinical vocabulary to facilitate reliable and accurate electronic communication of clinical information and enable consistent activity analysis. The NHS has made considerable investment in the Read Codes and the subsequent Clinical Terms project to produce Version 3, which extends the vocabulary from a medical to a clinical thesaurus. This development of the Read Codes as the NHS standard terminology is supported by the clinical professional bodies, including the Royal College of Nursing, the Royal College of Midwives, the Community Practitioners and Health Visitors Association (through the Strategic Advisory Group for Nursing Information Systems – SAGNIS). The group, which was set up to develop the coding for nursing, midwifery and health visiting, produced their final report in August 1995, although, like the development of all of the Read Codes, development will be ongoing. The report nevertheless provides the basis for the development of an EPR for health visiting.

Defined aggregations of clinical terms, agreed at national and local levels as appropriate, are also required to ensure the development of good-quality data for statistical use. Health care resource groups (HRGs) are useful tools, but to date they have been developed mainly in the acute inpatient care setting. HRGs are used to group together similar conditions that have similar resource implications. Community HRGs are defined as 'descriptions of care given by community professionals' and 'activity is described in groupings which are comparable in terms of costs and resources used' (NHS Executive 1997). However, this may need revisiting, as their groupings are at a very high level (e.g. individual case management). Within this there is likely to be wide variation in the amount of resources required, depending on the circumstances.

As all NHS clinicians, including health visitors, address the obligation to continually review and improve personal effectiveness through evidence-based practice and clinical audit, they face several problems:

- the variable quality and reliability of information
- a dearth of local clinical informatics expertise
- a lack of personal keyboard skills
- pressure on their time
- poor access to computers at their base
- the fact that health visitors operate at many different locations.

So far we have concentrated on individual care records and their use in the management of individual patients. However, there are many other areas where IM&T can be utilized. The next section considers the use of information management in a wider context.

THE VISION

The vision that is proposed is not new. The Chief Nursing Officer and Director of Nursing at the Department of Health, in her address to the British Computer Society Nursing Specialist Group, spoke of the importance for strategy, organizational structure and information technology to be managed together (Moores 1991) and at the same conference the following year stated that 'the integration of compatible and accessible data is essential for the future' and that 'a workforce capable of using information to manage both clinical care and the nursing resource is essential' (Moores 1992).

These three ideals – the full integration of information alongside strategic and organizational development, the accessibility and compatibility of data regardless of source and the ability to use information effectively to improve patient care and service delivery – still form the basis for the vision, with the addition of the use of the NHS Net, the 'information superhighway', to provide a private network with speed, reliability and security for the transfer of clinical information, links to other NHS sites and organizations from the desktop, and access to the Internet and sites containing rich sources of health information (including the National Electronic Library for Health).

In the not too distant future, all health visitors should have access to a computer at their main place of work, which will allow:

- use of e-mail as a quick and efficient means of communication to liaise with other professionals, e.g. to inform a GP of concerns about a particular client
- use of an electronic appointment system to make appointments for the client with self and other health professionals across organization boundaries
- easy and rapid access to current and standardized guidelines
- access to evidence-based data
- continual update of knowledge by access to electronic textbooks and journals
- input of clinical information to support client care at point-of-delivery
- the use of this clinical database in different views to produce information for other purposes such as management information, rather than collecting it separately
- use of an up-to-date multidisciplinary information base to inform programmes of care
- continual monitoring of processes and outcomes at the individual and caseload level

- automatic aggregation of clinical information across the service for audit purposes.

Once the information needed is available and the benefits can be demonstrated, this will provide the basis for a business case to support the investment required to allow health visitors to be provided with the equipment to enable them to access this type of information in their clients' homes.

USES OF INFORMATION IN HEALTH VISITING

Managing clients, measuring effectiveness and managing caseloads have all been discussed in the preceding sections by Charles.

SUPPORTING CLINICAL GOVERNANCE

A First Class Service (Department of Health 1998a) highlighted the fundamental importance of improving the quality of care throughout all areas of the NHS. This is because performance management processes designed simply to target outliers will eventually eliminate the extremes of poor performance but may not improve mediocre or average performance, and will therefore fail to benefit the vast majority of patients. There is another aspect of this: simple identification of outliers is a very simplistic assessment of quality – once identified, a 'drill-down' procedure into the underlying data is required to explore possible reasons for being in that position, particular aspects of the community to which the data is referring, interventions that may themselves be more time consuming or expensive but that may in fact relieve the burden from another area of the service. A more comprehensive database would allow these other possibilities to be explored.

Continual improvement of clinical service quality across the NHS must be supported by information on current comparative effectiveness and outcomes. It also requires a culture among clinical staff where the obligation on individuals to assess personal performance

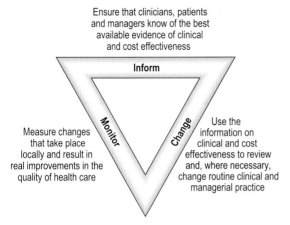

Ensure that clinicians, patients and managers know of the best available evidence of clinical and cost effectiveness

Inform

Monitor

Change

Measure changes that take place locally and result in real improvements in the quality of health care

Use the information on clinical and cost effectiveness to review and, where necessary, change routine clinical and managerial practice

Figure 15.7   Clinical effectiveness

is continually accepted as a natural and important element of being a professional. This is an area with which health visitors can be seen to be already conversant in terms of their reflective practice; however, what they have not developed is a culture of developing the information flows to support it in a coherent way.

Implementing a framework for clinical governance requires a comprehensive programme of quality improvement such as clinical audit, evidence-based practice and processes for monitoring clinical care using effectiveness information and clinical records systems (Fig. 15.7).

To achieve this, information must be drawn from:

- local clinical audit data
- national comparative data
- local care pathways and clinical protocols
- national best practice guidelines
- National Institute for Clinical Excellence evidence
- international research evidence.

This requires statistical data to be linked to textual reference material. For further discussion on the economic perspectives see Chapter 16.

REFERENCE MATERIAL

The rapid expansion of the use of electronic media has revolutionized the storage and

exchange of information, and access to the World Wide Web provides vast amounts of material available directly on to the desktop. In relation to the professional knowledge base, it is growing ever faster, and clinicians and managers find it impossible to keep abreast of the vast amounts of information available.

There is a need to critically appraise the growing body of medical literature and evidence to ensure that clinicians receive fast and convenient access to appropriate knowledge bases to provide real-time support to their care of individual patients.

There is now an opportunity to begin to use in earnest the NHS-accredited National Electronic Library for Health (NELH). Once placed here, the material may be regarded as 'official'. The National Institute for Clinical Excellence (NICE), established by *The New NHS* (Department of Health 1997a), has a remit to 'produce and disseminate clinical guidelines based on relevant evidence'. NICE will therefore be one of the major sources of accredited material placed in the NELH.

Senior managers in the NHS must lead their organizations into the Information Age 'from the front' (NHS Executive 1998a). They too have a need for access to up-to-date accredited information and so an 'NHS Information Zone' containing on-line reference material for the NHS management community is also planned.

Information for Health (NHS Executive 1998a) states that 'the NHS must have accurate and reliable data to support:

- local clinical governance
- National Service Frameworks, local care pathways and clinical protocols
- Health Improvement Programmes
- the national 'Framework for Assessing Performance'.

RISK MANAGEMENT

Risk analysis can be defined from a number of perspectives. The strategic guidance on effective use of information to support the management and delivery of nursing and midwifery care (NHS Executive 1995) states that the management of risk can be broken down into four stages – identification, analysis, control and cost:

- Identification: What can go wrong?
- Analysis:
  - How will it go wrong?
  - How severely?
  - How frequently?
  - How likely?
- Control:
  - What changes can be made to prevent it?
  - What will reduce the effect?
- Cost: How will any loss be paid for?

Information is required to manage risk effectively, but collecting too much data, or the wrong data, or not using it, wastes resources and time.

SUPPORTING THE NATIONAL SERVICE FRAMEWORKS (NSFs)

Gathering the best evidence of clinical and cost-effectiveness and relating that to the views of service users to determine the best ways of configuring the provision of particular services is an important new approach that relies on information. Successful delivery of the recently published NSF for Children *Every Child Matters* (Department for Education and Skills 2004b) and other NSFs which have issues related to children and young people is dependent on information sharing both within and between organizations.

While technology is not a solution in itself, in some circumstances it will enable change, e.g. through the introduction of systems to collect and audit data along a care pathway and share information between organizations.

DEVELOPING LOCAL CARE PATHWAYS AND CLINICAL PROTOCOLS

There is a need for those involved in planning and managing services to have ready access to a wide range of other information to support the best use of the national evidence base. Locally, there needs to be agreed guidance on service delivery in the form of local care pathways and protocols that can be accessed on an internal 'Intranet'.

HEALTH IMPROVEMENT PROGRAMMES

The three major functions of health improvement programmes are health needs assessment for a population, planning interventions to address those needs and monitoring their outcome. These are distinctly similar to those outlined by the Public Health Information Specification Project (PHIS), which was commissioned by the National Health Service Management Executive to develop the public health aspect of the common basic specification (CBS) data model. This project produced a model comprising three views. In the functional view, health needs assessment, intervention planning to address identified health needs and outcome monitoring are disaggregated into their elementary processes (Fig. 15.8).

The other two views are the entity model, which shows the data used and produced by the processes and the relationship between the data; and the behavioural view, the sequence in which processes may be carried out. There is an infinite variety of behavioural views since processes may be continuously reiterated, in any order. The whole model can be seen as a planning cycle in which activities can be continuously influenced by feedback of

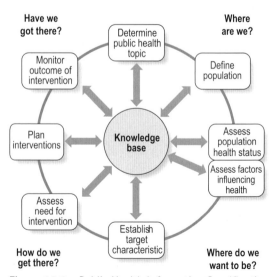

Figure 15.8 Public Health Information Specification model (redrawn from Wain & Holton 1993)

information and, as such, its use enhances the effectiveness and efficiency with which resources are used.

The New NHS and *Our Healthier Nation* (and other recent initiatives), have created a substantial information agenda for the collation and interpretation of information to support the local health improvement programme and the commissioning priorities of primary care groups in identifying the needs and measuring the health of different local communities to support the provision of more effective health care. All of these are an important part of the public health function, so it is not surprising that this model remains relevant.

HEALTH NEEDS ASSESSMENT

The public health function is also central to the role of the health visitor. Health needs assessment has been part of their role since the new syllabus for health visitors was introduced in 1965 and they have become increasingly proficient in the development of community and caseload profiles that include 'bottom-up' approaches to the epidemiological assessment of need. 'Through their contribution to the delivery of local health care and by the application of epidemiological, psychosocial and social science principles and knowledge, they act both as community participants and local researchers' (Robinson & Elkan 1996). Their broad knowledge base and their intimate knowledge of the local community makes their contribution invaluable and complementary to the 'top-down' approach to health needs assessment carried out at PCT level. Of particular value is the fact that health visitors are in a position not only to identify needs from a professional viewpoint but also to engage their clients in the process of negotiating care packages to meet their individual needs and to amass collective views on clients' perceptions of their health needs. 'The communication skills which many nurses, midwives and health visitors acquire during their professional education can equip them to participate in consultation with groups and individuals about their health needs' (NHS Executive 1993).

The national framework for assessing performance

Accurate and timely data are essential for management purposes, if actions are to be appropriate and evidence based. The reasons for poor data quality are:

- a backlash against the collection of information that supports only management needs

- a failure to feed back useful analyses to those from whom the information is collected

- no incentives to collect good quality data and in some cases perverse incentives to provide inaccurate and untimely data to avoid censure for poor performance.

The introduction of the national framework for assessing performance focusing on service quality and effectiveness offers the opportunity to create a new attitude in the NHS to information quality, especially if:

- a responsive and credible benchmarking service can be delivered locally, to support clinical governance and health planning, that is respected and valued by the clinical community

- there are inclusive processes for local staff, especially clinicians, to own the information and make active use of it to promote local clinical improvements.

THE KNOWLEDGE BASE

All the above functions require a vast knowledge base to support them. The new IM&T strategy states the government's commitment to providing information at a national level but there is a pressing need for information to be collected locally. There is much information already available that has been collected by individual health visitors, but a local strategy needs to be developed for making it available to all.

The knowledge base will be used to inform decisions made in the various ongoing developments, and these will feed back into the knowledge base, making it continually richer. Figure 15.9 shows the flow of information.

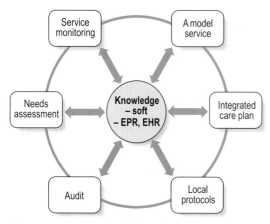

Figure 15.9 The knowledge wheel

THE COMMUNITY INFORMATION AGENDA

There is no doubt that the new information strategy is ambitious for all parts of the NHS, but nowhere more so than for community and primary care. The inadequacies of health systems to support community health staff have been apparent for many years and, as stated in *Information for Health* (NHS Executive 1998a), 'Even without the organisational changes signalled in the new NHS, the development of integrated primary community care systems would have been sensible. The new NHS proposals make this inevitable.'

The agenda therefore is to:

- develop a knowledge base to support all aspects of care provision
- modernize primary care information systems
- integrate primary and community care information systems
- use information captured in operational clinical systems to provide secondary data flow
- develop primary and community care effectiveness indicators for local and national performance management
- develop the means to extract the information needed automatically from primary and community care information systems to meet the needs of the national framework for assessing performance.

MAKING INFORMATION WORK – IMPLEMENTATION ISSUES FOR HEALTH VISITING

INFORMATION FRAMEWORK

The first building block in providing appropriate information and information systems for health visiting is to agree a robust information framework that adequately describes the range and complexity of services provided and supports the development of a health visiting patient record, which will form an integral part of a multi-agency child health record and support a cradle-to-grave electronic health record. The framework will need to contain elements that can be recorded consistently by different professionals so that information will be valid and comparable irrespective of where or by whom it was recorded. *Information for Health* and the discussion paper on case-mix groupings for community services both view information collection as focused upon that which is needed to support a full clinical record supporting clinical service delivery and used by clinicians as the prime information source. Specific extracts and aggregation of information from these records will be used for costing, planning and commissioning (Fig. 15.10).

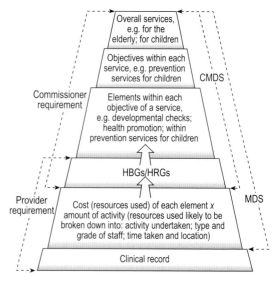

Figure 15.10 Levels of detail for commissioners and providers

The Community Health Care Resource Group's consultation document released in April 1997 used the four principles of health visiting underpinning all health visitor activity – the search for health needs, the stimulation of the awareness of health, the influence of policies affecting health and the facilitation of health enhancing activities – and from these identified the following groupings and elements.

GROUPINGS

A. Individual case management
B. Assessment
C. Health education/health promotion
D. A programme of monitoring individual health and development with associated health promotion
E. Parenting/caring skills
F. Child protection – on the Register
G. Protection of individuals or families at risk
H. Counselling/psychological support including bereavement
I. Management of diagnosed condition/problem
J. Nutritional guidance
K. Public health function.

CORE ELEMENTS OF HEALTH VISITING THAT UNDERPIN THEIR ACTIVITIES

- Advocacy/empowerment
- Caseload management
- Clinical supervision
- Formal communication
- Interagency working
- Liaison
- Management
- Prioritization of work and workloads
- Professional development
- Record keeping
- Referrals
- Reflective practice
- Research and development
- Systems management and management
- Teaching of other grades and professions.

The Information Framework exercise was focused specifically on unidisciplinary care, although it was acknowledged that it could be applied to multidisciplinary care. It aimed to include all activities, including those that were not necessarily patient related. It was acknowledged that there was a need to identify the key activity where several activities occurred as part of a single contact. This issue, however, is not new to health visiting and, although the need to identify the key activity or service recipient is similarly essential to ensuring comparable and consistent data collection, it has not been an area that has been successfully addressed. The model described in the Community Health Care Resource Group's consultation document was very complex. Each of the 11 groupings identified was defined and a range of activities included in the grouping was identified or details of the tools used were given. Items identified as a grouping can also occur at a lower level as an activity under another grouping heading. For example, 'assessment' is identified as a grouping in itself but also as an activity in six other groupings. Although the model reflects the range of health visiting services, it is perhaps too complex to be achieved in one move from existing information recording. It relies heavily on concepts that were proposed within the Community Minimum Data Set. This has not been implemented, possibly because of issues of user acceptability and ability of existing systems to collect the information. In addition this model has not resolved many of the issues regarding clear identification of the key activity and key recipient of the service that currently cause difficulties in collecting high-quality information.

The model for deriving information indicated by *Information for Health* proposes that the core building block would be the EHR. By means of common record structures and headings and use of standard clinical terms, information could be derived that was standardized and comparable. However, the current situation for health visiting seems to be a long way from achieving this, even in a paper-based system.

To make progress it may be advantageous to begin by defining a simpler model than that identified in the Community Health Care Resource Group proposals and Community

Minimum Data Set, while incorporating some of the features of these proposals that clinicians find easy to apply with some consistency and set about implementing them. This will ensure that health visitors will have more confidence in discussing and owning informatics issues and the quality of existing data will begin to improve. This must form a safer platform from which to embark on more ambitious information developments in the future.

WHAT INFORMATION TO COLLECT

The complexity of the health visitor's workload results in lack of consistency when trying to describe the services they deliver. A distinction can be made between the generic basic package of care, comprising advice, surveillance and immunization, that is delivered to every child and the additional services that may also be required relating to special needs, behaviour management, child protection, etc. However, in practice, elements of two or more different care packages may be delivered as part of an integrated care plan during a single contact. There are differences in how this information is currently recorded on diary sheets, which can result in double counting in terms of contacts. This complexity is also mirrored in attributing the recipient of the contact. Although a specific child may be the reason for a visit, advice may still be given even if the child is not present, e.g. if a child is exhibiting a specific behaviour problem that the health visitor feels is related to parental management or behaviour. There is often a difference of opinion among health visitors as to whether the contact is attributed to the adult, the child or both. Although data definitions allow recording of a proxy contact this often does little to illuminate the decision regarding recording of contacts. Advice may also be given regarding another child or to an adult relative or even a visiting friend. These opportunistic contacts are not always recorded in the same way by different health visitors, even those working within the same Trust. Even where definitive written guidance is provided to ensure consistency of data collection this is often not felt by professionals to be helpful, as it does not accord with how they view their service provision.

The introduction of the parent-held record, often known as 'the Red Book', meant that the records became the joint responsibility of the parent and the professional. Parents were encouraged to make entries in the book and it was envisaged that it would be taken along to GP visits and that the GP would make relevant entries, although there has been a reluctance among some GPs to participate in this joint record keeping. Most of the information held here, except for the child health surveillance record, is not replicated elsewhere. The health visitor only keeps additional information where there are specific concerns about child protection issues or where it is necessary to retain information about other family members. The only other record kept by the health visitor is what is known as the 'tracer card', which contains minimal details of care pathway contacts. This lack of uniformity and consistency in the manual records supporting health visitors is another factor contributing to the difficulty in providing good information to support service delivery.

This confusion is frequently mirrored in the provision of computerized information systems for health visitors. Typically the generic surveillance and immunization elements are supported by a version of the national Child Health System. These were often the earliest systems implemented and therefore the information collected on them was often extended as far as possible to capture other elements of the service. In many Trusts a community information system was introduced at a later date in addition to the Child Health System. This type of system would be structured in line with data manual guidance to provide information to support Korner returns. This entails a distinction between advice and support contacts, which are related to individuals, and health education and surveillance contacts, which are related to specific groups and tend not to be related to individuals. However, the fact that both types of contact are frequently fused within a single time-slot has led to considerable disparity in the information provided on these returns and recorded on the systems. The advent of GP fundholding caused a further twist when it became apparent that health education and surveillance contacts for a specific practice not delivered at the practice premises were not identifiable unless assigned to an individual client, i.e. as part of the advice and support recording mechanism.

METHODS OF DATA COLLECTION

Another problem is the fact that health visiting services are typically delivered in the client's home, a busy baby clinic or GP surgery. Although some Primary Care Trusts have gone some way to provide appropriate technology, such as palm-top computers, to allow use of information in the workplace, frequently this level of investment has not been possible. Most trusts have provided clinic-based computer access, with information input by clerical or clinical staff. Both approaches have their defenders. Clerical input is seen to be more cost effective, can ensure that information is recorded in a fairly consistent way and can be more timely and accurate than input by less computer-literate clinicians. However, as the need to record more clinical information to develop a full health record including assessments and care plans develops, the use of clerical staff becomes less appropriate. Clinical input can improve ownership, data quality (and quantity) and the use of information. However, this may not be an automatic result of installing computers for use by clinicians, as without significant staff support and organizational development programmes clinicians may revert back to using manual information sources. Birth books, clinic books and address books are often retained in tandem with computerized systems and are often maintained and consulted as the prime information source, to the detriment of computerized data quality.

INFORMATION SYSTEMS

There are major decisions to be made by health communities as to the development of information systems to support the collection of clinical information. In securing integrated care records services, a number of different scenarios for the use of existing systems may result. These include:

- existing systems, such as current GP systems and the Child Health System, being removed and replaced by entirely new systems
- basic existing administrative systems being retained and operated by incumbent suppliers with new suppliers adding clinical solutions on top of them
- basic existing administrative systems being retained but operated by new prime contractors who would also add clinical solutions on top of them
- retention of existing clinical systems which work effectively and which have the support of current users.

Although some GP system suppliers have developed community service modules, this may not in reality be the best way forward. It may be more beneficial for systems to be developed to meet the needs of specific professional groups, with interfaces being created that will enable them to be seamlessly linked. This would have several advantages. It would allow information to be more readily available to all the relevant teams, some of which are not primary care based. For example, although it is clearly beneficial to have the information within the primary care record for services that are part of primary health care, there is a risk that for other services provided by other organizations, such as those supporting children with special educational needs or district specialist services, linking this information directly to GP systems would mean that it could not be shared with all of those needing it. The most important criteria for the development of this new generation of systems is that they should enable multidisciplinary clinical information to be available to the professional at the point of contact with the client and be fully integrated with each other. The only way forward is for clinicians and IM&T specialists to work together in their development to ensure that everyone's needs are met. Health visitors need to be very actively involved in this process. John Badham, Head of Nursing for the National Programme for IT, stated that nurses and allied health professionals 'just don't know enough about the changes that are going to shake up the way they work following on from the introduction of new technology to the NHS' and he goes on to state that he is adamant that the involvement of nurses and allied health professionals is critical to take forward the development of new information systems as they are the ones who are going to be using the new information. He sees it as 'a once in a lifetime opportunity to make a difference' and urges members of these groups to become involved in the National Advisory Group which he set up in September 2004.

CONCLUSIONS

It can be seen that the implementation of the national IM&T strategy, which is the largest ever undertaken, is an ambitious one. It will have a particularly large impact on services such as health visiting, which along with other community based services is coming from an extremely low baseline in the use of information management and technology in supporting both client/patient care and service delivery. However, in some ways this can be seen as a challenge, as it gives an opportunity to start with a clean sheet of paper. This has to be an advantage for health visitors, as more recently there has been a definite move to involve clinicians from the outset and this gives a wonderful opportunity for them to set the agenda and make sure that the systems work for them, that data collection is manageable and that access to the information they need is available where and when they need it, whether in the client's home or in remote clinics. By making this information readily available to them, data quality will improve and so will patient care.

ACKNOWLEDGEMENT
We would like to thank Judith Bates, Independent Consultant in IM&T, for her comments on previous drafts of this chapter.

Chapter **16**

The health economics of public health practice

Jane Powell

CHAPTER CONTENTS

THE ROLE OF ECONOMICS IN 21st-CENTURY PUBLIC HEALTH

A little knowledge of some of the key concepts, thinking and techniques of health economics, and the limits of economic evaluation, can be viewed as an important part of professional development in specialist community public health practice. Economic evaluation encompasses a well-established set of techniques in forming part of the evidence base for health care, but the evidence from economic evaluations for public health policy and practice is scant in most areas of wider health care practice (Sefton et al 2002, Byford et al 2003). In recent years the demand for such evaluation has risen in response to the modernization agenda of government and the focus upon research aimed at reducing health inequalities (Miller 2003, Evans 2003). In order to encourage greater use of economic evaluation of programmes, interventions and care pathways in health visiting, there is a need for economists to better understand the nature of public health *as action or intervention* in order to ensure that the approaches they suggest that public health specialists and practitioners adopt, are useful and feasible.

THE STRUCTURE OF THIS CHAPTER

The first section of the chapter will focus on economics as a discipline, outlining economists' approaches to thinking about problems of resource allocation. It will outline key concepts from the perspective of public health professionals and tools and techniques that are closely associated with the work of health economists. The second section will outline the evaluation techniques in health economics, and their usefulness for health visiting practice, giving examples of the various types of economic evaluation study and an outline of 'how to do' the various stages of an economic evaluation of public health interventions in health visiting. The third section will summarize the economic evidence for specialist community public health–health visiting.

ECONOMICS – A DISCIPLINE

A definition of economics by Paul Samuelson (1976) provides a broad summary of the main concerns of economics. Economics is:

> the study of how men and society end up choosing with and without the use of money, to employ [allocate] scarce productive resources, [which may have alternative uses] for production and distribute them for consumption [efficiently and equitably], now and in the future, among various groups and people in society. It analyses the costs and benefits of improving patterns of resource allocation.

Economics is a discipline or a way of thinking (Cohen et al 1988). A number of tools and techniques, such as economic evaluation and appraisal, are associated with economics as a discipline. Orthodox economics can be applied to any system in which inputs have to be converted to outputs. In orthodox economics all systems are subject to 'scarce' resources, in which the term 'scarce' refers not to shortage, but to a limit on all resources. Economic agents or people in systems including the health care system have unlimited wants or infinite demands. The combination of scarcity of resources and unlimited demands creates a need to make choices about allocating resources. Alternatives for allocating resources are weighed up by taking account of opportunity costs. Efficiency and equity are two of the criteria for choice in allocation and distribution of resources.

ECONOMICS AND HEALTH VISITING

The purpose and function of health visiting relate directly to this definition of economics. Resources are scarce or finite. Health visitors cannot do everything they would wish to for the people they visit, as resources will not allow for this. Therefore, health visitors have to make choices about how to allocate scarce resources at their disposal. Efficiency is a criterion for sharing out or allocating resources amongst all competing uses in health visiting. Resources should be allocated in order to obtain the maximum 'health improvement' from the finite amount of resources. However, most health visitors would be concerned to allocate resources equitably as well, in order to reduce health inequalities. Unfortunately, it is very unlikely that an efficient allocation of resources will also be an equitable allocation of resources. However, this fact does not detract from the potential usefulness of economic techniques in any activity where scarce resources have to be employed and distributed efficiently.

THE DEVELOPMENT OF HEALTH ECONOMICS AS A BRANCH OF ECONOMICS

Monetarist ideology is particularly associated with Margaret Thatcher's time in government and was at the forefront of the creation of the quasi-market in health care in 1991. Monetarist economic theory is particularly concerned with efficiency, as opposed to equity, being the criterion for allocation of scarce health care resources. In the UK National Health Service, the proliferation of policy connected with monetarist economic theory created a false and damaging impression that health economists have much in common with accountants and were concerned merely with costs and prices.

At the end of the 19th century, the basis for the orthodox, modern economic theory was developed. Mathematical developments in the physical sciences were utilized by economists with engineering and science training. They sought to lift economics to the same status as the physical sciences. These early mathematical economists viewed the world as a smoothly functioning machine in which the relationships between a small number of key economic variables could be determined and reveal to us how the world in all its complexity works (Ormerod 1994).

'Marginal economics' resulted from the combination of theory about economic relationships, assumptions to reduce the complexity of the real world into manageable chunks and reduced form mathematical expressions to test these theories. The 'margin' was and still remains a key concept at the core of modern orthodox economics and health economics (Marshall 1936).

A subdiscipline of health economics developed in the late 1970s from the main discipline of economics and coincided with the creation of Archie Cochrane's evidence base movement for health care. Health economics is rooted mostly in micro (small) as opposed to macro (large) economics. As a branch of micro-economic theory, it is concerned with the behaviour of individual people and organizations, as opposed to the behaviour of aggregate, macro or whole economies. The approach to solving real world problems or way of thinking and tools and techniques of health economics arise from the mother discipline.

Some economists have openly criticized the ideologies of leading monetarist and Keynesian economists of the past as fundamentally flawed and too orthodox to explain the operation of complex economies (Ormerod 1994). In addition, criticisms of micro-economic theory have been directed at its shortcomings. In particular, the assumption of rational behaviour on the part of economic agents or people, pervasive in micro-economic theory, has been questioned forcefully. Assumptions that people behave rationally are often made in economic theorizing and empirical work, as this type of assumption allows economists to proceed to the neat solutions and answers that are required in empirical and evaluative work. Economists argue that assumptions can be relaxed later once an answer has been arrived at to imagine what difference this would have made. These criticisms have important implications for health economists as the foundations of health economics are firmly rooted in orthodox micro-economic theory and its focus on 'rational economic man'. In public health care the appearance of 'rational economic man' in economic evaluation frameworks is most unhelpful to public health policy makers, even if he is male and we are meant to ignore him or his presence is intended to kick-start upstream economic measures on tax that might discourage use of hazardous goods, for example, alcohol and cigarettes (Wanless 2004).

KEY CONCEPTS IN HEALTH ECONOMICS

Orthodox economic theory is founded on numerous principles and is full of jargon. Fortunately, for those in health visiting who have not had a thorough grounding in economic theory, explanation of a few key concepts will cover a substantial amount of what is needed to get by.

Opportunity cost

The value of a good or service as measured by the next best alternative foregone. Resources are limited and if they are used in one way they are not then available to be used again in another way. Very few activities are costless and costs can be incurred without money necessarily changing hands. For example, if a health visitor foregoes the opportunity to take a day's leave in order to attend to an urgent case then there is a cost, which is the benefit foregone in not enjoying the day's leave. The value of the best opportunity foregone as a result of undertaking an activity or the sacrifice involved is the opportunity cost. Usually money is used as a means of measuring opportunity cost. Definitions of cost in economics and accounting are different. The economist's notion of cost extends beyond the cost falling on the health service. All sacrifices involved in pursuing a particular policy are relevant, including those on other agencies, service users, patients and their families.

The margin

Marginal analysis is used to evaluate the change in costs and benefits produced by a change in production or consumption of one extra unit. Less formally it is often used to refer to the change in costs and benefits produced by increases or decreases in resources under consideration.

Efficiency

Allocative efficiency is concerned with objectives to be met and to what extent to meet them, when not all objectives can be met. Technical or X efficiency is about how best to meet a given objective at least cost.

Equity

Equity is the criterion concerned with the fairness of the distribution of resources. 'Fairness' is a value judgement and so greater equality may not necessarily mean greater equity.

Quality adjusted life year (QALY)

QALYs are indicators of the benefit or outcome of a treatment or service. They can be calculated by multiplying the changes in individual ratings of quality of life, with and without treatment, by the number of years of life for which the change is experienced. Health-related quality of life can be measured by presenting people with a scale, in which 0 is equivalent to being dead and 1 equivalent to perfect health or well-being. People can indicate at which point on the scale they perceive their current quality of life to be. For example, an improvement of 0.1 on a quality of life scale that measures quality of life before and after treatment for 1 year is equal to 0.1 of a QALY gained.

Economic evaluation and economic appraisal

Economic appraisal is a retrospective activity. Conversely, economic evaluation is prospective and can take place as a new health visiting programme is being rolled out and adapted through experience. Let us imagine that all activities undertaken by health visitors are under review in order to increase effective use of resources. A number of techniques from the same family can be applied in order to view systematically the costs and benefits of alternative ways of allocating resources. The technique chosen would depend on the precise objective of any review of health visiting activities, and the units in which outcomes of the different alternatives are measured must relate to this objective. If this is not the case, it is not possible to make comments about effective use of resources.

There are a number of different potential evaluative methods within the family of approaches available to an economist to design an economic evaluation. At present this analytic framework reflects the fact that most economic evaluation to date has been applied to evaluative acute health care interventions of the kind that take place in a hospital. This analytic framework is reflected in a major textbook on economic evaluation 'the blue book' by Drummond (Drummond et al 1997), guidelines for economic evaluation from the National Institute for Clinical Excellence (2004) and the Treasury Green Book (HM Treasury 2002). It can be argued that the economic framework reflected in these publications is very much suited to evaluation of individual interventions (in health care); rather than the complex programmes often found in public health practice. Within this analytic framework there are several types of economic evaluation, each of which has a different scope and suitability for evaluative tasks. These 'types' are outlined in the next section.

Cost-offset studies

The simplest economic studies are concerned only with costs. Such studies may be conducted as health and quality of life outcomes, and have already been established from other research, or are not measurable because of conceptual difficulties or research funding limitations. *Cost-offset studies* compare costs incurred with other costs saved. A health visiting programme might have high start-up costs, but might reduce the need for in-patient admissions and will create cost savings downstream. The limitation of this type of study is that it does not look at the alternative use of resources.

Cost minimization analysis

This type of economic evaluation study allows alternative uses of resources to be considered by evaluators. It is predicated on the knowledge that previous research has shown outcomes of various interventions to be similar. Well-conducted cost minimization analysis can be thought of as being a special type of cost-effectiveness analysis; however, evidence of similar outcomes is not available for interventions in some areas of public health practice. Indeed some areas of public health practice, for example the health of prisoners, has a dearth of information on both effectiveness and cost-effectiveness of public health care. Cost minimization analysis is not really a suitable technique for much of the activity that occurs in health visiting as part of public health practice, as it cannot deal with the complexity of outcome inherent in the programmes and care pathways implemented by health visitors in their work.

Cost-effectiveness analysis

Cost-effectiveness analysis is the most common approach used in economic evaluation and synthesizes single outcomes and costs, for example increase in life years gained from a health promotion intervention (Kelly et al 2004). An obvious weakness with strict cost-effectiveness methodology is enforced focus on a single outcome in order to compute ratios. Public health programmes or interventions usually have layered, multidimensional outcomes. Carrying multiple outcomes forward in an economic analysis is not easy analytically and the methodology of economics is concerned with the reduction of complexity into manageable chunks so that comparisons across alternative programmes can be made. Economists do not favour the notion of multiple outcomes in an economic evaluation. Economists believe it is impossible to compute ratios from multiple outcomes, so they tend to favour single outcomes,

for example the QALY, to facilitate like-for-like comparisons across the breadth of all spending by the Department of Health.

In terms of carrying multiple outcomes from a programme forward through an economic evaluation one option is available from three further types of economic evaluation. This option, cost-consequences analysis, is to retain all or most outcome dimensions using standard scales and a mix of process and final outcome measures and not to summarize these into one final outcome measure. The other two options weight outcomes in terms of money through cost–benefit or in terms of utility or cost–utility.

Cost–utility analysis (CUA)

In this type of analysis the evaluator measures and then values the impact of an intervention in terms of improvements in preference-weighted, health-related quality of life such as the QALY. CUAs allow comparisons to be made across all areas of health intervention aiding in resource allocation decision-making. However, this type of analysis does not capture broader non-health consequences and opportunity costs of public health programmes.

Cost–benefit analysis (CBA)

CBA values all costs and benefits in monetary units. If benefits exceed costs, investing in a programme would be worthwhile and vice versa. CBAs are theoretically an ideal approach; but conducting them can be problematic because of the difficulties associated with valuing outcomes, including public acceptability, in monetary terms. This in part explains the fact that NICE guidance on submissions of economic evaluations; as part of the technology appraisal process, explicitly excludes CBA (NICE 2004). Given the nature of public health interventions and their impact across many other sectors of the State there is a strong case for more cost–benefit analysis. NICE guidance currently only recommends a health and personal social services perspective, although costs to patients and families may also be reported.

Valuation methods used by health economists in CBA studies have concentrated on direct valuations by either asking individuals to state the amount they would be prepared to pay to achieve a given health state or health gain, or through observation of actual behaviour and by applying implicit values. More recently though, an approach first developed in marketing, has been used to value health interventions. This approach is known as *'conjoint analysis'* or *'discrete choice experiment'*. Conjoint analysis allows individuals to rank different real world scenarios, which may consist of several dimensions, to establish their valuations. Although its use in health promotion and public health has been limited thus far, conjoint analysis has scope to reveal the individual characteristics and environmental factors that may influence the uptake of interventions and initiate change in behaviour. By including cost as one of the dimensions in a discrete choice experiment, monetary values can also be elicited. Although complex, in that the scenarios need to be carefully devised, conjoint analysis has the advantage of not specifically asking individuals to value health states or health gains in monetary terms. This can mean conjoint analysis is easier to administer than traditional willingness-to-pay study designs, which increases its acceptability with policy makers. For a full description of conjoint analysis and discrete choice experiments readers are referred to research studies conducted by Mandy Ryan at the Health Economics Research Unit, University of Aberdeen.

Cost–consequences analysis

This is similar to cost-effectiveness analysis in terms of the questions addressed, but it is applied to evaluate interventions with more than one multidimensional outcome. In *cost-consequences analysis* for each alternative the evaluator would compute total costs and measure change along the relevant outcome dimensions. The cost and outcome results would need to be reviewed by decision makers and the different outcomes weighed up to compare with costs. While this approach has some limitations, as it does not synthesize benefits and costs, it can be used to look at the issue of changing behaviour that is so crucial to public health interventions. For example, a study seeking to improve compliance with medication might consider costs, insight, attitudes to medication, attitudes to health visitor, global functioning, symptoms and compliance as part of the cost-consequences analysis.

In cost-consequences analysis the evaluator does not attempt to combine measures of benefit into a single measure of effectiveness, so it cannot be used to rank interventions. Nevertheless it is a systematic technique that allows decision makers to weight and prioritize the outcomes of an evaluation. The analysis involves focusing on a particular problem, for example teenage pregnancy, and then considering two or more possibilities: to make one or more interventions or to do nothing; then, using either existing available data post hoc, or more prospectively, deriving new data, establishing an appropriate method for an analysis of costs and outcomes in a common currency. The evidence collected would need to relate to four questions: What works to improve health? What works to reduce inequalities in health? What works in changing behaviour? What works in promoting take-up of behaviour change interventions?

The sources of evidence for these different questions will be different. Outcomes can be measured in terms of quality adjusted life years (QALYs), healthy year equivalents (HYEs) or disability adjusted life years (DALYs). Common currency estimates would be compiled in order to capture a wide range of consequences, both good and bad, and the potential costs to the initial provider, partner organizations and other services. A cost-effectiveness ratio for every intervention would compare cost (minus the saving in resources) with a unit of outcome, for example a QALY.

ECONOMIC APPRAISAL AND OTHER EVALUATION STUDIES IN HEALTH VISITING

A QUESTION OF ECONOMIC EVALUATION

Many health visitor interventions take place every day. Some of these interventions are more beneficial than others and it is vital to appreciate the status of health visitor interventions, particularly when resources are cut or expanded. There is no point in attempting to establish the economic effectiveness of efficiency of an intervention that is not beneficial. Non-efficacious interventions consume resources in the same way as efficacious interventions and so clinical or technical appraisal of interventions must always precede economic evaluation. All interventions with positive outcomes are of course beneficial, but in economic evaluation we wish to establish through clinical evaluation the most efficacious interventions.

By making some assumptions with a hypothetical example, the above points can be clarified. Let us assume a clinical evaluation of two health visiting interventions: rehabilitation of elderly stroke victims in their homes and advice to the elderly to prevent fractures in the home are rated similarly in a clinical evaluation. Furthermore, assume that a later economic evaluation based on these findings reveals the benefits of both interventions are not large, but of similar size and the cost of advice from health visitors to prevent fractures in the elderly is much lower than rehabilitation of elderly stroke patients. An economic evaluation would conclude that prevention of fractures is a more efficient intervention (technically) than rehabilitation of elderly stroke victims, as the ratio of benefit to cost is larger for the former intervention than the latter.

FRAMEWORK FOR ECONOMIC EVALUATION OF PUBLIC HEALTH INTERVENTIONS

This section focuses on an economic framework for evaluating public health interventions that has been developed by the Centre for Social Exclusion (CASE) at the London School of Economics and the Health Economics Unit at the Institute of Psychiatry. This approach is outlined in a very thoughtful and practical textbook (Sefton et al 2002) and all readers are referred to this excellent source for more detailed exposition of this framework. Sefton et al (2002) argue that many public health interventions are more

complex and multi-level than interventions in health care, introducing problems for the application of 'traditional' economic evaluation techniques favoured by health economists. Readers are referred to the blue book by Drummond et al (1997) and Drummond & McGuire (2001) for exposition of the traditional framework for economic evaluation in health care.

THE STAGES OF PUBLIC HEALTH ECONOMIC EVALUATION

There are four stages in a thorough economic evaluation of public health interventions (Powell, 2003).

STAGE 1: PRE-IMPLEMENTATION
Define intervention(s) to meet need and consider service user perspectives

Economic evaluation in public health is about the design of effective programmes or interventions that meet the needs of individuals, population groups, communities and wider society. Economic evaluation is not meant to rubber-stamp decisions concerning resources that have already been made, or consist of a proposal to spend resources in a certain way. New interventions might be considered within an economic framework, as well as 'stay-the-same' or 'do nothing' options. Political motivations should not be part of economic evaluation.

The *thinking* stages of economic evaluation are crucial to its final quality. Time should be allocated during the thinking stage for consultation with everyone concerned with the options or alternatives in the evaluation, including all stakeholders and service users. Economists in the past have been reluctant to embrace the consultation stage, as they often wished to remain impartial in completing economic evaluation. In fact it is vital that economists take a hands-on approach at both Stage 1 and Stage 2 of an economic evaluation in order to get a feel for the factors and inputs that might be of importance at Stage 3. Economists' involvement with pre-implementation is needed in order to capture the variables relevant to the questions: What works to improve health? What works to reduce inequalities in health? What works in changing behaviour? What works in promoting take-up of behaviour change interventions?

Identify key components of an intervention

In order to determine the outcome of an economic evaluation, objectives must be set. Health visiting interventions are likely to have many outcomes at various levels. For example, interventions to prevent domestic violence will almost certainly benefit individuals abused by their partners. At one level quality of life, employment status and self-esteem might be improved and each of these could be a designated objective of these programmes. In addition, communities might also benefit from prevention of domestic violence at another level of outcome.

STAGE 2: PILOTING

Redefinition of problem and testing of intervention

At the piloting stage of a health visiting intervention, it is important to clarify the original objectives of a programme, particularly a new programme, as it is possible that the objectives could change. This might be because the objectives have developed (or failed to develop) and improvements have been seen (or not seen). For example, health visitor programmes that seek to increase support for ex-offenders with drug and alcohol problems in the community, might ask how such support is viewed by various probation services, counselling services and treatment centres. It might be relevant to consider whether support for drug and alcohol problems of ex-prisoners in the community relates to an overall government objective, for example, reduction of health inequalities in deprived or marginalized communities. Exploratory testing of a social intervention of this nature would examine how the specific elements of support for drug and alcohol problems operate while noting emergent 'best practice' in reducing health inequalities (Wanless 2004).

Research design, costs and outcome measures

Control or comparison groups

Economists take the view that an economic evaluation study design should demonstrate effectiveness of any programme or intervention with respect to another programme or intervention. There are numerous methods for achieving a comparison group, for example outcomes in one group that have received a programme compared with another group that has not, or the same group compared 'before' and 'after' a programme intervention.

Costs

There are four broad categories of cost that should be considered in economic evaluation:

- Programme costs arise from the direct cost of providing a public health intervention.
- Direct costs include all the individual elements of an intervention, such as staff, volunteer time, buildings, equipment, transport and support services.
- Non-programme intangible costs (or savings) arise from resultant programme effects, such as the savings that may result due to a reduction in the need for alternative programmes.
- Indirect costs, such as child, family and wider agency costs (or savings): for example, the salary of carers should also be included in economic evaluation.

Benefits

Economic evaluation should be wide ranging and have a societal perspective that includes savings (opportunity costs) to other parts of the public sector from implementation of a public health programme. Evaluators should therefore consider outcomes that may not be referred to in the objectives of a programme, including impact upon parties other than the main target group and the savings to wider society and other government departments from improved health or reduced health inequalities.

Outcome measures

Specialist community public health programmes impact on different levels of outcome. It is important to evaluate the impact of programmes on communities and organizations in which the programme is set, as well as on individuals, in order to capture the full impact of a programme.

There are two types of outcomes to be evaluated:

- Final outcomes arise from the populations impacted by health visitor programmes.
- Process outcomes arise from achievement of potential and actual joint working processes and partnership arrangements that arise from a public health programme.

Process outcomes relating to the manner in which an organization and its workers implement a programme are not part of traditional economic evaluation and the focus upon inputs and outputs. However, it is difficult to ignore process outcomes within public health programme evaluation as good process is an essential ingredient for success or failure in targeted public health programme implementation (Sefton et al 2002).

STAGE 3: MAIN EVALUATION
Measure costs and outcomes

In the past, economists favoured measurement of final outcomes, for example QALYs. In public health intervention, however, there are very likely to be process variables that arise from the impact of the intervention on the community and the existence of organizations or networks that facilitate success of an intervention.

In addition, capture of multi-layered outcomes at different levels requires 'hard' and 'soft' information to be incorporated into the measurement stage of economic evaluation.

Much effort should be made within public health economic evaluations to ensure appropriate costing methodology is applied. Resources used and their unit costs should be considered separately, following Beecham (2000). Readers are referred to Sefton et al (2002) for an excellent summary of the relevant considerations in measuring costs and outcomes and some excellent suggestions of ways to capture 'hard' and 'soft' information to incorporate within an economic evaluation.

STAGE 4: IMPLEMENTATION
Generalizability

It is important to consider the context of an economic evaluation and to decide if there is anything about the particular context that might be generalized to other settings. Particular groups in a community may achieve better outcomes and others worse from public health intervention. Time differences in the occurrence of costs and outcomes can be reflected with discounting by the public sector discount rate. Sensitivity analysis can be applied to test the robustness of any data to assumptions that might underlie the production of cost and outcome information. This is important in economic evaluation because assumptions will most probably have to be made during the course of an economic evaluation.

Assessing equity and user perspectives

It might be the case that costs and outcomes and the interaction effects between organizations, individuals, communities and society may not be apparent at first or may quickly fall off. Evaluation should continue to take place once a public health intervention is in place to inform improvement and evaluation of interventions.

Again, at this final stage it is important that economic evaluators embrace the users of services and become involved with the data generated, as it is then much more meaningful and provides richness to the process of interpreting the data generated.

An economist's first 'natural' instinct is to use quantitative data, but in public health interventions the usefulness of qualitative data should not be overlooked. It is usually a good source for trying to tease out what people actually mean by what they are saying and for gauging how and why public health programmes work as opposed to 'what works' in evidenced-based public health.

Strengths of economic evaluation

The great strength of economic evaluation as a technique is that it follows a systematic, rational and logical approach that leads enticingly to an answer; or in public health, to a range of answers that can be applied with other types of analysis and information in decision-making processes. It is, when conducted as it should be, much more transparent than deployment of 'expert judgement' as a basis for making decisions about public health resource allocation. Decision-making processes in public health may still be very cloudy, but the evidence from economic evaluation should at least act to create some discussion about values, viewpoints and judgements before decisions are made.

The thinking, problem definition time of economic evaluation, is also extremely worthwhile. If deficiencies in services and need have not been identified correctly or at all, then it becomes what it is not meant to be: a rubber-stamping exercise to support vested interests.

THE EVIDENCE BASE FOR EFFECTIVENESS AND COST-EFFECTIVENESS OF SPECIALIST COMMUNITY PUBLIC HEALTH PRACTICE

The aim of this section is to consider the evidence from systematic review and RCTs for public health interventions in health visiting. Conclusions are drawn concerning the relative effectiveness and cost-effectiveness of specialist health and home visiting. Effectiveness is considered in the first part of this section and cost-effectiveness in the latter part.

SYSTEMATIC REVIEW AND RANDOMIZED CONTROLLED TRIALS (RCTs)

Effectiveness evaluations of health visiting and home visiting are categorized. RCTs are discussed by client group category: the family, including young mothers and children; adults (after acute intervention); the elderly and mental health in the fourth category; and the whole population in the fifth category.

Categorization of the evidence base can help to focus on areas of priority in health and home visiting. However, quality of findings is dependent upon quality of research methodology and this has to be considered. All RCT studies included below applied random allocation of subjects and controls.

Families, parents and children

The findings of all but one of the RCTs concerning the family are positive for health visitor interventions. Health visitor intervention of the information and support variety has been recognized as beneficial in reducing health inequalities. In the one RCT study in which the findings are negative, the intervention was provision of information on the impact of smoking behaviour on preschool children (Eriksen et al 1996). Gephens et al (1996) demonstrated that interventions concerned with information only were less effective than those employing information and support. Consequently, the balance of evidence from RCTs reflecting positive outcomes for health visitor interventions with the family, seems to indicate this area as a priority for specialist health visitors.

Reilly et al (2004) assessed the impact of a health advocacy intervention for homeless patients ($n = 400$) using a quasi-experimental, 3-armed control trial research design. Data on health service utilization over a 3-month period was collected for all clients recruited to the study and direct health service costs were measured. The results demonstrated that health advocacy is cost neutral and can alter the pattern of help seeking by temporarily homeless, symptomatic adults (Reilly et al 2004).

A recent US review of the 'state of the science' with respect to effectiveness of professional versus lay home visits during pregnancy, is tackled in a study by Armstrong Persily (2003). The author draws attention to weaknesses in the studies available, including use of descriptive or quasi-experimental research designs, and/or clearly described interventions in most studies. She concludes that gaps in our knowledge of the impact of lay home visitors on pregnancy outcomes persist (Armstrong Persily 2003). Another review of the literature (English language publication) on primary care services promoting optimal child development from birth to 3 years, by Regalado & Halfon (2001) concludes that many primary care activities promoting the optimal development of children are efficacious. In general, the review supported efficacy of primary care educational efforts toward promoting optimal parent–child interaction, parents' understanding of child temperament, book-sharing activities and approaches to healthy sleep habits and office interventions, such as counselling for the management of excessive infant crying and sleep problems. This review recommends that evaluations of developmental assessment and services in primary care should be expanded in depth and breadth.

A prospective cohort study by Owen et al (2001) demonstrated that health visitors are able to perform oto-acoustic testing in the neonatal period ($n = 683$) at home and in local health centre clinics. The study demonstrated health visitors ($n = 12$) were able to achieve high population coverage rates and low false positive rates. The authors recommended that universal neonatal hearing screening by health visitors using OAE testing is feasible, well received and could be less demanding of health visitor time than current distraction testing.

Kendrick et al (2000) in a systematic review and meta-analysis of RCTS and quasi-experimental studies of the impact of at least one home visit on parenting and the home environment concluded that it is associated with improvement in both. The authors note the lack of UK evidence and suggest further work is needed before the results of this systematic review and meta-analysis can be extrapolated to UK health visiting. The review also advocates comparisons with paraprofessional and community mothers' delivery of similar programmes. Roberts et al (1996) investigated home visiting in prevention of childhood injury and child abuse in the UK by conducting a systematic review of RCTs. 3433 subjects included in the review were the parents of disadvantaged children from 11 RCTs. The follow-up period was between 8 months and 4 years. Extensive searching of MEDLINE, EMBASE and BIDS was conducted. In addition, the reference lists of all relevant

articles and textbooks were reviewed and the *Journal of Child Abuse and Neglect* was hand-searched from 1977 to 1995 using the terms social support, family support, home and health visitors, home and health visitations, child abuse and child neglect. Experts in the field were contacted and asked about published and unpublished work they were aware of. The quality of trials was assessed independently by two reviewers and agreement on methodological criteria was evaluated. Disagreements were settled by collaborative review. The review concluded that home visiting programmes have the potential to reduce significantly rates of childhood injury. However, the use of self reported abuse as an outcome instrument in RCTs of home visiting has questionable validity. The relative effectiveness of professional versus non-professional home visits is a question that remains unanswered on the basis of this study.

Deaves (1993) assessed the value of health education in the prevention of childhood asthma. Subjects were three groups of children examined over 2 years. Both groups demonstrated a good improvement in knowledge of asthma and its treatment. Health education has a significant positive impact on morbidity indicators related to night symptoms and restricted activities. Qualitative analysis also highlighted the value parents of asthmatic children place on counselling.

A study of risk status and home intervention among children with failure to thrive by Hutcheson et al (1997) highlights the importance of follow-up assessments in the evaluation of home intervention services by lay home visitors. The results suggest home visitors are most productive among mothers with low negative affectivity in families of low socio-economic status with children demonstrating failure to thrive. Differences in motor development, cognitive development and behaviour during play among children of mothers who reported low negative affectivity was demonstrated at 1 year.

A study supporting home visitor programs by community health nursing professionals was conducted by Starn (1992). Support for community health visits for at-risk women and infants was established by allocating 30 subjects to one of three groups. The Barnard Model of parent–infant interaction was utilized in the study. A third of participants were under 19 years of age and 20% abused alcohol, cigarettes or illicit drugs during early pregnancy. Counselling and supportive interventions were shown to establish rapport and encourage women to develop and maintain healthy lifestyles. Results indicated substance abuse stopped or substantially decreased during the intervention. Mothers in the intervention groups had fewer perinatal complications and better parent–infant interaction scores than controls. Healthy pregnancies and improved child development were the main outcomes of the study.

A study by Oeller & Vileisis (1990) demonstrated the effect of early visitation of siblings whose new brothers and sisters were in an intensive care nursery. The intervention group demonstrated a significant decrease in negative behaviours on a specific subset of Missouri Behavioural Checklist (MBCL) items.

Larson (1980) demonstrated in a longitudinal follow-up study the efficacy of prenatal and postpartum home visits on child health and development in working-class families. Significant differences between subjects and controls were established for accident rates, assessments of home environment and maternal behaviour, lower prevalence of mother–infant interaction or feeding problems and of non-participant fathers. The results support the efficacy of home visits, but only if a prenatal visit is included. Furthermore, the authors suggest that a relationship between mother and home visitor is sensitive to the timing of the initial encounter between them.

Eriksen et al (1996) examined the effect of information on smoking behaviour in families with preschool children. 443 consecutive families with one or two smoking parents, attending mother and child health centres in Oslo, Norway, were allocated randomly to an intervention group ($n = 221$) and a control group ($n = 222$). Communication between the health visitor and the family was prolonged at one well-child visit with a brief session on smoking and the parents were given three brochures.

There were no significant differences between the groups with respect to change in smoking behaviour.

Adults

The context of studies in this category is variable and it is not easy to establish the positive effects health visitors might have in interventions with adults. A recent study by Pritchard & Kendrick (2001) concluded that with suitable training practice nurses and health visitors can successfully manage patients with a range of conditions in primary care: reducing GP workload at no cost to patient satisfaction.

Earlier evidence seemed to suggest the rehabilitation of stroke victims with remedial therapy from health visitors is of limited benefit (Smith et al 1981). The findings of this study must be qualified as only a few stroke patients are suitable for intensive outpatient rehabilitation and so other professional health care groups might have achieved similar outcomes in this instance. Other professional groups are more suited to interventions with adults in need of rehabilitation. A study by Mor et al (1983) of the impact of follow-up surveillance by a friendly visitor to discharged rehabilitation patients indicates that the need to alert the medical system to impending patient problems occurs rarely. These findings suggest that informal support systems and regular use of medical services may be sufficient to monitor rehabilitation patients' progress.

Older people

A study of the effectiveness of health visitor-controlled 'telemedicine' for over-65s in Hamlet, north-east Scotland, concluded that specialist prescriber health visitors now have the opportunity to use telemedicine for the benefit of their patients in rural communities (MacDuff et al 2001).

Burridge (1988) canvassed health visitor opinion concerning priorities in urban and rural areas. Her small study sample demonstrated that health visitors considered visiting the elderly a low priority. Health visitor opinion supported strongly the employment of specialist health visitors as a more appropriate way of fulfilling elderly needs in the community. These findings are supported by the balance of evidence concerning the outcome of health visitor interventions with the elderly.

A study by Dunn et al (1994) considered health visitor intervention in the reduction of unplanned hospital readmission in patients recently discharged from geriatric wards. 204 subjects were allocated randomly to normal follow-up services and normal services including a health visitor on the third day after discharge. Findings indicated that a visit by a health visitor to elderly patients after discharge from geriatric wards is unlikely to be of sufficient benefit to the patients for the service to be funded from a saving in unplanned re-admissions.

Vetter et al (1992) investigated the ability of health visitors to prevent fractures in elderly people. Their subjects were 674 patients aged 70 plus on general practice records in a market town. Subjects were interviewed and 350 assigned to an intervention group and 324 to a control group. Health visitor intervention over 4 years concerned nutrition, referral of medical conditions, correction of environmental hazards in the home and fitness. The fracture rate over 4 years was measured. The incidence of fractures was insignificant at 5% in the intervention group and 4% in the control group. Health visitors were concluded to have no significant effect on the incidence of fractures in the elderly (70 years and over).

Williams et al (1992) evaluated the care of people aged over 75 years by health visitor assistants (HVAs) after discharge from hospital. A group of patients was allocated randomly to a programme of visiting and compared with an equally sized group of controls having no visits.

A process evaluation examined the actions taken by HVAs during their visits and related the actions taken to patients' measured health status and other characteristics. No overall benefit from the programme of visiting was found in the outcome evaluation. There was a wide variation in the numbers of actions recorded for different patients. Numbers of HVA actions were related to patient health status and sex,

with more actions being initiated for those in poorer health and women. Neither age nor whether the patient lived alone was found to be related to number of HVA actions. It was concluded that the lack of demonstrated overall benefit and the wide variation in actions suggests this type of service cannot be recommended for all discharged patients over 75 years.

However, a few studies have demonstrated positive outcomes in health visitor interventions with the elderly. Runciman et al (1996) evaluated health visitor follow-up in the discharge of elderly people from an accident and emergency department; 222 intervention patients and 192 controls were compared. Intervention patients received more services and were significantly more independent at 4 weeks. Consequently, health visitor assessment was seen as helpful.

Vetter et al (1984) considered the effect of health visitors working with elderly patients in general practice. A random sample of patients in general practice aged 70 and over was investigated. Independent assessments made at the beginning and end of the study showed that the health visitor in an urban practice has some impact on the caseload of patients. More services were provided for them, their mortality was reduced and their quality of life improved, though the last measure just failed to be statistically significant. The health visitor working in a rural practice, however, had no such effect.

A study by Hendrikson et al (1989) of coordinated contributions of home care personnel in admission to and discharge of elderly people from hospital in Denmark, demonstrated improved outcome for home visits. An intervention group ($n = 135$) had an average hospital stay of 11 days compared with 14.3 days in the control group ($n = 138$). The total number of bed-days was 1490 and 1970 respectively. No differences were observed with respect to number of diagnostic procedures during hospitalization, number of deaths, diagnoses on discharge and functional capacity.

The influence of a 'friendly visitor' programme on the cognitive functioning and morale of elderly persons was studied by Reinke et al (1981). 49 nursing home residents were assigned randomly to a group focusing on conversational interaction, a group in which the playing of cognitively challenging games supplemented conversation or a no-treatment control group. Each subject was visited by a student twice per week for 8 weeks. Subjects were given four tests of cognitive functioning (vocabulary, matrices, memory, problem solving) and three tests of morale (Life Satisfaction Index A, Philadelphia Geriatric Center Morale Scale and self-perceived health). They were rated by nursing home activity directors on morale, programme participation, alertness, sociability and physical condition. A multivariate analysis of covariance in which age, education and length of nursing home residency were covariates revealed a reliable overall effect for the treatment. Subjects in both groups demonstrated improved performance relative to control subjects. Furthermore, subjects in the conversation plus games condition demonstrated the greatest improvement. The findings above, particularly in the last study (Reinke et al 1988), support the notion of home visiting as opposed to health visiting conferring relatively greater benefit in the elderly when compared to other categories above.

Mental health

An RCT was conducted to evaluate an integrated model of primary care for a cohort of patients with serious mental disorders ($n = 120$) at a Veterans Affairs (VA) mental health clinic. The subjects were randomized to receive primary medical care through an integrated care initiative (on-site primary care, case management, patient education and close collaboration with mental health providers) located in the mental health clinic ($n = 59$) or through the VA general medicine clinic ($n = 61$). The authors conclude that on-site, integrated primary care was associated with improved quality and outcomes of medical care (Druss et al 2001). The area of health visitor interventions for families and clients with mental health problems is very under-researched. There is one other RCT included in the Cochrane database for health visitor interventions and this had a positive outcome. Holden et al (1989) investigated whether counselling and support

by health visitors is helpful in managing postnatal depression. 60 women identified as depressed by screening at 6 weeks post partum and by psychiatric interview at 13 weeks post partum were allocated randomly to an intervention and control group. Eight weekly counselling visits by health visitors were conducted. After 3 months 18 (69%) of the 26 women in the treatment group had fully recovered, compared with 9 (38%) from 24 in the control group. The study concluded that counselling by health visitors is valuable in managing non-psychotic postnatal depression. However, as these results were not compared with those for other health and social care professionals the findings cannot provide a benchmark for service provision.

Reduction in health inequalities – whole population

The role of health visitors as the professional group of health care experts in the community most able to reduce health inequalities has been long suspected. Gephens et al (1996) conducted an international review of interventions to reduce socio-economic health differences (SEHD) and found evidence to support this view. Specific interventions related to health visiting were included in this review containing 405 studies. Interventions aimed at specific age groups, prenatal care, infant care, preventive care for young children, child development, nutrition, tooth decay prevention, child safety at home, general health promotion, licit and illicit drugs, adolescent mothers and adult women were reviewed. In addition, 25 publications concerning cardiovascular disease, cancer in adults and smoking screening were included in the review. A further 26 publications concerning interventions aimed at unemployment, health care accessibility, general, financial and cultural differences were also included. Finally, 31 interventions described in the 'grey' literature were reported in little detail as they related to local health education interventions. MEDLINE was searched and recent journals consulted, and experts in the field of SEHD were approached for published and unpublished material.

The numbers and the brief and incomplete reporting in most studies made only a narrative review possible. However, some clear findings emerged from the collective evidence. Interventions were classified into three groups: effective, ineffective and dubious. An effective intervention demonstrated positive outcomes and was at least as effective for the lowest socio-economic social groups (SES groups) as for the highest. In most of the studies included in this review, efficacy was assessed in terms of the targeted outcome of the intervention (performance indicator) over social groups and not in terms of the reduction in health inequalities.

The findings of this review demonstrate the effectiveness of the health visiting profession in reducing SEHD. Interventions to reduce inequality in health can be effective if they either address structural determinants of health or include both information and personal support. Provision of information alone is not likely to reduce socio-economic differences in health (Gephens et al 1996). Health education approaches in the community which provide only information seem to be effective in higher SES groups, but are not as effective as interventions by health visiting professionals in providing information alongside personal support, in reducing socio-economic health differences. These findings suggest the input of health visitors may be crucial to government programmes such as Sure Start. Sure Start is aimed at supporting families and one of its aims is to reduce social inequalities in health. On the basis of this wide-ranging review, it appears that health visitors are the professionals uniquely placed to reach all groups in the population with a similar degree of effectiveness.

These findings suggest that information and personal support are very important factors in the reduction of health inequality. This implies that health inequalities can be further reduced with better information and more personal support. It is unlikely that any other group of health care professionals is better placed than health visitors to play a role in the further reduction of health inequalities.

These are favourable findings for health visiting, but this review has a few limitations. First, the authors have not searched the Social Sciences Citation Index (SSCI) or PSYCLIT for suitable RCTs to include in their review. Inclusion or exclusion criteria for RCTs in the review have

not been stated and intervention designs have not been described. Nevertheless, this review contains suitably presented data in narrative form and clear results and implications for each study (Cochrane Reviews Database www. cochrane.org).

ECONOMIC EVALUATION STUDIES IN HEALTH VISITING

Economic appraisal can be applied to allocate resources amongst competing treatments and settings. A search of the Health Management Database of Data, Helmis and Kings Fund databases (HMIC database www.ovid.com) in May 2004 revealed 35 studies with home visits or health visits and cost-effectiveness as key words. The most scientifically valid evidence is presented here.

Lee et al (2004) asked whether the role of community health practitioners ($n = 272$) in Korea was economically viable in a recent cost minimization study.

This study demonstrated a significant difference in average costs of care between a model based on CHP services and one including no CHP services, in which equivalent care was provided by physicians ($t = -6.833, p < 0.001$). The average costs ratio was 2.16 (SD = 1.24), with a range of 0.09–9.63, indicating that CHP services were almost half the price of the 'no CHP services' model. The evaluation provides evidence of the economic validity of CHP's role in the public sector, where there is no net income to serve as a policy guideline. The authors conclude that CHP services are more effective than physician services (or 'no CHP services').

Another economic evaluation sought to estimate the financial cost to the NHS of infant crying and sleeping problems in the first 12 weeks of age and assessed the cost-effectiveness of behavioural and educational interventions aimed at reducing infant crying and sleeping problems relative to usual services (Morris et al 2001). The authors estimated that the annual total NHS cost of infant crying and sleeping problems was £65 million. Incremental costs per interruption-free night gained for the behavioural intervention relative to control were

£0.56. For educational intervention relative to the control, they were £4.13. The authors concluded that the behavioural intervention incurred a small additional cost and produced a small significant benefit at 11 and 12 weeks of age. The educational intervention incurred a small additional cost without producing a significant benefit.

A cost-effectiveness study of a district programme for screening infants for hearing loss was conducted by Brown (1992). Three main alternatives were costed using the methods of decision analysis (Gravelle 1982) in one district health authority. These were no screening, the current, conventional policy, or a change-nothing option and one alternative option. The conventional policy included health visitor screening at 8–9 months plus development assessment and a hearing screen if necessary at 10 months by a clinical medical officer. The alternative option was to miss out health visitor screening and to offer screening by a clinical medical officer at 10 months, only if concern was expressed or from clinical indications during developmental assessment. The introduction of a clue-list or check-list of the general signs indicating that a baby is hearing normally during the first year of life, issued to families at the initial health visitor visit, was considered (Brown 1992).

According to the author, the annual expected cost per unit of output was £20.57 for the conventional policy, between £11.13 and £11.23 for the alternative and £11.27 for no screening. Introducing the clue-list under the alternative policy was likely to raise the cost per unit of output, but the effects were uncertain. Consequently, it appeared the alternative option which removes health visitors from the screening of infants for hearing loss was more cost effective than the conventional policy, but also had little advantage over not screening at all (Brown 1992).

CONCLUSIONS

Economics is relevant to specialist community public health–health visiting practice. In the first section of this chapter, the link between economics and the commodity 'health visiting interventions' is explained. Economic thinking and techniques can help whenever resources are scarce and demands are unlimited. All health visitors are familiar with these constraints from their everyday work. Often the need to extract better outcomes from dwindling resources can become overwhelming and economics can help with the process of deciding how priorities for purchasing should be established. In common with other areas of health care, some health visiting activities confer more benefits for a given cost than others. Economic evaluation studies can help to identify these activities to achieve efficient allocation of resources. Naturally, the incorporation of economic thinking and techniques in these areas is conditional upon overcoming the jargon barrier. This chapter has attempted to clarify the meanings of the key terms and concepts necessary to get by as a public health professional.

The value of information and support from health visitor professionals so vital in reducing health inequalities seems to be clear from review evidence. In addition, the role of economic factors, such as growth, inflation, unemployment and income in health outcomes in conjunction with health visitor interventions needs to be better understood. More economic evaluations of health visiting interventions are recommended. The quality of the current stock of clinical evaluations of health visiting interventions, apart from a number of reviews of RCTs, is poor. A number of areas, for example mental health, have been neglected badly. In addition, the distinction between benefits of health visiting and other home visiting activities and relative benefits of specialist and generalist health visitors with various client groups has not been adequately researched. More research to quantify the benefits of health visiting for individuals, families and society is needed for the true worth of the profession of health visiting to be reflected in future economic evaluations.

Chapter **17**

Specialist community public health nursing – opportunities and challenges for the health visiting profession

Marion Frost

There is nothing permanent except change
Heraclitus

INTRODUCTION

This chapter will draw together some of the key issues previously discussed in this book, focusing on recent changes in government, nursing and education policy and the implications for health visiting practice. Changes in the delivery of primary health care services and the development of a new professional register have heralded a process of modernization that has presented both opportunities and challenges for the health visiting profession. Health visitors are encouraged to strengthen the public health aspect of their role, including health promotion and prevention, working in partnership with individuals, families and communities with the goal of improving the health and well-being of the population (Department of Health 1999c, 2003c). While it is recognized that a wide range of individuals across a variety of sectors contribute actively to the public health agenda, public health practitioners such as health visitors are considered to be an essential component of the workforce (Wanless 2004). However, there is some confusion about the future role of the health visitor and whether the title of 'health visitor' will continue to be used. These issues will be discussed in relation to the implications for health visiting practice.

It is suggested that health visitors need to harness the opportunities provided by the changing primary care arena to work collaboratively with appropriate agencies and across all sectors to search for health needs, raise awareness of the implications for individuals and organizations, influence policy decisions that affect health and facilitate the development of health-enhancing activities, taking on a leadership role where appropriate. These principles of health visiting (CETHV 1977) have been used as the basis for developing the new educational standards for Specialist Community Public Health Nursing (although interestingly their source has not been acknowledged in the standards document). Health visitors must value their knowledge base and experience advocating for improving the health of populations with which they work and marketing their expertise to commissioners of services, education and training. As Wanless (2004) suggests, individuals may be responsible for their own and their children's health, but it is claimed that it is often health visitors who are most aware of the nature of the social networks and environment in which people's lives are experienced. It is people's 'lived' experience that enables or inhibits healthy choices to be made.

THE POLITICAL CONTEXT OF HEALTH VISITING AND PUBLIC HEALTH NURSING PRACTICE

Investing in health and reforming what is perceived to be an outdated health service is a key aspect of government rhetoric. The *NHS Improvement Plan* (Department of Health 2004b) reaffirms earlier policy directives to change from 'a sickness service' to a 'health service', with a greater emphasis being placed on public health strategies that promote health and prevent illness rather than focusing on treatment. NHS frontline staff are required to become increasingly creative, working more flexibly to support people in choosing healthier lifestyles.

Improving health, reducing inequalities in health and providing high-quality health care for clients and communities is at the heart of *The NHS Plan* (Department of Health 2000c). Changing practice is integral to this process of modernization, driven by a government keen to respond to public demand, changing health and social needs, technological advances and finite resources. All practitioners working in primary care are required to question professional boundaries redesigning their services around the needs of the patient as opposed to being service defined. 'Our objective is to liberate the talents and skills of all the workforce so that every patient gets the right care in the right place at the right time' (Department of Health 2002b, p. 34).

A vital part of this programme of reform is for nurses, midwives and health visitors to set up new services, working collaboratively across organizational boundaries and with local communities to support the developing public health strategy. Access to good-quality primary health care services has been poor for many of the most disadvantaged communities, with evidence suggesting that living in materially deprived neighbourhoods in poor-quality housing contributes to worse health for individuals (Acheson Report 1998), as discussed in Chapter 6. Despite increased national prosperity and an overall improvement in health during the last 20 years, striking inequalities remain linked to social circumstances, geographical location, employment, parental income, ethnicity and gender (HM Treasury/Department of Health 2002). The achievement of national targets to narrow the gap in infant mortality between socio-economic groups and increase life expectancy between the most deprived areas and elsewhere by 2010 requires coordination at government level, collaboration at Primary Care Trust level and partnership working in practice.

The theme of collaborative working across government, and between government and local communities, is central to the new approach to mainstream work on health inequalities, keeping it at the heart of policy developments. Objectives to improve health outcomes and tackle risk factors such as smoking and obesity are to be considered as important in terms of performance management as waiting times. The message for the primary care workforce is clear: there must be improved access and better-quality services for disadvantaged groups, particularly in relation to preventive services. However, the number and diversity of organizations and individuals responsible for improving health and reducing inequalities in health, as identified by Porter in Chapter 2, creates a challenge for nurses and health visitors working in the field of public health to engage with contributors across all relevant sectors. *Securing Good Health for the Whole Population* (Wanless 2004) identifies the complexity of establishing shared targets for public health work and of the need for adequate resourcing of activities at a local level in order to develop long-term sustainable action to improve population health. Short-term funding of projects creates uncertainties for the staff planning and managing services and disadvantages service users and their carers.

The change from a 'sickness' service to a 'health' service needs to be supported by strong leadership in the development of national and local priorities and a robust evidence base on the cost-effectiveness of interventions. However, as Frost suggests in Chapter 7, there are many barriers which prevent health visitors and other community nurses from developing a leadership role, including lack of support from management. It is imperative that health visitors further develop their negotiating and lobbying skills in order to influence service provision and key policy decision making at all levels. Being proactive at the strategic level is as important as responding to demands at the individual level if the health of vulnerable populations is to be improved.

In addition, Wanless (2004) identifies that the information base for public health work is lacking. Although there may be scientific justification for public health action there is little supporting research evidence for the practical implementation of preventive strategies. A key issue in terms of evaluating the outcomes of public health work is that improvements in health and health status take time to achieve and may vary between individuals and populations in spite of similar services being implemented. Research may be costly to resource and often requires a variety of approaches to data collection, including incorporating the user viewpoint. Health visitors may need training and support to enable them to identify service users' views, especially with groups such as children and young people, people with learning disabilities and mental health problems, and people from black and ethnic minority groups (Department of Health 2002b).

The measurement of health outcomes is also fraught with problems depending on whether public health is defined from a health promotional, preventive perspective linked to the behavioural sciences, biomedicine and epidemiology or from a social health perspective linked to social justice and social inclusion, which as Poulton (2003) suggests are the two emerging strands. While previous government documentation, *Tackling Health Inequalities: A Programme for Action* (Department of Health 2003c), endorsed a broad approach to public health encompassing both perspectives, the more recent public health white paper *Choosing Health?* (Department of Health 2004c) appears to focus more on the individual behavioural approach of healthier lifestyles, with limited emphasis on a sense of social justice through organized social and political effort.

Failing to take account of the structural influences on people's lives ignores the reality of experiencing poverty. The current government emphasis on individually focused health promotion programmes such as smoking cessation views smoking as an irrational, unhealthy behaviour. However, as Graham (1987) identified some years ago, women surviving on a low income may use smoking as a means of coping with the demanding task of caring for their children. Public health campaigns aimed at achieving behavioural change through health education activities may therefore be counterproductive and 'victim-blaming' unless there is an understanding of the environmental and social factors that shape people's lives. Daykin & Naidoo (1995) suggest that the lifestyle approach to promoting health offers most to those with access to economic and political resources.

The challenge for health visitors is therefore to raise awareness of the importance of considering the wide range of factors that influence health potential when identifying health needs, influencing policy and planning strategies to support clients. Health visitors (and all those involved in health and social care) will need to advocate for the vulnerable and disempowered to ensure equity in service planning and provision.

GOVERNMENT POLICY AND MODERNIZING HEALTH VISITING PRACTICE

The government has clearly stated the importance of health visitors working with other agencies and the public to achieve their plans for improving people's health and tackling the root causes of ill health through developing a 'family-centred public health role' (Department of Health 1999c, para. 11.17). As a result of this modern role:

- Parents will receive improved support including parenting education, health advice and information.

- Individuals and families will be able to have a tailored family health plan agreed in partnership with the health visitor to address their parenting and health needs.

- The health needs of families will be met by a team led by a health visitor including nurses, nursery nurses and community workers.

- Health visitors will initiate and develop programmes for peer support, based on the experience of organizations such as Home Start, Newpin and 'community mothers', where local parents use their experience to support others.

- Neighbourhoods or special groups such as homeless people within a practice or Primary Care Trust will have their health needs identified by health visitors, who will lead public health practice and agree local health plans.

- Local communities will be helped to identify and address their own health needs, for example accident prevention for older people.

Improving support to families, mothers and children is a key theme of the government's *Programme of Action* (Department of Health 2003c), which aims to tackle health inequalities through ensuring the best possible start in life in order to improve the health of future generations. Health visitors therefore have a key role in responding to this aspect of the public health agenda with their expert knowledge of child and family health promotion and protection.

This directive to change practice was followed by the publication of a resource pack (Department of Health 2001e) advising health visitors on ways in which their new role could be developed without clearly defining the concept of a 'family-centred public role'. Giddens (2001, p. 669) suggests that a family is 'a group of individuals related to one another by blood ties, marriage or adoption, who form an economic unit, the adult members of which are responsible for the upbringing of the children'. In relation to matters which influence its health and welfare, a family has both rights and responsibilities in terms of making choices both for the individual members and for the wider community. The role of the health visitor is to empower individual members of the group to engage in healthier lifestyles through identifying and minimizing internal and external stressors that inhibit change and strengthening resources that promote change.

However, Millar (1997) argues that in traditional family-centred care community nurses may view the family as a passive unit, reinforcing the role of the nurse as 'the professional expert'. This has the potential to disempower clients and their carers, leading to dependency and increased vulnerability. A contrasting paradigm recognizes the family as a dynamic unit that is valued and listened to by health professionals. Understanding the client's experiences and meanings of health facilitates the development of options for improving health (CETHV 1977). This latter view appears to sit more comfortably with government policy that demands client-centred care and public involvement and is central to the philosophy and values which underpin health visitor education and practice (NMC 2002c). Competencies for professional practice require health visitors to develop and sustain relationships with groups and individuals as part of the search for actual and potential health needs; for example (NMC 2002c, p. 11):

- listening to what people are saying and doing

- enabling people to think through their feelings about their health and social well-being

- actively encouraging people to think about their own health and social well-being and that of others in their group

- giving people sufficient time and space to think about and say what they want to say

This building of trusting relationships is an essential aspect of health visiting practice, which has been previously discussed by Robotham in Chapter 4.

As key public health and primary care practitioners, the Department of Health (2001e, p. 8) has also challenged health visitors to 'reclaim their public health roots' and work with groups other than young children. Public health has been defined as 'the art and science of preventing disease, prolonging life and promoting health through the organised efforts and informed choices of society, organisations, public and private, communities and individuals' (Wanless 2004, p. 3). This acknowledges the responsibility of the state, private and voluntary sectors, professionals and the public both as individuals and collectively in improving health. However, there may be conflicting viewpoints between these differing groups as to the importance of identified issues that need to be tackled. For example, government's proposals to tackle obesity as a key issue identified through the analysis of epidemiological data may be of less importance to a local community experiencing high levels of noise pollution. Health visitors are in a prime position to work with local communities and other public health workers to identify issues that affect the lives of local populations and raise awareness of their

importance to local commissioners of relevant services such as environmental health, transport and housing departments.

The debate about the future role of the health visitor has become more complex following a recent review of services for vulnerable children and young people by the Chief Nursing Officer (CNO) of England (2004) and the long awaited publication of the *National Service Framework for Children, Young People and Maternity Services* (Department for Education and Skills/Department of Health 2004). Both documents identify that improving the health and welfare of children and safeguarding vulnerable children is essential for the future health of the nation (and has been previously discussed in Chapters 8 and 9). Health visitors have traditionally focused their service on young children and their families, providing support and interventions that aim to promote health, prevent illness and tackle inequalities in health.

The CNO's report identifies that while the services of nurses and midwives and health visitors are highly valued, the Laming 2003 inquiry into the death of Victoria Climbié reports that further work is required to reduce the gaps and omissions in service delivery in order to provide better health care for vulnerable children. Nurses and health visitors need to develop better skills in identifying and supporting vulnerable children and families, and safeguarding those at risk. It is concerning to note that the report suggests that 'there is a mismatch between the needs and expectations of vulnerable children, young people and families' and the skills and knowledge of the professionals who work with them.

The report recognizes that it is becoming increasingly difficult for health visitors to work across all population groups and suggests that the way forward is to distinguish between those working with a wider public health remit and those responsible for the public health of children. To some extent this has already happened in the practice arena with the development of Sure Start initiatives and Children's Trusts. However, it continues to be important for the child to be viewed as a member of a family, and the family as part of the community, in order for child health initiatives to be effective. Health visitors are therefore required to have knowledge of both child and family health issues as well as knowledge of factors affecting the health of the community. Current training programmes predicated on the Nursing and Midwifery Council (2002) competency framework for health visiting practice prepare practitioners to work in both of these arenas, although reports from practice teachers suggest that practice experience in a community development approach to public health work may be more difficult to access than work experience with individuals and families.

A tripartite model of health visiting practice has developed in the Stockport area in response to the varied health needs of its diverse population that appears to fit well with the CNO's vision (Swann & Brocklehurst 2004). The service comprises (p. 251):

- a generic primary care health visiting service based on GP attachment

- a first parent visitor programme providing a dedicated service to first-time parents in deprived communities in Stockport

- a health visitor-led team of community development workers located in the most deprived areas of Stockport, none of whom holds a client case-load.

The decision to separate the population and family support functions of the health visiting service occurred in the 1990s in response to the unequal distribution of health and wealth across the borough and the difficulties health visitors faced in becoming experts in family support as well as competent community development workers. Many generic health visitors were also involved in postnatal support groups and other initiatives such as Book Start. A key element of the development programme has also been strong public health leadership with health visitors, nurses, doctors and other public health workers collaborating with operational service leaders for health gain. The provision of high-quality family support and effective leadership in community development by the health visiting service has been

enabled through proper training programmes and the setting of realistic targets based on sound evidence.

As well as the Stockport model of health visiting another response to the modernization programme has been the concept of corporate working, where individual practitioner caseloads are shared by a team of skill mix workers in order to facilitate the undertaking of public health activities (Brocklehurst & Adams 2004). This method of working has been developed and evaluated in four pilot sites funded by the Department of Health to explore changes in service delivery that may promote public health practice. Reported benefits of corporate working for clients include a greater pool of experience to access and improvement in the consistency of service provision. Practitioners benefit in terms of sharing knowledge and skills and morale is improved through team cohesion and support. The main concern that has arisen related to this method of working is the potential lack of continuity for vulnerable clients. This can be dealt with by ensuring continuity of practitioner during the assessment process and at times of stress, supported by rigorous communication and record-keeping systems.

Further recommendations from the CNO's report (2004, section 3.1) include identifying the need to 'move away from planning based on title or traditional role to one based on the needs of children, young people and families where their views and choices are taken into account'. The emphasis is on the provision of services that 'follow the child', with the avoidance of gaps through co-location in integrated teams that span health, social care and education boundaries. In addition, the CNO suggests that the role of health visitor and school nurse should become integrated into a specialist community public health nurse with a particular child and family focus who is able to work both in schools and communities. These statements clearly indicate a loss of role and title for both health visitors and school nurses, contradicting earlier comments made by the CNO earlier in 2004 during a reported conversation with Mark Jones, Director of CPHVA (Mullally & Jones 2004, p. 47): 'It is important to have a professional identity . . . we will still see district nurses, practice nurses and health visitors because that's what often motivates people to do what they do and these roles are meaningful to the public'.

It is no wonder that health visitors are confused about the future of their profession. As Brocklehurst (2004) suggests, health visiting has the opportunity to organize itself in response to these changes but this will be dependent on a number of factors, including:

- central government developing a more coordinated approach as to where specialist community public health nursing, health visiting and school nursing sit within its public health strategy

- health visiting being supported in a similar manner to other professions, with direct entry to the profession being actively debated as part of the recruitment strategy

- health visiting and other specialist community public health practitioners being allowed to develop national educational standards for initial training and ongoing professional development

- health visitors identifying opportunities for change and seeking support from managers to develop new ways of working in response to identified needs

- health visitors articulating more clearly to commissioners what it is they can offer as part of the modernization programme.

The combined role of health visitor and school nurse also poses a challenge for educational establishments who are charged with preparing practitioners who are 'fit for practice, fit for purpose, fit for award and fit for professional standing' (NMC 2004a). There are doubts as to whether this can be achieved within the designated 52-week programme, of which only 45 are programmed weeks, with 50% being theory and 50% of the time spent in practice. It should be noted that for a practitioner to qualify within a defined area of practice such as health visiting they are required to spend 16.3 weeks in settings and with clients central to their specialism.

The danger seems to be that courses may struggle to qualify specialist community public health practitioners who are sufficiently knowledgeable and skilled to work effectively with a vulnerable population unless commissioners are either prepared to purchase longer training programmes or invest in a more robust programme of continuing professional development.

The rapidly changing nature of health care reflects the need to develop programmes of education that prepare practitioners with the ability to respond proactively to change, initiate and lead developments where appropriate and work across professional boundaries to provide clinically effective services (NMC 2004a). Central to this process is the requirement for a mentor/practice teacher who is qualified to an appropriate level to support and assess the students they teach. Educationalists and those in practice have expressed concerns about the standards for the preparation of mentors and teachers of nursing and midwifery (ENB/Department of Health 2001). In response to this the NMC (2004b) have produced a consultation document proposing new standards to support learning and assessment in practice which suggests a new recordable practice teacher qualification for specialist practice. The outcome of this consultation is awaited and it can only be hoped that the result supports the recent development of the new NMC register, with a part for registered specialist community public health nurses which requires practice teachers able to support learning at a minimum of degree level, with many students likely to opt for a postgraduate route.

CONCLUSION

The government has clearly identified that all nurses, midwives and health visitors must respond to the modernization agenda and change ways of working to develop services that are responsive to client need. However, the future for health visiting is unclear, with what appear to be confusing messages being delivered in government, professional and education documents. The two strands which are emerging in England suggest that health visiting (along with school nursing and occupational health nursing) is being viewed as a defined pathway within a specialism of specialist community public health nursing that is central to the developing public health strategy or, alternatively, the profession of health visiting will be subsumed within a specialist community public health nurse role that incorporates both health visiting and school nursing.

Health visiting has much to learn from its past history in relation to the manner in which it has responded to change. It must once again decide what it wants for the future. Health visitors must value their knowledge and skills and have the confidence to seek out opportunities to initiate, develop and lead new approaches to practise in consultation with the public. In order to remain a viable part of the workforce it is argued that health visiting needs to be clear about its role and make a sound business case to the commissioners of services. The way forward is for health visiting to identify and harness the opportunities offered by the developing public health agenda, utilizing the principles to promote its own health. The profession needs to identify what it wants, raise awareness at appropriate levels, influence the policy agenda and then facilitate its own future development.

References

Acheson D 1988 Public health in England. HMSO, London

Acheson D 1998 Independent inquiry into inequalities in health. HMSO, London

Action on Elder Abuse 2000 Briefing notes

Acton T 1974 Gypsy politics and social change. Routledge & Kegan Paul, London

Acton T 1994 Gender issues in accounts of gypsy health and hygiene as discourses of social control. Medical Sociology Group, paper 24.10.94

Adams D, Channi Kumar R, Glover V, Modi N, Onogawa K 2003 Improving mother–baby interaction for mothers with post natal depression. Journal of Affective Disorders 63:201–207

Adams P, Conway M, Owens N 1992 The strategic use of information systems and technology: an overview for NHS chief executives and senior managers of the management in the 90s research programme. NHS Training Directorate, Bristol

Adoption and Children Act 2002 HMSO, London

Ainsworth M 1965 Further research into the adverse effects of maternal deprivation. In: Bowlby J (ed) Child care and the growth of love, 2nd edn. Penguin Books, St Ives

Akinsanya J, Cox G, Crouch C, Fletcher L 1994 The Roy adaptation model in action. Macmillan, Basingstoke

Aldgate J, Jones D, Rose W, Jeffery C 2004 The developing world of the child. Jessica Kingsley Publishers, London

Aldridge D, Pietroni P 1987 Clinical assessment of acupuncture in asthma therapy: discussion paper. Journal of Royal Society of Medicine 80:222–224

Allan G, Crow G 2003 In Watkins D, Edwards J, Gastrell P 2003 Community health nursing. Baillière Tindall, London

Allan P, Jolly M, 1982 Nursing midwifery and health visiting since 1900. Faber & Faber, London

Allmark P 1992 The ethical enterprise of nursing. Journal of Advanced Nursing 17:16–20

Amina Mama 1996 The hidden struggle: statutory and voluntary sector responses to violence against black women in the home. Whiting & Birch, London

Anderson E, Anderson P 1987 GPs and alternative medicine. Journal of the Royal College of General Practitioners 37:52–55

Appleton J 1994 The concept of vulnerability in relation to child protection: health visitors' perceptions. Journal of Advanced Nursing 20:1132–1140

Argyris C 1982 Reasoning, learning and action: individual and organisational. Jossey-Bass, San Francisco, CA

Argyris C, Schön D A 1974 Theory into practice, increasing professional effectiveness. Jossey-Bass, San Francisco

Armstrong Persily C 2003 Lay home visiting may improve pregnancy outcomes. Holistic Nurse Practice 17(5):231–238.

Arnold P 2004 Time for health gentleman. Primary Health Care 14(3):23–24

Ashby H T 1922 Infant mortality. Cambridge University Press, Cambridge

Ashton J, Seymour H 1988 The new public health. Open University Press, Milton Keynes

Audit Commission 1997 Comparing notes: a study of information management in Community Trusts. Audit Commission, London

Aukett A 1990 The Schedule of Growing Skills. Recorded interview at Carnegie Institute of Child Health, Birmingham

Austerberry H, Watson S 1982 Women on the margins. City University Housing Research Group, London

Baird A 2001 Diagnosis and prescribing: the impact of nurse prescribing on professional roles. Primary Health Care 11(5):24–26

Baird A 2003 Nurse prescribing: how did we get here? Journal of Community Nursing 17(4):4–10

Baird A 2004 Focus on … the consultation. Online. Available: www.nurse-prescriber.co.uk/Articles?The-Consultation.htm 23 April 2004

Baker M 2000 Making sense of the NHS White Papers, 2nd edn. Radcliffe Medical Press, Oxford

Baldry M, Cheal C, Fisher B 1985 Giving patients their own records in general practice. British Medical Journal 292:595–598

Bandura A 1973 Aggression: a social learning analysis. Prentice-Hall, Englewood Cliffs, NJ

Bandura A 1977a Self-efficacy: toward a unifying theory of behaviour change. Psychological Review 84:191–215

Bandura A 1977b Social learning theory. Prentice-Hall, Englewood Cliffs, NJ

Bandura A 1986 Social foundations of thought and action: a social cognitive theory. Prentice-Hall, Englewood Cliffs, NJ

Bandura A, Taylor C B, Williams S L et al 1985 Catecholamine secretion as a function of perceived coping self-efficacy. Journal of Consulting and Clinical Psychology 53:406–414

Banning M 1999 Education, education, education. In: Jones M (ed) Nurse prescribing: politics to practice. Baillière Tindall, Edinburgh, ch 6

Baraclough J, Damant M, Metcalfe D et al 1983 Statement on the interprofessional education and training for members of Primary Health Care Teams. Central Council for Education and Training in Social Works/Panel of Assessors for District Nurse Training/Royal College of General Practitioners/Council for the Education and Training of Health Visitors, London

Barber B 1963 Some problems in the sociology of the professions. Daedalus 92:669–688

Barker W 1984 Child development programme. Early Childhood Development Unit, University of Bristol, Bristol

Barker W 1985 The Körner Community Report: medical or prevention model? Evidence to Körner Working Group D

Barker W 1988 Child development programme. Early Childhood Development Unit, University of Bristol, Bristol

Barker W 1991 Is Monitor worth the time and effort? University of Bristol Early Childhood Development Unit, Bristol

Barlow J 1997 The effectiveness of parenting training programmes in improving behaviour problems in children aged 3–10 years. In: National Screening Committee/Royal College of Paediatrics and Child Health Proceedings: evolution or revolution? Systematic reviews of screening in child health, 17 December 1997 and 18 January 1998. Child Growth Foundation, London, p 19

Barna D 1995 Working with young men. Health Visitor 68:185–187

Barr H, Hammick M, Koppel I Reeves S 1999 Evaluating interprofessional education: two systematic reviews for health and social care. British Educational Research Journal 25:533–544

Basford L 2003 Maintaining nurse prescribing competence: experiences and challenges Nurse Prescribing 1(1):40–45

Bass B M 1990 Bass and Stogdill's Handbook of leadership: theory, research and management applications, 3rd ed. Free Press, New York

Bassuk E L, Weinreb L F, Ree Dawson S et al 1997 Determinants of behaviour in homeless and low-income housed preschool children. Paediatrics 100:92–100

Baumrind D 1967 Current patterns of parental authority. Developmental Psychology Monographs 4:1–103

Bax M, Hart H, Jenkins S 1990 Child development and child health. Blackwell Scientific, Oxford

Bayley N 1933 Mental growth during the first three years: a developmental study of sixty-one children by repeated tests. Genetic Psychology Monographs 14:1–92

Bayley N 1940 Mental growth in young children. Yearbook of the National Society for the Study of Education 39:11–47

Beattie A 1979 Social policy and health education: the prospects for a radical practice. Paper for the National Deviancy Conference, Edgehill College

Beattie A 1984 The price of political awareness. Paper for the Challenge of Choice. Conference, St Bartholomew's Hospital, London

Beattie A 1991 Knowledge and control in health promotion: a test for social policy and social theory. In: Gabe J, Calnan M, Bury M (eds) The sociology of the health service. Routledge, London, ch 7

Beattie A 1993 Sociopolitical philosophy of dimensions of conflict. In: Beattie A, Gott M, Jones L, Sidell M (eds) Health and wellbeing: a reader. C B Slack, London

Beattie A 1996 Knowledge and control in health promotion: a case study in social policy and social theory. In: Calman M, Gabe J (eds) The sociology of the Health Service. Routledge, London

Beauchamp T, Childress J 1989 Principles of biomedical ethics, 3rd edn (1991). Oxford University Press, Oxford

Becker M 1974 The Health Belief Model and personal health behaviour. C B Slack, Thorofare, NJ

Becker M H, Drachman R H, Kirscht J P 1974 A new approach to explaining sick role behaviour in low income populations. American Journal of Public Health 64:205–216

Bedford H E et al 1992 Use of an East End children's Accident and Emergency Department for infants: a failure of primary health care. Quality in Health Care 1:29–33

Beecham J 2000 Unit costs not exactly child's play: a guide to estimating unit costs for children's social care. Department of Health, London

Begg N, Ramsey M, White J et al 1998 Media dents confidence in MMR vaccine. British Medical Journal 316:561

Beitler B, Tkachuck B, Aamodt A 1980 The Neuman model applied to mental health, community health and medical–surgical nursing. In: Riehl J P, Roy C (eds) Conceptual models for nursing practice, 2nd edn. Appleton-Century-Crofts, New York

Belbin R M 1993 Team roles at work. Butterworth-Heinemann/British Medical Journal, Oxford

Bellman M H 1984 Serious acute neurological diseases of childhood: a clinical and epidemiological study with special reference to whooping cough disease and immunization. Unpublished MD thesis, University of London

Bellman M, Cash J, 1987 The Schedule of Growing Skills in practice. NFER-Nelson, London

Bellman M, Lingam S, Aukett A 1996 Schedule of Growing Skills II. NFER-Nelson, London

Benedict M M, Behringer Sproles J 1982 Application of the Neuman model to public health nursing practice. In: Neuman B (ed) Neuman systems model: application to nursing education and practice. Appleton-Century-Crofts, Norwalk, CT

Benjamin M, Curtis J 1992 Ethics in nursing. Oxford University Press, Oxford

Benner P 1984 From novice to expert: excellence and power in clinical nursing practice. Addison-Wesley, Menlo Park, CA

Benner P, Tanner C 1987 Clinical judgement: how expert nurses use intuition. American Journal of Nursing 23–31

Bennett G 1990 Action on elder abuse in the '90s: a new definition will help. Geriatric Medicine April:53–54

Bennett G, Kingston P, Penhale B 1997 The dimensions of elder abuse: perspectives for practitioners. Macmillan, Basingstoke

Bennett G D 1992 Handbook of clinical dietetics. Matthew Price, London

Bennett R 1997 Organisational behaviour, 3rd edn. Financial Times/Pitman Publishing, London

Bergman R 1981 Accountability: definition and dimensions. International Nursing Review 28(2):53–59

Bernice J 1986 Evaluation of a developmental screening system for use by child health nurses. Archives of Disease in Childhood 61:340–341

Betts T 1995 How we use aromatherapy. University of Birmingham

Biggs S, Phillipson C, Kingston P 1995 Elder abuse in perspective. Open University Press, Buckingham

Billingham K 1991 Public health and the community. Health Visitor 64:371–372

Binet A, Simon T 1915 A method of measuring the development of intelligence in young children. Medical Book Co, Chicago, IL

Birchall E, Hallett C 1995 Working together in child protection. HMSO, London

Birmingham FHSA 1993 Public health report, Ch 3: Traveller families' health

Birmingham Health Authority 1990 Child health surveillance policy. Birmingham Health Authority, Birmingham

Black D 1980 Inequalities in health: report of a research working group. Department of Health, London

Blackburn C 1991 Poverty and health: working with families. Open University Press, Milton Keynes

Blackburn C 1993 Gender, class and smoking cessation work. Health Visitor 66(3):83–85

Blakemore K, Boneham M 1994 Age, race and ethnicity. Open University Press, Buckingham

Blau P M 1964 Exchange and power in social life. John Wiley, New York

Blaxter M 1990 Health and lifestyles. Tavistock, London

Bliss H A 1982 Primary care in the emergency room: high in costs and low in quality. New England Journal of Medicine 306:998

Blumer H 1969 Symbolic interactionism: perspective and method. Prentice-Hall, Englewood Cliffs, NJ

BMA 2004 Asylum seekers and their health. BMA, London

Boardman A 1998 The use of emollients in dry skin conditions. MeReC Bulletin 9(12), National Prescribing Centre, Liverpool

Boardman A 1999 Management of head louse infection. MeReC Bulletin 10(5), National Prescribing Centre, Liverpool

Bolton P 1986 Developmental screening for children aged two. Health Visitor 59:149–151

Bond C 2003 Concordance: is it a synonym for compliance or a paradigm shift? Pharmaceutical Journal 271:496–497

Bond M, Holland S 1998 Skills of clinical supervision for nurses. Open University Press, Buckingham

Boston M 1997 Preventing teenage pregnancies. Community Nurse 3(4):18–20

Bower H 1998 MMR vaccine policy is backed. British Medical Journal 316:955

Bowlby J 1953 Child care and the growth of love, 2nd edn (reprinted 1990). Penguin, St Ives

Bowling A 1991 Measuring health: a review of quality of life measurement scales. Open University Press, Buckingham

Boyd E, Fales A W 1983 Reflective learning. Journal of Human Psychology 23:99–117

Brady-Wilson C 1991 US businesses suffer from workplace trauma. Personnel J July: 47–50

British National Formulary 2004 British Medical Association and Royal Pharmaceutical Society of Great Britain. Pharmaceutical Press, Oxford

Britt D W 1997 A conceptual introduction to modeling: qualitative and quantitative perspectives. Lawrence Erlbaum, Mahwah, NJ

Brocklehurst N 1998 Clinical supervision. West Midlands Clinical Supervision Learning Set, Birmingham

Brocklehurst N, Adams C 2004 Embodying modernization: corporate working. Community Practitioner 77(8):292–296

Brody S 1977 Screen violence and film censorship. Home Office Research Unit Report No 40. HMSO, London

Brookfield S 1990 Using critical incidents to explore learners' assumptions. In: Mezirow J et al (eds) Fostering critical reflection in adulthood. Jossey-Bass, San Francisco, p 177–193

Broome A 1989 Health psychology processes and applications. Chapman & Hall, London

Broome AK and Llewellyn S 1994 Health psychology: process and application. Chapman & Hall, London

Brotherson J 1988 Health Service Journal 7509:759

Broudy H S, Smith B D, Burnett J 1964 Democracy and excellence in American secondary education. In Eraut M 1985 Knowledge creation and knowledge use in professional contexts. Studies in Higher Education 10:117–133

Brown J 1992 Screening infants for hearing loss: an economic evaluation. Journal of Epidemiology and Community Health 46:350–356.

Browne K, Davies C, Stratton P 1988 Early prediction and prevention of child abuse. John Wiley, Chichester

Buggins E 2000 People as partners: adopting the 'crabmatic vision' approach. Community Practitioner 73(3):525–526

Buhler C, Hetzer H 1935 Testing children's development from birth to school age. Allen & Unwin, London

Bunton R, Macdonald G 1992 Health promotion: disciplines and diversity. Routledge, London

Burns J M 1978 Leadership. Harper & Row, New York

Burridge R 1988 The role of the health visitor with the elderly. Health Visitor 61:20–21

Burrows D E, McLeish J 1995 A model for research-based practice. Journal of Clinical Nursing 4:243–247

Butterworth T, Faugier J 1992 Clinical supervision and mentorship in nursing. Chapman & Hall, London

Byford S, McDaid D, Sefton T 2003 Because it's worth it: a practical guide to conducting economic evaluations in the social welfare field. York Publishing Service, York

Byrne P S, Long B E L 1976 Doctors talking to patients. HMSO, London

Caldwell P 1998 Re. MMR revisited hastily! Online. Available http://www.mailbase.ac.uk/liss-f/gp-uk/1998

Calman K 1998 Government declares MMR triple vaccine safe. Online. Available: www.itn.co.uk/Britain/brit0312/031206.htm

Cameron-Blackie G, Mouncer Y 1992 Complementary therapies in the NHS. NHS Confederation, London

Caplan G 1966 Principles of preventive psychiatry. Basic Books, New York

Care Standards Act 2000 HMSO, London

Carnwell R 1998 Conceptual models for practice. In: Blackie C (ed) Community health care nursing. Churchill Livingstone, Edinburgh

Carnwell R, Daly W M 2003 Advanced nursing practitioners in primary care settings: an exploration of developing roles. Journal of Clinical Nursing 12:630–642

Carper B 1978 Fundamental patterns of knowing in nursing. Advances in Nursing Science 11:13–23

Carr S, Procter S, Davidson A 2003 Models of public health nursing. Community Practitioner 76(3):96–99

Carroll I, Coll T, Underhill D 1974 Retarded brain growth in Irish itinerants. Journal of the Irish Medical Association 67:33–36

Carr-Saunders A 1928 Professions: their organisation and place in society. Clarendon Press, Oxford

Carr-Saunders A, Wilson P 1933 The professions. Frank Cass, London

Carter Y H, Bannon M J, Jones P W 1992 Health visitors and child accident prevention. Health Visitor 65(4):115–117

Cash J 1991 Recorded interview. Birmingham Children's Hospital

Catford J 2001 Illicit drugs: effective prevention requires a health promotion approach. Health Promotion International 16:107–110

Cattell P 1940 The measurement of intelligence of infants and young children. Psychological Corporation, New York

Caulfield H 2004a Legal aspects, responsibility, accountability in nurse prescribing. Prescribing Nurse Spring:20–22

Caulfield H 2004b Responsibility, accountability and liability in nurse prescribing. Prescribing Nurse Summer:18–20

Centers for Disease Control 1999 Mumps, measles and rubella vaccine (MMR). About the diseases. Internet.

CETHV 1965 Guide to syllabus of training. CETHV, London

CETHV 1973 The health visitor functions and implications for training. CETHV, London

CETHV 1977 An investigation into the principles of health visiting. Council for the Education and Training of Health Visitors, London

Chalmers K I 1992 Giving and receiving: an empirically derived theory on health visiting practice. Journal of Advanced Nursing 17:1317–1325

Chalmers K, Kristajanson L 1989 The theoretical basis for nursing at the community level: a comparison of three models. Journal of Advances in Nursing 14:569–574

Charles R P 1994 An evaluation of parent-held child health records. Health Visitor 67:270–272

Charles R P 1996 Reforming health visitor records. Health Visitor 69:101–102

CHI 2004 Key findings from the self-audits of NHS organisations, social services department and police forces. Online. Available: http://www.dh.gov.uk/assetRoot/04/06/95/45/04069545.pdf 24 Dec 2004

Child Accident Prevention Trust 1989 Preventing accidents to children: a training resource for health visitors. Health Education Authority, London

Child protection responsibilities of primary care trusts 2002 (Jacqui Smith MP). Department of Health, London, 28 January 2002

Children Bill 2004 Published by authority of the House of Lords. HMSO, London

Churchman C W 1971 The design of inquiring systems: basic concepts of systems and organisations. Cited in Kitchener K S, King P M 1990 The reflective judgement model: transforming assumptions about knowing. In: Mezirow J et al (ed) Fostering critical reflection in adulthood. Jossey-Bass, San Francisco

Clarke C 1999 Low self-esteem: a barrier to health promoting behaviour. Journal of Community Nursing. 13(1):4–10

Clarke C, Davidson A, Gibb C, Hart J 2003 Infant massage: developing an evidence base for health visiting practice. Journal of Community Practice 76(40):138–142

Clark J 1973 A family visitor: a descriptive analysis of health visiting in Berkshire. Royal College of Nursing, London

Clement S 1995 Listening visits in pregnancy: a strategy for preventing postnatal depression? Midwifery 11:75–80

Cody A 1999 Health visiting as therapy: a phenomenological perspective. Journal of Advanced Nursing 29:119–127

Cohen D R, Henderson J B 1988 Health prevention and economics. Oxford Medical Publications, Oxford

Cohen J 1987 Accident and emergency services and general practice: conflict of co-operation. Family Practitioner 4:81–83

Coit Butler F 1978 The concept of competence, an operational definition. Educational Technology 18:7–16

Cole A 2003 Dealing with diversity. Health Development Today April/May

Collins G, George K 2003 Development and support of community nurse prescribers. Primary Health Care 13(2):38

Colver A 1983 Home is where the damage lies. Health and Social Service Journal 2 June:662–663

Commission for Racial Equality 2004 Strategy for working with gypsies and travellers. CRE, London

Coney S 1995 The menopause industry. Women's Press, London

Conger R D, Conger K J, Elder G H et al 1992 A family process model of economic hardship and adjustment of early adolescent boys. Child Development 63:526–541

Cook A, James J, Leach P 1991 Positively no smacking. In Twinn S, Cowley S (eds) 1992 The principles of health visiting: a re-examination. HVA/UKSC, London

Council for the Education and Training of Health Visitors 1977 An investigation into the principles of health visiting. CETHV, London

Court S D M 1976 Fit for the future. Report of the Committee on Child Health Services. Cmnd 6680. HMSO, London

Courtenay M, Butler M 1999 Nurse prescribing: principles and practice. Greenwich Medical Media, London

Cowley S 1991 A grounded theory on situation and process in health visiting. Unpublished PhD Thesis, Brighton Polytechnic

Cowley S 2002 Public health in policy and practice: a source book for health visitors and community nurses. Baillière Tindall London

Cowley S, Billings J 1999 Resources revisited: salutogenesis from a lay perspective. Journal of Advanced Nursing 29(4):994–1004

Cox J, Holden J (eds) 1994 Perinatal psychiatry, use and misuse of the Edinburgh Postnatal Depression Scale. Gaskell, London

Cox J L, Holden J M, Sagovsky R 1987 Detection of postnatal depression: development of the 10-item Edinburgh Postnatal Depression Scale. British Journal of Psychiatry 150:782–786

CPHVA 1997 Professional briefing 9: integrated nursing teams. Health Visitor 70:229–231

CPHVA 1999 Keeping the record straight. Community Practitioner and Health Visitor Association. London

Craig P 1998 A description of the public health role for health visitors Unpublished MSc thesis, University of Glasgow

Creedon T, Corbay A, Keveney J 1975 Growth and development in travelling families. Journal of the Irish Medical Association 68:473–477

Crisis (2003) Statistics about homelessness. Online. Available: www.crisis.org.uk

Crittenden P 1988 Family and dyadic patterns of functioning in maltreating families. In: Browne K, Davies C, Stratton P (eds) Early prediction and prevention of child abuse. John Wiley, Chichester

Crout E 1988 Have health care will travel. Health Services Journal 98:48–49

Curtis H 1993 The schedule of growing skills in child protection work. In: The Schedule of Growing Skills: facilitating child surveillance. NFER-Nelson, London, p 5

Curtis H 1995 Letter to researcher (Reynolds M)

Dale J 1992 Primary care: the old bugbear of accident and emergency services. British Journal of General Practice 42:90–91

Daly W M 1998 Critical thinking as an outcome of nursing education. What is it? Why is it important to nursing practice? Journal of Advanced Nursing 28:323–331

Daly W M, Carnwell R 2003 Nursing roles and levels of practice: a framework for differentiating between elementary, specialist and advanced nursing practice. Journal of Clinical Nursing 12:158–167

Dalziel Y 2002 Community development as a public health function, In: Cowley S (ed) Public health policy and practice. Baillière Tindall, London

Daniel K 1999a Working in partnership. Community Practitioner 72(5):117–118

Daniel K 1999b Banking on success. Community Practitioner 72(12):390–391

Davies W, Frude N 1995 Preventing face-to-face violence: dealing with anger and aggression at work. APT, Leicester

Davis A, Bamford J, Wilson I et al 1997 A critical review of the role of neonatal hearing screening in the detection of congenital hearing impairment. Health Technology Assessment 1(10):1–177

Day J 2003 How reflections on concordance in mental health can affect research and clinical practice in adherence. Pharmaceutical Journal 271:505–507

Day M 1998 This won't hurt ... New Scientist 7 March

Daykin N, Naidoo J 1995 Feminist critiques of health promotion. In: Bunton R, Nettleton S, Burrows R (eds) The sociology of health promotion: critical analyses of consumption, lifestyle and risk. Routledge, London

de la Cuesta C 1994 Marketing: a process in health visiting. Journal of Advanced Nursing 19:347–353

Deaves D M 1993 An assessment of the value of health education in the prevention of childhood asthma. Journal of Advanced Nursing 18:354–363

Dennett L 1998 A sense of security. Granta, Cambridge

Department for Education and Employment 1999a Making a difference for children and families: Sure Start. DFEE, London

Department for Education and Employment 1998 Education for citizenship and the teaching of democracy in schools, Crick Report QCA, London

Department for Education and Employment 1999b Sure Start, a guide for trailblazers. DfEE Publications, Sudbury

Department for Education and Skills 2003 Keeping children safe: the government's response to the Victoria Climbié enquiry report and joint chief inspector's report. Safeguarding children. Cmnd 5861. HMSO, London

Department for Education and Skills 2004a Five year strategy for children and learners: putting people at the heart of public services. DfES, London

Department for Education and Skills 2004b Every child matters: next steps. HMSO, London

Department for Education and Skills/Department of Health 2004 National Service framework for Children. Young people and maternity services executive summary. HMSO, London

Department of the Environment 1994 Gypsy sites policy and unauthorised camping. Circulars 18/94, 76/94. Welsh Office

Department of Environment, Transport and the Regions 1998 A new deal for transport: better for everyone. HMSO, London

Department of the Environment, Transport and the Regions, Women's Unit and Department of Health 1999 Relationship breakdown: a guide for social landlords. DETR, London

Department of Health 1968 HMG Medicines Act. HMSO, London

Department of Health 1987 Promoting better health: the government's programme for improving primary health care. Cmnd 249. HMSO, London

Department of Health 1989a An introduction to the Children Act 1989. HMSO, London

Department of Health 1989b Report of the Advisory Group on Nurse Prescribing (Crown Report). HMSO, London

Department of Health 1989c Caring for people. HMSO, London

Department of Health 1989d Working for patients. Cmnd 555. HMSO, London

Department of Health 1991 The patient's charter. HMSO, London

Department of Health 1992a Medicines Products: Prescribing by Nurses etc., Act. HMSO, London

Department of Health 1992b The health of the nation: a strategy for health in England. HMSO, London

Department of Health 1992c Primary care: the future. HMSO, London

Department of Health 1993a The health of the nation: HIV/AIDS and sexual health. HMSO, London

Department of Health 1993b The health of the nation: targeting practice. The contribution of nurses, midwives and health visitors. HMSO, London

Department of Health 1995a The challenge of partnership in child protection: practice guide. HMSO, London

Department of Health 1995b Health of the young nation: your contribution counts. HMSO, London

Department of Health 1995c Weaning and the weaning diet: report of the working group on the weaning diet of the committee on medical aspects of food policy. HMSO, London

Department of Health 1995d Making it happen: public health – the contribution, role and development of nurses, midwives and health visitors. Report of the SNMAC. HMSO, London

Department of Health 1996a Primary care: the future: choice and opportunity. HMSO, London

Department of Health 1996b A new partnership for care in old age. Cmnd 3242. HMSO, London

Department of Health 1996c Regulation of nursing homes and independent hospitals. HSG(95)41. HMSO, London

Department of Health 1997a The new NHS – modern, dependable. Cmnd 3807. HMSO, London

Department of Health 1997b Report on supply and administration of medicines under group protocols (Crown Part 1). HMSO, London

Department of Health 1998a A first class service: quality in the new NHS. HMSO, London

Department of Health 1998b Our healthier nation: a contract for health. Cmnd 3852. HMSO, London

Department of Health 1999a Making a difference: strengthening the nursing, midwifery and health visiting contribution to health and healthcare. HMSO, London

Department of Health 1999b Review of prescribing, supply and administration of medicines. Final report (Crown Part 2). HMSO, London

Department of Health 1999c Saving lives: our healthier nation. HMSO, London

Department of Health 1999d Working together to safeguard children: a guide for interagency working to safeguard and promote the welfare of children. HMSO, London

Department of Health 1999e A national service framework for mental health. HMSO, London

Department of Health 2000a Domestic violence: a resource manual for health professionals. HMSO, London

Department of Health 2000b Framework for the assessment of children in need and their families. HMSO, London

Department of Health 2000c The NHS plan: a plan for investment. A plan for reform. HMSO, London

Department of Health 2000d Continuing professional development: quality in the new NHS. Department of Health, London

Department of Health 2000e National service framework for coronary heart disease. HMSO, London

Department of Health 2000f The NHS cancer plan. HMSO, London

Department of Health 2001a Care homes for older people, 1st edn (2002 2nd edn, 2003 3rd edn). HMSO, London

Department of Health 2001b National service framework for older people. HMSO, London

Department of Health 2001c The NHS plan: an action guide for nurses, midwives and health visitors. HMSO, London

Department of Health 2001d The Health and Social Care Act. HMSO, London

Department of Health 2001e Health visitor practice development resource pack. HMSO, London

Department of Health 2001f Shifting the balance of power within the NHS: securing delivery. HMSO, London

Department of Health 2001g The national strategy for sexual health and HIV. HMSO, London

Department of Health 2001h Governmental response to the House of Commons Select Committee on Health's Second Report on Public Health. Cmnd 5242. HMSO, London

Department of Health 2001i Working together, learning together: a framework for lifelong learning in the NHS. Department of Health, London

Department of Health 2001j Establishing the new Nursing and Midwifery Council. HMSO, London

Department of Health 2001k Diabetes service standard. HMSO, London

Department of Health 2002a Delivering 21st century IT support for the NHS: national strategic programme. HMSO, London

Department of Health 2002b Liberating the talents: helping primary care trusts and nurses to deliver the NHS Plan. HMSO, London

Department of Health 2002c Promoting the health of looked after children. HMSO, London

Department of Health 2002d Safeguarding children in whom illness is fabricated or induced: a joint Chief Inspector's report on arrangements to safeguarding children. HMSO, London

Department of Health 2002e National Service Frameworks: a practical aid to implementation in primary care. HMSO, London

Department of Health 2002f Delivering the NHS Plan: next steps on investment, next steps on reform. HMSO, London

Department of Health 2002g Diabetes service delivery strategy. HMSO, London

Department of Health 2002h National service framework for acute children's services. HMSO, London

Department of Health 2003a Every child matters. Cmnd 5861. HMSO, London

Department of Health 2003b Liberating the public health talents of community practitioners and health visitors. HMSO, London

Department of Health 2003c Tackling health inequalities: a programme for action. HMSO, London

Department of Health 2003d Supplementary prescribing by nurses and pharmacists within the NHS in England: a guide for implementation. HMSO, London

Department of Health 2003e What to do if you're worried a child is being abused. HMSO, London

Department of Health 2003f Getting the right start: national service framework for children, young people and maternity services: standards for hospital services. HMSO, London

Department of Health 2004a National specification for integrated care records service. HMSO, London

Department of Health 2004b The NHS improvement plan: putting people at the heart of public services. HMSO, London

Department of Health 2004c Choosing health: making healthier choices easier. HMSO, London

Department of Health 2004d National service framework for children, young people and maternity services. HMSO, London

Department of Health and Social Security 1986 Neighbourhood nursing: a focus for care (Cumberlege Report). HMSO, London

Department of Health and Social Services Inspectorate 1993 No longer afraid: the safeguard of older people in domestic settings. HMSO, London

Department of Health Specialist Clinical Services Division 1996 Child health in the community: a guide to good practice. HMSO, London

Department of Health/Department for Education and Skills 1999 National healthy school standard. DfES, Nottingham

Department of Health/Department of Education and Science/Welsh Office 1991 Working together under the Children Act 1989: a guide to arrangements for inter-agency co-operation for the protection of children from abuse. HMSO, London

Department of Health/Home Office/Department for Education and Employment 2000 Working together to safeguard children: a guide to inter-agency working to safeguard and promote the welfare of children. HMSO, London

Department of Health/Home Office/Department for Education and Skills 2003 Keeping children safe: the government's response to the Victoria Climbié Inquiry report and Joint Chief Inspectors' report safeguarding children. HMSO, London

Department of Health/Department of Education and Employment 2000 Framework for the assessment of children in need and their families. HMSO, London

Department of Health/User Experience and Involvement/Professional Leadership Branch 2004 The Chief Nursing Officers review of the nursing, midwifery and health visiting contribution to vulnerable children and young people. HMSO, London

Department of Health/Welsh Office 1995 Child protection: clarification of arrangements between the NHS and other agencies. HMSO, London

Department of Social Security 1999 Supporting people: a new policy and funding framework for support services. HMSO, London

Deshler D 1990a Metaphor analysis: exorcising social ghosts. In: Mezirow J et al (eds) Fostering critical reflection in adulthood. Jossey-Bass, San Francisco

Deshler D 1990b Conceptual mapping: drawing charts of the mind. In: Mezirow J et al (eds) Fostering critical reflection in adulthood. Jossey-Bass, San Francisco

DeVille-Almond J 2000 A community development project. In: Robotham A, Sheldrake D (eds) Health visiting: specialist and higher level practice, 1st edn. Churchill Livingstone. Edinburgh

Dewey J 1933 How we think. Cited in Palmer et al (eds) 1994 Reflective practice in nursing: the growth of the professional practitioner. Blackwell Science, Oxford

Dezateux C et al 1997 Screening for congenital dislocation of the hip: a cost effective analysis. In: National Screening Committee/Royal College of Paediatrics and Child Health Proceedings: evolution or revolution? Systematic reviews of screening in child health, 17 December 1997 and 8 January 1998. Child Growth Foundation, London, p 22–23

Dezateux C, Brown J, Godward S et al 1998 Systematic reviews in child health. Royal College of Paediatrics and Child Health, London

Diment Y 1991 Routine health visiting of a family based upon Becker's health belief model. In: While A (ed) Caring for children: towards partnership with families. Edward Arnold, Sevenoaks, UK

Dimond B 2005, Legal aspects of nursing, 4th edn. Pearson Longman, London

Dingwall R 1989 Some problems about predicting child abuse and neglect. In: Stevenson O (ed) Child abuse: public policy and professional practice. Wheatsheaf, London

Dingwall R, Rafferty M, Webster C 1988 An introduction to the social history of nursing. Routledge, London

Dobash R E, Dobash R 1980 Violence against wives. Open Books, London

Dobby J 1986 The development and testing of a method for measuring the need for, and value of, routine health visiting within a District Health Authority. Health Promotion Research Trust, London

Doering C H, Brodie H K H, Kraemer H C et al 1974 Plasma testosterone levels and psychologic measures in men over a two month period. In Owens R G, Ashcroft J B 1985 Violence, a guide for the caring professions. Croom Helm, London

Donabedian A 1980 Explorations in quality assessment and monitoring: 1. The definition of quality and approaches to its assessment. Health Administration Press, Ann Arbor, MI

Donaldson D 2001 The report of the Chief Medical Officer's project to strengthen the public health function. Department of Health, London

Downey G, Coyne J C 1990 Children of depressed parents. Psychological Bulletin 108:50–76. In Shaw D S, Vondra J I 1995 Infant attachment security and maternal predicators of early behaviour problems: a longitudinal study of low-income families. Journal of Abnormal Child Psychology 23(3):335–357

Downie R S, Calman K C 1989 Healthy respect: ethics in health care. Faber & Faber, London

Drennan V 1985 Working in a different way. Paddington and North Kensington Health Authority, London

Dreyfus H, Dreyfus S 1980 A five-stage model of the mental activities involved in directed skill acquisition. Unpublished report. University of California, Berkeley

Drillien C, Drummond D 1983 Developmental screening and the child with special needs. Heinemann, London

Drummond M F, O'Brien B, Stoddart G, Torrance G 1997 Methods for the economic evaluation of health care programmes, 2nd edn. Oxford Medical Publications, Oxford

Drummond M, McGuire A 2001 Economic evaluation in health care: merging theory with practice. Oxford University Press, Oxford

Druss B G, Levinson C, Rosenheck R 2001 Integrated medical care for patients with serious psychiatric illness. Archives of General Psychiatry 58(9):861–868

Duckett H, Macfarlane E 2003 Emotional intelligence and transformational leadership in retailing. Leadership and Organisation Development Journal 24(6):309–317

Dudley Area Child Protection Committee 2004 Child protection procedures: a framework for inter-agency working to safeguard and promote the welfare of children. Dudley Area Child Protection Committee, Dudley

Dudley J 1994 The stage model of reflection. Unpublished paper, University of Wolverhampton

Duncan P 1990 To screen or not to screen? Health Education Journal 49:120–122

Dunn M 1970 Development of an instrument to measure nursing performance. Nursing Research 19:502–503

Dunn W R, Hamilton D D 1986 The critical incident technique: a brief guide. Medical Teacher 8(3):207–215

Dunn W R, Hamilton D D, Harden R M 1985 Techniques of identifying competencies needed of doctors. Medical Teacher 7:15–25

Dunn R B, Lewis P A, Vetter N J et al 1994 Health visitor intervention to reduce days of unplanned hospital re-admission in patients recently discharged from geriatric wards: the results of a randomised controlled study. Archives of Gerontological Geriatrics 18:1523

Durward L 1990. Traveller mothers and babies: who cares for their health? Maternity Alliance, London

Dwivedi K, Varma V 1996 Meeting the needs of ethnic minority children. Jessica Kingsley, London

Dyson S 1995 Whooping cough vaccine: historical, social and political controversies. Journal of Clinical Nursing 4(2):125–131

Eastman M 1984 Old age abuse. Age Concern, Mitcham

Easy F 1995 Letter. Vaccine debate inflames reaction. Health Matters Autumn(23)

Eaton M 1994 Abuse by any other name: feminism, difference and intralesbian violence. In: Fineman MA, Mykitiuk R (ed) The public nature of private violence. Routledge, New York

Edet E E 1991 The role of sex education in adolescent pregnancy. Journal of the Royal Society of Health Febrary:17–18

Edwards S 1985 A socio-legal evaluation of gender ideologies in domestic violence, assault and spousal homicides. Victimology 10:186–205

Egan G 1982 The skilled helper, 2nd edn. Brooks/Cole, Pacific Grove, CA

Egan G 1986 The skilled helper, 3rd edn. Brooks/Cole, Pacific Grove, CA

Egeland B 1988 Breaking the cycle of abuse: implications for prediction and intervention. In: Browne K, Davies C, Stratton P (eds) Early prediction and prevention of child abuse. John Wiley, Chichester

El Ansari W, Phillips C J, Hammick M 2001 Collaboration and partnerships: developing the evidence base. Health and Social Care in the Community 9(4):215–227

Elkan R, Blair M, Robinson J J A 2000a Evidence-based practice and health visiting: the need for theoretical underpinnings for evaluation. Journal of Advanced Nursing 31(6):1316–1323

Elkan R, Kendrick D, Hewitt M et al 2000b The effectiveness of domiciliary health visiting: systematic review of international studies and a selective review of British literature. Health Technology Assessment 4(13)

Elliott P 1996 Shattering illusions: same-sex domestic violence. In: Renzetti C M, Miley C H (eds) Violence in gay and lesbian domestic partnerships. Harrington Park Press, New York

Ellis R (ed) 1988 Professional competence and quality assurance in the caring professions. Chapman & Hall, London

Enabling People Programme 1997 Information for caring. NHS Management Executive, London

ENB/Department of Health 2001 Preparation of mentors and teachers: a new framework for guidance. English National Board Nursing, Midwifery and Health Visiting, London

Eraut M 1985 Knowledge creation and knowledge use in professional contexts. Studies in Higher Education 10:117–133

Eraut M 1994 Developing professional knowledge and competence. Falmer Press, London

Eriksen W, Sorum K, Bruusgaard D 1996 Effects of information on smoking behaviour in families with preschool children. Acta Paediatrica 85:209–212

Etzioni A 1969 The semi-professions and their organization: teachers, nurses and social workers. Free Press, New York

Evans R 2001 Children living with domestic violence. Emergency Nurse 9(6):22–26

Evans D 2003 New directions in tackling inequalities in health. In: Orme J, Powell J, Taylor P et al (eds) Public health for the 21st century: new perspectives on policy participation and practice. Open University Press, Milton Keynes

Ewles L, Simnett I 2003 Promoting health: a practical guide. Baillière Tindall, London

Eysenck H J 1983 Current theories of crime. In: Karas E (ed) Current issues in clinical psychology, vol 1. Plenum Press, New York

Faculty of Family Planning and Reproductive Health Care 2003 Service standards for sexual health services. Online. Available: http://www. ffprhc. org.uk March 2004

Fagan J 1997 Clients' views of health visitors and child health surveillance. Health Visitor 70:146–147

Fawcett J 1985 Analysis and evaluation of conceptual models of nursing. F A Davis, Philadelphia, PA

Fawcett J 1992 Conceptual models and nursing practice: the reciprocal relationship. Journal of Advanced Nursing 17:224–228

Feather N T (ed) 1982 Expectations and actions: expectancy–value models in psychology. Lawrence Erlbaum, Hillsdale, NJ

Feder G 1990 The politics of traveller health research. Critical Public Health (3)

Fiedler F E 1967 A theory of leadership effectiveness. McGraw-Hill, New York

Fielder A 1997 Pre-school vision screening: discussion. In: National Screening Committee/Royal College of Paediatrics and Child Health Proceedings: evolution or revolution? Systematic reviews of screening in child health, 17 December 1997 and 8 January 1998. Child Growth Foundation, London, p 11–12

Finkelhor D 1986 A sourcebook on child sexual abuse. Sage, Beverly Hills, CA

Fischbach F T 1991 Documenting care. F A Davis. Philadelphia, PA

Flanagan J C 1954 The Critical Incident Technique. Cited in Dunn W R, Hamilton D D 1986 The Critical Incident Technique: a brief guide. Medical Teacher 8(3)

Flanagan J C 1963 Cited in Dunn W R, Hamilton D D 1986 The Critical Incident Technique: a brief guide. Medical Teacher 8(3)

Fletcher L Buka P 1999 A legal framework for caring. Macmillan, London

Focault M 1979 Power and knowledge. Harvester Press, Brighton

Forester S 2002 An exploration of the factors that influence the adoption of community development approaches within health visiting. Unpublished

MSc thesis, St George's Hospital Medical School, University of London

Forester S 2004 Adopting community development approaches. Community Practitioner 77(4):140–145

Frankenburg W, Dodds J 1967 The Denver Developmental Screening Test. Journal of Paediatrics 71:181–191

Frankenburg W, Dodds J, Fandal A 1973 Denver Developmental Screening Test. Test Agency, High Wycombe

Frank-Stromborg M, Pender N J, Walker S N 1990 Determinants of health-promoting lifestyles in ambulatory cancer patients. Social Science and Medicine 31:1159–1168

Frazer W 1950 A history of English public health 1834–1939. Baillière Tindall & Cox, London

French P 1999 The development of evidence-based nursing. Journal of Advanced Nursing 29:72–78

Friend B 1999 Power to the people. Community Practitioner 72(4):81–82

Friere P 1972 The pedagogy of the oppressed. Penguin, London

Frodsham C, Jones M 2004 Evaluation of nurse practitioner role at a homeless centre: interim report. South Birmingham PCT (unpublished report)

Frude N 1996 Abuse within families. In: Gastrell P, Edwards J (eds) Community health nursing: frameworks for practice. Baillière Tindall, London

Fulder S J, Munro R E 1985 Complementary medicine in the United Kingdom: patients, practitioners, and consultations. Lancet ii:542–545

Fullerton R, Dickson R, Sheldon T 1997 Preventing and reducing the adverse effects of teenage pregnancy. Health Visitor 70(5):197–199

Fung S F 1998 Factors associated with breast self-examination behaviour among Chinese women in Hong Kong. Patient Education and Counseling 33:233–243

Gallant M H, Beaulieu M C, Carnevale F A 2002 Partnership: an analysis of the concept within the nurse–client relationship. Journal of Advanced Nursing 40(2):149–157

Gallie W B 1955 Essentially contested concepts. In: Glen S 1995 Developing critical thinking in higher education. Nurse Education Today 15:170–176

Garcia A, Norton-Broda M A, Frenn M et al 1995 Gender and development differences in exercise beliefs among youth and prediction of their exercise behaviour. Journal of School Health 65:213–219

Gardiner E 1999 In: Jones M (ed) Nurse prescribing: politics to practice. Baillière Tindall, Edinburgh, ch 1

Garside M 2000 Developing a family health plan. Institute of General Practice, Sheffield

Garside M 2002 An evaluation of family health plans. Institute of General Practice and Primary Care, Sheffield

Gask L, Usherwood T 2002 ABC of psychological medicine: the consultation. British Medical Journal 324:1567–1569

Gephens A, Gunning-Schepers L J 1996 Interventions to reduce socio-economic health differences: a review of the international literature. European Journal of Public Health 6(3):218–226

Gesell A 1925 The mental growth of the pre-school child. Macmillan, New York

Gesell A 1948 Studies in child development. Harper, New York

Gesell A, Amatruda C S 1947 Developmental diagnosis. Hoeber, New York

Gesell A, Amatruda C S, Castner B M et al 1930 Biographies of child development. Hamish Hamilton, London

Gibb C, Randall P E 1989 Professionals and parents: managing children's behaviour. Macmillan, London

Gibbs G 1988 Learning by doing: a guide to teaching and learning methods. Further Education Unit, Oxford Polytechnic, Oxford

Gibson C H 1991 A concept analysis of empowerment. Journal of Advanced Nursing 16:354–361

Giddens A 2001 Sociology, 4th edn. Polity Press/Blackwell, Oxford

Gilbert A, Banks J 1997 30 degrees westward: a case study in making it happen. Ivybridge Public Health Project, unpublished report

Gillon R 1989 Philosophy and practice of medical ethics. John Wiley, Chichester

Girot E A 1993 Assessment of competence in clinical practice: a phenomenological approach. Journal of Advanced Nursing 18:114–119

Girvin J 1998 Leadership and nursing. Palgrave, Basingstoke

Glass N 1998 Origins of the Sure Start programme. In: Children and Society, vol 13. John Wiley, Chichester

Glen S 1995 Developing critical thinking in higher education. Nurse Education Today 15:170–176

Goffman E 1961 Encounters, two studies in the sociology of interaction. Bobbs-Merrill, New York

Gogna S, Hari T 2000 Public health needs of South Asians in Britain. In: Robotham A, Sheldrake D (eds) Health visiting: specialist and higher level practice, 1st edn. Churchill Livingstone, Edinburgh

Goldstone L A et al 1983 Monitor: an index of the quality of nursing care for acute medical and surgical wards. Newcastle upon Tyne Polytechnic Products, Newcastle upon Tyne

Goodman J 1984 Reflection and teacher education: a case study and theoretical analysis. Interchange 15:9–26

Goodwin S 1988 Whither health visiting? Health Visitor 61:379–382

Goudie H, Redman J 1996 Making health services more accessible to younger people. Nursing Times 92(25):45–46

Graham H 1987 Women's smoking and family health. Social Science and Medicine 25(1):47–56

Gravelle H S E, Simpson P R, Chamberlain J 1982 Breast cancer screening and health service costs. Journal of Health Economics 1:185–207

Green C 1999 Toddler taming, a parent's guide for the first four years. Vermillion, London

Green J, Dale J 1992 Primary care in accident and emergency and general practice: a comparison. Social Science and Medicine 35:987–995

Green J M, Murray D 1994 The use of the Edinburgh Postnatal Depression Scale in research to explore the relationship between antenatal and postnatal dysphoria. In: Cox J, Holden J (eds) 1994 Perinatal psychiatry, use and misuse of the Edinburgh Postnatal Depression Scale. Gaskell, London

Green L W, Kreuter M W, Deeds S F et al 1980 Health education planning: a diagnostic approach. Mansfield, Palo Alto, CA

Greer S, Bauchner H, Zucherman B 1989 The Denver Developmental Screening Test: how good is its predictive validity? Developmental Medicine and Child Neurology 31:774–781

Griffiths R 1954 The abilities of babies. University of London Press, London

Griffiths R 1970 The abilities of young children. Test Agency, High Wycombe

Griffiths Report 1988 Community Care: agenda for action. HMSO, London

Groves E 2002 In: Humphries J L, Green J (eds) Nurse prescribing, 2nd edn. Palgrave, Basingstoke, ch 2

Guillebaud J 1993 Contraception: hormonal and barrier methods. Martin Dunitz, London

Haggart M 1993 A critical analysis of Neuman's systems model in relation to public health nursing. Journal of Advanced Nursing 18:1971–1922

Haggstrom W C 1970 The psychological implications of the community development process. In: Carcy L J (ed) Community development as a process. University of Missouri Press, Columbia, MO

Hall D 1986 Developmental tests and scales. Archives of Disease in Childhood 61:213–215

Hall D (ed) 1989 Health for all children: a programme for child health surveillance. Report of the Joint Working Party on Child Health Surveillance. Oxford University Press, Oxford

Hall D (ed) 1991 Health for all children: a programme for child health surveillance. Report of the Joint Working Party on Child Health Surveillance, 2nd edn. Oxford University Press, Oxford

Hall D (ed) 1996 Health for all children: a programme for child health surveillance. Report of the Joint Working Party on Child Health Surveillance, 3rd edn. Oxford University Press, Oxford

Hall D B M, Elliman D (eds) 2003 Health for all children, 4th edn. Oxford University Press, Oxford

Hamer S, Collinson G 1999 Achieving evidence-based practice. Baillière Tindall/Royal College of Nursing, London

Hampshire and Isle of Wight Public Health Network 2003 Developing the workforce in Hampshire and the Isle of Wight to specialist level. Workforce Development Paper, January 2003

Handy C 1999 Understanding organisations, 4th edn. Penguin, London

Hanks H, Stratton P 1988 Family perspectives in early sexual abuse. In: Browne K, Davies C, Stratton P (eds) Early prediction and prevention of child abuse. John Wiley, Chichester

Hanlon G 1998 Professionalism as enterprise: service class politics and the redefinition of professionalism. Sociology 32(1):43–63

Hanlon G 2000 Sacking the New Jerusalem? The new right, social democracy and professional identities. Sociological Research Online 5(1)

Harding S, Pandya N 1995 The role of health advocates in health visiting teams. Health Visitor 68:192–193

Harris J 1985 The value of life. Routledge, London

Harter S 1983 Developmental perspectives on the self-system. Cited in Sarafino E 1994 Health psychology, 2nd edn. John Wiley, New York

Hatchwell P K 1992 Genetic research: implications for workplace screening. Occupational Health Review April/May:8–11

Hatton P 1990 Measles/mumps/rubella vaccine (MMR): an audit of Leeds Health professionals' knowledge of contraindications and intention to vaccinate assessed by postal questionnaire. Journal of Public Health Medicine 12(2):124–130

Hawskley B, Carnwell R, Callwood I 2003 A review of the public health roles of health visitors and school nurses. Journal of Community Nursing 8(10):447–454

Haynes R, Sackett D, Taylor D et al 1978 Increased absenteeism from work after detection and labelling of hypertensive patients. New England Journal of Medicine 299

Health Development Agency 2000 Participatory approaches in health planning: a literature review. Health Development Agency, London

Health Education Authority 1995 Black and minority ethnic groups in England: health and lifestyles. HEA, London

Health Education Authority 1997 Promoting health through primary care nursing. Health Education Authority, London

Health Protection Agency 2003 Renewing the focus: HIV and other sexually transmitted infections in the United Kingdom in 2002. Online. Available: http://www.hpa.org.uk March 2004

Health Resources and Service Administration (HRSA) 1997 National vaccine injury compensation program: vaccine injury table. Online. Available: http://www.hrsa.dhhs.gov/bhpr/vic/table.htm

Health Visitor Association 1994 Mix and match. HVA, London

Heath H 1998 Reflections and patterns of knowing in nursing. Journal of Advanced Nursing 27:1054–1059

Heider J 1992 The tao of leadership. Gower, Aldershot

Hendriksen C Stromgard E, Sorensen K H 1989 Co-operation concerning admission to and discharge of elderly people from the hospital: the coordinated contributions of home care personnel. Ugeskrift for laeger 151:1531–1534

Hennessy D A 1985 Mothers and health visitors. In: Twinn S F 1991 Conflicting paradigms of health visiting: a continuing debate for professional practice. Journal of Advanced Nursing 16:966–973

Heron J 1986 Six category intervention analysis, 2nd edn. Human Potential Research Project, University of Surrey, Guildford

Herzberg F 1966 Work and the nature of man. World Publishing, New York

Hickman D J, Thomas M W 1969 Professionalisation in Britain: a preliminary measurement. Sociology III:37–53

Hinde R A, Tamplin A, Barret J 1993 A comparative study of relationship structure. British Journal of Social Psychology 32:191–207

HM Treasury 1998 Comprehensive spending review: cross departmental review of provision for young children: supporting papers, vols 1 and 2. HMSO, London

HM Treasury 2002 The Green Book: appraisal and evaluation in central government. HMSO, London

HM Treasury/Department of Health 2002 Tackling health inequalities: summary of the 2002 cross-cutting review. HMSO, London

HMSO 1968 Seebohm Report: report of the committee on local authority and allied personal Social Services. Cmnd 3703. HMSO, London

HMSO 1989 The Children Act: guidance and regulation. HMSO, London

Hoghughi M 1998 The importance of parenting in child health. British Medical Journal 316:1545–1550

Hoghughi M, Speight A 1998 Good enough parenting for all children: a strategy for a healthier society. Archives of Disease in Childhood 78:293–296

Holden J 1994 Using the Edinburgh Postnatal Depression Scale in clinical practice. In Cox J, Holden J (eds) Perinatal psychiatry, use and misuse of the Edinburgh Postnatal Depression Scale. Gaskell, London

Holden J M, Sagovsky R, Cox J L 1989 Counselling in a general practice setting: controlled study of health visitor intervention in treatment of postnatal depression. British Medical Journal 298:223–226

Homans G 1961 Social behaviour: its elementary forms. Harcourt Brace Jovanovich, New York

Home Office 1997 Witness in Court – a leaflet for witnesses in court. Home Office pubs

Home Office 1998 Government policy around domestic violence. HMSO, London

Home Office 1999 Supporting families, a consultation document. HMSO, London

Home Office 2000 Domestic violence: break the chain. Multi-agency guidance for addressing domestic violence. HMSO, London

Home Office 2002 Achieving best evidence in criminal proceedings: guidance for vulnerable or intimidated witnesses, including children. Home Office Communication Directorate, London

Home Office 2003 Witness in Court – a leaflet for witnesses in court. Home Office pubs

Home Office/Cabinet Office 1999 Living without fear: an integrated approach to tackling violence against women. HMSO, London

Hooper J, Longworth P 1998 Health needs assessment in Primary Care Teams. Calderdale and Kirklees Health Authority, Huddersfield

Hooper J, Longworth P 2002 Health needs assessment workbook. Health Development Agency London

House of Commons 2004 Bichard Inquiry Report. London: The Stationary Office

House of Lords Select Committee on Science and Technology 2000 Complementary and alternative medicine 6th report, Session 1999–2000. HL Paper 123. London

House of Lords 2004 Children Bill. London: The Stationary Office

Houston A 2003 Sure Start: a complex community initiative. Community Practitioner 76(7):257–260

HSC 1974 The Health and Safety at Work Act. HMSO, London

Hudson R 1997 Demonstrating effectiveness: compiling the evidence. Health Visitor 70:459–461

Hulse J A et al 1997 Population growth analysis using the Child Health Computing System: a method of assessing the value of child health surveillance. In: National Screening Committee/Royal College of Paediatrics and Child Health Proceedings: evolution or revolution? Systematic reviews of screening in child health, 17 December 1997 and 8 January 1998. Child Growth Foundation, London, p 21

Hulse J A, Schilg S, Blount J et al 1998 Systematic reviews of child health. Royal College of Paediatrics and Child Health, London

Human Rights Act 1998 HMSO, London

Humphries E 1989 An evaluation of the developmental examination programme used in Halesowen by audit of the medical records of children statemented between January 1988 and December 1989 to determine if children with learning difficulties could have been identified before. Unpublished PGD thesis

Hunt J M 1996 Guest editorial. Journal of Advanced Nursing 23:423–425

Hutcheson J J, Black M M, Talley M et al 1997 Risk status and home intervention among children with failure to thrive: follow-up at age 4. Journal of Pediatric Psychology 22:651–668

Hutton J 2002 Helping frontline nurses deliver the NHS plan. Press release 15 November 2002 (2002/0471)

Hyett E 2003 What blocks health visitors from taking on a leadership role? Journal of Nursing Management 11:229–233

Illich I 1977 Disabling professions. Marion Boyars, London

Illingworth R S 1987 The development of the infant and young child, 9th edn. Churchill Livingstone, Edinburgh

Independent Review of Residential Care 1988 Residential care: a positive choice. Report of the Independent review of residential care chaired by Gillian Wagner. HMSO, London

Information on local provision of health care can be found on www.NHSGateway. Another good source of information for the health care professional is www.harpweb.org

Ingalsbe N, Spears M C 1979 Development of an instrument to evaluate critical incident performance. In: Dunn W R, Hamilton D D 1986 The Critical Incident Technique: a brief guide. Medical Teacher 8(3)

Ingram D R, Clarke D R, Murdiq R A 1978 Distance and the decision to visit an emergency department. Social Science and Medicine 12:55–62

Integrated Care Network 2004 Integrated working and children's services: structures, outcome and reform. http://omni.ac.uk

Integrated Children's system 2002 DfES, London

Inter-agency Group 2004 From vision to reality: transforming outcomes for children and families. IGA, London

Irish College of General Practitioners 1995 Quality in practice programme. Irish College of General Practitioners, Dublin

Iyer P W, Camp N H 1991 Nursing documentation. Mosby Year Book, Chicago, IL

Jacks H 2004 Consent to treatment: workshop and training. Mills & Reeve, Stoke on Trent

Jackson C 1992 Trick or treat. Health Visitor 656:199–201

Jackson P, Plant Z 1996 Youngsters get an introduction to sexual health clinics. Nursing Times 92(21):34–36

Jarman B 1983 Identification of underprivileged areas. British Medical Journal 286:1705–1709

Jarvis P 1983 Professional education. Croom Helm, London

Jarvis P 1987 Adult learning in the social context. Croom Helm, London

Jarvis P 1992 Reflective practice and nursing Nurse Education Today 12:174–181

Jarvis P 1999 The way forward for practice education. Nurse Education Today 19:269–273

Jarvis P, Gibson S 1985 The teacher practitioner in nursing, midwifery and health visiting. Croom Helm, London

Jeffreys M 1965 An anatomy of social welfare services. Cited in Robinson J 1982 An evaluation of health visiting. CETHV, London

Jenkins G, Asif Z, Bennett G 2000 Listening is not enough. Journal of Adult Protection 2:1

Jezierski M 1992 Guidance for intervention by ED nurses in cases of domestic violence. Journal of Emergency Nursing 18:28A–30A

Jinks A, Smith M, Ashdown-Lambert J 2003 The public health roles of health visitors and school nurses: a survey. British Journal of Community Nursing 8(11):496–501

Johns C 2000 Becoming a reflective practitioner, Blackwell Science, Oxford

Johns C C 1992 The Burford Nursing Development Unit holistic model of nursing practice. Journal of Advanced Nursing 16:1090–1098

Johnson M R D 1996 Ethnic minorities, health and communication. Research paper in ethnic relations no. 24. NHS Executive and West Midlands Regional Health Authority Centre for Research in Ethnic relations, Birmingham

Johnson M R D 2003 The provision of healthcare services for asylum seekers. Home Office, London

Johnson T J 1972 Professions and power. Macmillan Education, London

Johnson Z, Howell F, Molloy B 1993 Community mothers' programme: randomised controlled trial of non-professional intervention in parenting. British Medical Journal 306:1449–1452

Jones J S 1990 Geriatric abuse and neglect. In Bennett G, Kingston P, Penhale B 1997 The dimensions of elder abuse: perspectives for practitioners. Macmillan, Basingstoke

Jones M 1996 Clients express preference for one-step sexual health shop. Nursing Times 96(21):32–33

Jones M (ed) 1999 Nurse prescribing: politics to practice. Baillière Tindall, Edinburgh

Jordan S, Griffiths H 2004 Nurse prescribing: developing the evaluation agenda. Nursing Standard 18(29):40–44

Kant I 1964 Groundwork of the metaphysics of morals. Paton H J (transl). Harper & Row, New York, p 90–91

Kelly A, Symonds A 2003 The social construction of community nursing. Palgrave Macmillan, Basingstoke

Kelly M, McDaid D, Ludbrook A et al 2004 Economic appraisal of public health interventions. Health Development Agency, London

Kendrick D, Bakewell S 1995 On the verge: the gypsies and England. University of Hertford Press, Hatfield

Kendrick D, Elkan R, Hewitt M et al 2000 Does home visiting improve parenting and the quality of the home environment? A systematic review and meta analysis. Archives of Disease in Childhood 82(6):443–451

Kennedy C 2004 Healthcare Commission to inspect NHS and private health. Press release, 1 April 2004. Online. Available: www.healthcarecommission. org.uk

Kenny T 1993 Nursing models fail in practice. British Journal of Nursing 2(2):133–136

Kerr S, Jowett S, Smith L 1997 Education to help prevent sleep problems in infants. Health Visitor 70:224–225

Kessen W 1965 The child. John Wiley, New York

Kiln M R 1998 Those giving MMR vaccine had no input into it. Letter. British Medical Journal 316(7147):1824

King I 1981 A theory for nursing. John Wiley, New York

King M D 1968 Science and the professional dilemma. In: Gould J (ed) Penguin social sciences survey. Penguin, Harmondsworth, p 34–73

Kitchener K S 1983 Educational goals and reflective thinking. In Kitchener K S, King P M 1990 The reflective judgement model: transforming assumptions about knowing. In Mezirow J et al (ed) Fostering critical reflection in adulthood. Jossey-Bass, San Francisco

Kitchener K S, King P M 1990 The reflective judgement model: transforming assumptions about knowing.

In: Mezirow J et al (eds) Fostering critical reflection in adulthood. Jossey-Bass, San Francisco

Kitson A, Ahmed L B, Harvey G et al 1996 From research to practice: one organisational model for promoting research-based practice. Journal of Advanced Nursing 23:430–440

Kivel P 1996 Uprooting racism: how white people can work for racial justice. New Society, Philadelphia, PA

Klaus D, Gosnell D, Jacobs A et al 1966 Controlling experience to improve nursing efficiency: background and study plans. Report 1. American Institute for Research, Pittsburgh

Klaus D, Reilly P, Taylor J 1968 Controlling experience to improve nursing efficiency: categories of nursing performance. Report no 2. American Institutes for Research, Pittsburgh

Kogan M, Redfern S 1995 Making use of clinical audit: a guide to practice in the health professions. Open University Press, Buckingham

Labonte R 1998 A community development approach to health promotion. Health Education Board for Scotland, Edinburgh

Laidman P 1987 Health visiting and preventing accidents to children. Research report no 12. Child Accident Prevention Trust, Health Education Authority, London

Laming Report 2003 The Victoria Climbié Inquiry (Command Paper). Cmnd 5730. HMSO, London

Lancet 1986 Developmental surveillance. Lancet 26(April):950–952

Larson C P 1980 Efficacy of prenatal and postpartum home visits on child health and development. Pediatrics 66:191–197

Latter S, Courtenay M 2004 Effectiveness of nurse prescribing: a review of the literature. Journal of Clinical Nursing (13):26–32

Law J et al 1997 Child health surveillance: an evaluation of screening for speech and language delay (executive summary). In: National Screening Committee/Royal College of Paediatrics and Child Health Proceedings: evolution or revolution? Systematic reviews of screening in child health, 17 December 1997 and 8 January 1998. Child Growth Foundation, London

Lawton E 1996 Leader of the pack. Health Visitor 69:198

Le May A 1999 Evidence-based practice. Nursing Times clinical monographs no 1. NT Books, London

Lee T, Ko I S, Jeong S H 2004 Is an expanded nurse role economically viable? Journal of Advanced Nursing 46(5):471–479

Leon D A, Watt O, Gibson L 2001 International perspectives to health inequalities and policy. British Medical Journal 322:691–694

Letellier P 1996 Twin epidemics: domestic violence and HIV infection among gay and bisexual men. In: Renzetti C M, Miley C H (eds) Violence in gay and lesbian domestic partnerships. Harrington Park Press, New York

Lewin K 1935 A dynamic theory of personality. McGraw-Hill, New York

Lewin K 1951 Field theory in social science. Harper, New York

Lewis C 2004 Screening for Chlamydia. Community Practitioner 77(2):44

Lewis M 1988 What can child development tell us about child abuse? In: Browne K, Davies C, Stratton P (eds) Early prediction and prevention of child abuse. John Wiley, Chichester

Lightfoot J 1994 Demonstrating the value of health visiting. Health Visitor 67:19–20

Ling M S, Luker K A 2000 Protecting children: intuition and awareness in the work of health visitors. Journal of Advanced Nursing 32(3):572–579

Little L 1997 Teenage health education: a public health approach. Nursing Standard 11(49):43–46

Lloyd N, O'Brien M, Lewis C 2003 Fathers in Sure Start programmes: national evaluation summary. DfES, London

London Borough of Wandsworth 2002 Sure Start Roehampton: delivery plan. Unpublished

Long N 1996 Parenting in the USA. Clinical Child Psychology and Psychiatry 1:469–453

Luker K A 1978 Goal attainment: a possible model for assessing the work of the health visitor. Nursing Times 75:1488–1490

Luker K A 1982 Evaluating health visiting practice: an experimental study to evaluate the effects of focused health visitor intervention on elderly women living alone at home. Royal College of Nursing, London

Luker K A 1985 Evaluating health visiting practice. In: Luker K A, Orr J (eds) Health Visiting. Blackwell Scientific, Oxford

Luker K A 1997 Evaluation of nurse prescribing. Final Report, University of Liverpool/University of York, Liverpool/York

Luker K, Orr J 1992 Health visiting towards community health nursing, 2nd edn. Blackwell Scientific, Oxford

Luker K A, Austin L, Willock J et al 1997 Nurses' and GPs' views of the nurse prescribers' formulary. Nursing Standard 11(22):33–38

Luker K A, Hogg C, Austin L et al 1998 Decision making: the context of nurse prescribing. Journal of Advanced Nursing 27:657–665

Lusk S L, Ronis D, Kerr M J et al 1994 Test of the health promotion model as a causal model of workers' use of hearing protection. Nursing Research 43:151–157

Lynn M 1987 Update: Denver Developmental Screening Test. Journal of Paediatric Nursing 2:348–351

MacDuff C, Harvey S 2001 Telemedicine in rural care. Part 2: Assessing the wider issues. Nursing Standard 15(33):33–37

Macfarlane A, Sefi S, Cordeiro M 1990 Child health: the screening tests. Oxford University Press, Oxford

MacFarlene J A Saffin K 1990 Do general practitioners and health visitors like parent held child health records? British Journal of General Practice 40:106–108

Mack P, Trew K 1991 Are fathers' views important? Health Visitor 64:257–258

Mackereth C 1999 Joined up working: community development in primary care. CPHVA, London

Marcé Society 1994 The emotional effects of childbirth: distance learning course. H Wharton, Doncaster

Marley L 1995 Setting up a duty health visitor rota. Health Visitor 68:456

Marris T 1971 The work of health visitors in London: a Department of Planning and Transportation survey, 1969. Research report 12. Greater London Council, London

Marshall A 1936 Principles of economics, 8th edn. Macmillan, London

Marteau T M 1989 Psychological costs of screening: may sometimes be bad enough to undermine the benefits of screening British Medical Journal 299:527

Marteau T M 1990 Reducing the psychological costs. British Medical Journal 301:26–28

Matthews E 1986 Can paternalism be modernised? Journal of Medical Ethics 12:133–135

Maxwell R 1984 Quality assurance in health. British Medical Journal 12 May:1470–1472

Mayall B, Foster C D 1989 Child health care, living with children, working for children. Heinemann Nursing, Oxford

McClymont M, Thomas S, Denhamm M J 1991 Health visiting and elderly people: a health promotion challenge. Churchill Livingstone, Edinburgh

McConnaughy E A, Procaska J O, Velicer W F 1983 Stages of change in psychotherapy: measurement and sample profiles. Psychotherapy: Theory, Research and Practice 20:368–375

McFarlane J 1986 The value of models for care. In: Kershaw B, Salvage J (eds) Models for nursing. John Wiley, Chichester

McKee C M, Gleadhill D N S, Watson J D 1990 Accident and emergency attendance rates: variation among patients from different general practices. British Journal of General Practice 40:150–153

McMullan M, Endacott R, Gray M A et al 2003 Portfolios and assessment of competence: a review of the literature. Journal of Advanced Nursing 41(3):283–294

Mead G H 1934 Mind, self, and society. University of Chicago Press, Chicago, IL

Meade T W, Dyer S, Browne W et al 1990 Low back pain of mechanical origin: randomised comparison of chiropractic and hospital outpatient treatment. British Medical Journal 300:1431–1437

Meerabeau E 1992 Tacit nursing knowledge: an untapped resource or a methodological headache? Journal of Advanced Nursing 17:108–112

Megargee E I 1966 Undercontrolled and overcontrolled personality types in extreme anti-social aggression. In Owens R G, Ashcroft J B 1985 Violence, a guide for the caring professions. Croom Helm, London

Meleis A I 1985 Theoretical nursing: development and progress. Lippincott, Philadelphia

Merrill J 1989 Attempted suicide by deliberate self-poisoning amongst Asians. In Smaje C 1995 Health, race and ethnicity: making sense of the evidence. King's Fund Institute/Share, London

Messages from Research 1995 Studies in child protection. HMSO, London

Mezey G 1997 Domestic violence in pregnancy. In: Bailey S et al (eds) Violence against women. RCOG, London

Mezirow J 1981 A critical theory of adult learning and education. Adult Education 32(1)

Mezirow J et al 1990 Fostering critical reflection in adulthood. Jossey Bass, San Francisco

Miles M, Huberman A 1994 Qualitative data analysis, 2nd edn. Sage, London

Millar B 1997 Family nursing and community nursing practice. In: Gastrell P, Edwards J (eds) Community Health Nursing Frameworks for Practice. Baillière Tindall, London

Miller C 1975 American Rom and the ideology of defilement. In: Rehfisch F (ed) Gypsies, tinkers and other travellers. Academic Press, London, p 41–54

Miller C 2003 Public health meets modernisation. In: Orme J, Powell J, Taylor P et al (eds) Public health for the 21st century: new perspectives on policy participation and practice. Milton Keynes, Open University Press

Miller D, Madge N, Diamond J, Wadsworth J, Ross E 1993 Pertussis immunisation and serious acute neurological illnesses in children. BMJ 307:1171–1176

Millerson G 1964 Dilemmas of professionalism. New Society 4:15

Milligan F 1998 Defining and assessing competence: the distraction of outcomes and the importance of the educational process. Nurse Education Today 18:273–280

Ministry of Agriculture, Fisheries and Food 1989 Manual of nutrition. HMSO, London

Ministry of Health 1956 An inquiry into health visiting. HMSO, London

Minugh P A, Rice C, Young L 1998 Gender, health beliefs, health behaviours, and alcohol consumption. American Journal of Alcohol Abuse 24:483–497

Mitchell J H 1969 Compliance with medical regimens: an annotated bibliography. Department of Medical Care and Hospitals, School of Hygiene and Public Health, Johns Hopkins University, Baltimore, MD

Moch S 1990 Personal knowing: evolving research and practice. Cited in Heath H 1998 Reflections and patterns of knowing in nursing. Journal of Advanced Nursing 27:1054–1059

Moores Y 1991 Nursing and IT: issues and opportunities. Information Technology in Nursing 3(3)

Moores Y 1992 The nursing profession's contribution to the strategy for NHS information management and technology. Information Technology in Nursing 4(4)

Mor V, Granger C V, Sherwood C C 1983 Discharged rehabilitation patients: impact of follow-up surveillance by a friendly visitor. Archives of Physical and Medical Rehabilitation 64:346–353

Morgan W, Walker J H, Holohan A M, Russell I T 1974 Casual attenders: a socio medical study of patients attending accident and emergency departments in the Newcastle upon Tyne area. Hospital and Health Services Review 70:180–194

Morris S, St James-Roberts I, Gillham P 2001 Economic evaluation of strategies for managing crying and sleeping problems. Archives of Disease in Childhood 84:15–19

Mullally S 2003 Chief Nursing Officers' Report. HMSO, London

Mullally S, Jones M 2004 A conversation with … Community Practitioner 77(2):47–49

Mullins L 1999 Management and organisational behaviour, 5th edn. Financial Times/Pitman Publishing, London

Murphy A, Tallis R 2003 How to achieve concordance through ethnic sensitivity and lateral thinking: a case study. Pharmaceutical Journal 271:511–512

Murrey L, Cooper P J 1997 Effects of postnatal depression on infant development. Archives of Disease in Childhood 77(2):99–102

Myers P 1982 Management of minor medical problems and trauma: general practice or hospital. Journal of the Royal Society of Medicine 75:875–883

Naidoo J, Wills J 1994 Health promotion: foundations for practice. Baillière Tindall, London

Naidoo J, Wills J 2000 Health promotion: foundations for practice (2nd edn). Baillière Tindall, London

Naish J, Kline R 1990 What counts can't always be counted. Health Visitor 63:421–422

National Assembly for Wales 2001 Improving health in Wales: structured changes in the NHS in Wales. National Assembly for Wales, Cardiff

National Audit Office 1992 Report of the Comptroller and Auditor General: NHS accident and emergency departments in England. HMSO, London

National Health Service Executive 1994 Nurse prescribing guidance. HMSO, London

National Institute for Clinical Excellence 2004 Guide to the methods of technology appraisal. Online. Available: http://www.nice.org.uk/page.aspx?o=201974 11 Jun 2004

National Prescribing Centre 1998 The use of emollients in dry skin conditions. MeReC Bulletin vol 9(12). National Prescribing Centre, Liverpool

National Prescribing Centre 1999 Signposts for prescribing nurses: general principles of good prescribing. Prescribing Nurse Bulletin 1(1)

National Prescribing Centre 2001 Maintaining competency in prescribing: an outline framework to help nurse prescribers. National Prescribing Centre, Liverpool

Neighbour R 1987 The inner consultation: how to develop an effective and intuitive consultation style. LibraPharm, Reading

NESS (National Evaluation of Sure Start) 2002 National evaluation: early experiences of implementing Sure Start. DfES, London

Neuman B 1989 The Neuman systems model. Appleton & Lange, Norwalk, CT

NHS Confederation, British Medical Association 2003 The new GMS contract investing in General Practice. NHS Confederation, London

NHS Executive 1993 New world, new opportunities: nursing in primary health care. HMSO, London

NHS Executive 1995 Planning guidelines. NHS Executive, London

NHS Executive 1996 Promoting clinical effectiveness. NHS Executive, Leeds

NHS Executive 1997 Priorities and planning guidance for the NHS: 1997/98. NHS Executive, Leeds

NHS Executive 1998a Information for health: an information strategy for the modern NHS 1998–2005. HMSO, London

NHS Executive 1998b In the public interest: developing strategy for public participation in the NHS. HMSO, London

NHS Leadership Centre 2001 Online. Available: www.NHSLeadershipQualities.nhs.uk

Nicoll A, Elliman D, Ross E 1998 MMR vaccination and autism. British Medical Journal 316:715–716

Nolan M 1996 The Blenheim Harding Trust: meeting the needs of young women who become pregnant. Modern Midwife 6(11):22–24

Norris C (ed) 1982 Concept clarification in nursing. Aspen Systems, Germantown, MD

North Staffs Combined Healthcare Trust 1996 Promoting health visiting, May 1996

Northern Ireland Office 1999 Partnership for equality: White Paper (CM3890). Belfast Annual Report

Novak J D, Gowan D B 1984 Learning how to learn. Cambridge University Press, New York

Nurse Prescribers' Formulary 1994 British Medical Association/Royal Pharmaceutical Society of Great Britain. Pharmaceutical Press, Oxford

NMC 2002a Code of professional conduct. Nursing and Midwifery Council, London

NMC 2002b Guidelines for records and record keeping. Nursing and Midwifery Council, London

NMC 2002c Requirements for pre-registration health visitor programmes. Nursing and Midwifery Council, London

NMC 2002d Scope of professional practice. Nursing and Midwifery Council, London

NMC 2003a Third part of the new register: specialist community public health nursing. Proposed competency framework. Nursing and Midwifery Council, London

NMC 2003b Radical restructure: a new look register. NMC News Autumn (3):4

NMC 2004a Standards of proficiency for specialist community public health nurses. Nursing and Midwifery Council, London

NMC 2004b The third part of the register in N&MC. Nursing and Midwifery Council, London

NMC 2004c News July 2004

Nursing and Midwifery Council for England 2002a The NMC standards for medicines management. Nursing and Midwifery Council, London

Nursing and Midwifery Council for England 2002b The NMC code of professional conduct: standards for conduct, performance and ethics, Nursing and Midwifery Council, London

Nursing and Midwifery Council for England 2002c The NMC standards for records and record keeping. Nursing and Midwifery Council, London

Oakeshott M 1962 Rationalism in politics: and other essays. In Eraut M 1985 Knowledge creation and knowledge use in professional contexts. Studies in Higher Education 10:117–133

ODPM 2002 Homelessness statistical release. Office of the Deputy Prime Minister, London

ODPM 2003 Guidance on managing unauthorised camping. ODPM, London

ODPM 2004a Homelessness and health information sheet no. 1: personal medical services. Office of the Deputy Prime Minister, London

ODPM 2004b Homelessness and health information sheet no. 2: health visiting services. Office of the Deputy Prime Minister, London

ODPM 2004c The impact of overcrowding on health and education: a review of evidence and literature. Office of the Deputy Prime Minister, London

Oehler J M, Vileisis R A 1990 Effect of early sibling visitation in an intensive care nursery. Journal of Developmental and Behavioural Pediatrics 11:7–12

Office of National Statistics 1997 General household survey. Office of National Statistics, London

Office of National Statistics 2000 Abortion statistics, Series AB 28, TSO, London. Online. Available: http://www.statistics.gov.uk Mar 2004

Okely J 1975 Gypsy women: models in conflict. In: Ardener S (ed) Perceiving women. Malaby, London, p 55–86

Okely J 1983 The traveller gypsies. Cambridge University Press, Cambridge, UK

Olds D, Henderson C, Cole R 1998 Long-term effects of nurse home visitation on children's criminal and anti-social behaviour. Journal of the American Medical Association 280(14):1238–1244

Olson D H, Russell C S, Sprenkle D H 1979 Circumplex model of marital and family systems. II: Empirical studies and clinical intervention. Cited in Gastrell P, Edwards J 1996 Community health nursing: frameworks for practice. Baillière Tindall, London

O'Neill P 1990 State health plan for the poor stalls. The Oregonian 15 June

Ong B N 1986 Women in the transition to socialism in Sub-Saharan Africa. In: Munslow B (ed) Africa's problems in the transition to socialism. Zed Books, London

Open University 1998 Clinical supervision: a development pack for nurses, K509. Open University Press, Buckingham

Orem D E 1985 Nursing: concepts of practice, 3rd edn. McGraw-Hill, New York

Orem D E 1991 Nursing concepts of practice, 4th edn. Mosby Year Book, St Louis, MO

Orlando I 1961 The dynamic nurse–patient relationship. Putnams, New York

Ormerod P 1994 The death of economics. Faber & Faber, London

Ottewill R, Wall A 1990 The growth and development of the community health services. Business Education Publishers, Sunderland

Owen M, Webb M, Evans K 2001 Community based universal neonatal hearing screening by health visitors using otoacoustic emissions. Archives of Disease in Childhood, Fetal and Neonatal Edition 84:F157–F162

Owens R G, Ashcroft J B 1985 Violence, a guide for the caring professions. Croom Helm, London

Padgett K 1991 Correlates of self-efficacy beliefs among patients with non-insulin dependent diabetes mellitus in Zagreb, Yugoslavia. Patient Education and Counseling 139–147

Pahl J, Vaile M 1986 Health and health care among travellers. University of Kent Health Services Research Unit, Canterbury

Parsons T 1954 The professions and social structure. In: Essays in sociological theory. Free Press, Glencoe, IL, ch 2

Parton N 1990 Taking child abuse seriously. In: The Violence against Children Study Group. Taking child abuse seriously, contemporary issues in child protection theory and practice. Unwin Hyman, London, ch 1

Pearson P, Waterson T 1992 Newcastle parent held record: report of a pilot study. Newcastle upon Tyne Health Authority, Newcastle upon Tyne

Pender N J 1987 Health promotion in nursing practice, 2nd edn. Appleton & Lange, Norwalk, CT

Pender N J 1996 Health promotion in nursing practice, 3rd edn. Appleton & Lange, Stamford, CT

Pender N J, Walker S N, Sechrist K R et al 1990 Predicting health-promoting lifestyles in the workplace. Nursing Research 39:326–332

Peninsula Medical School 2003 Complementary medicine: the evidence so far (a documentation on clinically relevant research 1993–2003) University of Exeter

Pennebaker J W 1990 Opening up: the healing power of confiding in others. In Sarafino E P 1994 Health psychology. John Wiley, New York

Peplau H 1952 Interpersonal relations in nursing. G P Putman, New York

Phillipson C 1992 Confronting elder abuse: fact and fiction. Generations Review 2:2–3

Pietroni P M 1987 Holistic medicine: new lessons to be learned. The Practitioner 231:1386–1390

Pilgrim D, Rogers A 1995 Mass childhood immunisation: some ethical doubts for primary health care workers. Nursing Ethics 2(1):63–70

Pitts M, Phillips K 1991 The psychology of health. Routledge, London

Plant A 1992 Health visitor performance indicators. Unpublished paper. North Staffordshire Combined Healthcare NHS Trust

Polanyi M 1958 Personal knowledge: towards a post critical philosophy. Routledge & Kegan Paul, London

Polanyi M 1967 The tacit dimension. Routledge & Kegan Paul, London

Police Reform Act 1998 Home Office, London

Polit D, Hungler B 1995 Nursing research: principles and methods, 5th edn. Lippincott, Philadelphia

Pollak K I, Carbonari J P, DiClemente C C et al 1998 Causal relationships of processes of change and decisional balance: stage-specific models for smoking. Addictive Behaviors 23:437–448

Pollitt E 1994 Poverty and child development: relevance of research in developing countries to the United States. Child Development 65:283–295. In Shaffer D R 1996 Developmental psychology: childhood and adolescence, 4th edn. Brooks/Cole, Stamford, CT

Porter S, Ryan S 1996 Breaking the boundaries between nursing and sociology: a critical realist ethnography of the theory practice gap. Journal of Advanced Nursing 24:413–420

Poulton B 1999 User involvement in identifying health needs and shaping and evaluating services: is it being realised? Journal of Advanced Nursing 30(6):1289–1296

Poulton B 2003 Putting the 'public' back into public health. Community Practitioner 76(3):88–91

Powell M, Moon G 2001 Health Action Zones: the third way of a new area based policy. Health and Social Care in the Community 9(1):43–50

Powell J E 2003 Economics and public health. In: Orme J, Powell J, Taylor P et al (eds) Public health for the 21st century: new perspectives on policy participation and practice. Open University Press, Milton Keynes

Preece S 2002 Nurse prescribing, accountability and legal issues. In: Humphries J L, Green J (eds) Nurse prescribing, 2nd edn. Palgrave, Basingstoke, ch 3

Price B 2004 Conducting sensitive patient interviews. Nursing Standard 18(38):45–52

Prime R & D Ltd for Skills for Health 2003 Functional map for the practice of public health. November 2003

Pringle M K 1975 The needs of children. In Straw J, Anderson J 1996 Parenting: a discussion paper. Hutchinson, London

Pritchard A, Kendrick D 2001 Practice nurse and health visitor management of acute minor illness in a general practice. Journal of Advanced Nursing 36(4):556–562

Procaska J, DiClemente C 1984 The transtheoretical approach: crossing traditional boundaries of therapy. Dow Jones-Irwin, Homewood, IL

Procaska J, DiClemente C 1988 Treating addictive behaviours: processes of change. Plenum Press, New York

Protection of Children Act 1999 Department of Health list. HMSO, London, ch 14

Public Health Development 2001 Hampshire and Isle of Wight conference report, December 2001. Hampshire and Isle of Wight Public Health Development Project, Winchester

Quigley R, Cavanagh S, Harrison D et al 2004 Clarifying health impact assessment, integrated impact assessment and health needs assessment. Health Development Agency, London

Randall P 1997 Adult bullying: perpetrators and victims. Routledge, London

RCN 1996 Clinical effectiveness: a Royal College of Nursing guide. Royal College of Nursing, London

RCN 1990 Dynamic standard setting system. Royal College of Nursing, London

RCN 1996 National health manifesto. Royal College of Nursing, London

RCN 1998 Guidance for nurses on clinical governance. Royal College of Nursing, London

Regalado M, Halfon N 2001 Primary care services promoting optimal child development from birth to age 3 years: review of the literature. Archives of Pediatric Adolescent Medicine 155:1311–1322

Rehfisch F (ed) 1975 Gypsies, tinkers and other travellers. Academic Press, London

Reilly D T 1983 Young doctors' views on alternative medicine. British Medical Journal 287:337–339

Reilly S, Graham-Jones S, Gaulton E et al 2004 Can a health advocate for homeless families reduce workload for the primary healthcare team? A controlled trial. Health and Social Care in the Community 12(1):63–74

Reinke B J, Holmes D S, Denney N W 1981 Influence of a 'friendly visitor' program on the cognitive functioning and morale of elderly persons. American Journal of Community Psychology 9:491–504

Renzetti C M, Miley C H (eds) 1996 Violence in gay and lesbian domestic partnerships. Harrington Park Press, New York

Reynell J 1969 Reynell developmental language scales. NFER, London

Reynolds M 1992 Developmental screening: the need for change. Unpublished BSc project, University of Wolverhampton

Reynolds M 1999 A study to explore the usefulness of the Schedule of Growing Skills in enabling health visitors to fulfil their role of promoting the child's health and development in child protection work. Unfinished MPhil dissertation, University of Wolverhampton

Richardson D, Robinson V (eds) 1993 Introducing women's studies. Macmillan, London

Riding H 1985 Serological surveillance of herd immunity to various infectious agents and the investigation of some rapid viral diagnostic techniques. MSc thesis, University of Glasgow

Roberts H 1990 Women's health counts. Routledge, London

Roberts I, Kramer M, Suissa S 1996 Does home visiting prevent childhood injury: a systematic review of randomised controlled trials. British Medical Journal 312:29–33

Roberts J 1988 Why are some families more vulnerable to child abuse? In: Browne K, Davies C, Stratton P (eds) Early prediction and prevention of child abuse. John Wiley, Chichester, p 43–56

Roberts K, Ludvigsen C 1998 Project management for health care professionals. Butterworth-Heinemann, Oxford

Roberts M M 1989 Breast screening: time for a rethink? British Medical Journal 299:1153–1155

Robinson J 1982 An evaluation of health visiting. CETHV, London

Robinson J 1992 Problems with paradigms in a caring profession. Journal of Advanced Nursing 17:632–638

Robinson J 1998 The effectiveness of domiciliary health visiting: a systematic review of the literature commissioned from the University of Nottingham by the NHS R & D Technology Assessment Programme. Conference paper presented to the RCN, London

Robinson J, Elkan R 1996 Health needs assessment: theory and practice. Churchill Livingstone, Edinburgh

Robotham A 1994 Are academic levels in health visiting theory discernible in practice? Unpublished dissertation for Masters in Education, University of Wolverhampton

Robotham A 2000 Assessment of competence to practice. In: Sines D, Appleby F, Raymond E (eds) Community health care nursing, 2nd edn. Blackwell Science, Oxford

Robotham A 2001 The grading of health visitor fieldwork practice. Unpublished PhD thesis, University of Wolverhampton

Robotham A, Harvey J 2000 Clinical and corporate governance and the health visiting service. In: Robotham A, Sheldrake D (eds) Community health care nursing, 2nd edn. Blackwell Science, Oxford

Robotham A, Sheldrake D (eds) 2000 Health visiting: specialist and higher level practice, 1st edn. Churchill Livingstone. Edinburgh

Rogers C 1967 On becoming a person: a therapist's view of psychotherapy. Constable, London

Rogers C R 1951 Client-centred therapy. Constable, London

Rose R M, Holaday J W, Bernstein I S 1971 Plasma testosterone, dominance rank and aggressive behaviour in male rhesus monkeys. In Owens R G, Ashcroft J B 1985 Violence, a guide for the caring professions. Croom Helm, London

Rosenstock I M 1966 Why people use health services. Milbank Memorial Fund Quarterly 44:94

Rosenstock I M 1974 Historical origins of the Health Belief Model. In: Becker M H (ed) The Health Belief Model and personal health behaviour. C B Slack, Thorofare, NJ

Rossman G B, Wilson B L 1991 Numbers and words revisited: being 'shamelessly eclectic'. Evaluation Review 9:627–643

Roter D, Hall J, Merisca R et al 1998 Effectiveness of interventions to improve patient compliance: a meta-analysis. Medical Care 36:1138–1161

Roter J B 1966 Generalized expectancies for the internal versus external control of reinforcement. Cited in Sarafino E P 1994 Health psychology. John Wiley, New York

Rotter D 1977 Patient participation in the patient–provider interaction: the effect of patient question asking on the quality of interaction, satisfaction and compliance. Health Education Monographs 5:281–315

Rowntree D 1987 Assessing students: how shall we know them? Kogan Page: London

Roy C 1970 Adaptation: a conceptual framework for nursing. Nursing Outlook 18:42–45

Roy C 1975 A diagnostic classification system for nursing. Nursing Outlook 23:90–94

Roy C, Andrews H 1991 The Roy Adaptation Model: the definitive statement. Appleton & Lange, Norwalk, CT

Royal College of General Practitioners 2003 The role of primary care in the protection of children from abuse and neglect. Royal College of General Practitioners, London

Royal College of Obstetricians and Gynaecologists 2001 Why mothers die 1997–1999: confidential enquiries into maternal deaths in the United Kingdom. London

Runciman P 1990 Competence-based education and the assessment and accreditation of work-based learning in the context of P2000 programmes of nurse education: a literature review. National Board for Nursing, Midwifery and Health Visiting for Scotland, Edinburgh

Runciman P, Currie C T, Nicol M et al 1996 Discharge of elderly people from an accident and emergency department: evaluation of health visitor follow-up. Journal of Advanced Nursing 24:711–718

Rutter D, Quine L 2002 Changing health behaviour. Open University Press, Buckingham, UK

Sackett D L, Richardson W S, Rosenburg G W et al 1997 Evidence based medicine: how to teach and practice EBM. Churchill Livingstone, New York

Sadler P 1998 Leadership. Kogan Page, London

Safe Childbirth for Travellers 1992 Joint action to stop eviction of traveller mothers and babies. Information Pack, June 1992

Safety and Justice 2003 The government's proposals on domestic violence. HMSO, London

Sampson J 1930 The wind on the heath: a gypsy anthology. Chatto & Windus, London

Samuelson P A 1976 Economics. McGraw-Hill, Tokyo

Sanderson D 1997 Cost analysis in child health surveillance. In: National Screening Committee/Royal College of Paediatrics and Child Health Proceedings: evolution or revolution? Systematic reviews of screening in child health, 17 December 1997 and 8 January 1998. Child Growth Foundation, London, p 20–21

Sanz E J 2003 Concordance and children's use of medicine. Pharmaceutical Journal 271:858–860

Sarafino E P 1994 Health psychology. John Wiley, New York

Save the Children Fund 1993 Bringing up children in a traveller community. Leeds Traveller Project, Leeds

Saylor C R 1990 Reflection and professional education: art, science, and competency. Nurse Educator 15:8–11

Schering A 1987 Schering Report IX: The forgetful patient: the high cost of improper patient compliance. Pharmaceutical Journal 271

Schneider A 1979 Evaluation of nursing competence. Little Brown, Boston

Schön D A 1983 The reflective practitioner. Basic Books, New York

Schön D A 1987 Educating the reflective practitioner: towards a new design for teaching and learning in the professions. Jossey-Bass, San Francisco, CA

Schutz A 1972 The phenomenology of the social world. Heinemann, London

Scottish Executive 1999 Towards a healthier Scotland: a White Paper on health (CM4269). HMSO, Edinburgh

Scott-Samuel A 1984 Identification of underprivileged areas. British Medical Journal 287:130

Seedhouse D 1988 Ethics: the heart of health care. John Wiley, Chichester

Sefton T, Byford S, McDaid D et al 2002 Making the most of it: economic evaluation in the social welfare field. York Publishing Services, York (for the Joseph Rowntree Foundation)

Seligman M E P 1975 Helplessness: on depression, development and death. Freeman, San Francisco

Settersten L, Lauver D R 2004 Critical thinking, perceived health status, and participation in health behaviours, Nursing Research 53(1):11–18

Seyle H 1956 The stress of life. McGraw-Hill, New York

Shariatmadari D, Miller P 2003 Health needs assessment tool. Sure Start South Fenland. Presentation material

Sharples H 2004 Detection of autism in pre-school children: what's needed? Community Practitioner 77(6):219–223

Shaw D S, Vondra J I 1995 Infant attachment security and maternal predicators of early behaviour problems: a longitudinal study of low-income families. Journal of Abnormal Child Psychology 23(3):335–357

Sheldrake D, Sillman C, Notter J 1997 Developing partnerships in practice: using the Edinburgh Postnatal Depression Scale in health visiting. Report produced for Southern Birmingham Community Health NHS Trust. University of Central England, Birmingham

Sheldrake D, Sillman C, Notter J 1998 Developing partnerships in practice: using the Edinburgh Postnatal Depression Scale. Journal of Community Health Nursing 1:50–54

Sheridan M 1960 The developmental progress of infants and young children. HMSO, London

Sheridan M 1975 From birth to five years: children's developmental progress, 3rd edn. NFER-Nelson, London

Shickle D, Chadwick R 1994 The ethics of screening: is 'screeningitis' an incurable disease? Journal of Medical Ethics 20(1):12–18

Shinitzky H E, Kub J 2001 The art of motivating behaviour change: the use of motivational interviewing to promote health. Public Health Nursing 18(3):178–185

Sieghart P 1982 Professional ethics: for whose benefit? Journal of the Society of Occupational Medicine 32:4–14

Simpson L, Stockford D 1979 Gypsy children and their health needs. Save the Children Fund, London

Sims R 1999 In: Jones M (ed) Nurse prescribing: politics to practice. Baillière Tindall, Edinburgh, ch 1

Sinclair R, Bullock R 2002 Learning from past experience: a review of serious cases reviews. Department of Health, London

Skills for Health 2004 National occupational standards for public health. Online. Available: http://www.skillsforhealth.org.uk 16 Nov 2004

Skinner B F 1938 The behaviour of organisms. Appleton-Century-Crofts, New York

Skrabanek P 1990 Why is preventative medicine exempted from ethical constraints? Journal of Medical Ethics 16:187–190

Slater R 1995 The psychology of growing old: looking forward. Open University Press, Buckingham

Smith D S, Goldenburg E, Ashburn A et al 1981 Remedial therapy after stroke : a randomised controlled trial. British Medical Journal: Clinical Research Education 282:517–520

Smith M A 2004 Health visiting: the public health role. Journal of Advanced Nursing 45(1):17–25

Smith S, Baker D, Buchan A et al 1992 Adult domestic violence. Health Trends 24:97–99

SNMAC 1995 Making it happen: public health – the contribution, role and development of nurses, midwives and health visitors. Report of the Standing Nursing and Midwifery Advisory Committee. HMSO, London

Snowdon S K, Stewart-Brown S L 1997 Pre-school vision screening: results of a systematic review. CRD Report 9. NHS Centre for Reviews and Dissemination, York

Snowdon S, Stewart-Brown S 1998 Systematic reviews of child health. Royal College of Paediatrics and Child Health, London

Snyder J A 1994 Emergency department protocols for domestic violence. Journal of Emergency Nursing 20:65–68

Social Exclusion Unit 1998 Bringing Britain together: a national strategy for neighbourhood renewal. HMSO, London

Somers-Smith M J, Race A J 1997 Assessment of clinical skills in midwifery: some ethical and practical problems. Nurse Education Today 17:449–453

Southall D, Samuels M P, Golden M H 2003 Classification of child abuse by motivation and degree rather than by type of injury. Archives of Diseases of Childhood 88:101–104

Starey N 2003 What is clinical governance? Health Economics Unit, HEO 060902

Starn J R 1992 Community health nursing visits for at risk women and infants. Journal of Community Health Nursing 9:103–110

Steehan M P et al 1992 Efficacy of traditional Chinese herbal therapy in adult atopic dermatitis. Lancet 340:13–17

Stewart M 1995 Effective physician–patient communication and health outcomes: a review. Canadian Medical Association Journal (152):1423–1433

Stoate H G 1989 Can health screening damage your health? Journal of the Royal College of General Practitioners May:193–195

Stop it now UK & Ireland Annual Review 2002–2003 (a project of the Lucy Faithful Organisation Registered Charity No. 1013025), Birmingham

Stop it now! 2001 Together we can prevent child sexual abuse. Leaflet. Birmingham

Stotts A L, DiClemente C C, Carbonari J P, Mullen P D 1996 Pregnancy smoking cessation: a case of mistaken identity. Addictive Behaviors 21:459–471

Stratton P (ed) Early prediction and prevention of child abuse. John Wiley, Chichester

Streiner D, Norman G 1995 Health Measurement Scales: a practical guide to their development and use, 2nd edn (reprinted 2001). Oxford University Press, New York

Stutsman R 1931 Mental measurement of pre-school children. World Book Co, New York

Suppiah C 1994 Working in partnership with community mothers. Health Visitor 67:51–53

Supporting families 1998 A consultation document. HMSO, London

Sure Start Unit 2003a Sure Start guidance: 2004–2006 delivery guidance. DfES, London

Sure Start Unit 2003b Planning and delivering Sure Start, 6th wave edn. DfES, London

Sure Start Unit 2003c National evaluation report: fathers in Sure Start local programmes. DfES, London

Suris A M, Trapp M C, DiClemente C C et al 1998 Application of the transtheoretical model of behavior change for obesity in Mexican American women. Addictive Behaviors 23:655–668

Sutherland A 1987 The body as symbol among the ROM. In: Blacking J (ed) The anthropology of the body. Academic Press, London

Sutton J C, Jagger C, Smith U K 1995 Parents' views of health surveillance. Archives of Disease in Childhood 73:57–61

Swage T 2000 Clinical governance in health care practice. Butterworth-Heinemann, Oxford

Swann B, Brocklehurst N 2004 Three in one: the Stockport model of health visiting. Community Practitioner 77(7):251–256

Swayne J 1989 Survey of the use of homeopathic medicine in the UK health system. Journal of Royal College of General Practitioners 39:503–506

Symposium 1990 The Practitioner 234:111–125

Taylor L, Gowman N, Quigley R 2003 Addressing inequalities through health impact assessment. Health Development Agency, London

Teenage Pregnancy Unit 2003 Teenage pregnancy: report by Social Exclusion Unit. Online. Available: http://www.teenagepregnancyunit.gov.uk Apr 2004

Tejero A, Trujols J, Hernandez E et al 1997 Processes of change assessment in heroin addicts following the Procaska & DiClemente transtheoretical model. Drug and Alcohol Dependence 47:31–37

Thomas J Research-based anger management strategies Medsurg Nursing 12(2):103–110

Thomas J D 1985 Gypsies and American medical care. Annals of Internal Medicine 102:842–845

Thomas J D, Douecette M M, Stoeckle J D 1987 Disease, lifestyle and consanguinity in 58 American gypsies. Lancet ii: 377–379

Thomas J, Wainwright P 1996 Community nurses and health promotion: ethical and political perspectives. Nursing Ethics 3(2):97–107

Thomas K J, Carr J, Westlake L et al 1991 Use of non-orthodox and conventional healthcare in Great Britain. British Medical Journal 302:207–210

Thomason J et al 1997 Neonatal screening for inborn errors of metabolism. In: National Screening Committee/Royal College of Paediatrics and Child Health Proceedings: evolution or revolution? Systematic reviews of screening in child health, 17 December 1997 and 8 January 1998. Child Growth Foundation, London, p 13–15

Thompson T W 1929 The uncleanness of women among English gypsies. Journal of the Gypsy Lore Society (third series) 1(102):15–43

Tisserand R, Balacs T 1995 Essential oil safety. Churchill Livingstone, Edinburgh

Tizzard B 1997 Adopting older children. In Hoghughi M and Speight A. *op cit.*

Tones K 1991 Health promotion, empowerment and the psychology of control. Journal of the Institute of Health Education 29:17–26

Tones K, Tilford S 1994 Health education: effectiveness, efficiency and equity. Nelson Thornes, Gloucester

Tones K, Tilford S 2001 Health promotion: effectiveness, efficiency and equity, 3rd edn. Nelson Thornes, Cheltenham

Torrington D, Weightman J, Johns K 1989 Effective management. Prentice-Hall, Englewood Cliffs, NJ

Townsend P, Davidson N (eds) 1982 Inequalities in health: the Black Report. Penguin, Harmondsworth

Townsend P, Davidson N, Whitehead M 1988 Inequalities in health and the health care divide. Penguin, Harmondsworth

Traveller Law Reform Coalition and The Institute for Public Health Policy 2004 Moving forward. Online. Available: http://www.centralbooks.com

Tschudin V, Marks-Maran D 1993 Ethics. Baillière Tindall, London

Tsoneva J 2004 Understanding patients' beliefs and goals in medicine-taking. Professional Nurse 19(8): 466–468

Tuckman B 1965 Development sequence in small groups. Psychological Bulletin 63:384–399

Tudor-Hart J 1971 The inverse care law. Lancet i:405–412

Turner T 1998 Parenting: off to a Sure Start? Community Practitioner 71:278–280

Twinn S 1989 Change and conflict in health visiting practice: dilemma in assessing professional competency of student health visitors. Unpublished PhD thesis, University of London

Twinn S F 1991 Conflicting paradigms of health visiting: a continuing debate for professional practice. Journal of Advanced Nursing 16:966–973

Twinn S, Cowley S (ed) 1992 The principles of health visiting: a re-examination. HVA/UKSC, London

Twinn S, Roberts B, Andrews S 1996 Community health care nursing. Butterworth-Heinemann, Oxford

UKCC 1992 The scope of professional practice. United Kingdom Central Council for Nursing, Midwifery and Health Visiting, London

UKCC 1994a The future of professional practice: the Council's standards for education and practice following registration. United Kingdom Central Council for Nursing, Midwifery and Health Visiting, London

UKCC 1994b Professional conduct: occasional report on standards of nursing in nursing homes. United Kingdom Central Council for Nursing, Midwifery and Health Visiting, London

UKCC 1996 Guidelines for professional practice. United Kingdom Central Council for Nursing, Midwifery and Health Visiting, London

United Nations Convention on the Rights of the Child 1989 UN Assembly document

Upton D J 1999 How can we achieve evidence-based practice if we have a theory–practice gap in nursing today? Journal of Advanced Nursing 29:549–555

Urey B 1968 A method for analysis of nursing tasks. EdD dissertation, Columbia University

Utting Report 1997 Review of the inadequacy of safeguards against the abuse of children living away from home. HMSO, London

Vetter N J, Jones D A, Victor C R 1984 Effect of health visitors working with elderly patients in general practice: a randomised controlled trial. British Medical Journal 288:369–372

Vetter N J, Lewis P A, Ford D 1992 Can health visitors prevent fractures in elderly people? British Medical Journal 304:888–890

Wakefield A J, Murch S H, Linnell A A J et al 1998 Ileal–lymphoid–nodular hyperplasia, non-specific colitis and pervasive developmental disorder in children. Lancet 351:637–641

Wagner Report 1988 See Independent Review of Residential Care

Wain R, Holton S 1993 Conference Proceedings, Current Perspectives in Healthcare Computing. BHJC Ltd

Wanless D 2002 Securing our future health: taking a long term view. HMSO, London

Wanless D 2004 Securing good health for the whole population. HMSO, London

Warner N 1992 House of Commons Second Report on child adoption: choosing with care. HMSO, London

Warner Report 1997 Report of the committee of inquiry into the selection, development and management of staff in children's homes. HMSO, London

Watson G, Glaser E A 1964 Watson–Glaser critical thinking appraisal manual. Harcourt Brace & World, New York

Watson P 1994 The organisation and delivery of health care services for Gypsy and Traveller families in the West Midlands. Report for the Association of West Midlands Community Health Councils Surveys and Information Committee

Watts A 1992 A tool for profiling. North Staffordshire Combined Healthcare NHS Trust, unpublished paper

Weaver R 1996 Localities and inequalities. In: Bywaters P, McLeod E (eds) Working for equality in health. Routledge, London

Weinstein N D 1980 Unrealistic optimism about future life events. Journal of Personality and Social Psychology 39(5):806–820

Weiss M, Britten N 2003 What is concordance? Pharmaceutical Journal 271:493

Wharton R, Lewith G 1986 Complementary medicine and the general practitioner. British Medical Journal 1986; 292:1498–1500

While A (ed) 1986 Research in preventive community nursing care: 15 studies in health visiting. John Wiley: Chichester

While A 1991 Health teaching in a primary school using Becker's health belief model. In: While A (ed) Caring for children: towards partnership with families. Edward Arnold, London

While A E, Biggs K S M 2004 Benefits and challenges of nurse prescribing. Journal of Advance Nursing 45(6):559–567

While A F, Rees K L 1993 The knowledge of health visitors and district nurses regarding products in the proposed formulary for nurse prescription. Journal of Advanced Nursing 18:1573–1577

Whittington D, Boore J 1988 Competence in nursing. In: Ellis R (ed) Professional competence and quality assurance in the caring professions. Chapman & Hall, London

Wilensky H 1964 The professionalisation of everyone? American Journal of Sociology 70:137–159

Williams E I Greenwell J & Groom L M 1992 The care of people over 75 years old after discharge from hospital: an evaluation of time tabled visiting by health visitor assistants Journal of Public Health Medicine 14:138–144

Wilson G 1987 Background information (unpublished report)

Wilson J, Tingle J (eds) 1999 Clinical risk modification: route to clinical governance? Butterworth-Heinemann, Oxford

Wilson J, Jungner G 1968 Principles and practice of screening for disease. WHO, Geneva

Windsor B 1990 The Coalpool Project: health visiting, a corporate caseload. Unpublished paper, Walsall Health Authority

Winnicott D 1965 The maturational process and the facilitative environment. International Universities Press, New York

Winstanley J 2000 Manchester Clinical Supervision Scale. Nursing Standard 14(19):31–32

Wood P K 1983 Inquiring systems and problem structure: implications for cognitive development. Cited in Kitchener K S, King P M 1990 The reflective judgement model: transforming assumptions about knowing. In: Mezirow J et al (ed) Fostering critical reflection in adulthood. Jossey-Bass, San Francisco

Woodhead D 2000 The health and well being of asylum seekers and refugees. Kings Fund, London

World Health Organization 1978 Alma-Ata declaration primary health care. WHO, Geneva

World Health Organization 1981 Global strategy for health for all by the year 2000. WHO, Copenhagen

World Health Organization 1985 Targets for health for all. WHO Regional Office for Europe, Copenhagen

World Health Organization 1997 The Jakarta Declaration on leading health promotion into the 21st century. Health Promotion International 12:261–264

World Health Organization 1999 Health 21: health for all in the 21st century. European Health for all series No 6. WHO, Copenhagen

Wright S 1998 Developing health visiting practice using action research. Community Practitioner 71: 337–339

Wyatt J 1996 Medical informatics, artefacts or science? Methods of Information in Medicine 35:197–200

Young D 1998 re MMR revisited hastily! www.mailbox.ac.uk/lists-f-j/gp-uk/1998-03/0132.htm

Index

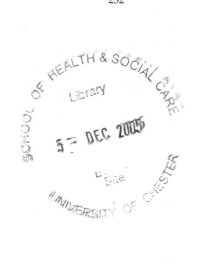